Lithium in Neuropsychiatry

The Comprehensive Guide

Lithium in Neuropsychiatry
The Comprehensive Guide

Editors

Michael Bauer MD PhD
Professor of Psychiatry, Charité University Medicine Berlin,
Berlin, Germany

Paul Grof MD PhD FRCP
Director of the Mood Disorders Center of Ottawa and Professor of Psychiatry,
University of Toronto, Canada

Bruno Müller-Oerlinghausen MD
Professor Emeritus of Clinical Psychopharmacology, Freie Universität Berlin,
Chairman of the Drug Commission of the German Medical Association, Germany

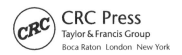
CRC Press
Taylor & Francis Group
Boca Raton London New York

CRC Press is an imprint of the
Taylor & Francis Group, an **informa** business

CRC Press
Taylor & Francis Group
6000 Broken Sound Parkway NW, Suite 300
Boca Raton, FL 33487-2742

First issued in paperback 2018

© 2006 by Taylor and Francis Group, LLC
CRC Press is an imprint of Taylor & Francis Group, an Informa business

No claim to original U.S. Government works

ISBN-13: 978-1-84184-515-9 (hbk)
ISBN-13: 978-1-138-38129-2 (pbk)

A CIP record for this book is available from the British Library.

Library of Congress Cataloging-in-Publication Data available on application

**Visit the Taylor & Francis Web site at
http://www.taylorandfrancis.com**

**and the CRC Press Web site at
http://www.crcpress.com**

Contents

Special populations and applications in medicine

Effects on body systems

Dedication

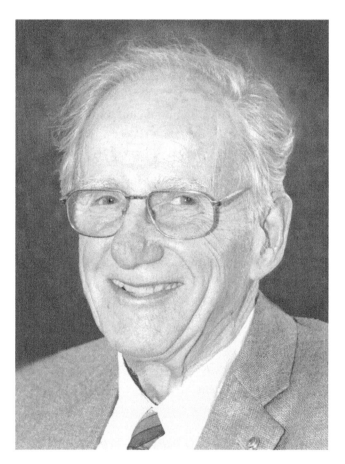

Prof Dr Dr hon MOGENS SCHOU (1918–2005)

This book is dedicated to MOGENS SCHOU who taught all of us how to use lithium in neuropsychiatry. Once he discovered lithium's prophylactic action in mood disorders, he researched tirelessly all its aspects and did not spare any effort to make the treatment available to all those in need, the millions of patients with recurrent mood disorders.

Contributors

Editors

Michael Bauer, MD PhD
Professor of Psychiatry
Department of Psychiatry and Psychotherapy
Charité University Medicine Berlin
Campus Charité Mitte
Berlin
Germany

Paul Grof, MD, PhD, FRCP
Director, Mood Disorders Center of Ottawa
Ottawa, Ontario
Canada
and
Professor of Psychiatry
University of Toronto
Toronto, Ontario
Canada

Bruno Müller-Oerlinghausen, MD
Professor Emeritus of Clinical
  Psychopharmacology
Freie Universität Berlin
and
Chairman, Drug Commission of the German
  Medical Association
Berlin
Germany

Contributors

Mazda Adli, MD
Supervising Psychiatrist
Department of Psychiatry and Psychotherapy
Charité University Medicine Berlin
Campus Charité Mitte
Berlin
Germany

Bernd Ahrens, MD
Privatdozent
Arcus Institute for Disease Management
Office Luebeck
Luebeck
Germany

Gisela Albrecht, MD
Vivantes Clinic Spandau
Director, Clinic for Dermatology and
  Allergology
Berlin
Germany

Jochen Albrecht, MD
Head,
Department of Psychiatry and Psychotherapy
Charité University Medicine Berlin
St. Hedwig Krankenhaus
Berlin
Germany

Martin Alda, MD, FRCPC
Professor of Psychiatry and Canada Research
    Chair
McGill University
Montreal, Quebec
Canada

Christopher Baethge, MD
Deutsches Ärzteblatt
50859 Köln
Germany
and
Klinik für Psychiatrie und Psychotherapie
Universität zu Köln
Köln
Germany

Ross J Baldessarini, MD
Professor of Psychiatry and Neuroscience
Harvard Medical School
Boston, Massachusetts
Director, Psychopharmacology Program
McLean Division, Massachusetts General
    Hospital
Belmont, Massachusetts
USA

Margaret G Baudhuin, MLS
Madison Institute of Medicine, Inc
7617 Mineral Point Road, Suite 300
Madison, Wisconsin
USA

Robert H Belmaker, MD
Stanley Research Center
Faculty of Health Sciences
Ben Gurion University of the Negev
Beer-Sheva
Israel

Anne Berghöfer, MD
Institute for Social Medicine, Epidemiology
    and Health Economics
Charité University Medical Center
Berlin
Germany

Yuly Bersudsky, MD, PhD
Stanley Research Center
Faculty of Health Sciences
Ben Gurion University of the Negev
Beer-Sheva
Israel

Jeffrey Bierbrauer
Department of Psychiatry and Psychotherapy
Charité University Medicine Berlin
Campus Charité Mitte
Berlin
Germany

Nick J Birch, BSc, PhD, CBiol, FIBiol, MEWI
Consulting Pharmacologist, Emeritus
    Professor
Academic Consultancy Services Ltd
Codsall
Staffordshire
UK

Irene M Bratti, MD
Chief Resident in Psychiatry
Semel Institute for Neuroscience and Human
    Behavior
University of California
Los Angeles, California
USA

Tom Bschor, MD, Associate Professor
Director, Jewish Hospital Berlin
Department of Psychiatry and Psychotherapy
Berlin
Germany

Joseph R Calabrese, MD
Professor of Psychiatry
Co-Director, Bipolar Disorder Research Center
Case University School of Medicine
Director, Mood Disorders Program
Director, Division of Ambulatory Care
University Hospitals of Cleveland
Cleveland, Ohio
USA

De-Maw Chuang, PhD
Chief, Section on Molecular Neurobiology
Biological Psychiatry Branch
National Institute of Mental Health
National Institutes of Health
Bethesda, Maryland
USA

Philip H Cogen, MD, PhD
Semel Institute for Neuroscience and Human
    Behavior
Department of Psychiatry and Biobehavioral
    Sciences of the David Geffen School of
    Medicine
University of California
Los Angeles, California
USA

Nicolas Andres Crossley, MD
Department of Psychiatry and Psychotherapy
Charité University Medicine Berlin
Campus Charité Mitte
Berlin
Germany

Chad Daversa, MA
Executive Director
International Society for Bipolar Disorders
Pittsburgh, Pennsylvania
USA

John M Davis, MD
Gilman Professor of Psychiatry
Psychiatric Institute
Department of Psychiatry
University of Illinois at Chicago &
    University of Maryland Psychiatric Research
    Center
Chicago, Illinois
USA

Dorian Deshauer, MD
Mood Disorders Research Unit
Royal Ottawa Hospital
Ottawa, Ontario
Canada

Anne Duffy, MD, MSc, FRCP
Canada Research Chair in Child Mood
    Disorders
Associate Professor of Psychiatry
McGill University
Montreal, Quebec
Canada

Gianni L Faedda, MD
Director, Lucio Bini Mood Disorders
    Center
New York
USA

Werner Felber, MD
Professor of Psychiatry
Department of Psychiatry
University of Dresden Carl Gustav Carus
Dresden
Germany

Malte Folkerts
Department of Psychiatry, Division of Clinical
    Neurobiology
Ludwig-Maximilians-University of Munich
Munich
Germany

Vincent S Gallicchio, PhD, MT(ASCP), DP(Hon),
    FRSA, FASAHP
Endowed Professor of Clinical Sciences and
    Internal Medicine
Chandler Medical Center
University of Kentucky
Lexington, Kentucky
USA

John R Geddes, MD
Professor of Epidemiological Psychiatry
Department of Psychiatry
University of Oxford
Warneford Hospital
Oxford
UK

Sonja Gerber, MD
Department of Psychiatry and Psychotherapy
University of Freiburg
Freiburg
Germany

Samuel Gershon, MD
Professor Emeritus
Western Psychiatric Institute and Clinic
University of Pittsburgh Medical Center
Pittsburgh, Pennsylvania
USA

Tasha Glenn, PhD
ChronoRecord Association, Inc.
PO Box 3501
Fullerton, California
USA

Frederick K Goodwin, MD
The Center for Neuroscience, Medical
   Progress and Society at the George
   Washington University Medical Center
Bethesda, Maryland
USA

Guy M Goodwin, DPhil, FRCPsych
WA Handley Professor of Psychiatry
Department of Psychiatry
University of Oxford
Warneford Hospital
Oxford
UK

John H Greist, MD
Madison Institute of Medicine, Inc
Madison, Wisconsin
USA

Laszlo Gyulai, MD
Associate Professor of Psychiatry
Director, Bipolar Disorders Program
University of Pennsylvania Medical
   Center
Philadelphia, Pennsylvania
USA

Brian B Harris, BSc, MB, FRCPsych
Senior Lecturer in Psychiatry
Department of Psychological Medicine
Cardiff University School of Medicine
University Hospital of Wales
Heath Park
Cardiff
UK

Bette L Hartley, MLS
Madison Institute of Medicine, Inc
Madison, Wisconsin
USA

Ulrich Hegerl, MD
Professor of Psychiatry
Department of Psychiatry
Ludwig-Maximilians-University of Munich
Munich
Germany

John Hennen, PhD
Deceased 2005

Mohammed S Inayat, MS
Chandler Medical Center
University of Kentucky
Lexington, Kentucky
USA

James W Jefferson, MD
Madison Institute of Medicine, Inc.
Madison, Wisconsin
USA

Georg Juckel, MD
Director
Westfälisches Zentrum Bochum
Psychiatrie – Psychotherapie – Psychosomatik
Kinik der Ruhr-Universität Bochum
Bochum
Germany

Dieter Kampf, MD
Associate Professor Emeritus of Internal
  Medicine
Freie Universität
Berlin
Germany

David J Katzelnick, MD
Madison Institute of Medicine, Inc.
Madison, Wisconsin
USA

George Kirov, PhD, MRCPsych
Senior Lecturer in Genetics
Department of Psychological Medicine
Cardiff University School of Medicine
University Hospital of Wales
Heath Park
Cardiff
UK

John H Lazarus, MA, MD, FRCP, FACE, FRCOG
Professor of Clinical Endocrinology
Centre for Endocrine and Diabetes
  Sciences
Cardiff University School of Medicine
University Hospital of Wales
Heath Park
Cardiff
UK

Ute Lewitzka, MD
Department of Psychiatry and Psychotherapy
Technische Universität Dresden
Dresden
Germany

Rasmus W Licht, MD, PhD
Associate Professor of Psychiatry and Clinical
  Pharmacology
Director, Mood Disorders Research and
  Clinical Unit
Aarhus University Psychiatric Hospital
Risskov
Denmark

Daniel Z Lieberman, MD
Associate Professor of Psychiatry and
  Behavioral Sciences
Director of the Clinical Psychiatric Research
  Center
George Washington University
Washington, DC
USA

Mario Maj, MD
Professor of Psychiatry and Chairman
Department of Psychiatry
University of Naples
Naples
Italy

Frank Martens, MD, PhD
Charité University Medicine Berlin
Department of Nephrology and Medical
  Intensive Care
Campus Virchow-Klinikum
Poison Information Center
Berlin
Germany

Paraskevi Mavrogiorgou, MD
Department of Psychiatry and Psychotherapy
Charité University Medicine Berlin
Campus Charité Mitte
Berlin
Germany

E Serap Monkul, MD
Department of Psychiatry
Dokuz Eylul University School of Medicine
Izmir
Turkey

David J Muzina, MD
Director, Adult Inpatient Psychiatric Services
Director, Bipolar Disorders Research Unit
The Cleveland Clinic
Cleveland, Ohio
USA

Agneta Nilsson, MD
The Sahlgrenska Academy of Göteborg
  University
Institute of Clinical Neuroscience, Psychiatry
  Section
Sahlgrenska University Hospital
Göteborg
Sweden

Andrea Pfennig, MD
Department of Psychiatry and Psychotherapy
Charité University Medicine Berlin
Campus Charité Mitte
Berlin
Germany

Oliver Pogarell, MD
Department of Psychiatry, Division of Clinical
  Neurobiology
Ludwig-Maximilians-University of Munich
Munich
Germany

Josef Priller, MD
Professor of Molecular Psychiatry
Department of Psychiatry and
  Psychotherapy
Charité University Medical Center
Campus Charité Mitte
Berlin
Germany

Janusz K Rybakowski, MD, Prof Dr
Head, Department of Adult Psychiatry
Poznan University of Medical Sciences
Poznan
Poland

Jaclyn Saggese, BA
The Center for Neuroscience, Medical
  Progress and Society at the George
  Washington University Medical Center
Bethesda, Maryland
USA

Paola Salvatore, MD
Assistant Professor of Psychiatry
University of Parma, Italy
and
Research Associate in Psychiatry
Harvard Medical School
Boston, Massachusetts
USA

Johanna Sasse, MD
Department of Psychiatry and Psychotherapy
Charité University Medicine Berlin
Campus Charité Mitte
Berlin
Germany

Christof Schaefer, MD
Pharmakovigilanz- und Beratungszentrum für
  Embryonaltoxikologie
Berlin
Germany

Bettina Schmitz, MD
Professor of Neurology
Neurologische Klinik und Poliklinik
Charité University Medicine Berlin
Campus Virchow-Klinikum
Humboldt-University Berlin
Berlin
Germany

Mogens Schou, MD, Dr med sci, Dr honoris causa
Dr Schou died on the 29th September 2005

Marylou Selo
15 West 72nd Street – Apt. 21N
New York
USA

Alona Shaldubina M Med Sc
Stanley Research Center
Faculty of Health Sciences
Ben Gurion University of the Negev
Beer-Sheva
Israel

Christian Simhandl, MD
Professor of Psychiatry
Psychiatrische Abteilung, Krankenhaus
  Neunkirchen
Neunkirchen
Austria

Jair C Soares, MD
Krus Associate Professor and Chief
Director, MOOD-CNS Program
Chief, Division of Mood and Anxiety
  Disorders
Department of Psychiatry
The University of Texas Health Science Center
  at San Antonio
San Antonio, Texas
USA

Krista Nielsen Straarup
Aarhus University Psychiatric Hospital
Risskov
Denmark

Aleksandra Suwalska, MD
Lecturer, Department of Adult Psychiatry
Poznan University of Medical Sciences
Poznan
Poland

Kenneth Thau, MD
Professor, Medizinische Universität Wien
Universitätsklinik für Psychiatrie
Vienna
Austria

Leonardo Tondo, MD, MS
Associate Professor of Psychology
University of Cagliari
Cagliari
Italy
and
Lecturer in Psychiatry
Harvard Medical School
McLean Hospital
115 Mill Street
Belmont, Massachusetts
USA

Dietrich van Calker, MD, PhD
Professor of Psychiatry
Department of Psychiatry and
  Psychotherapy
University of Freiburg
Freiburg
Germany

Per Vestergaard, DrMedSc
Professor of Psychiatry
Aarhus University Psychiatric Hospital
Risskov
Denmark

Adele C Viguera, MD, MPH
Assistant Professor of Psychiatry
Associate Director, Perinatal and Reproductive
  Psychiatry Program
Massachusetts General Hospital
Harvard Medical School
Boston, Massachusetts
USA

Jun-Feng Wang, MB, PhD
Assistant Professor
The Vivian Rakoff Mood Disorders Laboratory
Centre for Addiction and Mental Health
Department of Psychiatry
University of Toronto
Toronto, Ontario
Canada

Peter C Whybrow, MD
Professor of Psychiatry
Director, Semel Institute for Neuroscience and
  Human Behavior
Chairman, Department of Psychiatry and
  Biobehavioral Sciences of the David Geffen
  School of Medicine
760 Westwood Plaza
University of California
Los Angeles, California
USA

Robert C Young, MD
Professor of Psychiatry
Institute of Geriatric Psychiatry
Weill Medical College of Cornell University,
   White Plains
New York
USA

L Trevor Young, MD, PhD
Professor of Psychiatry
The Vivian Rakoff Mood Disorders
   Laboratory Centre for Addiction and Mental
   Health
Department of Psychiatry
University of Toronto
Toronto, Ontario
Canada

Petr Zvolsky, MD, DrSc
Professor Emeritus
Charles University
Prague
Czech Republic

Foreword

Lithium is nothing if not fascinating. Created in the first minutes after the Big Bang, it was discovered nearly 15 billion years later, in 1817, by a chemist analyzing minerals excavated from an island cave off the coast of Sweden. Within the year, lithium had been isolated by English chemists William Thomas Brande and Sir Humphry Davy. Because it was not found free in nature – existing instead in igneous rocks and mineral springs – it was given the Greek name *lithos*, for stone.

Within 75 years of its discovery, lithium had been utilized to treat a variety of medical conditions, including periodic depression and mania. Its therapeutic uses in these disorders of mood is the primary focus of *Lithium in Neuropsychiatry: The Comprehensive Guide*. This excellent book gives an outstanding and comprehensive overview of the history of lithium's use in the treatment of affective illness, including early controversies and the increasingly sophisticated experimental paradigms developed to test both its efficacy and its safety. Leading clinical researchers give the evidence for lithium's effectiveness in acute mania, depression, mixed states and rapid cycling, as well as in prophylaxis. The use of lithium in special clinical populations, such as children, the elderly and pregnant women, is covered in detail, as is its singularly important role in the prevention of suicide. Lithium's demonstrated ability to decrease the mortality rate in high-risk patients makes the book's emphasis upon lithium – still the gold standard of care for bipolar disorder, despite disturbingly effective promotional campaigns on behalf of medications that have demonstrated much less efficacy – all the more important. The role of lithium in non-psychiatric illnesses such as leukopenia, viral infections and thyrotoxicosis is also discussed, as are the potential therapeutic implications of recent research into lithium-induced neurogenesis. The effects of lithium on kidney, cardiovascular, metabolic and thyroid functioning are covered at length, in addition to findings from more basic research fields such as pharmacokinetics, studies of cellular signal transduction pathways, brain imaging and immunology. The last section of the book deals with highly practical issues involved in clinical practice, namely, drug interactions, medication adherence and toxicity.

I cannot pretend to be entirely objective about lithium. I have taken it, except for an initial period of intermittent, and quite damaging non-compliance, for the better part of 30 years. I owe my life to lithium, as do many hundreds of thousands of patients with manic-depressive illness. I also owe my life to the research done by several of those who contributed to this book. Lithium is not an easy drug, but neither are mania and depression easy illnesses to have, or to treat. This book gives to lithium the seriousness and importance it deserves.

Kay Redfield Jamison, PhD
Professor of Psychiatry
The Johns Hopkins School of Medicine

Preface

Lithium in Neuropsychiatry offers a comprehensive outline of the many uses of lithium in neuropsychiatric disorders as well as indications for its use in internal medicine. We intended it primarily for use by clinicians – physicians and other health-care workers who use lithium to treat patients suffering from these disorders. Thus, it addresses various aspects of effective and safe use of lithium in clinical practice. But, because the book also provides an up-to-date description of basic neuroscience relevant for the use of lithium and of the variety of lithium's effects in the brain and human body, it will also serve interested researchers. The contributors to this book are all experts in their fields and internationally recognized for their significant contributions to lithium research.

Lithium was discovered almost 200 years ago and has been used in medicine in one form or another for almost 150 years. Since its introduction into psychiatry in 1949, many new aspects of its use in psychiatry and the neurosciences have been discovered in basic and clinical research.

Lithium is intriguing for several reasons. It is a simple element easily found in the periodic table, yet it has demonstrated a unique, striking efficacy in many patients with bipolar and unipolar mood disorders. Although its value has now been established for several decades, its clinical use varies markedly among different countries. Its value as a suicide-preventing agent is being increasingly recognized and has spurred new interest in lithium's use. The ability of lithium to significantly reduce suicidal risk distinguishes it from other mood-stabilizing agents that are available today. Furthermore, basic research has recently revealed that lithium may possess demonstrable neuroprotective properties. These new data suggest that lithium may become useful in the prevention and treatment of dementia and other neurodegenerative disorders.

We are very grateful to the authors, who with their contributions to this book have provided clinicians and patients with a rich source of knowledge and experience. We would also like to thank Catherine Aubel, Arlene Fox and Anke Schlicht for their general and editorial assistance.

THE INTERNATIONAL GROUP FOR THE STUDY OF LITHIUM-TREATED PATIENTS (IGSLI)

Over the past 17 years IGSLI has worked in, and significantly contributed to, the core areas of lithium research. This book was therefore written in close collaboration with IGSLI. The group was founded in 1988 by Mogens Schou (Risskov/Aarhus, Denmark), Bruno Müller-Oerlinghausen (Berlin, Germany) and Paul Grof (Ottawa, Canada). The main goal of this cooperation has been to conduct systematic work on those important problems of lithium treatment that can be resolved only in an international joint effort. Unified designs have been created and scientific data from the IGSLI member centers linked for the purpose of shared analyses. This approach allowed us to work with large numbers of prospectively followed patients – something that could be accomplished only within a multicenter approach. Centers in Vienna, Prague, Zürich and Dresden quickly joined the group. All these centers had longstanding experience in the long-term lithium treatment of patients with mood disorders. Overall, the research is based on shared, standardized, computer-based documentation of the diagnosis, family history,

course of illness before and during treatment, and on modalities of treatment that are comparable. The group meets regularly at research conferences to plan and discuss joint projects and to prepare publications. In 2002, the group converted to a registered association and launched its own homepage (www.igsli.org).

The most recent 19th IGSLI meeting took place in Poznan, Poland, in September 2005. At this gathering Mogens Schou presented a new project testing the efficacy of lithium in unipolar patients with unrecognized bipolar propensity ('hidden bipolars'). He passed away 3 days after this meeting, a few weeks short of his 87th anniversary. The picture of him on the dedication page was taken just before the IGSLI meeting in September 2005.

Michael Bauer
Paul Grof
Bruno Müller-Oerlinghausen

IGSLI Members 2006

Adli, Mazda (Treasurer), Berlin, Germany
Ahrens, Bernd, Lübeck, Germany
Alda, Martin, Montreal, Canada
Angst, Jules (Honorary Member), Zurich, Switzerland
Baethge, Christopher, Cologne, Germany
Bauer, Michael (President), Berlin, Germany
Berghöfer, Anne (Secretary), Berlin, Germany
Bschor, Tom (Secretary), Berlin, Germany
Deshauer, Dorian, Ottawa, Canada
Duffy, Anne, Montreal, Canada
Felber, Werner, Dresden, Germany
Glenn, Tasha, Fullerton, CA, USA
Grof, Paul, Ottawa, Canada
Gyulai, Laszlo, Philadelphia, USA
Lewitzka, Ute, Dresden, Germany
Licht, Rasmus Wenzer, Risskov, Denmark

Müller-Oerlinghausen, Bruno, Berlin, Germany
Paclt, Ivo, Prague, Czech Republic
Pfennig, Andrea, Berlin, Germany
Priller, Josef, Berlin, Germany
Rybakowski, Janusz K, Poznan, Poland
Sasse, Johanna, Berlin, Germany
Selo, Marylou, New York, USA
Simhandl, Christian, Neunkirchen, Austria
Smolka, Michael, Mannheim, Germany
Suwalska, Aleksandra, Poznan, Poland
Thau, Kenneth, Vienna, Austria
Van Calker, Dietrich, Freiburg, Germany
Vestergaard, Per, Risskov, Denmark
Young, L Trevor, Toronto, Canada
Zvolsky, Petr, Prague, Czech Republic

Part A

INTRODUCTION AND HISTORY

1 Lithium: a fascinating element in neuropsychiatry

Philip H Cogen, Peter C Whybrow

'Everything Old is New Again'

What accounts for the fascination with lithium in neuropsychiatry? The role of the guinea pig in its serendipitous discovery as an antimanic agent, the subsequent establishment of lithium as the 'gold standard' of treatment in bipolar disorder in humans and the protean neuroendocrine manifestations of treatment are well supported by the breadth of material in this monograph. Perhaps more than any of these, however, it is the fact that a naturally occurring element rather than an engineered biopharmaceutical remains the first-line treatment for patients with bipolar disorder. This is truly remarkable in this age of 'designer drugs'.

Indeed, that lithium is derived from a natural source and continues to play a pivotal role in psychiatry many years after its discovery invites a comparison with digitalis, which for many decades was considered the most valuable drug for the treatment of cardiac failure[1]. As with digitalis, lithium therapy mandates determination of the appropriate balance between insufficient dosing with suboptimal efficacy and overdosing with considerable toxicity. Both medications are titrated by combining clinical status with blood level determinations. Thus, in many ways, although digitalis has now lost its pri-

macy, that it once had for the heart, lithium now has it for the brain.

As with digitalis, first identified by William Withering in 1741 from the foxglove plant[1], attention has been given to treatments containing lithium since ancient times. Mineral springs, recognized as having therapeutic value as early as the 5th century, have subsequently been found to contain lithium[2]. Although in most instances the content of lithium in such therapeutic waters was later found to be meager, a fashion for mineral spas and bottled lithium water was initiated that has continued into modern times.

A brief review of the identification and subsequent medical use of lithium serves to highlight this fascinating history. The element now called lithium was first obtained from the mineral petalite that was discovered in 1800 by Jorge Bonifacio de Andrada e Silva, a Brazilian scientist and nobleman, on Uto, an island off the Swedish coast[2]. The initial chemical analysis of petalite by the Reverend Edward Clarke revealed that 1.75% of the sample was unaccounted for by previously identified elements[2]. In 1818 additional studies by Arfwedson, a Swede working in the laboratory of Berzelius, successfully isolated the new element, which he named lithion as it came from a mineral sample[2] (Figure 1.1).

The name was later changed to lithium. As early as 1843 Alexander Ure proposed that lithium carbonate could be used to dissolve urinary calculi, owing to its affinity for uric acid[3]. Similarly, gout being known to be the result of an increase in uric acid, Alfred Garrod in 1859 proposed that lithium could be dissolved in water to treat gouty phalanges by topical application. It was around this time that a 'uric acid diathesis' was proposed as the root cause of certain mood disorders[4]. Professor A. Trousseau thus believed that 'folie' – specifically mania – was the result of excessive uric acid when 'gout retroceded to the head'[2].

In 1870 the pioneer neurosurgeon S. Weir Mitchell published a paper in the *American Journal of Medicine* proposing the use of lithium bromide as an antiepileptic medication[2]. In 1884 Alexander Haig proposed that the 'uric acid diathesis' accounted for gout, headache, digestive diseases and depression, and in 1888 supported his thesis by demonstrating that oral lithium citrate decreased uric acid excretion[5]. Haig suggested that this offered a new therapy

for the various maladies then attributed to an excess of uric acid[5].

Such an attempt to describe a unifying therapeutic concept for a myriad of maladies, including those of the brain, strongly parallels the history of digitalis. Following the initial use of preparations of digitalis designed to treat dropsy (edema), it was proposed that similar treatment might be useful for maladies as variable as epilepsy, hydrocephalus and even insanity[1]. In the late 1880s foxglove was widely used as a remedy for psychiatric disease, and the artist Vincent Van Gogh, who famously suffered with bipolar disorder, was treated with a preparation containing foxglove by Dr Gachet, his personal physician and friend[6]. Van Gogh immortalized Gachet in two well-known portraits in which the doctor is shown holding the foxglove plant as a representation of his 'melancholy nature'[6]. That Van Gogh was prescribed foxglove rather than lithium is especially ironic, given the medical history of the times. In 1889, as Van Gogh lay dying in Auvers from his self-inflicted wounds, he was only a few hundred miles from Munich, where Emil Kraepelin was busily developing the modern classification of manic-depressive illness, and contemporaneously the physician Karl Lange had begun to explore the use of lithium as a treatment for affective illness.

It was Karl Lange, indeed, who first showed the value of lithium in the treatment of depression. A Danish internist, he found that patients with depression and gout treated with lithium showed an improvement in their mood. He published these results in a monograph[2]. His brother Fritz Lange, also a physician, subsequently published a monograph in 1894 entitled *The Most Important Groups of Insanity* in which he listed lithium carbonate as an antidepressant[2].

The late 19th century also saw the rise of mineral spas as a fashionable health-promoting activity in both Europe and North America. As

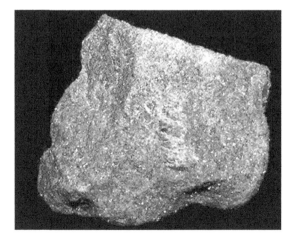

Figure 1.1 Lithium-containing lepidolite

early as 1824 Berzelius described the mineral springs in Bohemia as a source of lithium[2]. In concert with the times Willard Morse, a physician, proposed in 1887 that these mineral waters could be used to treat gout and rheumatism because of lithium's action on uric acid[2]. By 1889, however, analysis of the mineral springs showed that these waters actually contained very little lithium. For example, the commercially sold Londonderry Lithium Water had only 4 ppm of lithium[2]. Thus, to achieve a physiologic lithium effect, one would have to drink 150 000–200 000 gallons! In fact, water from the Potomoc River was shown to have a content of lithium five times that of these bottled waters (one wonders what the content is today). As the results of these analyses became better known, the uric acid hypothesis fell into disrepute and a waning of popularity for lithium ensued.

Half a century later, the first experimentally based use for lithium in medicine arose from the work of the Australian psychiatrist John Cade. In 1946 Cade obtained urine samples from patients with mania, depression and schizophrenia, and injected them intraperitoneally into guinea pigs, looking for the elusive substance causing these mental disorders. The urine from the manic patients killed the animals most easily, and Cade once again entertained the old idea that urea might have an important role in triggering this increased mortality. He added lithium to the preparation to render the urea more soluble. In the experiments that followed, Cade observed that the guinea pigs treated with this urea–lithium solution became docile and lethargic approximately 2 hours after injection for a period of approximately 1–2 hours. This behavioral change suggested to Cade that patients exhibiting manic symptoms might benefit from lithium treatment. On 3 September 1949, in his classic article in *The Medical Journal of Australia*, Cade reported the treatment of ten patients who suffered chronic mania; all received a beneficial effect from

either 1200 mg of lithium citrate or 600 mg of lithium carbonate[7]. It is of interest that six patients with mania and schizophrenia were also treated, and each showed improvement in their mood with no change in their psychotic symptoms[7]. While the first patient treated later died from toxicity, the last patient died in 1980, some 31 years later, at age 76, of a myocardial infarction[2].

In the USA, the widespread use of lithium as a treatment for mania was hampered initially by an earlier effort to replace sodium with lithium salts in hypertension. Lithium had been shown to have a salty taste as early as 1936, and it was marketed as a salt substitute in 1948, only to be withdrawn in 1949 after several deaths from toxicity[2]. Physicians were therefore reluctant to recommend lithium treatment, and patients similarly were reluctant to try it. Outside the USA, however, after careful scrutiny, lithium was shown to be an effective agent in mania and in the prophylaxis of manic-depressive illness. Work by Ron Young in England demonstrated positive results in the treatment of mania, albeit with little effect on depression[2]. Safety further increased with the advent of the spectrophotometer, when lithium levels could be monitored to avoid toxicity. Samuel Gershon worked on lithium in Australia, and subsequently had a major role in bringing lithium treatment to the USA[8]. The widespread clinical use of lithium, however, is mostly associated with the pioneering work of the Danish physician Mogens Schou. (Remarkably, Dr Schou's father, also a physician, had previously written a negative critique of the Lange brothers' work on lithium and its effect on mood disorders[2].) Mogens Schou's first reported trial, in 1953, consisted of 35 manic patients treated with both lithium citrate and lithium carbonate. All these patients showed improvement in their manic states[9]. Flow spectrophotometry was used to obtain lithium levels, which were targeted to the 0.5–2.0 mmol/l range. There was one patient death, due to a pontine infarction, which was attributed to vascular disease, although the patient had a serum lithium level of 4.5 mmol/l. In a subsequent study in 1955, of 48 patients, 81% showed improvement in their illness, and demonstrated lithium's potential as a prophylactic agent[9].

In subsequent years, lithium use was expanded, particularly in France and England. GP Hartigan showed a positive treatment effect of lithium for both mania and depression, suggested routine monitoring of serum lithium levels and published treatment guidelines in the *British Journal of Psychiatry* 1954[10]. Despite the growing evidence of the effect of lithium on patients with mood disorders, there remained skeptics. Perhaps most notable was Barry Blackwell, who wrote a paper entitled 'Prophylactic lithium – another therapeutic myth?'[11]. He suggested that prior studies had targeted inappropriate patients such as those who had received electroconvulsive therapy, and that follow-up was insufficient. Additional studies proved this to be untrue. In 1968, Nathan Kline, one of the main proponents of the use of lithium in the USA, wrote an opposing monograph entitled 'Lithium comes into its own'[2]. Baastrup and Schou, who in 1969 reported the outcome of a double-blinded study of the effect of lithium treatment on mood disorders showing clearly positive results, provided further evidence of efficacy[12]. However, in the USA, widespread acceptance of lithium came only after a Veterans Administration–National Institute of Mental Health (VA-NIMH) study run by Samuel Gershon showed positive results for lithium treatment of patients with acute bipolar disorder. In 1974 lithium was also shown to be effective in the prophylaxis of patients with bipolar disorder in another combined VA-NIMH study, and the Food and Drug Administration (FDA) released it for widespread use, some 21 years after its initial proposal as an effective antimanic agent[2].

Lithium has an effect on multiple systems, and metabolic balance is paramount in the successful use of lithium in the treatment of bipolar disorder. Common side-effects of lithium treatment include renal, endocrine, digestive and nervous system components[13]. Maintaining the balance between lithium use and thyroid function is particularly critical. As early as 1970 goiters were identified in up to 60% of patients treated with lithium[14], and subsequently both clinical and chemical hypothyroidism were reported[15]. The direct effect of lithium on the thyroid is multi-faceted: there is both a decreased uptake of iodine into the gland and possibly an increase in antithyroid antibodies[13]. Thyroid biopsy specimens from some patients treated with lithium assume the pathologic appearance of Hashimoto's thyroiditis[13]. This alteration of thyroid function by lithium use creates a paradoxical situation. As hypothyroidism is associated with an increase in the severity of bipolar disorder, lithium treatment thus both improves and potentially worsens the condition of patients with this illness, should the thyroid axis prove vulnerable to lithium's antithyroid action. In a similar fashion, the improvement in nervous system function brought on by the control of the bipolar diathesis contrasts with the side-effects including tremor, distractibility, disorientation, and poor memory and judgment. The occurrence of these effects rests in part on the variation in distribution of lithium in different bodily organs. Thus, a serum lithium level of 1.0 mmol/l (the goal for optimal treatment) in nuclear magnetic resonance spectroscopic studies has been shown to result in brain lithium levels of only 0.2–0.3 mmol/l in the occipital pole[16].

Recently, lithium's role in modulating nervous system function has expanded with studies revealing its neuroprotective properties, specifically in the retardation of viral infection and against degenerative illness including Alzheimer's disease. There is evidence that lithium protects against N-methyl-d-aspartate receptor-mediated excitotoxic damage to rat cerebellar granule and cortical neurons in culture[17]. Such glutamate-mediated excitotoxicity has been linked to cellular damage in stroke, amyotrophic lateral sclerosis, and possibly neurodegerative diseases such as Alzheimer's dementia[17]. Pre-treatment with lithium has reduced quinolinic acid damage to striatal neurons in a model of cortical ischemia[17]. Lithium has also been shown to induce neurogenesis *in vivo* in rat hippocampal progenitor cells[18]. These observations further illustrate the myriad of functions attributed to this single element.

Hence, the story of lithium use in psychiatry is one of serendipity, international collaboration, miscommunication and finally vindication of a unique therapeutic role, now with established widespread use. This is not only a humanitarian triumph but also a remarkable economic achievement. It has been estimated that the use of lithium carbonate to treat bipolar disorder in the USA has reduced the costs of mental health care by 2.9 billion dollars over a 10-year period[19]. In combination with an additional estimate of savings of 1.3 billion dollars resulting from the return of patients to their functional productive lives, that results in cumulative savings of over 4 billion dollars[19]. Not a bad record for a simple salt!

REFERENCES

1. Aronson JK. An Account of the Foxglove and its Medical Uses 1785–1985. Oxford: Oxford University Press, 1985
2. Johnson FN. The History of Lithium Therapy. London: Macmillan, 1984
3. Ure A. Calculus in the bladder, treated by litholysis. Lancet 1860: 185–6
4. Garrod AB. The Nature and Treatment of Gout and Rheumatic Gout. London: Walton and Maberly, 1859
5. Haig A. Mental depression and the excretion of uric acid. Practitioner 1888; 41: 342–54
6. Ovcharov BW. Van Gogh in Provence and Auvers. New York: McClelland and Stewart, 1992
7. Cade JFJ. Lithium salts in the treatment of psychotic excitement. Med J Aust 1949; 36: 349–52
8. Gershon S. Lithium in mania. Clin Pharmacol Ther 1970; 11: 168–87
9. Schou M, Juel-Neilsen N, Stromgren E, et al. The treatment of manic psychoses by the administration of lithium salts. J Neurol Neurosurg Psychiatry 1954; 17: 250–60
10. Hartigan GP. The use of lithium salts in affective disorders. Br J Psychiatry 1963; 109: 810–14
11. Blackwell B, Shepherd M. Prophylactic lithium – another therapeutic myth? An examination of the evidence to date. Lancet 1968; 1: 968–71
12. Schou M, Baastrup PC, Grof P, et al. Pharmacological and clinical problems of lithium prophylaxis. Br J Psychiatry 1970; 116: 615–19
13. Lazarus JH. Endocrine and Metabolic Effects of Lithium. New York: Plenum, 1986
14. Schou M, Amdisen A, Jensen SE. Occurrence of goiter during lithium treatment. Br Med J 1968; 3: 710–13
15. Rogers MP, Whybrow PC. Clinical hypothyroidism occurring during lithium treatment: two case histories and a review of thyroid function in 19 patients. Am J Psychiatry 1971; 129: 50–5
16. Gyulai L, Wicklund SW, Greenstein R, et al. Measurement of tissue lithium concentration by lithium magnetic resonance spectroscopy in patients with bipolar disorder. Biol Psychiatry 1991; 29: 1161–70
17. Chuang DM. The antiapoptotic actions of mood stabilizers: molecular mechanisms and therapeutic potentials. Ann NY Acad Sci 2005; 1053: 195–204
18. Lograce DC, Eisch AJ. Mood-stabilizing drugs: are these neuroprotective agents clinically relevant? Psych Clin North Am 2005; 28: 399–414
19. Reifman A, Wyatt RJ. Lithium: a brake in the rising cost of mental illness. Arch Gen Psychiatry 1980; 37: 385

2 History of lithium treatment

Mogens Schou, Paul Grof

Contents   Introduction • Early uses in medicine • Early uses in psychiatry • John Cade's contribution • Groundwork for prophylaxis • Opposition: the therapeutic myth • Irrefutable proof • Acceptance and widespread use of lithium • Further problems • Is there a renaissance of lithium treatment? • Impact of lithium treatment on psychiatry

INTRODUCTION

The history of the introduction of lithium into psychiatry is intriguing. It offers insights both into the way in which new ideas originate and develop in medicine and into the social and historical forces that help to mold them and to promote or oppose their acceptance.

This cursory account of the history deals only with the main points and tells only part of the story. For more details the reader must turn to publications where the history has been outlined more fully[1–5].

The acceptance in the 1970s of lithium as an effective prophylactic agent prompted a sudden increase of interest in its past. Many fascinating links to its early use in medicine and psychiatry were uncovered. A checkered history emerged.

EARLY USES IN MEDICINE

Lithium salts were observed to dissolve urate deposits on cartilage in a test tube, and this gave rise to the assumption that they might remove gouty deposits *in vivo* as well. In 1859 Garrod[6] introduced lithium salts for the treatment of gout and urinary calculi. Lithium was thereafter given as a treatment of rheumatism, uremia, renal calculi and a large variety of related disorders, but without confirmation of effect in these diseases.

Several other uses were proposed, for example lithium as a stimulant, as a sedative, for the treatment of diabetes and infectious diseases, or as a caries-preventive additive to toothpaste. Lithium was also thought to be an active ingredient of spring waters used medicinally, even though they contained only minimal amounts. For decades lithium continued to be utilized for such varied purposes without scientific verification.

EARLY USES IN PSYCHIATRY

Nineteenth century physicians used lithium salts for what they called 'folia', 'mania', 'gouty mania' and 'mental derangement', but apparently their clinical descriptions had only transitory effects on lithium usage. In 1886 the Danish neurologist and physiologist Carl Lange published a monograph entitled 'On Periodical Depressions and their Pathogenesis'[7]. It was published in Danish and German, and it has lately been translated into English and supplemented with a biographical portrait of the author[8]. In this publication Lange gave the first report of his and his brother's use of a lithium-containing mixture for the prevention of recurrences of periodic depressions. Lithium was given in accordance with Lange's belief in 'the uric acid diathesis' – a chimera that nevertheless had an extraordinary resilience.

This hypothesis was eventually given up, and lithium treatment was abandoned. The evidence of its effect had been based on clinical impressions and not on systematic trials.

JOHN CADE'S CONTRIBUTION

In the late 1940s the Australian psychiatrist John Cade was searching for a treatment of 'psychotic excitement', i.e. manic-depressive illness. He suspected that a normal metabolite circulating in excess in the body was the cause of the illness. On the basis of a reasoning that is not easy to follow, Cade injected lithium urate intraperitoneally into guinea pigs and saw that they became calmer and less responsive to stimuli but without becoming drowsy.

He further found that lithium carbonate had the same effect on the guinea pigs. The lithium ion, not uric acid, must accordingly have been what produced an effect. The idea then dawned on Cade that lithium might be used in the treatment of agitated psychiatric patients.

Before Cade used lithium carbonate on his patients he tried it on himself for a few weeks. He observed no ill effects and embarked on a clinical trial in groups of psychiatric patients. The ten manic patients responded, their symptoms disappeared and the symptoms returned on discontinuation of lithium. This dramatic finding was reported in the September 1949 issue of *The Medical Journal of Australia*[9]. Cade later experimented with the therapeutic potential of elements resembling lithium such as rubidium, cesium and strontium, but, although some of his observations seemed promising, they were not followed up.

Unexpected obstacle: toxicity panic

An obstacle that delayed the introduction of lithium treatment in psychiatry was a panic that erupted in the late 1949s in the USA. Within that context the timing of Cade's discovery was inopportune. A solution of lithium chloride has a salty taste and was sprinkled on the almost tasteless low-salt diet of cardiac and hypertensive patients. When lithium was given in this uncontrolled way, it produced a number of intoxications, some of them lethal. Although Talbott[10] showed that lithium intoxication could be avoided by monitoring the serum lithium concentration, this unfortunate incident left many physicians leery of any medical use of lithium.

Confirmation of the antimanic effect

Cade's discovery should eventually lay the foundation of modern lithium therapy, but Cade did not extend his observations beyond the ten patients described in his paper. The torch was fortunately carried on, and his findings were soon supported by Noack and Trautner[11] and by clinical reports from France. Names such as Despinois, Reyss-Brion, Deschamps, Duc, Lafon, Passouant and Carrère could be mentioned. In these studies there were no control groups.

It was in 1952 that professor Erik Strömgren in Risskov, Denmark, drew the attention of Mogens Schou to the Australian reports, and Schou designed a protocol for a partly open and partly double-blind trial, which he carried out in collaboration with Strömgren and two other clinicians. Serum lithium levels were monitored systematically throughout the trial. The study was published in 1954[12], and it confirmed Cade's clinical findings of a therapeutic effect of lithium in mania. During the following years observations similar to those from Risskov were made elsewhere in Denmark and in England, France and Australia. The vast majority of the patients improved when they were treated with lithium.

GROUNDWORK FOR PROPHYLAXIS

In the following decades lithium was used to treat manic episodes, but an effect on depressive episodes was also noted[13]. The possibility of a long-term, stabilizing treatment in bipolar and depressive disorder was nevertheless not explicitly considered, and the concept of any maintenance treatment emerged only against much opposition.

In 1956 Schou[14] had noted that a patient stopped having manic and depressive recurrences when he was given lithium also during the intervals between episodes. Some years later Hartigan in England[15] and Baastrup in Denmark[16], similarly observed that manic patients continued on lithium showed a marked reduction of the frequency of both manic and depressive recurrences. These parallel observations encouraged Baastrup and Schou to undertake a longitudinal study of patients with many recurrences. Baastrup selected and treated the patients in Glostrup, and Schou, working in Risskov some distance from Glostrup, collected and analyzed the data and wrote the final paper. The findings were published 1967[17] and showed that recurrences were significantly less frequent and severe during long-term lithium treatment than before such treatment, or they remitted fully.

Schou and Baastrup then joined forces with Angst and Grof and published their prospective observations of 250 lithium-treated patients. Their study led to the same result[18]. By the end of the 1960s there was a sizeable body of observations demonstrating lithium as a useful drug in both acute and long-term treatment of mood disorders. The potential importance of lithium in psychiatry finally dawned for the psychiatric profession.

OPPOSITION: THE THERAPEUTIC MYTH

While the data supporting a prophylactic effect of lithium were accumulating, so was criticism of the evidence. Psychiatrists who had never tried to treat patients with lithium were skeptical of such novelty.

Blackwell and Shepherd[19] felt that the evidence did not support the notion of a prophylactic effect. They claimed that some of the patients had had a 'fragmented' rather than a recurrent course of illness, that the follow-up period had been too short, that the statistical method chosen weighted the facts in favor of the hypothesis, and finally that the non-blind evaluation of recurrences was biased. In a subsequent letter to the editor, Lader[20] argued that patients selected for having had frequent episodes for some years must be expected to have fewer episodes during the following years. Baastrup and Schou refuted these criticisms[21,22].

Views about the evidence and about the prophylactic usefulness of lithium became sharply divided. Based on their own clinical observations many psychiatrists came out strongly in favor of prophylaxis, but there were several aspects to this controversy. The underlying difficulty was that a generally accepted methodology of prophylactic trials had not been available before 1970, and it is in fact still being perfected[23]. Systematic research on the natural history and course of mood disorders was still at an early stage. The historical development of lithium treatment has served to illustrate the methodological and ethical issues involved in the testing and documentation of drug effects, particularly during long-term treatment.

IRREFUTABLE PROOF

The controversy created uncertainty among British and American psychiatrists, who hesitated to start prophylactic lithium treatment, and it became clear that more than verbal refutation was needed. What was required was new evidence entirely free of methodological weaknesses.

However, a painful ethical problem was involved, namely that of switching some patients from lithium to placebo in order to place them in a control group. Since Baastrup and Schou's data strongly indicated that lithium is effective against recurrent depressions, giving patients placebo might expose them to further suffering and perhaps suicide.

Schou therefore designed a trial protocol that took the special ethical problems into consideration. It was blind to the observers, but a non-blind outsider could transfer a patient to lithium if she or he relapsed during the trial, and he did not tell the blind observers whether that patient had been on lithium or on placebo. The trial accordingly remained double-blind.

A sequential analysis terminated the trial as soon as the difference between lithium- and placebo-treated patients had reached statistical significance ($p < 0.01$). In this way as few patients as possible were exposed as briefly as possible to placebo. The trial lasted less than 6 months[24], and the final analysis showed high significances, namely in the group of patients with depressive disorder ($p < 0.001$) and in the group with bipolar disorder ($p < 0.00001$).

The Danes had proved their point, and psychiatrists in other countries such as Ireland, England, Scotland and the USA thereafter validated the findings in a series of double-blind studies. It became clear that lithium does have a prophylactic effect against both manias and depressions, and that it acts in both bipolar and depressive disorder.

ACCEPTANCE AND WIDESPREAD USE OF LITHIUM

Now psychiatrists had an effective tool to stave off recurrences of manic-depressive illness in most patients. At long last a useful remedy had been found for a protracted, devastating and potentially fatal disease.

Psychiatrists in many countries gratefully accepted these important advances, but there were marked geographic differences. In Scandinavia the acceptance of prophylactic lithium was relatively rapid and with limited dissent. Lithium also continued to spread in Australia and in most of continental Europe, for example in Germany, Switzerland, Czechoslovakia, Italy and Greece. In Canada, Kingstone[25] published the first North American paper.

In England and the USA the spread of lithium treatment was more uneven. In the early days the introduction of lithium treatment in England was associated with the names of Rice, Maggs and Coppen. Particularly convincing and elegant was a double-blind lithium trial performed by Alec Coppen and his co-workers[26]. In the USA there was initially much enthusiasm and much opposition. Kline[27] and Gershon and Shopsin[28] played particularly important roles in the expansion of lithium treatment and the acceptance of lithium as a prophylactic drug. Lithium was also increasingly used in Third World countries. It should have helped that it is inexpensive in comparison with other psychotropic drugs, but its use was hampered by the marked lack of psychiatric services.

In addition to manic-depressive illness the use of lithium expanded to other indications: schizoaffective conditions, cycloid psychoses, aggressive states, alcoholism, potentiation of antidepressants and several others. In some of these conditions lithium had an effect, in others not.

FURTHER PROBLEMS

Problems did not stop with criticism from the Maudsley hospital. In 1995 Moncrieff[29] claimed that a prophylactic effect of lithium had not been proved, but she mixed data of different kinds and from different eras, and careful analyses showed that lithium remains effective in those patients and those types of mood disorder for which it was proved to work in the first place.

Repeated challenges came particularly from those who evaluated the treatment in naturalistic studies, from a broadening of the diagnostic criteria for bipolar disorder, and from concern about side-effects.

The efficacy of treatment is always less in naturalistic studies than the efficacy in research studies. Naturalistic studies involve a broader patient selection and may be conducted without sufficient attention being paid to compliance and monitoring.

Broadening of diagnostic criteria beyond those that originally constituted indications for prophylactic lithium treatment[30,31] led to introduction of competing drugs from the pharmaceutical industry. Lithium is produced from the mineral spodumene in North Carolina or extracted from brine pumped up from a salt desert in Chile. As a product found in nature it cannot be patented and is therefore relatively inexpensive. While this could be seen as an advantage, it became a problem when lithium had to compete with manufactured, patented medications after 1990. Probably the best example of this paradox was the case of advertising divalproex. Without solid evidence of a prophylactic effect, divalproex became the most dispensed drug for the treatment of bipolar patients in the USA. This was also the case in Canada, but is no longer.

Side-effects of long-term treatment led, at times, to warnings against lithium. In 1977 the observation of morphological changes in the kidneys of lithium-treated patients generated serious concern among psychiatrists. Many asked themselves whether the patients' mental health was bought at the expense of their kidney function, and whether patients given lithium treatment would eventually develop uremia and require dialysis or kidney transplant. The number of patients who started lithium treatment dropped drastically, ongoing treatments were interrupted, patients had recurrences and suicides are known to have occurred. Some patients objected violently to being deprived of the treatment that had changed their lives, but protests were overruled, and the patients were left in a miserable state[32]. Chapter 21 deals in detail with lithium and the kidneys. As with any long-term treatment, our profession is only gradually learning to assess the degree of such adverse effects and to balance pros and cons of prophylactic lithium treatment for each patient.

IS THERE A RENAISSANCE OF LITHIUM TREATMENT?

Despite overwhelming evidence of the efficacy of prophylactic lithium, continuing debates are likely to occur and are perhaps unavoidable between opponents who incorrectly believe that they are discussing the same issue. The correct evaluation of the outcome of stabilizing treatment in recurrent mood disorders is much more challenging than one would assume. Capricious course, fluctuating compliance, differently responding subtypes of bipolar disorder and in some cases only gradual improvement all make it difficult to evaluate the relationship between medication and a change in the course of illness in any individual patient.

However, there has recently been a trend to return to evidence-based medicine; interest in and use of lithium have revived. We owe this change to the demonstration of lithium's unique antisuicidal properties in affective disorders[33], to laboratory indications of a neuroprotective action of lithium[34] and to its special value as a research tool in neurobiology.

It has also been important that Canadian observations showed different indications for prophylactic treatment with lithium and for long-term treatment with competing drugs[35,36]. In patients with typical bipolar disorder, those with fully remitting, episodic bipolar disorder, lithium is clearly the best prophylactic agent. In patients with atypical bipolar disorder such as 'bipolar spectrum disorder' many patients with mood-incongruent symptoms and co-morbidity are included. Lithium may be of partial help, but then one can see rebound and low or unstable effects. In such patients anticonvulsant drugs and atypical neuroleptics are better.

IMPACT OF LITHIUM TREATMENT ON PSYCHIATRY

Until 1967 no medication had seemed capable of averting recurrences of bipolar disorder. The introduction of prophylactic treatment with lithium changed things radically. Lithium probably provides the most interesting and cogent example of the effect drugs have had upon the practice and research in psychiatry.

In practice it has primarily been lithium's ability to prevent recurrences that changed treatment fashions. In research the introduction of lithium has been a major stimulus for neurobiology, demonstrating that a simple element can produce major neurobiological changes. Lithium became the focus of attention of psychiatrists, psychologists, pharmacologists, biochemists, geneticists and many others. It was probably the advent of lithium treatment that made psychiatric research truly interdisciplinary. Research on all aspects of the affective disorders has been greatly stimulated by demonstration of the efficacy of lithium treatment. Lithium may well become one of the clues to our understanding of mood disorders.

In academic psychiatry the acceptance of lithium treatment led to the important recognition that mood disorders are much more common than was previously presumed. The existing classification systems had to be reconsidered. As the past four decades have shown, prophylactic lithium treatment has made a significant contribution to modern psychiatry, both because of its specific use in alleviating recurrent affective disorders and because of its stimulation of psychiatric research and conceptual thinking.

REFERENCES

1. Gattozzi AA. Lithium in the Treatment of Mood Disorders. NIMH Publication 5033, National Clearing House for Mental Health Information, 1970
2. Johnson FN, Cade JFJ. The historical background to lithium research and therapy. In Johnson FN, ed. Lithium Research and Therapy. London: Academic Press, 1975: 9–22
3. Johnson FN. The History of Lithium Therapy London: MacMillan, 1984
4. Schou M. Phases in the development of lithium treatment in psychiatry. In Samson F,

Adelmann G, eds. The Neurosciences: Paths of Discovery. II. Boston: Birkhäuser, 1992: 148–66

5. Healy D. Lithium. Interview with Mogens Schou. In Healy D. The Psycho-pharmacologists II. London: Chapman & Hall, 1997: 259–84

6. Garrod AB. The Nature and Treatment of Gout and Rheumatic Gout, 1st edn. London: Walton and Maberly, 1859

7. Lange C. Om Periodiske Depressionstilstande og deres Patogenese. Copenhagen: Jens Lunds Forlag, 1886

8. Schioldann J. In commemoration of the centenary of the death of Carl Lange. The Lange theory of 'Periodical Depressions'. A landmark in the history of lithium therapy. Adelaide: Adelaide Academic Press, 2001

9. Cade JFJ. Lithium salts in the treatment of psychotic excitement. Med J Aust 1949; 36: 349–52

10. Talbott JH. Use of lithium salts as a substitute for sodium chloride. Arch Intern Med 1950; 85: 1–10

11. Noack C, Trautner E. Lithium treatment of maniacal psychosis. Med J Australia 1951; 38: 219–22

12. Schou M, Juel-Nielsen N, Strömgren E, Voldby H. The treatment of manic psychoses by the administration of lithium salts. J Neurol Neurosurg Psychiatry 1954; 17: 250–60

13. Vojtěchovský M. Zkusenosti s lecbou solemi lithia. Problemy Psychiatrie v Praxi a ve Vyzkumu. Prague: Czechoslovak Medical Press, 1957: 216–24

14. Schou M. Litiumterapi ved mani: Praktiske retningslinier. Nord Med 1956; 55: 790–4

15. Hartigan GP. The use of lithium salts in affective disorders. Br J Psychiatry 1963; 109: 810–14

16. Baastrup PC. The use of lithium in manic-depressive psychosis. Compr Psychiatry 1964; 5: 396–408

17. Baastrup PC, Schou M. Lithium as a prophylactic agent: its effect against recurrent depression and manic-depressive psychosis. Arch Gen Psychiatry 1967; 16: 162–72

18. Angst J, Weis P, Grof P, et al. Lithium prophylaxis in recurrent affective disorders. Br J Psychiatry 1970; 116: 604–14

19. Blackwell B, Shepherd M. Prophylactic lithium: another therapeutic myth? An examination of the evidence to date. Lancet 1968; 1: 968–71

20. Lader M. Prophylactic lithium. Lancet 1968; 2: 103

21. Baastrup PC, Schou M. Prophylactic lithium. Lancet 1968; 1: 1419–22

22. Baastrup PC, Schou M. Prophylactic lithium. Lancet 1968; 2: 349–50

23. Grof P. Designing long-term clinical trials in affective disorders. J Affect Disord 1994; 30: 243–55

24. Baastrup PC, Poulsen JC, Schou M, et al. Prophylactic lithium: double-blind discontinuation in manic-depressive and recurrent-depressive disorders. Lancet 1970; 2: 326–30

25. Kingstone E. The lithium treatment of manic and hypomanic states. Compr Psychiatry 1960; 1: 317–30

26. Coppen A, Peet M, Bailey J, et al. Double-blind and open studies of lithium prophylaxis in affective disorders. Psychiatr Neurol Neurosurg 1973; 76: 501–10

27. Kline NS. Lithium: The History of its Use in Psychiatry. Basel: Karger, 1969

28. Gershon S, Shopsin B. Lithium: Its Role in Psychiatric Research and Treatment. New York: Plenum, 1973

29. Moncrieff J. Lithium revisited. A re-examination of the placebo-controlled trials of lithium prophylaxis in manic-depressive disorder. Br J Psychiatry 1995; 167: 569–74

30. Baldessarini RJ. Frequency of diagnoses of schizophrenia versus affective disorders from 1944 to 1968. Am J Psychiatry 1970; 127: 759–63

31. Grof P, Fox D. Admission rates and lithium therapy [Letter]. Br J Psychiatry 1987; 150: 264–5

32. Kassirer JP. Adding insult to injury. Usurping patients' prerogatives. N Engl J Med 1983; 308: 898–901

33. Müller-Oerlinghausen B, Ahrens B, Grof E, et al. The effect of long-term lithium treatment on the mortality of patients with manic-depressive or schizoaffective illness. Acta Psychiatr Scand 1992; 86: 218–222

34. Manji HK, Moore GJ, Rajkowska G, et al. Neuroplasticity and cellular resilience in mood disorders. Mol Psychiatry 2000; 5: 578–93

35. Grof P. Selecting effective long-term treatment of bipolar disorders. J Clin Psychiatry 2003; 64 (Suppl 5): 53–61.

36. Alda M. The phenotypic spectra of bipolar disorder. Eur Neuropsychipharmacol 2004; 14 (Suppl 2): S94–9

3 The lithium story: a journey from obscurity to popular use in North America

Samuel Gershon, Chad Daversa

Contents   Introduction • Early Investigations and Background • Australian work • Lithium outside Australia • Spread into North America • Mounting evidence • FDA approval • VA-NIMH study • Lithium in North America today • Conclusion

INTRODUCTION

Lithium entered into significant therapeutic usage in the USA in the late 1940s. Lithium chloride became a popular salt substitute for patients on sodium-free diets. It was being taken by patients with heart and kidney disease, and some fatalities and serious poisonings resulted[1]. These events and the history of lithium in 'therapeutic' spa waters for the treatment of a multitude of disorders would not appear to be auspicious for its re-entry into modern therapeutics.

In this chapter we present a historical travelog of some dramatic medical events leading to the therapeutic investigation of lithium in North America circa 1960. This episode began in a remote location in times distant from those of our new century. These clinical events occurred in Australia, which at that time was geographically and scientifically distant from the main stage of activities in this field. The time was also different in many regards, as my*

colleague, Dr Mark Bauer, has recently referred to this aspect of scientific communication as a Third Force for the New Millennium – our current e-savvy culture and electronic discourse having a tremendous impact on every aspect of our research communications. In order to present the story of lithium's re-entry into the USA, I propose to set the picture in the frame of my own experiences and work with it, in Australia prior to my first visit to the USA in 1959.

EARLY INVESTIGATIONS AND BACKGROUND

The setting was Melbourne, Australia: a remote and isolated part of the world. It was here that John Cade published his finding of the dramatic efficacy of lithium in an open trial in 10 hospitalized manic patients in 1949[2]. Cade was not a well-known scientific figure and did not fol-

---

*All first person references in this text refer to the first author, Samuel Gershon.

low up with any further clinical studies on lithium at all; nevertheless, this report suggested a remarkable effectiveness in that clear and marked improvement occurred in every one of the cases studied. Notably, the prior scientific work with lithium in animals did not really establish the underpinnings for this clinical report and also could hardly establish an appropriate clinically effective dose. It is also interesting to note that Cade's report appeared in *The Medical Journal of Australia*, a journal not at everybody's fingertips in 1949. Thus, it was these uncontrolled observations by an astute clinician on just ten manic patients that produced the platform for the launch of this new era.

The same year that Cade published his report, physicians in the USA learned mainly that lithium was a toxic and lethal substance. These cardiac patients were the ideal cases for lithium toxicity, as would be clearly demonstrated in later studies[3].

Cade also became concerned and insecure of its safe usage in his own cases reported in 1949. These observations on toxicity are reported in *The History of Lithium Therapy* by Neil Johnson[4], who had access to Cade's unpublished clinical notes. In fact, Cade's first case, WB, actually died of lithium toxicity. Toxicity also led to lithium discontinuation in some of his other cases and often treatment was started and then discontinued because of toxicity.

Toxicity presented other difficulties as no formal proposals for its treatment had been evaluated and presented. Thus, lithium toxicity had the potential for changing safe usage into a hazard and carried a potential risk of patient non-compliance. Toxicity and death continued to be reported in psychiatric patients in Australia and elsewhere, and the lithium poisonings in the USA created an inopportune backdrop for its reintroduction as a therapy in North America.

To comprehend how lithium survived the toxicity scare and to appreciate fully the impact of this story, one has to introduce the modern reader to the therapeutic void and nihilism that existed in psychiatry before 1950. With lithium, we suddenly had the possibility of successfully treating a major psychiatric disorder manic-depressive disease; initially, treatment centered on the manic episode. Furthermore, this claim was made for a non-sedative agent of very low cost; sedatives, electroconvulsive therapy and extensive use of restraints were the main alternatives in 1949–50. The therapeutic scope was expanded over the years to lay claim to prophylaxis for both the manic and the depressive phases of the disorder. The era of psychopharmacology had now begun, and the landscape of psychiatry slowly evolved into the profession that it is today. This was a very different picture from our current expectation that, if the patient has psychological distress, there is a medication that is expected to address it. It was in this environment that my experience with lithium began.

AUSTRALIAN WORK

I graduated from the University of Sydney medical school in 1950 and then continued with a medical internship in 1951. During this year I had the opportunity of trying lithium with manic in-patients in a setting essentially free of concomitant medication. In 1952 I moved to Melbourne to start my psychiatric residency at the Royal Park Receiving Hospital where John Cade was the superintendent. During this period, our contacts were simply those of resident and senior staff member. My research interests and activities were all associated with my teachers, mentors and colleagues at the University of Melbourne. My main supports there were in the Departments of Physiology and Pharmacology under the chairmanship of Professor RD

Wright and F Shaw, respectively. The most important and valuable relationship at a personal and professional level was with Dr EM Trautner. These relationships and my formal association with these departments, as well as my subsequent appointment in the Department of Pharmacology, gave me the opportunity to start a number of research endeavors. Here I will mention only those related to lithium.

The publications on lithium in Australia at the time were few. In 1950, Ashburner[5] reported on two cases of toxicity and Roberts[6] on 19 clinical cases. Then, in 1951, in what 'was probably as influential as Cade's original report in promoting lithium therapy more widely'[7], Noack and Trautner presented the largest clinical experience with lithium in over 100 mixed psychiatric subjects in a paper entitled 'the lithium treatment of maniacal psychosis', which appeared in *The Medical Journal of Australia*. This paper made a case for a high success rate in manic patients with little benefit in other psychiatric diagnoses and raised the issue of a specificity of therapeutic activity for lithium[8]. Another Australian report came in 1954 from Glesinger[9], who was located in the remote region of Western Australia. I was able to meet all these people and their efforts were, in retrospect, remarkable. They took some very daring steps and none (with the exception of Trautner) had the safety net of lithium assays.

It was during my first year at the University of Melbourne that I had the good fortune to seek out Trautner. Together, we published several other papers on lithium. One paper that presented a number of interesting issues was entitled 'The excretion and retention of ingested lithium and its effect on the ionic balance of man' (1955). It raised the proposition of a differential pattern of retention and excretion of lithium ion in manic and non-manic subjects[10]. The data showed an increased retention of lithium in the manic patients during the manic phase and flushing out of more lithium in the urine when the mania resolved. These observations tended to point in the direction of pharmacological specificity for lithium in so-called 'typical' manic cases. This paper also presented the details of the use of the spectrophotometric assay of lithium.

Unfortunately, the spectrophotometer was not used for plasma monitoring in the Australian studies until Trautner's extensive work was carried out on it. Even after this technology became available, and despite the deaths experienced by Cade and reported by Roberts in 1950, some clinicians felt that careful clinical observation was an adequate safeguard. My comments in Johnson's book[4] were 'It was Dr Trautner who first used plasma lithium assays in his studies. Altogether, Dr Trautner's exceedingly important role in the early studies on lithium has sadly been completely neglected.' This was echoed by Professor R Douglas Wright, Trautner's departmental chairman, who stated 'I believe that his [Trautner's] part in the lithium story has been overshadowed'[4]. It was Professor Wright who enabled Trautner and me to set up the first spectrophotometer for lithium assays in a mental hospital in Victoria. Its use was still ignored by many clinicians. Trautner was considered by many psychiatrists in Melbourne as a biochemist, with interests limited to this domain. However, he definitely was not looking for the limelight. He was not one to press his views in public, so much so that he never made a public presentation at any scientific or psychiatric meetings. Still, I worked with him for over 10 years, and he was directly involved with our patients and followed their clinical progress throughout our entire relationship.

Over the course of these 10 years, our continued collaboration produced several other reports. Notable among these was a report that touched on the prophylactic potential of lithium in bipolar disorder entitled 'The treatment of shock-dependency by pharmacological agents'[11], though its title gives no clue to this aspect of the issue. We also reported on the issues involved in lithium poisoning and presented a treatment plan for these cases[12]. In 1958 we attempted to address the issue of the teratology of lithium in a rat study[12]. That was my last lithium study in Australia, and the next was during my first stay in the USA in 1959–60[13].

In all, there were a total of eight papers published on lithium treatment worldwide in the first 5 years after Cade's publication in 1949. In the second 5 years there were a total of 19 clinical papers worldwide, including those of Schou and Gershon, and this number fell to 16 in the third 5 years. It is evident that during this 15-year period following the first report there was clearly no big bang. Thus, Cade's paper in 1949[2] produced only a tiny splash and a small ripple.

LITHIUM OUTSIDE AUSTRALIA

The first reports on the use of lithium in psychiatry, outside Australia, were purported to have been French publications in 1951 and 1952, after which sporadic reports appeared over the next 5 years, including a few other French articles, two Italian and two Czech articles and one English article[7]. The historical ties between Australia and Great Britain may account for the publication of the seminal reports coming out of Australia that would ultimately influence investigators such as David Rice, a British psychiatrist running his own study and whose work resulted in the first British report in 1956 on the antimanic effects of lithium[4].

Perhaps one of the most well-recognized figures to be influenced by the Australian reports was Mogens Schou, a Danish psychiatrist whose connection with the Australian work was via a fairly straight line. Schou's professor, Eric Strömgren, brought the Australian lithium work to Schou's attention. Further, it was specifically the paper by Noack and Trautner that first alerted Strömgren to

lithium, which in turn led to a review of the Cade article. The Noack and Trautner article was much more detailed than that of Cade and was the more effective stimulus for Strömgren and Schou's lithium usage. Schou then engaged in a correspondence with Trautner on the use of serum lithium evaluations. Thus, Schou used routine electrolyte estimations in his studies and consequently handled toxicity very successfully.

Although the body of evidence supported the initial reports of lithium's efficacy, these early investigators experienced varying degrees of opposition to the use and claimed efficacy of lithium. Baastrup, a close colleague of Schou in Denmark, wrote to N Johnson of 'considerable opposition to lithium, not least from academics, although this opposition was not supported by criticism of our work'. Trautner wrote to Schou that 'we were experiencing similar problems in Australia'. However, in our case we had the support of the chairmen of the Departments of Physiology and Pharmacology at the University of Melbourne, without which we would not have been able to continue. Fortunately, we could continue to conduct studies and report our work primarily with the participation of the faculty at the University. Nevertheless, we were never asked to present our findings anywhere in Australia other than at the University of Melbourne.

SPREAD INTO NORTH AMERICA

While the first published report of an open study on lithium in 17 manic patients came from Edward Kingstone in Montreal in 1960[4], the significant body of data came to the USA principally from knowledge transmitted from Mogens Schou and myself. Dr Heinrich Waelsch, the Chief Biochemist at the New York State Psychiatric Institute, had worked directly with Mogens Schou and communicated his interest in 1958 to Ronald Fieve, then a resident under Waelsch[4].

When I first came to the USA in 1959, an opportunity afforded by a Research Award, the climate was quite different at the University of Michigan. I spent the year at the recently established Schizophrenia and Psychopharmacology Research Project at the University of Michigan, a group that welcomed innovative studies. With my colleague there, Arthur Yuwiler, our first study was undertaken in 1959 and published in 1960. Our report was the first published in a US journal. This paper made a case for a special therapeutic effect of lithium in 'typical' mania and a marked decrease in activity in more atypical cases[13]. A differential effect was demonstrated and later studied with my colleagues at New York University[14]. These electroencephalogram (EEG) findings demonstrated lithium toxicity with brain changes seen in the EEG, and this correlated with associated side-effects and elevated blood plasma levels[14]. Another study demonstrated a poor effect of lithium in a schizophrenic population and demonstrated a clear differential effect between chlorpromazine (CPZ) and lithium in schizophrenic patients[15].

Although many people were uninterested and some justifiably skeptical, during this year between 1959 and 1960, much interest was demonstrated around the country. During this year, Arthur and I also met on several occasions with the remarkable Jonathan Cole, who was then the head of the Psychopharmacology Research Branch at the National Institute of Mental Health (NIMH). Even though I was a most junior fellow, I had the opportunity to present our material at the NIMH, a presentation facilitated by Dr Seymour Kety, the head of the NIMH Research Program. The climate for this presentation was fundamentally receptive, and whatever criticism was presented was directed towards moving research forward and not impeding a resolution of the issues raised. Thus, a very valuable link was developed with the US community in psychopharmacology and

an important link in the chain of transmission of information about lithium was afforded me. This transmission of information was rapid and resulted in the generation of many foci of contagion.

Nathan Kline was another powerful force in demanding attention to new ideas in psychiatry at this time, mainly because of his previous work with the introduction of reserpine and a monoamine oxidase inhibitor into psychiatry. He now took up the cause for studies with lithium and was responsible for helping create a responsive climate.

In 1963 I moved to the USA permanently and after a short but very active sojourn at the recently established Missouri Institute of Psychiatry in St Louis (here we had superb clinical and laboratory research facilities and with my colleagues carried out a number of studies on lithium), moved to New York University and there began an exceptionally productive period as head of the Neuropsychopharmacology Research Unit. Much of the work conducted at the New York University – Bellevue Hospital was translational, with colleagues involved in both the pre-clinical and clinical components of the project. A major contribution from this period was the significant work conducted with Baron Shopsin that explored the effect of synthesis inhibitors on the response of patients to antidepressant drugs. These studies led to the wide use of synthesis inhibitors in dissecting the role of serotonin in depression.

At this stage, it could be adduced that two pathways of transmission appear: one in the reports of Cade, Noack and Trautner transmitted to Mogens Schou via Strömgren and the other related to my contacts and travels in the USA. Both of these pathways were intersecting, and I came to know Mogens Schou very well after my stay in the USA. We maintained close contact on many occasions. The other set of contacts was with Gordon Johnson, another colleague from Australia, and Andrew Ho.

Both joined us at New York University and both contributed significantly to different aspects of work on lithium. Ho focused on animal studies of the anatomic distribution of lithium in the brain, as well as on studies of the effects of lithium on neurotransmitters.

MOUNTING EVIDENCE

In 1966, over 100 articles on the topic of lithium were published in a single year[16]. Savings related to direct costs such as lowered health-care costs and to indirect costs from increased productivity 'have led to the startling claim that about $4 billion was saved by lithium in the US economy in the decade 1969–79'[17]. Very limited information on lithium appeared until the 121st meeting of the American Psychiatric Association (APA) in New York in 1966, at which information on the use of lithium in the treatment of hypomania was presented. In this presentation by Jacobson he coined the term 'hypomanic alert'. Both this terminology and his application as an intervention strategy were ahead of the times and this early work contributed significantly to thinking about early intervention and the concept of prophylaxis.

Dr Joe Tupin and colleagues also presented a paper at this APA meeting on their experience in treating ten patients with mania. Tupin and his colleagues, Schlagenhauf and White, had earlier recommended a manic patient from Texas to Ronald Fieve, who successfully treated the patient with lithium and sent him back to Texas[4]. Tupin had been in touch with Ron Fieve and myself prior to this report and he was enthusiastic in trying the treatment and in collecting all the information he could get before going ahead. The patients in this trial had not responded well to previous intensive phenothiazine treatment, but all responded favorably to lithium with improvement noted by 4–5 days and always before the 10th day.

Their clinical description is in fact the classic response pattern seen in typical manic cases. The following year Wharton and Fieve reported a good response for 19 patients treated with lithium.

FDA APPROVAL

After gaining wider acceptance in the scientific community, a well-documented flood of applications to conduct further research on the therapeutic effects of lithium carbonate began to arrive at the doorstep of the Food and Drug Administration (FDA), creating an administrative burden for the US regulatory agency[18]. However, pharmaceutical companies were loath to become involved with the marketing of a 'money-losing drug' and it quickly became apparent that some sort of intervention would be necessary to accommodate the demand, prompting the American College of Neuropsychopharmacology (ACNP) to file its own new drug application (NDA) with the FDA to bring the disowned product to market[18].

In fact, it would not be until 1970 that the FDA would approve the use of lithium[19]; however, this was limited to treatment of acute mania only. The therapeutic use of lithium in North America, and more specifically in the USA, was slow to catch on; this can be to a large degree attributed to the poisonings that occurred there, but it may also have been a result of the fact that lithium was not available for patent and that there was an initially cautious stance from both investigators and regulatory bodies in the USA. This delayed development clearly defines a phenomenal lag time between discovery and usage and acceptance in the USA. Even after this there was little widespread clinical usage and very little commercial interest in it.

The dissemination of information and usage was formalized in the USA in a report commissioned by the National Institute of Mental Health (NIMH) on the status of lithium therapy, based on personal interviews and a review of work in both the USA and Europe in 1970[20]. All of these activities and contacts led me to publish the first textbook, entitled *Lithium: Its role in Psychiatric Research and Treatment* together with my colleague Baron Shopsin in 1973. It is our belief that this aided the distribution of information on lithium and supported the comfort of physicians in its more widespread usage.

VA–NIMH STUDY

Ultimately, in 1974 a decision to expand lithium's indication to cover prophylaxis was made by the FDA, although 'approval for unipolar recurrent depression was … still … withheld'[4]. This was due in no small measure to the Prien *et al.* Veterans Administration–NIMH Study.

Prior to the popular use of lithium, phenthiazines such as chlorpromazine were typically considered a staple in the psychiatrists' armamentarium; thus, it was not surprising that, after lithium was shown to be clearly efficacious for the treatment of mania, a large-scale, multicenter study comparing these two agents at 18 different sites was co-sponsored by the National Institute of Mental Health and the Veterans Administration, now known to posterity as the VA-NIMH study. I was fortunate to be associated with this study as a consultant. This study, which included 255 manic-depressive patients, would ultimately show chlorpromazine to be more effective than lithium in a group dubbed 'highly active'. The findings of this study also revealed that highly active patients responded more quickly to chlorpromazine than to lithium. This is inherent in lithium's rate of onset and it affected the outcome of these studies as well, resulting in early terminations in the lithium group because of behavioral overactivity.

However, when viewed in the context of the existing body of data on lithium in manic patients, some were inclined to believe that the nature of the multicenter site opened the study up to criticism on the basis of diagnostic imprecision. As the study was open to patients presenting with schizoaffective disorder, it was hypothesized by the study's detractors that many in the 'highly active' group may have displayed symptoms that were more readily aligned with the atypical forms of the affective illness and would therefore predictably show a poorer response to lithium[7].

LITHIUM IN NORTH AMERICA TODAY

Although it is still considered first-line treatment for bipolar disorder in the USA today, the legacy of lithium is a mixed bag. With little interest from corporate entities, and newer, profitable drugs entering the research pipeline, it is likely that lithium's role in the landscape of pharmacotherapy for affective illness will continue to evolve. Pharmaceutical industry involvement at all levels of research, including sponsorship of drug trials run at major research universities, has raised the question of bias in study design and reporting, as well as in the publication of new drug research. Even regulatory agencies such as the FDA, once inclined to take a cautious stance on new drugs, have been accused of 'sleeping on the job'. As a result of this environment, many young clinicians now view lithium as outdated 'older generation' pharmacotherapy.

CONCLUSION

Lithium sparked a psychopharmacological revolution in psychiatry, or could be considered to be the breeder core. It dramatically and clearly wrought much good, but, like all revolutions, also created adverse effects. These have involved a wide swathe of clinical, medical, social and economic issues, and we will have to attain a larger perspective to evaluate the total effects of these events. I enjoyed traveling this road of discovery and have been privileged to meet many fellow travelers on the way. The most rewarding aspect of the journey was the opportunity to have new colleagues join the caravan. This caravan has traveled a long and tortuous course but in the end has traversed the world and changed the face of psychiatry.

REFERENCES

1. Corcoran AC, Taylor RD, Page IH. Lithium poisoning from the use of salt substitutes. JAMA 1949; 139: 685

2. Cade JF. Lithium salts in the treatment of psychotic excitements. Med J Aust 1949; 2: 349

3. Coats DA, Trautner EM, Gershon S. Treatment of lithium poisoning. Aust Ann Med 1957; 1: 11–15

4. Johnson FN. The History of Lithium Therapy. London: Macmillan, 1984

5. Ashburner JV. A case of chronic mania treated with lithium chloride and terminating fatally. Med J Aust 1950; 2: 386

6. Roberts EL. A case of chronic mania treated with lithium citrate and terminating fatally. Med J Aust 1950; 2: 261–2

7. Johnson G, Gershon S. Early North American research on lithium. Aust NZ J Psychiatry 1999; 33: S48–S53

8. Noack HC, Trautner EM. The lithium treatment of manical psychosis. Med J Aust 1951; 2: 219

9. Glesinger B. Evaluation of lithium in treatment of maniacal psychotic excitement. Med J Aust 1954; 1: 277

10. Trautner EM, Morris R, Noack CH, Gershon S. The excretion and retention of ingested lithium and its effect on the ionic balance of man. Med J Aust 1955; 2: 42

11. Gershon S, Trautner EM. The treatment of shock-dependency by pharmacological agents. Med J Aust 1956; 1: 783–7

12. Trautner EM, Pennycuik PR, Morris RJH, et al. The effects of prolonged sub-toxic lithium ingestion on pregnancy in rats. Aust J Exp Biol Med Sci 1958; 36: 305–21

13. Gershon S, Yuwiler A. Lithium ion: a specific psychopharmacological approach to the treatment of mania. J Neuropsychiatry 1960; 1: 229–41

14. Shopsin B, Johnson G, Gershon S. Neurotoxicity with lithium: differential drug responsiveness. Int Pharmacopsychiatry 1970; 5: 170–82

15. Shopsin B, Kim SS, Gershon S. A controlled study of lithium vs. chlorpromazine in acute schizophrenics. Br J Psychiatry 1971; 119: 435–40

16. Jefferson JW, Greist JH, Baudhuin MG, Hartely BI. The lithium literature, an evolutionary tree reflecting scientific advances and pseudoscientific retreats. In Birch NJ, Gallicchio VS, Becker RW, eds. Lithium: 50 years of Psychopharmacology. Weidner Cheshire, CT: Publishing Group, 1999: 22–7

17. Birch NJ. The inorganic biochemistry and pharmacology of lithium: overview, background, and a novel idea. In Birch NJ, Gallicchio VS, Becker RW, eds. Lithium: 50 years of psychopharmacology. Cheshire, CT: Weidner Publishing Group, 1999: 234–6

18. Kline NS. A narrative account of lithium usage in psychiatry. In Gershon S, Shopsin B, eds. Lithium: Its Role in Psychiatric Research and Treatment. New York: Plenum Press, 1973: 5–13

19. Soares JC, Gershon S. The psychopharmacologic specificity of the lithium ion: origins and trajectory. J Clin Psychiatry 2000; 61 (Suppl 9): 16–22

20. Goodwin FK, Ebert MH. Lithium in mania: clinical trials and controlled Studies. In Gershon S, Shopsin B, eds. Lithium: Its Role in Psychiatric Research and Treatment. New York: Plenum Press, 1973: 245–7

4 Different views on the use of lithium across continents

Daniel Z Lieberman, Jaclyn Saggese,
Frederick K Goodwin

Contents   Introduction • History • Economics • Prescribing • Advantages

INTRODUCTION

Comprehensive management of bipolar disorder requires treatment of acute mania and depression, as well as the prevention of mania and depression during the maintenance phase. The most stringent definition of a mood stabilizer would require efficacy in all phases; however, these conditions are not easily met. A review undertaken by Bauer and Mitchner designed to evaluate how well specific agents met more or less stringent definitions of mood stabilizer concluded that only lithium, which has some degree of efficacy in all phases, is a true mood stabilizer based on the most restrictive definition[1]. Despite the fact that there is more evidence available on the use of lithium than any other drug in maintenance treatment of bipolar disorder[2], there has been a fairly marked shift away from the prescription of lithium in the USA compared to Europe and the rest of the world.

HISTORY

As discussed in Chapter 2, lithium's efficacy in the treatment of mania was first reported in Australia by Cade in 1949. Controlled trials carried out by Schou and colleagues in Denmark in the 1950s were the beginning of a broader recognition of lithium as an effective treatment for bipolar disorder. In the USA, however, there was more concern about the safety of lithium. Around the same time that Cade was observing therapeutic effects of lithium in Australia, physicians in the USA were reporting several deaths caused by unrestricted use of lithium as a salt substitute for cardiac patients, giving it a reputation as a dangerous and toxic substance. As a result of these experiences, lithium was virtually neglected in the USA until the early 1960s.

ECONOMICS

Another reason for the slow acceptance of lithium in the USA was economic. Drugs typically are introduced by pharmaceutical companies, which invest in the studies necessary for US Food and Drug Administration (FDA) approval. A pharmaceutical company receives a patent on a new drug (15 years of exclusivity at that time), which allows it to recoup its investment. Lithium salts, of course, could not be patented, and therefore lacked a pharmaceutical company as an advocate for FDA approval. It was not until 1970, when the National Institute of Mental Health and the Lithium Task Force of America (William Bunney, Irvin Cohen, Jonathan Cole, Ronald Fieve, Samuel Gershon, Robert Prien and Joseph Tupin) worked with Smith Kline and the FDA to facilitate the approval of lithium for the treatment of mania, that it became available to doctors and patients in the USA[3].

Although lithium subsequently became the first-line treatment for bipolar disorder in the USA, its use began declining relative to Europe and the rest of the world in the early to mid-1990s. A 5-year naturalistic study found that between 1989 and 1994 the portion of hospitalized patients receiving lithium monotherapy for bipolar disorder in the USA declined from 84% to 43%. During this same period the use of valproate (alone or in combination with lithium) increased from 0% to 38% of antimanic treatment regimens, while carbamazepine was decreasing from 24% to 18%[4]. More recently, Goodwin and his colleagues in two large research-oriented health maintenance organizations found that this trend continued after 1994[5]. Pharmacy data from a sample of 20 638 health plan members revealed that the distribution of first mood stabilizing drugs prescribed, based on the year of initial diagnosis, changed substantially over time. The ratio of initial filled prescriptions for lithium to that of divalproex

shifted from 6:1 in 1994 to 1:2 in 2001, while there was little change in the use of carbamazepine (Figure 4.1).

PRESCRIBING

There are multiple factors that contribute to prescribing decisions made by physicians. Some, such as the inherent efficacy and safety of a medication, are the same regardless of where the physician practices. Other factors, however, are dependent on social, cultural, economic and political characteristics that vary across countries. These factors include the perceived efficacy of the agent, education and training, regulatory agency decisions, medical-legal environment and marketing activity. These different variables are described in more detail below.

In recent years, an increase in the number of lithium-resistant cases has been seen in clinical practice in the USA, and reported in the academic literature[6]. Kukopulos *et al.* reported that, among rapid cyclers, bipolar patients who had previously been exposed to an antidepressant did not respond as well to lithium[7]. When the serotonin-specific reuptake inhibitors were introduced, they were believed to be safe and easy to use, and antidepressant prescriptions increased dramatically. Now the majority of antidepressant prescriptions are written by primary care physicians who do not have the necessary expertise to distinguish bipolar depression from major depressive disorder. Increasing rates of substance abuse in the 1970s and the cocaine epidemic that started in the 1980s have also become factors in lithium refractoriness in the USA.

Long-term prescribing habits are established during medical education and specialty training, and since an increasing proportion of this comes from industry-supported educational programs, lithium is covered briefly at best. Another key component of clinical education

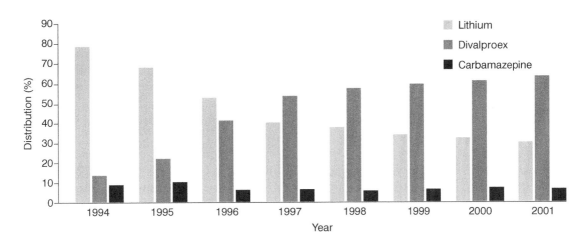

Figure 4.1 Distribution of initial mood stabilizer prescriptions according to year of initial bipolar disorder diagnosis

comes from individuals modeling themselves after mentors, teachers and supervisors. Thus new physicians who work with supervisors who have extensive experience with lithium will be more likely to develop their own expertise with this drug. This kind of education is all the more important for a generic drug like lithium, because it will never be adequately covered in the dominant industry-supported educational programs. However, if lithium use continues to diminish in the USA, it will gradually fade in this mentor-driven educational experience as psychiatrists trained since the early 1990s become tomorrow's mentors. Recommendations for training residents in the use of lithium include experience with large numbers of patients receiving lithium as monotherapy, and with long-term follow-up of at least 8–12 months[3]. Many US residencies no longer provide this type of training. Thus a vicious cycle is set in motion as lithium's increasing unfamiliarity feeds the misperception that it is too difficult to use, and has been replaced by newer agents.

The role of lithium in Europe has evolved in a way that has been very different from that in the USA. This is not to imply a monolithic approach to psychopharmacology in the European community. For example, a recent survey of psychotropic drug prescriptions given to patients with a variety of diagnoses in ten European countries found that patients in Spain were on the most drugs, and patients in Germany were on the fewest. Larger doses of antipsychotic medications were seen in Denmark, England, Germany and Spain, while higher doses of benzodiazepines were seen in Denmark, England, The Netherlands and Norway[8].

In spite of these differences, there exists a remarkable consensus on the use of lithium as the first-line agent in the treatment of bipolar disorder. A survey of 1041 patients with bipolar disorder in 11 European countries gathered information on demographics, history of illness and type of treatment received. The authors reported that the problems encountered by bipolar patients were similar throughout the European countries studied, regardless of cultural differences[9]. The most frequently prescribed medication for these bipolar patients was lithium in 9 of 11 countries consisting of Austria, France, Holland, Hungary, Italy,

Portugal, Spain, Sweden and the UK. In Finland typical neuroleptics were reported most frequently, and lithium was second. In Russia typical neuroleptics were also the most frequent, followed by amitriptyline, and then lithium[10].

Specialized lithium clinics are more common in Europe than in the USA, and they encourage lithium use in a number of different ways. The treatment environment in a lithium clinic is an intermediate step between the highly controlled setting of a clinical trial and routine clinical practice in which lithium treatment may not always be properly implemented. Because they are staffed by experienced clinicians who are sophisticated in the use of lithium, treatment is handled more skillfully, and better outcomes are possible. Furthermore, educational opportunities exist in these settings that would be hard to duplicate elsewhere.

Licht and colleagues described the treatment of the first 148 patients seen at the Aarhus University Psychiatric Hospital lithium clinic[11]. Although some patients in this clinic were treated with carbamazepine, oxcarbazepine, or valproate, 89% received lithium monotherapy. The authors stated that this was not unique to the lithium clinic environment, but reflective of the fact that lithium is the drug of first choice for maintenance treatment in Denmark[12]. The mean serum lithium level of patients in this study was 0.63 mEq/l. This level is lower than is typically seen in the USA. A consensus panel of US experts in bipolar disorder recommended a range of 0.7–1.2 mEq/l for acute mania, and 0.6–1.1 mEq/l for maintenance treatment[13]. Because many of lithium's adverse effects are related to the serum level, the common belief in the USA that lithium is associated with more severe side-effects than other mood stabilizers may be influenced by the use of higher doses.

Specialists who work in lithium clinics check levels more frequently, and are more likely to avoid levels that are too high. A lithium clinic in Somerset, UK, compared elevated lithium levels among their patients to two other groups: patients treated as psychiatric hospital outpatients, and patients treated by general practitioners (GPs)[14]. During the 3-month investigation period 1.2% of lithium clinic attendees had serum levels above 1.0 mEq/l, compared to 6.0% of the hospital outpatients, and 13.2% of the patients seen by a GP. Additionally, the mean serum lithium level was significantly lower in lithium clinic attendees (0.58 mEq/l) compared to psychiatric outpatients (0.67 mEq/l) and GP patients (0.69 mEq/l).

A hostile legal climate characterized by widespread medical malpractice litigation and increasing costs of malpractice insurance can influence prescribing patterns by forcing doctors to practice defensive medicine. The costs of medical malpractice premiums have risen rapidly in Europe, but even more in the USA. In the UK, for example, premiums have risen by 8% per year over the past 3 years, while in the USA premium increases have been approximately 30% per year[15]. An untoward fear of litigation can lead a physician to focus on the risks of a medication, while neglecting the benefits. The perception of lithium as a drug with greater risks than other mood stabilizers is a significant liability in this environment

Differing regulatory climates affect the way medications are used. Regulatory agencies grant permission for medications to be labeled for specific indications, and may require particular safety issues to be highlighted. In the USA, there are eight drugs that have been approved for the treatment of bipolar mania (lithium, aripiprazole, carbamazepine, olanzapine, quetiapine, risperidone, valproate and ziprasidone), and four drugs approved for maintenance (lithium, lamotrigine, olanzapine and aripiprazole, the last based on 6-month data). In other countries, there are fewer competitors that have regulatory approval. Although medications are routinely prescribed 'off label', regulatory approval confers important benefits. Relevant to the medical-legal issue discussed above, off label use of a medication carries greater malpractice risk in the case of a poor outcome. Third-party payers may deny reimbursement for medications when they are prescribed off label, and pharmaceutical companies can legally market a drug for a specific indication only if that indication has received formal approval.

Marketing efforts on behalf of a drug are directly related to its potential profitability. Unlike alternative mood stabilizers, lithium cannot be patented, and therefore generates a tiny amount of money compared to any of its 'competitors'. A part of the high earnings from a mood stabilizer that is proprietary is used to finance educational programs that increase physicians' confidence in using the medication, and consequently support sales of the product.

The disparity in profitability between lithium and patented medications is larger in the USA because of a lack of price controls on pharmaceuticals (which, incidentally, the authors believe are not desirable because they can discourage innovation). For example, a 500 mg tablet of divalproex generates 71% more revenue in the USA than in Canada (US dollars (USD) 2.00 vs. USD 1.17). By comparison, a 300-mg tablet of immediate release lithium sells for USD 0.19 in the USA and USD 0.12 in Canada. Olanzapine, another widely used mood stabilizer, costs 37% more for a 10-mg tablet in the USA compared to the UK, which represents a difference of USD 2.42 per pill for this medication (USD 9.00 vs. USD 6.58). As the top-selling drug of Eli Lilly & Co., sales of olanzapine reached USD 4.4 billion-a-year in 2005, and accounted for one-third of Lilly's total earnings[16].

Many of the educational programs funded by pharmaceutical companies provide useful information that increases psychiatrists' knowledge base, and familiarizes them with new developments in the field. One drawback, however, is that most presentations focus almost exclusively on the drug being promoted. In the USA this exclusive focus is ironically due to restrictions placed on pharmaceutical companies by the FDA. The FDA prohibits speakers at promotional programs from providing comparison data or other information about alternative pharmacologic agents.

In addition to promotional programs, pharmaceutical companies also sponsor a large number of continuing medical educational (CME) courses via unrestricted educational grants. CME speakers are free to present any material that they feel is appropriate, and there is an expectation that the programs be fair and balanced by including information on all relevant compounds. Even in these settings, however, the use of lithium is rarely the focus. Instead, there is generally an emphasis on new developments in the field related to research on recently introduced drugs. The net effect of these various industry-supported programs is that substantial resources are available to teach physicians about brand name drugs, while very little is available for programs on lithium.

Direct to consumer advertising (DTCA) of prescription drugs is currently allowed in only two countries: the USA and New Zealand. DTCA (which includes increasing use of the Web for this purpose) can help increase public awareness of health problems, and when certain illnesses, such as depression and bipolar disorder, are poorly recognized and undertreated, DTCA can help encourage a useful dialog between a doctor and a patient. In other circumstances, however, DTCA can lead to pressure on doctors to prescribe a drug that they do not believe is indicated, or is not the best choice for a patient's needs. In the USA all of the currently approved mood stabilizers, except lithium, have active DTCA campaigns.

Fewer data are available regarding the use of lithium outside the USA and Europe. In Japan lithium is identified as the first choice for the treatment of mania in a published algorithm for the treatment of bipolar disorder[17], and general agreement with this recommendation is seen among practicing psychiatrists. A survey of 298 Japanese psychiatrists found a broad consensus for the use of lithium as the first-line treatment of mania, though there was less agreement on the treatment of bipolar depression[18].

Mania was once believed to be rare in China compared to Western countries, and as a result lithium use was uncommon. A 1980 survey found that only about half of Chinese psychiatric hospitals were using lithium, and that prophylactic use of lithium was limited[19]. The author of this study speculated that the factors responsible for this limited use included the infrequency of the diagnosis of mania, fear of toxicity and lack of laboratory facilities for monitoring levels.

A similar survey in China, carried out 6 years later, found that significant gains had been made in the use of lithium[20]. The percentage of psychiatric hospitals using lithium had risen to 87%. Of those hospitals that continued to avoid lithium, many were located in rural areas. Typical neuroleptics were readily available in these areas, but patients had to travel hundreds of kilometers to obtain even small amounts of lithium, and the drug was more costly than neuroleptics.

None of the trends described above have yet shown clear signs of abating, and it is unlikely in the USA that the use of lithium will substantially increase relative to other mood stabilizers. The extent of this secular shift in prescribing practices is unfortunate, because for many patients the combination of a modest dose of lithium with an anticonvulsant is superior to the anticonvulsant alone, and for some patients, no alternative mood stabilizer is as effective as lithium monotherapy. Additionally, lithium is the only mood stabilizer shown to reduce the likelihood of suicide and this means that, on the whole, psychiatrists who do not know how to use it are exposing their patients and themselves

to greater risk. For all of these reasons a psychiatrist who does not know how to use lithium should not be considered competent to treat bipolar patients, and training programs responsible for this deficiency should not be accredited.

ADVANTAGES

Finally, new research suggests that lithium has neuroprotective effects that can reverse long-term loss of neuronal viability that can occur in patients with bipolar disorder[21]. While the clinical significance of this neuroprotective effect has not yet been determined, a better understanding of the ways in which lithium exerts its therapeutic effects via interaction with intracellular signaling mechanisms may nevertheless spur the development of new mood-stabilizing compounds. Even the most fervent advocates of lithium express disappointment that no alternative has become available that exceeds the efficacy of lithium in a way that other mood stabilizers fail to achieve[22]. Restoring the benefits of lithium to patients in the USA may paradoxically require the development of a completely new medication that duplicates and goes beyond the specific therapeutic effects of this unique element that launched the psychopharmacology revolution, a revolution that not only transformed our field but has allowed millions of patients around the world to lead essentially normal lives.

REFERENCES

1. Bauer MS, Mitchner L. What is a 'mood stabilizer'? An evidence-based response. Am J Psychiatry 2004; 161: 3–18
2. Baldessarini RJ, Tondo L, Hennen J, et al. Is lithium still worth using? An update of selected recent research. Harvard Rev Psychiatry 2002; 10: 59–75

3. Fieve RR. Lithium therapy at the millennium: a revolutionary drug used for 50 years faces competing options and possible demise. Bipolar Disord 1999; 1: 67–70

4. Fenn HH, Robinson D, Luby V, et al. Trends in pharmacotherapy of schizoaffective and bipolar affective disorders: a 5-year naturalistic study. Am J Psychiatry 1996; 153: 711–13

5. Goodwin FK, Fireman B, Simon GE et al. Suicide risk in bipolar disorder during treatment with lithium and divalproex. JAMA 2003; 290: 1467–73

6. Goodwin FK, Ghaemi SN. The impact of the discovery of lithium on psychiatric thought and practice in the USA and Europe. Aust NZ J Psychiatry 1999; 33 (Suppl): S54–64

7. Kukopulos A, Reginaldi D, Laddomada P, et al. Course of the manic–depressive cycle and changes caused by treatment. Pharmakopsychiatr Neuropsychopharmakol 1980; 13: 156–67

8. Bowers L, Callaghan P, Clark N, et al. Comparisons of psychotropic drug prescribing patterns in acute psychiatric wards across Europe. Eur J Clin Pharmacol 2004; 60: 29–35

9. Morselli PL, Elgie R, Cesana BH, et al. GAMIAN-Europe/BEAM survey II: cross-national analysis of unemployment, family history, treatment satisfaction and impact of the bipolar disorder on life style. Bipolar Disord 2004; 6: 487–97

10. Morselli PL. Elgie R. GAMIAN-Europe/BEAM survey I – global analysis of a patient questionnaire circulated to 3450 members of 12 European advocacy groups operating in the field of mood disorders. Bipolar Disord 2003; 5: 265–78

11. Licht RW, Vestergaard P, Rasmussen NA, et al. A lithium clinic for bipolar patients: 2-year outcome of the first 148 patients. Acta Psychiatr Scand 2001; 104: 387–90

12. Vestergaard P, Schou M. Lithium treatment in Aarhus. 1. Prevalence. Pharmacopsychiatry 1989; 22: 99–100

13. Sachs GS, Printz DJ, Kahn DA, et al. The Expert Consensus Guideline Series: medication treatment of bipolar disorder 2000. Postgrad Med Spec 2000: 1–104

14. Masterton G, Warner M, Roxburgh, et al. Supervising lithium. A comparison of a lithium clinic, psychiatric out-patient clinics, and general practice. Br J Psychiatry 1988; 152: 535–8

15. Kath J. Learning from mistakes: incident reporting, risk management, cost reduction. Lessons Learned in Medical Malpractice. University Hospital of Zurich, 2004

16. Bloomberg. Lilly wins ruling blocking generic forms of top-selling zyprexa. 2005 http://quote.bloomberg.com/apps/news?pid=10000006&sid=a0mDSx5emhzo&refer=home. 2005

17. Motohashi N. Algorithms for the pharmacotherapy of bipolar disorder. Psychiatry Clin Neurosci 1999; 53 (Suppl): S41–4

18. Oshima A, Higuchi T, Fujiwara Y, et al. Questionnaire survey on the prescribing practice of Japanese psychiatrists for mood disorders. Psychiatry Clin Neurosci 1999; 53 (Suppl): S67–S72

19. Shanming Y. Lithium therapy in China. Brief communication. Acta Psychiatr Scand 1981; 64: 270–2.

20. Shan-Ming Y, Schou M, Zhi-Hong T. Lithium therapy in China: 6 years later. Acta Psychiatr Scand 1987; 76: 219–20

21. Gould TD, Zarate CA, Manji HK, et al. Glycogen synthase kinase-3: a target for novel bipolar disorder treatments. J Clin Psychiatry 2004; 65: 10–21

22. Schou M. Forty years of lithium treatment. Arch Gen Psychiatry 1997; 54: 9–13, discussion 14–5

5 The position of lithium in international and national guidelines for the treatment of mood disorders

Nicolas Andres Crossley,
Bruno Müller-Oerlinghausen, Tasha Glenn,
Michael Bauer

Contents   Introduction • Review of guidelines • Lithium and acute mania • Lithium in acute bipolar depression • Lithium in the prophylaxis of bipolar disorder • Lithium augmentation for resistant unipolar depression • Lithium in the prophylaxis of unipolar depression • Guideline development • Conclusion

INTRODUCTION

In an effort to improve quality and cost-effectiveness, many insurance companies and medical associations promote the implementation into everyday practice of prescribing guidelines for both general practitioners and specialists. Guidelines should assist the practitioner with routine decision-making and be based on the best available evidence. Well-known experts or professional associations usually write these guidelines. Recently, many guidelines have been issued by specialists' associations (e.g. the American Psychiatric Association (APA), Deutsche Gesellschaft für Psychiatrie, Psychotherapie und Nervenheilkunde (DGPPN)), national institutions (e.g. the National Institute for Clinical Excellence (NICE), the Scottish Intercollegiate Guidelines Network (SIGN), Arzneimittelkommission der deutschen Ärzteschaft (AkdÄ)) and international organizations (e.g. the World Federation of Societies of Biological Psychiatry (WFSBP)).

Fifty years ago, lithium was the only drug available for the treatment of bipolar disorder, and lithium was also widely used for episode prevention in unipolar depression. Both the introduction of many new pharmacological agents and the evolving understanding of the classification of mood disorders have transformed treatment, as is reflected in recent guidelines. In this chapter, the recommendations for the use of lithium for bipolar disorder and unipolar depression in a sampling of well-known guidelines are compared. This chapter does not provide a systematic review of available international guidelines for mood disorders, nor does it consider how extensively treatment guidelines are implemented into routine practice.

REVIEW OF GUIDELINES

Table 5.1 contains recommendations from 11 major international and national guidelines that have been published since 2000 for both bipolar disorder and unipolar depression[1–17]. The guidelines are from Australia, New Zealand, Canada, England, Germany, Scotland, the USA and the WFSBP. Nine of these guidelines cover acute mania, ten cover acute bipolar depression, ten cover prophylaxis of bipolar disorder and seven cover unipolar depression.

LITHIUM AND ACUTE MANIA

As shown in Table 5.1, there is widespread agreement in the guidelines for the role of lithium in the treatment of acute mania. Lithium monotherapy has a primary role in the management of the 'classical' euphoric type of mania in all nine guidelines. Valproate (divalproate) and atypical antipsychotics are also noted as a treatment for euphoric mania in all nine guidelines, especially when the mania is severe. One benefit of valproate is that it can be used intravenously at a loading dose for a faster response[18]. There is also general agreement that lithium is less effective in mixed mania or rapid cycling. Eight guidelines provide a specific recommendation for mixed or dysphoric mania and all agree that lithium monotherapy is not a first-line treatment for dysphoric or mixed mania. Valproate, atypical antipsychotics

and carbamazepine are considered first-line choices. A specific recommendation for mania with rapid cycling is included in five guidelines and all mention lithium in combination with valproate or an antipsychotic as either a first- or a second-line choice, while one includes lithium monotherapy as a first-line choice (APA)[4]. None of the guidelines give specific recommendations for the treatment of hypomania.

Many recommendations for the treatment of acute mania have been derived from studies of patients with classical euphoric mania or from older studies with less rigorous standards than are found in modern clinical trials. As the concept of bipolar disorder is evolving from categorical to dimensional, new studies are required to delineate the treatments most suited for the subtypes of mania and hypomania. Thus, this lack of clear evidence for the treatment of specific subtypes of bipolar disorder makes it difficult to make firm recommendations for the treatment of subtypes of mania, and is reflected in the diverging recommendations.

LITHIUM IN ACUTE BIPOLAR DEPRESSION

There is also widespread agreement among the guidelines regarding the role of lithium in acute bipolar depression. Of the ten guidelines, eight recommend lithium in combination with an antidepressant (usually specifying a selective serotonin reuptake inhibitor (SSRI)) and five also suggest lithium monotherapy as an alternative monotherapy. Eight guidelines also state that lamotrigine can be used instead of lithium. Most guidelines recommend tailoring the treatment for each patient, balancing the stronger antidepressant potential of the combination therapy (mood stabilizer plus antidepressant) with the higher risk of switching into mania. The APA was particularly cautious about the use of antidepressants in bipolar depression, even in combination with a mood stabilizer, because of the lack of evidence of safety and efficacy at the time the guidelines were published[19]. A meta-analysis addressing this issue was available only after the APA guideline was published[20].

LITHIUM IN THE PROPHYLAXIS OF BIPOLAR DISORDER

All ten guidelines include lithium as a first-line choice of a prophylactic agent for bipolar disorder. There is a consensus that lithium is the drug with the best available evidence for efficacy in the prophylaxis of bipolar disorder and for the prevention of suicide. There is some variance, however, in the drugs recommended as alternatives to lithium, most of them including valproate, lamotrigine, carbamazepine or olanzapine (Table 5.1).

Although all guidelines include lithium as a first-line choice for the prophylaxis of bipolar disorder, it is expected that a patient survey would find considerable variability in the agents prescribed over the long term due to many factors, as described below.

Rationale for selection of the prophylactic agent

The guidelines provide different rationales for selection of the prophylactic agent. For example, the APA guidelines recommend continuing the drug that was successful in the acute manic period as the prophylactic agent[4]. In contrast, both the Danish[10] and German[11] guidelines propose that the preferred prophylactic agent for the patient determine the treatment selection for the acute manic episode.

Importance of the anti-suicide potential of the prophylactic agent

There is a different emphasis among the guidelines on the importance of the anti-suicidal potential of the prophylactic agent. With surprisingly homogeneous evidence available, lithium is undoubtedly the drug that has the greatest evidence supporting an anti-suicidal and thus mortality-reducing effect (see Chapter 15). According to a meta-analysis by Baldessarini et al.[21], one would need to treat only 125 patients with lithium over 1 year to save one patient per year. Yet, of the ten guidelines, only the two German guidelines recommend considering the suicidal risk when selecting an appropriate prophylactic treatment[11,15].

While the low frequency of suicidal events makes it methodologically difficult to use the reduction of suicidality as an outcome criterion in psychiatric drug trials, it is certainly an important factor to consider, especially when recommending treatments for mood disorders. To weight its epidemiological importance, one could consider that in Germany in the year 2000, suicide killed more people than did traffic accidents, drugs and violent acts together, and around 60% of these suicides were related to a depressive episode (Statistisches Bundesamt 2002, from reference 11). Long-term prophylactic treatment for bipolar disorder is certainly one of the areas in which these data should have the greatest impact.

Expanding the bipolar spectrum

With the expansion of the bipolar spectrum to include non-classical bipolar disorder, there is less evidence available as to which prophylactic agent is most efficacious. As more evidence is gathered in future studies, drugs other than lithium may be superior prophylactic agents for specific subtypes of bipolar disorder. It is particularly difficult to obtain a level of evidence that

Table 5.1 Summary of recommendations of different international and national guidelines concerning lithium prescription*

Guideline (in chronological order)	Bipolar depression	Mania – classical	Mania – rapid cycling	Mania – dysphoric/mixed	Hypomania	Bipolar disorder – prophylaxis	Unipolar refractory depression – augmentation	Unipolar depression – prophylaxis
Germany: DGPPN 2000[1]	Li, VAL, CBZ; if already on any of them, consider combination with SSRI or bupropion	1st Li, 2nd CBZ, VAL	1st VAL, 2nd CBZ, or Li + anticonvulsant	1st VAL, 2nd CBZ or Li	No explicit recommendations given	1st Li; alternatives: CBZ, VAL	Augmentation therapy with Li or THY considered between change of AD, AD combination, psychotherapy + AD or ECT	AD full doses or Li
UK: BAP 2000 and 2003[2,3]	SSRI + Li or VAL or antipsychotics; if less severe (although less evidence supporting), monotherapy with LAM, Li or possibly VAL	If severe aAP or VAL; if not severe, consider also Li or CBZ; if not responding, consider Li/VAL + antipsychotic or clozapine	No explicit recommendations for acute management; Li, VAL or LAM as initial treatment for prophylaxis	Li not mentioned unless previously on long-term treatment (1st VAL, antipsychotics)	No recommendations given, classification considered controversial	1st Li; 2nd options: VAL, olanzapine, CBZ or LAM	Augmentation with Li or THY recommended after failure to respond to two antidepressants; other options are adding psychotherapy or ECT (the latter both less strongly recommended)	1st AD full dose; 2nd Li
USA: APA 2002[4]	Li or LAM; refer lack of evidence to recommend combination with AD	Li or VAL, adding aAP if severe; aAP such as olanzapine are also an alternative for less ill patients as monotherapy	1st Li or VAL; 2nd LAM; combinations might be required between any of these drugs or with aAP	1st VAL + aAP; 2nd Li + aAP; monotherapy with aAP if less severe	No recommendations given	Li or VAL as first line	Augmentation therapy with Li, non MAOI-AD, THY, anticonvulsants or psychostimulants considered particularly for partial responders; other options are ECT, AD + psychotherapy or dose change of AD	Li not mentioned (treatment effective in acute phase, either AD full dose, psychotherapy, or periodic ECT)
WFSBP 2002, 2003 and 2004[5-9]	Li or LAM + SSRI	Li, VAL, olanzapine or risperidone	VAL or CBZ; Li + VAL or clozapine only for refractory cases	Li suggested not very effective (VAL, CBZ, olanzapine or risperidone)	Consider drug of choice for prophylaxis; if not intended, VAL or aAP	Li; if rapid cycling, Li+CBZ or VAL	Augmentation strategy (1st option Li, 2nd THY, pindolol, buspirone), switch to other AD (same or different class), or combine 2 AD	Li or AD full dose

continued over

continued

Guideline (in chronological order)	Bipolar depression	Mania – classical	Mania – rapid cycling	Mania – dysphoric/ mixed	Hypomania	Bipolar disorder – prophylaxis	Unipolar refractory depression – augmentation	Unipolar depression – prophylaxis
Denmark: DPA 2003[10]	Li or LAM, with or without AD	Li (if patient compliant and prophylaxis planned), VAL, antipsychotic	No explicit recommendations given	Li referred as having low response rate (VAL or olanzapine)	No explicit recommendations given	1st Li, unless side-effects, patients' preference, or uncooperative patient	Indication not target of guideline	Indication not target of guideline
Germany: DGBS (Weissbuch) 2003[11]	Li+SSRI or LAM+SSRI	Li, VAL, olanzapine or risperidone	Monotherapy with Li not recommended as first choice; 1st VAL or CBZ; 2nd Li+VAL or clozapine	VAL, CBZ or olanzapine; Li suggested less effective	Consider best treatment for prophylaxis; if not intended, VAL or aAP	Li, especially if suicidal; consider CBZ as first option if not suicidal and atypical presentation	Indication not target of guideline	Indication not target of guideline
Australia & New Zealand: RANZCP 2004[12,13]	Li or LAM or any of them + AD (1st SSRIs)	Li, VAL, CBZ, olanzapine	No explicit recommendations given	VAL or olanzapine; Li may be considered if response to anticonvulsants is poor	No explicit recommendations given	Li, VAL, LAM or CBZ; Li supported by the best evidence	1st CBT+AD, switch to other AD or increase in dose if on TCA or venlafaxine; 2nd augmentation with Li; venlafaxine high doses can also be considered (less evidence supporting)	Li not mentioned (AD or CBT)
UK: NICE 2004[14] (Recommendations for specialist mental health services)	Indication not target of guideline	Indication not target of guideline	Indication not target of guideline	Indication not target of guideline	Indication not target of guideline	Indication not target of guideline	If failure to two or more AD, Li augmentation or CBT + AD; venlafaxine or combination of 2 AD recommended with less supporting evidence	Li explicitly not recommended (expert opinion)

continued over

continued

Guideline (in chronological order)	Bipolar depression	Mania – classical	Mania – rapid cycling	Mania – dysphoric/ mixed	Hypomania	Bipolar disorder – prophylaxis	Unipolar refractory depression – augmentation	Unipolar depression – prophylaxis
Germany: AkdÄ 2006[15]	Li monotherapy sufficient for many patients	Indication not target of guideline	Indication not target of guideline	Indication not target of guideline	Indication not target of guideline	1st Li, 2nd CBZ; LAM considered if depressive episodes predominate	After rechecking compliance, diagnosis and evaluating changing AD consider 1st Li augmentation, 2nd THY augmentation	AD full dose or Li (especially for those with previous suicide attempts)
Canada: CANMAT 2005[16]	Li or LAM, or combinations with Li/VAL/ olanzapine + SSRI, Li+VAL or Li/VAL + bupropion	Li, VAL, aAP, or combination of Li/VAL with aAP	VAL, olanzapine or Li+VAL; Li monotherapy suggested not as effective as in patients without rapid cycling	VAL, olanzapine, CBZ, or aAP + Li/VAL; Li monotherapy suggested not as effective as in classical mania	Insufficient evidence for recommendations (only risperidone suggested useful)	Li, LAM (for those with mild manias), VAL, olanzapine	Indication not target of guideline	Not in scope
Scotland: SIGN 2005[17]	Li/VAL/ antipsychotic + AD or monotherapy with LAM	1st antipsychotic or VAL; Li can be used if combined with antipsychotic or no immediate control of the episode required	No definite recommendation; evidence for Li is inconclusive (anticonvulsants or antipsychotics)	No definite recommendation; Li regarded as less effective (VAL)	No recommendation; given	1st Li; CBZ if Li ineffective, unacceptable or bipolar II; LAM if depressive episodes important	Indication not target of guideline	Indication not target of guideline

* Care has been taken to maintain the language used in the recommendation

Li, lithium; VAL, valproate/divalproate; CBZ, carbamazepine; LAM, lamotrigine; AD, antidepressant; SSRI, selective serotonin reuptake inhibitors; TCA, tricyclic antidepressants; MAOI, monoamine oxidase inhibitors; CBT, cognitive-behavioral therapy; aAP, atypical antipsychotics; THY, thyroid hormone supplementation; ECT, electroconvulsive therapy will be accepted worldwide because of the many methodological challenges found in studies of prophylaxis, including ethical issues involving the use of placebos, study design and endpoint selection.

Side-effect profiles

All the available agents for prophylaxis of bipolar disorder may be associated with significant side-effects that require the substitution of alternative agents. Since the prophylaxis of bipolar disorder requires life-long therapy, the side-effect profile has a significant impact on the selection and continued use of the prophylactic agent.

Patient preference

High patient adherence is necessary for any prophylactic agent to be effective. With increasing worldwide emphasis on active participation in their care, patients may be directly involved in the selection among the agents available for prophylaxis.

LITHIUM AUGMENTATION FOR RESISTANT UNIPOLAR DEPRESSION

Today there is an active debate about the most appropriate treatment for patients with unipolar depression who do not respond to antidepressants, and this lack of consensus is reflected in guidelines. Most guidelines recommend a wide range of options after a re-evaluation of the diagnosis and optimization of the initial treatment (e.g. dose increase). If it is determined that the patient requires augmentation therapy, six of the seven guidelines list augmentation with lithium as a first-line choice, with the seventh showing lithium as a second-line choice. There is consistent scientific evidence to support the use of lithium augmentation in unipolar depression, particularly in the management of treatment-resistant depression (Chapter 11)[22].

LITHIUM IN THE PROPHYLAXIS OF UNIPOLAR DEPRESSION

There is inconsistency among the guidelines as to the use of lithium for the prophylaxis of unipolar depression. Of the seven guidelines, all recommend continuing the antidepressant used to treat the acute depression at the full dose for the prophylaxis of unipolar depression. Although the available evidence supports the anti-suicidal effect of lithium in unipolar depression as well as bipolar disorder[21] only four of the seven guidelines recommend lithium use for prophylaxis. The German[1,15], Scottish[17] and WFSBP[6] guidelines give special consideration to the anti-suicidal effect of lithium for the prophylaxis of unipolar depression, while the recent NICE guideline explicitly discourages its use[14].

GUIDELINE DEVELOPMENT

The general consensus for the need for critical, independent and systematic evaluation of published medical data has been a critical factor driving the development of practice guidelines. Nevertheless, many existing guidelines in all areas of medicine are far from rigorous in design[23]. Therefore, specialized independent institutions have been established in many countries to evaluate the quality of existing guidelines. Improving guideline quality also implies increasing the costs and time for their production. A reasonable balance should be sought between the high investment involved in the production of a guideline and its potential impact on medical practice. The Drug Commission of the German Medical Association considers an interval of 2–3 years for updating a guideline as appropriate in most cases. Since guideline committees take years to finish a report, the clinician will frequently have to consult an old and probably outdated guideline or be unable to find recommendations for the problem he or she is facing. New methods of developing guidelines have been proposed to solve this problem[24].

Even if the problem of evaluating the existing evidence in an objective and time/cost-effective way were solved, this would certainly not imply that every guideline would make identical and ideal recommendations. Studies are designed and performed in a very controlled environment where many potentially confounding variables are eliminated. The differences between clinical trials and clinical practice are taken into consideration when an expert panel interprets the 'current best evidence'. Other factors that may influence the recommendations include the interests of health system organizations, relationships between the guideline authors and the pharmaceutical industry[25] and social interactions that occur in the group[26]. Furthermore, the panels must consider complex methodological controversies such as the importance and validity of meta-analyses or Cochrane reviews (www.cochrane.org). Methods have also been developed internationally to assist with guideline development including the Agree Collaboration for the Evaluation of Guidelines[27] and the GIN Association for Helping Developing Guidelines[28]. Nevertheless, the clinician should be cautious when reading different guidelines, taking into account that recommendations reflect the influence of factors other than the best available evidence.

Finally, a caveat should be mentioned. The production of an independent and valid guideline is a difficult and challenging task. However, the implementation of a guideline into medical practice is even more difficult and the factors – positive or negative – influencing the transferral process from evidence to practice are still widely unknown. Perhaps the inclusion of more practicing clinicians in the process of guideline development would improve the acceptance by general practitioners and specialists.

CONCLUSION

Lithium still has a prominent role in current guidelines for both the acute and the long-term management of mood disorders. There is widespread agreement for the use of lithium in bipolar disorder and as an augmentation agent for unipolar depression. However, in the 'real therapeutic world' both individual clinical issues and differing prescribing rationales may result in the use of alternative agents, especially for long-term prophylaxis. When comparing international guidelines, focusing upon where recommendations diverge quickly highlights treatment areas in which convincing evidence may be lacking and further controlled studies are required. For example, in contrast to the use of lithium in acute classical mania, the lack of consensus in the selection of a prophylactic agent for subtypes of bipolar disorder, or of a prophylactic agent for unipolar depression may reflect a lack of sufficient evidence for multiple international guideline committees to reach the same conclusions.

REFERENCES

1. Deutsche Gesellschaft für Psychiatrie, Psychotherapie und Nervenheilkunde,

DGPPN. Gaebel W, Falkai P, eds. Praxisleitlinien in Psychiatrie und Psychotherapie. Behandlungsleitlinie Affektive Erkrankungen. Darmstadt: Steinkopff, 2000; 5

2. Anderson IM, Nutt DJ, Deakin JFW, on behalf of the Consensus Meeting and endorsed by the British Association for Psychopharmacology. Evidence-based guidelines for treating depressive disorders with antidepressants: a revision of the 1993 British Association for Psychopharmacology guidelines. J Psychopharmacol 2000; 14: 3–20.

3. Goodwin GM, for the Consensus Group of the British Association for Psychopharmacology. Evidence-based guidelines for treating bipolar disorder: recommendatins from the British Association for Psychopharmacology. J Psychopharmacol 2003; 17: 149–73

4. Amercian Psychiatric Association. Practice Guidelines for the Treatment of Psychiatric Diseases. Compendium 2002. Washington DC: American Psychiatric Association, 2002

5. Bauer M, Whybrow PC, Angst J, et al., WFSBP Task Force on Treatment Guidelines for Unipolar Depressive Disorders. World Federation of Societies of Biological Psychiatry (WFSBP) Guidelines for Biological Treatment of Unipolar Depressive Disorders, Part 1: Acute and Continuation Treatment of Major Depressive Disorder. World J Biol Psychiatry 2002; 3: 5–43

6. Bauer M, Whybrow PC, Angst J, et al., WFSBP Task Force on Treatment Guidelines for Unipolar Depressive Disorders. World Federation of Societies of Biological Psychiatry (WFSBP) Guidelines for Biological Treatment of Unipolar Depressive Disorders, Part 2: Maintenance Treatment of Major Depressive Disorder and Treatment of Chronic Depressive Disorders and Subthreshold Depressions. World J Biol Psychiatry 2002; 3: 67–84

7. Grunze H, Kasper S, Goodwin G, et al., WFSBP Task Force on Treatment Guidelines for Bipolar Disorders. World Federation of Societies of Biological Psychiatry (WFSBP) Guidelines for Biological Treatment of Bipolar Disorders, Part I: Treatment of Bipolar Depression. World J Biol Psychiatry 2002; 3: 115–24

8. Grunze H, Kasper S, Goodwin G, et al., WFSBP Task Force on Treatment Guidelines for Bipolar Disorders. World Federation of Societies of Biological Psychiatry (WFSBP) Guidelines for Biological Treatment of Bipolar Disorders, Part II: Treatment of Mania. World J Biol Psychiatry 2003; 4: 5–13

9. Grunze H, Kasper S, Goodwin G, et al., WFSBP Task Force on Treatment Guidelines for Bipolar Disorders. World Federation of Societies of Biological Psychiatry (WFSBP) Guidelines for Biological Treatment of Bipolar Disorders, Part III: Maintainance Treatment. World J Biol Psychiatry 2004; 5: 120–35

10. Licht RW, Vestergaard P, Kessing LV, et al., Danish Psychiatric Association and the Child and Adolescent Psychiatric Association in Denmark. Psychopharmacological treatment with lithium and antiepileptic drugs: suggested guidelines from the Danish Psychiatric Association and the Child and Adolescent Psychiatric Association in Denmark. Acta Psychiatr Scand 2003; 108 (Suppl 419): 1–22

11. Erfurth A, ed. Weissbuch. Bipolare Störungen in Deutschland. Deutsche Gessellschaft für Bipolare Störungen e.V. Germany, 2003

12. Royal Australian and New Zealand College of Psychiatrists Clinical Practice Guidelines Team for Bipolar Disorder. Australian and New Zealand clinical practice guidelines for the treatment of bipolar disorder. Aust NZ J Psychiatry 2004; 38: 280–305

13. Royal Australian and New Zealand College of Psychiatrists Clinical Practice Guidelines Team for Depression. Australian and New Zealand clinical practice guidelines for the treatment of depression. Aust NZ J Psychiatry 2004; 38: 389–407

14. NHS National Institute for Clinical Excellence. Depression. Management of depression in primary and secondary care. Clinical Guideline 23, December 2004. www.nice.org.uk/CG023 NICEguideline

15. Arzneimittelkommission der deutschen Ärzteschaft. Empfehlungen zur Therapie der

Depression, 2nd edn. Düsseldorf: Nexus-Verlag, 2006, in press. www.akdae.de

16. Yatham LN, Kennedy SH, O'Donovan C, et al. for Canadian Network for Mood and Anxiety Treatments. Canadian Network for Mood and Anxiety Treatments (CANMAT) guidelines for the management of patients with bipolar disorders: consensus and controversies. Bipolar Disord 2005; 7 (Suppl 3): 5–69

17. Scottish Intercollegiate Guidelines Network (SIGN). Bipolar Affective Disorder. A National Clinical Guideline. May 2005. www.sign.ac.uk

18. Keck PE Jr, McElroy SL, Bennett JA. Pharmacologic loading in the treatment of acute mania. Bipolar Disord 2000; 2: 42–6

19. Hirschfeld RM, Fochtmann LJ, McIntyre JS. Antidepressants for bipolar depression. Am J Psychiatry 2005; 162: 1546–7

20. Gijsman HJ, Geddes JR, Rendell JM, et al. Antidepressants for bipolar depression: a systematic review of randomized, controlled trials. Am J Psychiatry 2004; 161: 1537–47

21. Baldessarini RJ, Tondo L, Hennen J. Lithium treatment and suicide risk in major affective disorders: update and new findings. J Clin Psychiatry 2003; 64 (Suppl 5): 44–52

22. Bauer M, Döpfmer S. Lithium augmentation in treatment-resistant depression: meta-analysis of placebo-controlled studies. J Clin Psychopharmacol 1999; 19: 427–34

23. Grilli R, Magrini N, Penna A, et al. Practice guidelines developed by specialty societies: the need for a critical appraisal. Lancet 2000; 355: 103–6

24. Raine R, Sanderson C, Black N. Developing clinical guidelines: a challenge to current methods. BMJ 2005; 331: 631–3

25. Choudhry NK, Stelfox HT, Detsky AS. Relationships between authors of clinical practice guidelines and the pharmaceutical industry. JAMA 2002; 287: 612–17

26. Pagliari C, Grimshaw J, Eccles M. The potential influence of small group processes on guideline development. J Eval Clin Pract 2001; 7: 165–73

27. The AGREE Collaboration. Appraisal of Guidelines for Research and Evaluation (AGREE) Instrument. http://www.agree-collaboration.org/

28. http://www.g-i-n.net/

6 Facing two demons: lithium therapy from a patient's point of view

Marylou Selo

Contents   Bipolar illness strikes (demon 1) • How to solve the dilemma? Increase knowledge and decrease stigma • The patient returns home • Coming to terms with bipolar illness – finding equilibrium • Suicide • Doctor–patient relationship • Compliance • Dealing with the side-effects of lithium • What patients, parents/partners or relatives or other important others must know about lithium treatment • Self-help groups • New evidence on the power of peer support • Conclusion

BIPOLAR ILLNESS STRIKES (DEMON 1)

Imagine this scenario:

A psychotic episode takes hold of you with little or no warning. You begin acting irrationally and/or dangerously. You vaguely recognize that something is terribly wrong, but you can't put your finger on it. Panic sets in. You cannot rest and while you are trying to escape from the demons in your brain, the police arrest you. You fight like an animal. The police remain calm, put handcuffs on you and haul you off to the emergency room of the nearest hospital. Your brain now focuses on one thing only: escape!

You must outsmart the doctor who will interview you or else you will be locked up. So you put your best foot forward, calm yourself down and

indeed manage to convince the intake resident that the neighbors and the police overreacted and that yes, you were a little excited, but now you are perfectly fine and will go home and sleep. The doctor asks whether you have taken drugs. You convincingly shake your head in denial and say that you think that the anti-drug policy of the government should be much stricter. It works! The doctor sets you free.

The last thing you want to do is to go home. Freedom must be celebrated! You deserve a new car and now seems the perfect time to buy that exquisite little laptop you have seen advertised. As you are trying to pay with an already overdrawn credit card you get into such an irritated and threatening state that the cashier calls the police and off you go to the hospital again. This time you cannot calm yourself down. In anger you throw your shoes at the emergency room nurse who does not bring you the glass of water you demanded, fast enough. You climb on a chair and exclaim: 'With God and all of you as my witnesses, see how miserable the staff of this emergency room treats us. If John F. Kennedy were still alive, he would change this.'

Now it is serious. A ward door locks behind you. This is the end. You have gone too far. You are hospitalized and given an injection.

Upon waking up, you have not the faintest notion of where you are or how you got there. You are surrounded by weird people: some old, some young, some seemingly healthy and strong, some obviously insane.

Some person in regular clothing comes over and gives you pills to take. You don't even realize she is a nurse, since you are not aware that you are in a hospital. So you take the little paper cup with pills and throw them high up in the air screaming: 'You won't get me to take drugs! I am too smart for that!' You drink the little cup of water and toss it up in the air exclaiming 'Good to the last drop!' The staff does not take this lightly. Solitary confinement is the result. Total confusion sets in. Where have all the people gone? Where on earth are you? Maybe this is hell? Could be with some of these ugly, loud, smelly people. . . . . You scream and shout until you have no voice left and collapse on the mattress on the floor. You don't know what time of day it is. A male nurse with a flashlight comes in to check on you. It so happens that you have recently been given a similar flashlight. Now you think that man stole your flashlight and you jump up and grab him by the arm so as to retrieve what you think is your flashlight! However, the male nurse reports that the patient has assaulted him. Well: now his colleagues rush in in great numbers and next thing you know, you are subdued and thrown into a straitjacket. Somehow it feels welcome. You can't scream because you have lost your voice, you cannot move because you are tied down. The demons in the brain seem tied down too. Sleep is welcome. Somehow the straitjacket provides a womb-like safety. Much later some persons come in announcing that they will now exercise you. You become

extremely panicky and fearful because your mind does not hear 'exercise' but 'exorcise'! You have no voice, but as soon as the straitjacket is untied you start flailing around with your limbs, terror-stricken. Naturally the nurses get scared and tie you right back down again. Somehow, with the medications you were given you begin realizing that you are in a hospital. You still have no idea how you got there, but when you are walked out by two nurses into the corridor you recognize it as a hospital corridor and you recognize a nurse's station. Slowly but surely you are adjusting to life on the ward, participating in meals and planned activities. It still all seems very unreal. You learn your diagnosis and the names of your medications, but it is meaningless if you have no prior knowledge of mental illness. All you know is that you are not yourself, that you feel like someone hit you over the head with a hammer, that you are being given lithium (demon 2), some poison that makes your mouth dry, gives you a metallic taste, makes you dizzy, thirsty and hungry all the time, that you are gaining weight and that you couldn't care less about that or anything else for that matter.

Granted the above is fortunately no longer the typical introduction of a patient to bipolar disorder. However, against this background it is easy to imagine that a patient wants nothing more badly than to get away from the horror just experienced and pick up life where he left it. He will not be willing to take medications and certainly not lithium, a medication that he will possibly have to take every single day for the rest of his life.

There are other scenarios. For many patients the point of hospitalization signals reaching a haven and coming to rest. The hospital is the place where no demands are made on the patient and where he has no responsibilities for a while. Many patients return voluntarily to the hospital when they feel they are falling off the tightrope of their daily lives. It is fortunate that the threshold to hospitalization has been lowered in recent decades.

HOW TO SOLVE THE DILEMMA? INCREASE KNOWLEDGE AND DECREASE STIGMA

Ideally, every person would know the signs and symptoms of mental illness and recognize them when they strike. Most people know what to do if a person chokes in a restaurant or if a person has a heart attack. However, very few people know how to deal with one who has mental illness. Few people know what the symptoms of depression or mania are and even fewer people realize that they are experiencing signs of mania or depression. Ignorance, stigma and fear prevail. Encouragingly, the German city of Nürnberg, and the Swiss cities of Zug and Bern have started pilot programs to reduce suicide by educating journalists, teachers, nurses, social workers, police, clergy, pharmacists, etc. on depression and its most daunting side-effect: suicide.

It is helpful if the psychiatrist, the psychologist, the nurse, or a psychiatric social worker sits down with the patient and explains the illness and adds that it is quite possible to live and work with bipolar disorder once the illness has been brought under control with lithium. It would have even more impact if a former patient were to come to the hospital to talk at length with the patient. Former patients have been there, they can offer advice and they will be listened to more readily, because their credibility is greater than that of the professionals.

Unfortunately, in most places in the world there are too few competent psychiatrists. Often psychiatrists are quite expensive and many patients simply cannot afford psychiatric care. Moreover, in the USA, only a few psychiatrists under the age of 40 have learned how to prescribe and adjust lithium, which still is the gold standard for bipolar disorder. They ought to learn to prescribe and fine-tune lithium.

Social workers must be better educated too. It makes no sense for a social worker to prepare a bipolar patient for disability if he in fact should be quite able to return to work. It can be ruinous and devastating for a patient to hear that he shall never work again.

Everyone should make a point of educating the press and correcting journalists when they report incorrectly or in a sensational tone about suicides or mental illness. In America this has been done successfully by members of self-help groups.

Stigma must be reduced in the work place, in places of worship and in all areas of daily living.

THE PATIENT RETURNS HOME

Once the patient has been discharged from the hospital after an episode of mania or depression, he faces many problems. On the one hand nothing has changed and yet everything is different. How will he get through the day? In the beginning stages it is difficult to concentrate. Reading is next to impossible, owing to lack of concentration and sometimes blurred vision caused by antidepressants. There is a marked change in activity. Going out for a walk is unappealing. The prospect of being seen by neighbors is scary. It is impossible to watch television all day. Sitting in a chair and staring into space is disconcerting to others. If the patient is lucky to have a supportive family, they will rally around him and try to be helpful. If he lives alone, it will seem to him that someone hit him over the head and that he is just regaining consciousness.

Work and mail will have piled up. The answering machine is full and it is difficult to figure out where to start. Tomorrow is another day, and many tomorrows might follow without anything getting done. The patient will be lucky if someone did the dishes and took out the garbage during his stay in the hospital …

Here again, a social worker from the hospital or a former patient volunteer can be most helpful. At this point in time the patient is quite vulnerable and open to advice; unfortunately, he is also open to the wrong advice given by well-meaning friends and relatives. They may say things like: 'Oh well, the hospitalization was just a mishap. You look fine. You don't need all those pills. Try some "natural" medicines, maybe St John's Wort/if you pray/take vitamins/spend more time in nature/read more poetry/treat yourself to a wellness spa once in a while/take up sports, or whatever is in vogue at the time, you will be just fine'.

As the patient starts thinking about his diagnosis and tackling his tasks, he will regain some confidence in himself and eventually he will think that he can handle this illness on his own, that he does not need to take the horrible medications, and that he will be fine. He will get most annoyed at his parents or partner if they inquire about his taking the medication. His irritability will go up a notch if well-meaning relatives or parents or partner start treating him as an invalid, taking too much consideration, or, on the other hand, urging him to act 'normally' again. The latter will be the case if the parents/partner are in denial and convinced that, now the hospitalization is over, life will be back to normal forever.

As the bills start coming in for purchases made during (hypo) mania, the patient is faced with the reality of what he has done. He may be facing a person he barely recognizes as being the person he has always thought he was. During the period of increased libido he might have gone overboard not only with money, but also with sexual adventures. It is not unusual for patients to state that they have slept with seven different partners in seven nights.

Some patients seek thrills such as having sex in a car while their partner is driving. Others do things they might have fantasized about such as going skinny-dipping at a fashionable beach and shocking the prim and proper.

Such excesses are likely to ruin friendships and relationships. During (hypo) mania and sometimes even during depression patients will be uninhibited and say whatever comes to mind, often insulting and hurting the people they love.

It will be difficult for partners/family and for the patient himself to distinguish between the excesses caused by the illness and the actions taken based on the true character of a person. Here cognitive therapy is most helpful.

COMING TO TERMS WITH BIPOLAR ILLNESS – FINDING EQUILIBRIUM

It is hard to face the world and make decisions: to hide or not to hide your diagnosis and from whom; to make or not to make major life changes; perhaps to go back to school; perhaps to learn another profession. The most difficult thing is to learn to give meaning to life with a disability and make the best of it.

The worst form of the illness and the most difficult to medicate is rapid cycling. This is defined as having more than four episodes a year. However, there are patients who cycle several times during one day. Patients with this form of the illness often face worst-case scenarios. It is almost impossible for them to keep a job, to live in a family setting or to live on their own. The patient will need help from all the therapists: psychopharmacologists, psychologists, social workers, etc.

Despite all new medications, some depressions can be difficult to treat and they may last a long time. During a depression the life of a patient is on hold, but life outside is not. The depression may cause even a good relationship to flounder. Job loss is frequent. Financial problems may be enormous. The longer the episode the harder it gets to put life back on track or to start a new life. Lost time is an issue with most patients. Bipolar patients have an easier time making up for lost time when they are doing well. Another big issue is self-esteem. Most patients seem to have a lack of it. Some try to cover up the lack of self-esteem and appear cocky. Others have such a need to be liked that they cannot say no. Manipulative tendencies seem to be present in most persons suffering from bipolar illness. These issues can be dealt with in cognitive therapy and in self-help groups.

SUICIDE

Depression and bipolar illness are deadly diseases. More people worldwide commit suicide than die from traffic accidents and AIDS together. Most people who commit suicide suffer from clinical depression. Yet fewer funds are made available for suicide prevention than for AIDS prevention and traffic safety. Another troubling statistic: in the USA 30 000 people die of suicide each year; that is twice as many as of homicide.

If a patient can no longer bear being depressed, he will take no consideration of anyone. If he feels that there is no hope he will kill himself. Sometimes he will think his family/partner is better off without him, since he is such a burden.

The issue of suicide should be addressed by the doctor, the family/partner, clergyman, etc. A depressed patient who feels like killing himself frequently lacks the willpower and wherewithal to do it. The time when an antidepressant medication kicks in, is the time to be especially alert to the patient. The antidepressant may give the patient the drive to get up and do it, before his spirits are lifted.

DOCTOR–PATIENT RELATIONSHIP

A correct diagnosis and hitting upon the right combination of medications can be life-savers. Discouragement and lack of hope will frequently lead to suicide. Bipolar illness is a constant walk on the tightrope, seeking to stay in balance without falling into depression or soaring into mania.

Therefore, it is of the utmost importance for the patient to build up a relationship of trust and mutual respect with their therapists. It is difficult for the patient to report accurately what is happening to them when they are not themselves. It is important for the doctor to know them well enough to assess and treat their symptoms appropriately. In many cases it may be helpful for the psychiatrist to get an assessment of the partner/family. The goal is to find the patient's equilibrium and remain in balance.

To find that balance, medication is often not sufficient. Cognitive therapy and other therapies may be required. Support at home, at work, with peers, or in a self-help group are essential to getting better. So is educating yourself about the illness and gaining insight into what may trigger an episode.

Some doctors act as if they are doing one a favor by taking care of one and taking one's money! A psychiatrist who does not return a telephone call from a patient in a timely fashion is not acting in a professional manner. If a doctor fails to realize that a patient is suicidal and does not return a phone call the result may very well be fatal!

COMPLIANCE

Patients must learn to be compliant with their medications, to watch their diet, to exercise on a regular basis, and especially to make sure that they sleep regularly and sufficiently. A change in sleep patterns may be the first alarm signal indicating the start of an episode. It is quite helpful to keep a mood diary to keep track of major episodes and minor mood swings. It is important for the patient to learn to pace himself. This is quite difficult for most bipolar patients, many of whom have an exuberant character.

Research has shown that self-help groups are quite conducive to compliance. Like children, patients would rather listen to strangers than to their parents.

Every patient should keep a history of episodes and of medications that have helped in the past. A medication that helped in the past is likely to help again. This will save a considerable amount of time experimenting with medications when the doctor or the patient moves to a different part of the world.

DEALING WITH THE SIDE-EFFECTS OF LITHIUM

There are as many side-effects of any medication as there are people. Unfortunately, all medications have potential side-effects. Some patients can tolerate these better than others. All medications should be started low and increased gradually ('start low – go slow'). When discontinuing a medication, it should also be withdrawn gradually. A sudden stop of medications may bring about an episode and increase suicidal tendencies. Doctors and patients should work closely together to minimize the side-effects and fine-tune the medication to suit the needs of the patient. The most common side-effects of lithium are a slight hand tremor, thirst, increased urine production, weight gain, cognitive changes, gastrointestinal upsets and poor memory. Thyroid function may decrease and require supplemental thyroid medication. Some patients have no side-effects whatsoever. Almost all side-effects can be minimized if patient and psychiatrist work closely together.

Lithium during pregnancy requires special attention and cooperation by psychiatrist and gynecologist.

On the positive side: many patients report a decrease of headaches or migraines after going on lithium. There is no indication that lithium reduces creativity. On the contrary, artists have found that they can work more consistently when on lithium.

WHAT PATIENTS, PARENTS/ PARTNERS OR RELATIVES OR OTHER IMPORTANT OTHERS MUST KNOW ABOUT LITHIUM TREATMENT

Patients and persons living with the patient must familiarize themselves with the benefits and side-effects of lithium. They should know about the lithium serum levels and about the blood tests that must be done on a regular basis. They must know that blood tests must be done 12 hours after the last dose of lithium was taken. They must be aware about the implications of lithium on the thyroid and the kidneys. They must know that lithium makes one thirsty but that one should drink mostly water to quench that thirst; otherwise there might be considerable weight gain.

The book *Lithium Treatment of Mood Disorders* by Professor Mogens Schou, published by Karger, should be required reading for every patient and every caretaker of a person on lithium. Well-informed patients and partners/family make good partners for psychiatrists and benefit the patient. Knowledge is power! A good doctor–patient relationship is essential to treatment.

It is crucial that psychiatrist and patient develop a true partnership. The psychiatrist should speak with family members to find out what the patient was like before the illness struck. Doctor, partner/family and patient should work toward regaining the level of functioning that was there, before the illness struck. At all times the patient should be viewed as a whole person and not just as a person presenting with bipolar illness. Slowly but surely lithium will give the patient the stability to reorganize his life, if the patient takes the medication religiously as prescribed. The patient will learn that lithium will protect him from suicidal thoughts and from suicide attempts, that lithium is not addictive and that it can be safely taken during pregnancy if the obstetrician and the psychiatrist work together closely.

The patient and the people surrounding him will learn that the latest research shows that lithium may protect neurons in the brain and that it therefore may ward off senility and Alzheimer's disease. Similarly, there is evidence that the area of the brain affected by a stroke is smaller in persons on lithium.

Despite all efforts to educate the patient and his partner/family, etc. a time may come when the patient is fed up with it all and exclaims: 'Shut up, leave me alone. I won't listen to you anymore'. Then it is high time to find a self-help group.

SELF-HELP GROUPS

When the time has come for the patient and his partner/family to seek out a self-help group, they will find people who have had similar problems before and who are willing to help. They will tell the patient and his partner/family that they can overcome the condition but that they cannot do it alone. Lectures in the self-help group will provide valuable education.

While talking to other bipolar patients, patients will discover that here they are understood, that they fit right in. They are no longer isolated from the rest of the world. People attending support groups consist of fellow-patients, partners/spouses of patients, parents of patients, siblings of patients and children of patients. Depending on the number of persons who show up on any given group evening, all three generations may be in the same group, or they may meet in different groups such as youth group, postpartum depression women, friends and family, depressed group, job-seeking group, topic group (e.g. 'lithium'). Sometimes they start out in separate groups and come together for the second part of the evening. Meetings may take place in a hospital, in church buildings, in union halls, in the living room of the facilitator, or in any other office or other space available for free. Some groups organize hikes, outings to a movie, picnics and in some cases even 1-week vacations, where patients can, for example, hike, bike, swim, or ski in the daytime and be involved in group sessions in the evening.

The newly diagnosed bipolar patient will find encouragement from the examples the group members give. Recently diagnosed patients will find stabilized patients who will encourage them to continue the treatment plan. Patients in the self-help group in many cases have a family, job, children, a house, a car, etc. They will explain how the medication takes time to take effect. There will be an exchange of experiences regarding doctors, medications and side-effects. The recently diagnosed patient will see that all sorts of creative activities take place within the self-help group. Many self-help groups foster creativity by putting out a newsletter on a regular basis. Members may contribute poems, essays, photographs, drawings, etc.

The recently diagnosed person will find people in the group who will help with shopping or accompanying the patient on dreaded visits to the psychiatrist, the doctor or the dentist. A recently diagnosed bipolar patient might need and find help to consolidate debts incurred during the period of (hypo) mania. In addition, the self-help group will offer a social network to get together on holidays or weekends.

Likewise, the partner/family members will find support and consolation in talking to other partners/family members. They will learn that they are not alone in their concerns and they will learn how to address those concerns from those who have experienced similar problems. They will hear similar stories of dread and horror from the people who are attending the self-help groups. Shared grief is halved grief!

The worst story I ever came across as a facilitator in a family member self-help group is the story a distraught lady told one evening. Her son, a brilliant and gifted medical student, had been diagnosed as bipolar and put on medication. The medication worked well and he was able to complete his medical degree. He was well liked and respected by his fellow students. During his internship he experienced difficulties because of the lack of sleep. He decided to reduce and eventually quit his medications so that he would deal better with the sleep deprivation. He became slightly paranoid but continued to function well in his profession. He went out to buy a gun, which he kept on his nightstand to ward off a possible intruder. Next he bought another gun to keep in his car 'just in case'. One night, while at a gas station, he became suspicious of the gas station attendant, who had walked off with his credit card. When the gas station attendant returned together with a huge black man, the young doctor panicked and shot the gas station attendant dead. Upon his arrest, he was taken to prison. His mother could not convince the authorities that her son needed medication. The son became increasingly more paranoid and unruly. What was the poor mother supposed to do?

She received immense support and encouragement in the support group. A lawyer in the group offered her legal advice free of charge. Other members of the group related stories telling how they had narrowly escaped arrest and imprisonment by good fortune and the grace of God. A doctor was found to testify as an expert witness and convince the court that the young doctor needed to be put back on medication. Eventually, he was allowed to work as a doctor in the prison where he was serving his sentence.

Not quite a happy ending, but under the circumstances of the Rhode Island legal system, a bearable solution for both mother and son and a reminder of the fact that gun-laws are in dire need of revision.

The above story illustrates how essential it is to stay on lithium if it has shown benefits. Fortunately, only a few stories are quite this dramatic, but in almost every group it becomes evident that the family/partner suffers just as much as the patient, but in a different way.

NEW EVIDENCE ON THE POWER OF PEER SUPPORT

The winter 2004–2005 issue of the DBSA (Depression and Bipolar Support Alliance) reports that recent research in the USA suggests that service programs operated by and for people with mental illness can improve individual well-being in many ways. This confirms that services and support given and received by those with a shared experience of mental illness are critical to maintaining hope and health, building resilience and sustaining recovery. It improves recovery by helping people to rediscover their strengths and participate in their treatment. It assists with social inclusion by helping individuals to build or rebuild interpersonal skill through relating to others in support groups. By educating patients and families about depression and bipolar disorder, peer support increases empowerment. Earlier research has already shown that self-help groups do an excellent job in promoting compliance.

CONCLUSION

What is needed to tame the two demons (bipolar illness and medication) and co-exist with them

- A knowledgeable psychiatrist (psycho-pharmacologist)
- The right medication in the right dose
- Cognitive therapy with a competent therapist
- Education and insight (hard work on the patient's part)
- Support of family/partner, friends, colleagues, etc.
- Destigmatization of the illness by society

Summary of the steps to be taken by the patient

- Leave denial behind
- Gain acceptance of the illness and what it entails for you
- Seek the best possible treatment for you
- Learn to self-manage
- Use empowerment strategies
- Embark on the road to recovery
- Do whatever it takes for you to stay in equilibrium
- Most importantly: never give up; never ever give up!

Useful websites

Dr Ivan's Depression Central
DBSAlliance.org

DGBS.org
NARSAD.org
Changing moods.de
www.bsne.de (Bipolar Selbsthilfe Netwerk, e.v.)

Partial list of self-help groups dealing with depression and bipolar disorder

Australia

Bipolar Disorder Meetup
Perth
Website: bipolar.meetup.com/members/87

Fyreniycel (Fire and Ice)
E-mail: Fyrenicycel-subscribe@egroups.com

Mood Disorders Association (SA) (founded 1983)
Marleston, South Australia
Australia
Tel: 08 8221-5170
mda@mhrc.org.au
Contact: Carol Fuller
carolf@mhrc.org.au

Austria

SHG Neunkirchen
Peisinger Str. 19
A-2620 Neunkirchen, Austria
E-mail: psychiatrie@khneunkirchen.at

Club D&A (Depression and Anxiety) – Clubzentrum
Wien
Schottenfeldgasse 40/8
A-1080 Wien
Tel: + 43 407 7227-71
E-mail: office@club-d-a-a.at

Belgium

VVMD (Flemish Association of Manic Depressives)
Tel: +32 53 77 50 97
E-mail: vvmd.vzw@belgacom.net

Psychoarts 2000
E-mail: luc.leysen@klina.be

Brazil

ABRATA
Adriano Camargo
Sao Paolo,
E-mail: apersone@hotmail.com

APOLAR
E-mail: aplar@silvanprado.psc.br
Website: www.silvanprado.psc.br

Canada

Mood Disorders Society of Canada
3-304 Stone Road West
Guelph, Ontario, N1G 4W4, Canada
Tel: +1 519 824-5565
E-mail: washdown@shaw.ca
Website: mooddisorderscanada.ca

Denmark

Depressionsforeningen
Vendersgade 22
1363 Copenhagen
Tel: +45 3312 4727
Contact: Mrs Jette Balslev
E-mail: depression@inet.uni2.dk
Website: www.depressionforeningen.dk

France

ARGOS 2001
(Ass. d'aide aux personnes atteintes de troubles bipolaires
et a leur entourage)
E-mail: bianca.von.heiroth@club-internet.fr
Website: http://argos.2001.free.fr

France Depression
Association Francaise contre la dépression et la maladie
maniaco-dépressive
Association Loi 1901
4 rue Vigée Lebrun
F 75015 Paris
Tel: +1 4061 0566
E-mail: france.depression@libertysurf.fr

Germany

DGBS Deutsche Gesellschaft für Bipolare Störungen e.v.
PO Box 920249
D-21132 Hamburg
Tel: +49 40 40 85408883
E-mail: dgbs.ev@t-online.de
Website: www.dgbs.de (lists self-help groups in all of
Germany)
Bipolar Selbsthilfe Netzwerk e.V.
Am Schmidtgrund 43
D 50765 Cologne
E-mail: Michael-tillmann@bipolar-netzwerk.de
www.bsne.deX

Ireland

Aware
Contact: Mr. Fran Gleeson
E- email: aware@iol.ie and info@aware.ie

Mood Disorder Fellowship of Ireland
Fenian Chambers
3738 Fenian Street
Dublin 2
(May no longer exist; has no website)

Italy

Fondazione IDEA – Istituto per la ricerca e la preven-
zione della Depressione e dell' Ansia
Sede Nazionale: Via Statuto 8; Milano 20121;
Tel. 02-654126
Fax 02 654716
claracantarelli@yahoo.it
e-mail: ideaidea@tin.it
(per info, aiuto) e-mail: idearisponde@tin.it

The Netherlands

Nationaal Fonds Geestelijke Volksgezondheid
Depressiecentrum
PO Box 5103
3502 JC UTRECHT
Contact: Aly van Geleuken
a.vanGeleuken@nfgv.nl
info@depressiecentrum.nl.

VMDB (Association of Manic Depressives and Care-
Givers)
PO Box 24076
Kaap Hoorndreef 56-C
NL 3563 AV- Utrecht, The Netherlands
Tel: +31 30 260 3030
E-mail: mbakhuis@dds.nl
Website: www.vmdg.nl

South Africa

South African Bipolar Site
(lists self help groups)
www.bipolar.co.za

Spain

Associació de Bipolars de Catalunya (ABC)
C-Cuba, 2
Hotel d'Entitas 'CAN GUARDIOLA'
0830 BARCELONA, España
Tel: +34 93 27 41 460 and +34 93 274 93 38
E-mail: cen00abc@jazzfree.com

Allianza para la Depression
General Margallo 27
E-28020 Madrid
E-mail: smith@alianzadedepression.com

Switzerland

Equilibrium (founded 1994)
CH 6340 Baar
Tel: +41 848 143 144
Website: www.depressionen.ch
E-mail: info@depressionen.ch

United Kingdom

Manic Depressive Fellowship
Castle Works, 21 St George's Road
London SE1 6ES
Tel: +44 20 7793 260 0
E-mail: mdf@mdf.org.uk

Depression Alliance
Tel: +44 845 1232320
Website: www.depressionalliance.org

Manic Depressive Fellowship Scotland
Mile End Mill – Studio 10/9
Abbey Mill Business Centre

Seed Hill Rd.
Paisley, PA1 1TJ Scotland
E-mail: manic@globalnet.co.uk

USA

Child and Adolescent Bipolar Foundation
(On-line support and education for parents, teachers, and kids)
Chicago, Ill.
Website: www.bpkids.org

Depression and Bipolar Support Alliance (DBSA)
(founded 1986)
(Previously National DMDA (Depressive and Manic Depressive Association)
730 N. Franklin Street - #501
Chicago, Ill. 606 10v
Tel: +1 800 626-3632
Website: www.dbsalliance.org

Mood Disorders Support Group/New York (MDSG)
(founded 1980)
PO Box 30377
New York, N.Y. 10011
Tel: +1 212 533 MDSG
Website: www.mdsg.org

Partial list of celebrities having experienced depression and/or bipolar illness (compiled by Canadian Bipolar Association)

Alvin Ailey, dancer and choreographer
Edwin 'Buzz' Aldrin, astronaut
Louie Anderson, comedian, actor
Ann-Margaret, actress
Diane Arbus, photographer
Lionel Aldridge, football player
Alexander the Great, king
Hans Christian Anderson, author
Tai Babilonia, figureskater
Oksana Baiul, figureskater
Honore de Balzac, writer
Samuel Barber, classical composer
Roseanne Barr, actress
Drew Barrymore, actress
James M Barrie, writer
Rona Barrett, columnist
Charles Baudelaire, poet
Shelley Beattie, athlete and artist
Ned Beatty, actor

Samuel Becket, writer
Ludwig von Beethoven, composer
Menachem Begin, Prime Minister of Israel
Brendan Behan, poet
Irving Berlin, composer
Hector Berlioz, composer
John Berryman, poet
William Blake, poet
Charles Bluhdorn, executive, Gulf Western
Napoleon Bonaparte, emperor
Kjell Magne Bondevik, Prime Minister of Norway
Clara Bow, actor
Tommy Boyce, musician, composer
Cheyenne Brando, actor
Marlon Brando, actor
Richard Brautigan, writer
Van Wyck Brooks, writer

John Brown, abolitionist
Ruth Brown, singer
Anton Bruckner, composer
Art Buchwald, political humorist
John Bunyan, writer
Robert Burns, poet
Robert Burton, writer
Tim Burton, artist, movie director
Willie Burton, basketball player
Barbara Bush, former First Lady
Lord Byron, poet
Helen Caldicott, activist, writer
Donald Cammell, movie director, screenwriter
Robert Campeau, Canadian businessman
Albert Camus, writer
Truman Capote, writer
Drew Carey, actor and comedian
Jim Carrey, actor and comedian

Dick Cavett, broadcaster
CE Chaffin, writer, poet
Ray Charles, R&B performer
Thomas Chatterton, poet
Paddy Chayefsky, writer, movie director
Lawton Chiles, former governor of Florida
Frederic Chopin, composer
Winston Churchill, British Prime Minister
Sandra Cisneros, writer
Eric Clapton, blues-rock musician
Dick Clark, entertainer (American Bandstand)
John Cleese, actor
Rosemary Clooney, singer
Kurt Cobain, rock star
Tyrus Cobb, athlete
Leonard Cohen, poet and singer
Natalie Cole, singer
Garnet Coleman, Texas legislator
Samuel Coleridge, poet
Judy Collins, musician, writer
Shawn Colvin, musician
Jeff Conaway, actor
Joseph Conrad, author
Pat Conroy, writer
Calvin Coolidge, US president
Francis Ford Coppola, director
Billy Corgan, musician
Patricia Cornwell, writer
Noel Coward, composer
William Cowper, poet
Hart Crane, writer
Oliver Cromwell, soldier and statesman
Kathy Cronkite, writer
Dennis Crosby, actor
Sheryl Crow, singer and rock musician
Richard Dadd, artist
John Daly, athlete (golf)
Rodney Dangerfield, comedian
Charles Darwin, explorer and scientist
David, Israeli King
Ray Davies, musician
Thomas De Quincey, poet
Lenny Dee, musician
Sandra Dee, actor
Ellen DeGeneres, comedienne, actor
Sebastian Deisler, German soccer star
John Denver, singer and actor

Muffin Spencer Devlin, pro golfer
Diana, Princess of Wales
Paolo DiCanio, athlete (soccer)
Charles Dickens, writer
Emily Dickenson, poet
Isak Dinesen, author
Scott Donie, Olympic athlete (diving)
Terence Donovan, photographer
Michael Dorris, writer
Theodore Dostoevski, writer
Eric Douglas, actor
Tony Dow, actor, producer, director
Richard Dreyfuss, actor
Jack Dreyfus, manager, Dreyfus Fund
Kitty Dukakis, former First Lady, Mass.
Patty Duke, actress
Thomas Eagleton, lawyer, US Senator
Thomas Eakins, artist
Thomas Edison, inventor
Edward Elgar, composer
TS Eliot, poet
Queen Elizabeth I of England
Ralph Waldo Emerson, writer
Robert Evans, film producer
James Farmer, civil rights leader
Philo T Farnsworth, television pioneer
William Faulkner, writer
Jules Feiffer, cartoonist and satirist
Tim Finn, musician, composer
Carrie Fisher, actress and writer
F Scott Fitzgerald, writer
Larry Flynt, magazine publisher
Betty Ford, former First Lady
Harrison Ford, actor
James Forrestal, cabinet member
Steven Foster, writer
Michel Foucault, writer, philosopher
George Fox, Quaker
Connie Francis, entertainer
Andre Franquin, cartoonist
Albert French, writer
Sigmund Freud, psychiatrist
Brenda Fricker, actress
Peter Gabriel, rock star
John Kenneth Galbraith, economist
Judy Garland, singer, actor
James Garner, actor
Paul Gascoigne, athlete (soccer)
Paul Gauguin, artist
Harold Geneen, executive, ITT Industries

King George III of England
Stan Getz, musician
Kaye Gibbons, writer
Kendall Gill, athlete (basketball)
Kit Gingrich, Newt's mother
Johann Goethe, writer
Oliver Goldsmith, poet
Dwight Gooden, baseball player
George Gordon, poet
Tipper Gore, wife of US Vice-President
Arshille Gorky, artist
Francisco de Goya, painter
Phil Graham, owner, Washington Post
Graham Green, writer
Shecky Greene, comedian
Philip Guston, artist
Alexander Hamilton, politician
Linda Hamilton, actress
Georg Frederich Handel, composer
Pete Harnisch, baseball player
Mariette Hartley, actress
Juliana Hatfield, musician
Hampton Hawes, musician
Stephen Hawking, physicist
Nathaniel Hawthorne, writer
Lillian Hellman, writer
Ernest Hemingway, writer
Margaux Hemingway, actor
Audrey Hepburn, actress
King Herod, Biblical figure
Kristin Hersh, musician
Hermann Hesse, writer
Abby Hoffman, writer and activist
Sir Anthony Hopkins, actor
Gerard M Hopkins, poet
Edward Hopper, artist
Nick Hornby, British author
Howard Hughes, industrialist
Victor Hugo, author
Helen Hutchison, broadcaster
Henrik Ibsen, playwright
Jack Irons, musician
Eugene Izzi, writer
Andrew Jackson, US President
Janet Jackson, singer
Henry James, writer
William James, writer
Kay Redfield Jamison, psychologist, writer
Randall Jarrell, poet
Thomas Jefferson, US President

Jim Jenson, CBS News
Jeremiah, Biblical figure
Joan of Arc, French leader
Job, Biblical figure
Billy Joel, musician, composer
Elton John, musician, composer
Daniel Johns, musician
Samuel Johnson, poet
Daniel Johnston, musician
Ashley Judd, actor
Franz Kafka, writer
Karen Kain, prima ballerina
Danny Kaye, entertainer
John Keats, writer
Margot Kidder, actress
Larry King, talkshow host
Ernst Ludwig Kirchner, artist
Gelsey Kirkland, dancer
Heinrich von Kleist, poet
Percy Knauth, journalist
Joey Kramer, musician
William Kurelek, artist
Pat LaFontaine, hockey player
Charles Lamb, poet
Jessica Lange, actor
Peter Nolan Lawrence, English writer
Edward Lear, artist
Frances Lear, publisher
Robert E Lee, US general
Vivian Leigh, actress
John Lennon, musician
Rika Lesser, writer, translator
Primo Levi, chemist, writer
Bill Lichtenstein, producer (TV &
    radio)
Allie Light, director
Abraham Lincoln, US President
Vachel Lindsey, writer
Karl Paul Link, chemist
Ross Lockridge Jr, writer
Joshua Logan, producer
Jack London, writer
Rick London, cartoonist
Greg Louganis, US diver and Olympic
    gold medallist
Courtney Love, musician
James Russell Lowell, poet
Robert Lowell, poet
Malcolm Lowry, writer
J Anthony Lukas, writer
Salvador Luria, bacterial geneticist
Martin Luther, Protestant leader

Gustav Mahler, composer
Duke of Marlborough, soldier
Elizabeth Manley, Canadian
    figureskater
Camryn Mannheim, actor
Martha Manning, psychologist, writer
Imelda Marcos, Philippine dictator's
    wife
Jay Marvin, radio personality, writer
Masako, Crown Princess of Japan
Vladimir Mayakovsky, poet
Gary McDonald, Australian actor
Kevin McDonald, comedian, actor
Robert McFarlane, former United
States National Security Adviser
Rod McKuen, writer, poet, producer
Sarah McLachlan, singer, Lilith Fair
    creator
Kristy McNichol, actress
Peter McWilliams, writer
Herman Melville, writer
Burgess Meredith, actor
Robert Merrill, musician, lyricist
Paul Merton, British comedian
Conrad Meyer, writer
Michelangelo, artist
Dimitri Mihalas, scientist
John Stuart Mill, writer
Edna St Vincent Millay, poet
Kate Millet, writer and feminist
Spike Milligan, humourist
John Milton, poet
Charles Mingus, composer
Carmen Miranda, singer
Claude Monet, artist
Thelonious Monk, musician
Marilyn Monroe, actor
Alanis Morissette, Canadian singer
SP Morrissey, musician
John Mulheren, financier (US)
Edvard Munch, artist
Robert Munsch, writer
Les Murray, Australian poet
Modest Mussogorgsky, composer
Benito Mussolini, Italian dictator
Ilie Natase, tennis player, politician
Ralph Nader, US consumer rights
    advocate
Nebuchadnezzar, Biblical figure
Sir Isaac Newton, physicist
Florence Nightingale, British nurse
Vaslav Nijinksy, ballet dancer

Richard Nixon, US president
Deborah Norville, television journalist
Sinead O'Connor, musician
Georgia O'Keeffe, painter
Eugene O'Neill, playwright
John Ogden, pianist
Laurence Olivier, actor
Margo Orum, writer
Ozzie Osborne, rock star
Donny Osmond, musician
Marie Osmond, musician
Wilfred Owen, poet, soldier
Nicola Pagett, actor
Charles Parker, composer
Dorothy Parker, writer, poet, wit
Dolly Parton, singer
Boris Pasternak, writer
John Pastorius, composer
George Patton, soldier
Pierre Peladeau, publisher
Charley Pell, former coach, University
    of Florida
Teddy Pendergrass, musician
Walker Percy, writer
Murray Pezim, Canadian businessman
Jimmie Piersall, baseball player
William Pitt, Prime Minister
Sylvia Plath, poet
Edgar Allen Poe, writer
Jackson Pollock, artist
Cole Porter, composer
Ezra Pound, poet
Alma Powell, wife of General Colin
    Powell
Susan Powter, motivational speaker
Charlie Pride, country singer
Sergey Rachmaninoff, composer
Bonnie Raitt, singer
Mac Rebennack (Dr John), musician
Lou Reed, singer
Jeannie C Riley, singer
Rainer Maria Rilke, poet
Joan Rivers, comedian
Lynn Rivers, US Congresswoman
Alys Robi, Canadian vocalist
Norman Rockwell, artist
Theodore Roethke, poet
George Romney, artist
Theodore Roosevelt, US President
Axl Rose, rock star
Roseanne, actor, writer, comedienne
Amelia Rosselli, poet

Dante Rossetti, poet and painter
Gioacchimo Rossini, composer
Martin Rossiter, musician
Philip Roth, writer
Mark Rothko, artist
Gabrielle Roy, author
John Ruskin, writer
Winona Ryder, actor
Yves Saint Laurent, fashion designer
May Sarton, poet, novelist
Francesco Scavullo, artist, photographer
Lori Schiller, writer, educator
Charles Schulz, cartoonist (Peanuts)
Robert Schumann, German composer
Delmore Schwartz, poet
Ronnie Scott, musician
Alexander Scriabin, composer
Jean Seberg, actress
Monica Seles, athlete (tennis)
Anne Sexton, poet
Linda Sexton, writer
Mary Shelley, author
Percy Bysshe Shelley, poet
William Tecumseh Sherman, general
Frances Sherwood, writer
Dmitri Shostakovich, musician
Scott Simmie, writer, journalist
Paul Simon, composer, musician
Lauren Slater, writer
Christopher Smart, poet
Jose Solano, actor
Phil Specter, promoter and producer
Alonzo Spellman, athlete (football)
Muffin Spencer-Devlin, pro golfer

Vivian Stanshall, musician, writer, artist
Rod Steiger, actor
George Stephanopoulos, political advisor
Robert Louis Stevenson, writer
Sting, singer and musician
Teresa Stratas, opera singer
Darryl Strawberry, baseball player
William Styron, writer
Emmanuel Swedenbourg, religious leader
James Taylor, singer and musician
Kate Taylor, musician
Lili Taylor, actor
Livingston Taylor, musician
PI Tchaikovsky, composer
Alfred, Lord Tennyson, poet
Tracy Thompson, writer, reporter
Dylan Thomas, poet
Edward Thomas, poet
Leo Tolstoy, writer
Henri de Toulouse-Lautrec, artist
Spencer Tracy, actor
Ted Turner, founder, CNN Network
Mark Twain, author
Hunter Tylo, actress
Mike Tyson, prizefighter
Jean-Claude Van Damme, actor
Vincent Van Gogh, artist
Vivian Vance, actor
Victoria, British Queen
Mark Vonnegut, doctor, writer
Kurt Vonnegut, writer
Sol Wachtler, judge

Tom Waits, musician
Mike Wallace, broadcaster
Michael Warren, executive, Canada Post
George Washington, US President
Damon Wayans, comedian, actor, writer, director, producer
Walt Whitman, poet
Dar Williams, musician
Robin Williams, actor
Tennessee Williams, playwright
Brian Wilson, rockstar (Beach Boys)
William Carlos Williams, physician, writer
Bill Wilson, co-founder of Alcoholics Anonymous
Jonathan Winters, comedian
Hugo Wolf, composer
Thomas Wolfe, writer
Mary Wollstonecraft, writer
Ed Wood, movie director
Natalie Wood, actor
Virginia Woolf, writer
Luther Wright, basketball player
Elizabeth Wurtzel, writer
Tammy Wynette, singer
Bert Yancey, pro golfer
Boris Yeltsin, former President, Russia
Faron Young, musician
Robert Young, actor
William Zeckendorf, industrialist
Emile Zola, writer
Stefan Zweig, poet

Part B

CLINICAL APPLICATIONS

7 Lithium in the treatment of acute mania

Rasmus W Licht

Contents Introduction • Controlled studies on lithium in mania • Clinical aspects other than efficacy • Translating the evidence into clinical practice • Outlook

INTRODUCTION

Acute mania: a devastating condition requiring treatment

The lifetime risk for developing bipolar mania leading to hospitalization is around 1%[1], and the risk of recurrence is almost 90%. Untreated, the manic episode generally lasts for 2–8 months. The condition is almost invariably associated with substantial negative interpersonal and social consequences, and death from suicide or from physical breakdown may occur. Poor compliance with treatment constitutes a major problem, and side-effects of drugs may increase the risk of non-compliance. For these reasons, the acute treatment of mania should not only be effective and well tolerated, it should also anticipate the future course of this recurrent illness.

Has lithium still a role to play as an antimanic?

Considering all the agents available today for treating acute mania, a key question is whether lithium still has a role to play for this indication. Based on recent treatment guidelines for bipolar disorder[2–6], where lithium as monotherapy is recommended as first-line treatment for milder cases of acute, pure mania and in combination with an (atypical) antipsychotic for more severe cases, the answer to that is definitely yes. This positive position of lithium, despite its narrow therapeutic index, may partly be due to the fact that this drug has a combined property of well-established antimanic efficacy (reviewed below) and well-established prophylactic efficacy (reviewed in Chapter 8), implicating that an acute antimanic treatment with lithium at the same time can be considered as the initiation of a prophylactic treatment. Also, the acute antidepressant efficacy of lithium (reviewed in Chapter 11) may diminish the potential risk of a cycling into depression in the aftermath of a manic episode. There are other good reasons for keeping lithium in the armamentarium for the acute treatment of mania and therefore for educating and training doctors, nurses and others in its use. Besides being a first-line agent in certain cases as mentioned above, lithium seems a rational choice in cases where other agents such as antipsychotics or valproate have not been sufficient for managing a manic episode, which happens in more than 50% of cases. Despite the fact that such strategies for treating failures to first-line treatments have not been evaluated in randomized clinical trials (RCTs)[7], the rationale for using lithium as a second-step treatment is that this molecule pharmacodynamically acts on mania presumably through other mechanisms (at least in part) than the other available treatments. Unfortunately, the specific mechanisms of therapeutic action of lithium are far from fully understood (see Chapter 28).

The use of lithium as an antimanic agent

To what extent lithium is used in clinical practice worldwide for the treatment of acute mania is uncertain. At the Aarhus University Psychiatric Hospital (in Risskov, Denmark) serving a well-defined catchment area, only 14 (11%) out of 125 manic patients consecutively admitted over a 2-year period from 1990 to 1992 received lithium as the main antimanic treatment[8]. The remaining patients were treated primarily with typical antipsychotics. This relatively infrequent use of lithium as an antimanic agent under routine conditions cannot simply be explained as the doctors at this hospital being unaware of the drug, since the Aarhus University Psychiatric Hospital had a leading role in the early development of the clinical use of lithium, primarily initiated by Schou (see

Chapter 2) and the hospital has continued research on lithium[9]. Also, the scarce use of lithium in acutely manic patients at that time cannot be the result of heavy marketing from manufacturers of the alternative treatments for mania, i.e. valproate and the atypical antipsychotics, since the industrial interest for this indication did not start until later, i.e. starting in the mid-1990s with the industrial promotion of valproate, followed by olanzapine and the other atypical antipsychotics. In a more recent comprehensive survey, less than 10% of acutely manic patients were treated with a mood stabilizer alone (comprising lithium)[10].

Besides the lack of industrial backing, there may be several reasons for the seemingly low use of lithium under routine clinical conditions. One major reason is that it may not calm the highly active manic patients sufficiently. This clinical observation was demonstrated convincingly in the two large studies by Prien et al. in 1972[11,12] reviewed below. However, a commonly used strategy adopted since the late 1980s of combining lithium with a benzodiazepine may partly overcome this limitation[13]. Another limitation, and perhaps the major limitation, is the low therapeutic index of lithium, i.e. the ratio between the lowest doses causing toxicity and the lowest doses required for effect. The therapeutic index is particularly low when acute mania is the target, due to the relatively high serum concentrations of lithium required for treating this condition. This necessitates frequent measurements of the serum concentrations of lithium. Therefore, a considerable degree of patient cooperativeness is needed, which can far from be taken for granted in this patient population. Besides thereby reducing the effectiveness of the drug, i.e. the effect displayed under routine circumstances as opposed to the pharmacological efficacy per se, this requirement may also reduce the availability of the treatment, because many centers and doctors may not have easy access to laboratory facilities, in particular in developing countries.

CONTROLLED STUDIES ON LITHIUM IN MANIA

Trials driven by investigators versus trials driven by industry

Many earlier investigator-driven RCTs indicated that lithium worked in mania, but not until 1994, with the publication of the industry-driven study by Bowden et al.[14] aiming at drug approval of valproate for mania, was lithium shown to be better than placebo in a parallel-group designed study. Later on, the evidence for the acute antimanic efficacy of this drug was further substantiated in other similar industry-generated drug-approval multicenter trials, using lithium as an internal standard to validate assay sensitivity. After the clinical research in drug treatment of mania started to be dominated by industry, many of the earlier investigator-driven RCTs were often neglected. However, despite the fact that these trials had many methodological limitations[15], they still contain valuable clinical information on lithium. Also, it should not be forgotten that many of these single-site studies, although they had small sample sizes, may add to the evidence of an effectiveness of lithium (as opposed to the mere efficacy), since these investigators may have recruited more typical patients than those recruited for modern multicenter trials, with each site often recruiting only a very low number of highly cooperative patients, free of drug abuse and co-morbid conditions[7].

Early trials suggesting efficacy

The first evidence of lithium as a potential antimanic agent was published in 1949 by Cade[16], when he described the observation that lithium seemingly had tranquilizing properties in ten patients with what he called psychiatric excitement. At this time there were no other pharma-cological treatments available for this condition. The observation by Cade was confirmed by four placebo-controlled cross-over studies conducted between 1954 and 1971, as reviewed by Goodwin and Jamison[17]. Following these early placebo-controlled trials, the antimanic efficacy of lithium was evaluated in six randomized comparative trials conducted from 1970 to 1978, using chlorpromazine as the drug of reference (Table 7.1)[12,18–22]. Chlorpromazine had been introduced in the 1950s and was the drug of choice for mania until the late 1960s, when haloperidol was introduced[17]. In the majority of the lithium–chlorpromazine trials, comparable within-group declines in symptom scores were noted[18–21], but owing to small sample sizes, these between-group comparisons were essentially inconclusive. The two large RCTs found chlorpromazine to be superior[12] and inferior[22] to lithium, respectively. In the study by Prien et al.[12], the patients were divided into approximately two equal proportions based on their level of activity. In the highly active patients, who were also the most severely ill, chlorpromazine was superior to lithium, whereas in the less severely ill patients, lithium and chlorpromazine were comparable. In addition, the drop-out rates due to lack of effect were lower among patients allocated to chlorpromazine than among patients allocated to lithium. In contrast to these findings, Takahashi et al.[22] reported lithium to be superior to chlorpromazine with response rates of 68% and 47%, respectively. However, this may have been due to the use of relatively low doses of chlorpromazine. In a few of these reports, lithium was suggested to be potentially more specific in ameliorating manic core symptoms than chlorpromazine[18,21,22]. In 1980, Garfinkel et al.[23] found haloperidol to be superior to lithium, with the difference being statistically significant after 8 days of treatment, whereas in a previous comparison, lithium was comparable to haloperidol (and chlorpromazine)[20]. In three of

Table 7.1 Investigator-initiated parallel-group designed randomized controlled trials evaluating lithium in mania, published in peer-reviewed international journals, listed by year of publication

Authors and year of publication	Result of comparison[a]	n
Platman[19] 1970	Li = CPZ	23
Spring et al.[21] 1970	Li = CPZ	14
Johnson et al.[18] 1971	Li = CPZ	34
Prien et al.[12] 1972	Li < CPZ	255
Prien et al.[11] 1972	Li < CPZ	83
Takahashi et al.[22] 1975	Li > CPZ	80
Shopsin et al.[20] 1975	Li = HAL = CPZ	30
Biederman et al.[37] 1979	Li-HAL > P-HAL	36
Garfinkel et al.[23] 1980	HAL-Li = HAL-P	21
	HAL-P > Li-P	
Braden et al.[47] 1982	Li < CPZ	53[b]
Lenzi et al.[24] 1986	Li = CAR	22
Lerer et al.[25] 1987	Li > CAR	34
Lusznat et al.[26] 1988	Li = CAR	52
Johnstone et al.[38] 1988	PI-Li > LI[c]	22[be]
	PI-Li > PI[d]	
Okuma et al.[28] 1990	Li = CAR	105
Small et al.[27] 1991	Li = CAR	52
Freeman et al.[29] 1992	Li = VAL	27
Lenox et al.[35] 1992	LO-Li =	20
	HAL-Li	
Garza-Trevino et al.[33] 1992	Li = VER	20
Walton et al.[32] 1996	Li > VER	40
Gouliaev et al.[36] 1996	Li-CLO =	28
	ZU-CLO	
Clark et al.[34] 1997	Li = CLO	40
Segal et al.[30] 1998	Li = RIS = HAL	43
Berk et al.[31] 1999	OL = Li	30
Chou et al.[39] 1999	$HAL_{low dose}$-Li >	20[b]
	$HAL_{low dose}$-P;	
	$HAL_{low dose}$-Li =	19[b]
	$HAL_{high dose}$	
Kowatch et al.[40] 2000	Li = CAR = VAL	42

Li, lithium; CPZ, chlorpromazine; HAL, haloperidol; P, placebo; CAR, carbamazepine; VAL, valproate; PI, pimozide; LO, lorazepam; VER, verapamil; CLO, clonazepam; ZU, zuclopenthixol; RIS, risperidone; OL, olanzapine

[a] Any stated difference means a statistically significant difference at least at the 5% level

[b] Subsample of a larger sample of patients

[c] Pimozide combined with lithium superior to lithium regarding psychotic symptoms

[d] Pimozide combined with lithium superior to pimozide regarding manic symptoms

[e] One of four treatment groups contained pure placebo but was not analyzed separately

the RCTs comparing an antipsychotic with lithium, the antipsychotic seemed to have a more rapid onset of action than lithium[12,20,23].

In these earlier studies the use of unreliable criteria for mania creates difficulties in the evaluation of the generalizability. In addition, outcome measures specifically designed for mania were not used in these studies. Finally, with one exception[22], well-defined categorical response criteria were not applied.

More recent investigator-driven comparative monotherapy trials

Lithium versus antiepileptics

Carbamazepine has been compared with lithium in five RCTs[24–28] (Table 7.1), using lithium as the reference drug. However, large amounts of concomitant antipsychotics blurred the comparisons in three of the trials[24,26,28]. In one of the two trials not confounded by the use of antipsychotics, Lerer et al.[25] found a response rate of 29% with carbamazepine compared to 79% with lithium during 4 weeks. Contrasting with these findings, Small et al.[27] reported low response rates of around one-third in the lithium-treated as well as the carbamazepine-treated patients. However, this sample was dominated by patients who previously had responded insufficiently to lithium. In a small comparison of lithium against valproate in outpatients, response rates on valproate and lithium were 64% and 92%, respectively[29].

Lithium versus atypical antipsychotics

Segal et al.[30] showed risperidone to be comparable to haloperidol and to lithium. However, due to a small sample size (Table 7.1) and to achievement of only modest serum lithium levels, interpretations are difficult to make. Furthermore, no response rates were reported.

The same limitations apply to an investigator-initiated study by Berk et al.[31], finding no difference between lithium and olanzapine.

Lithium versus calcium channel blockers

One RCT found lithium to be superior to verapamil[32]. Another RCT was inconclusive due to a small sample size[33]. In both studies, additional antipsychotics were given.

Lithium versus and combined with benzodiazepines

Since earlier trials have suggested that clonazepam and lorazepam might have specific antimanic properties (see review by Licht[13]), Clark et al.[34] compared clonazepam with lithium in a 4-week trial. No differences were found but the sample size was small and concomitant treatment with antipsychotics was allowed. In another small 4-week study, Lenox et al.[35] found similar response patterns over time for a combination of lithium and clonazepam and a combination of lithium and haloperidol using survival analysis, suggesting that adding a benzodiazepine might compensate for the relatively slow onset of action that had been demonstrated in some comparisons against antipsychotics as reviewed above. Likewise, in a small RCT from our group comparing a combination of lithium and clonazepam with a combination of zuclopenthixol and clonazepam, the declines in mania rating scores over time were similar in the two groups[36].

Trials on combining lithium and a typical antipsychotic

In the aforementioned study by Garfinkel et al.[23] finding haloperidol to be superior to lithium, a combination of haloperidol and lithium was not superior to haloperidol alone. However, the patients were assessed solely by the Brief Psychiatric Rating Scale (BPRS). In contrast, Biederman et al.[37] found a combination of haloperidol and lithium to be modestly superior to haloperidol alone in schizomania, when comparing BPRS total scores. In an RCT with complex design, Johnstone et al.[38] observed an additive effect of pimozide and lithium in a subgroup of 22 patients with concomitant psychotic symptoms and elevated mood. In a more recent study in psychotic manic patients, low-dose haloperidol (5 mg) combined with lithium were more effective than low-dose haloperidol alone, but not more effective than high-dose haloperidol (25 mg) with or without lithium[39].

Lithium trials in younger populations with mania

In the only study evaluating the antimanic efficacy of lithium in young people, 42 outpatient manic patients aged between 8 and 18 years were randomized to 6 weeks of open treatment with either lithium, valproate or carbamazepine. Response rates were similar across treatments and comparable to those seen in adults[40].

Industry-generated placebo-controlled trials

Monotherapy trials

The drug approval trials using lithium as the reference drug or for validating the design are listed in Table 7.2. In the aforementioned trial by Bowden et al.[14], the response rate (response defined as a 50% reduction or more on the Mania Rating Scale (MRS)) was 49%, 48% and 25% for lithium, valproate and placebo, respectively, during 3 weeks. The proportions of pre-mature terminations on valproate and on lithium due to lack of effect also appeared similar. Of the patients allocated to lithium treatment, 42% had a history of lithium non-response or non-tolerance, clearly favoring valproate in the comparison. The changes over time in the MRS scores in the valproate- and in the lithium-treated patients were quite similar. In an older multicenter RCT, the antimanic efficacy of oxcarbazepine has been suggested to be equivalent to lithium. However, this study has only been published in summary form[41]. In a recent study, primarily testing quetiapine against placebo in pure mania, both quetiapine and lithium were superior to placebo in terms of response rates and remission rates, with response and remission defined as a 50% reduction or more on the Young Mania Rating Scale (YMRS) and as a score below 13 on the YMRS, respectively[42]. In addition, the response and remission rates of quetiapine and lithium were found to be similar. Thus, the response rates after 3 weeks were 53%, 53% and 27% for lithium, quetiapine and placebo, respectively, which is comparable to the rates in other similar studies in acute mania. The remission rates were 49%, 47% and 22% rates for lithium, quetiapine and placebo, respectively. Interestingly these rates were also compared after 12 weeks, where almost the same ratios between the effect sizes of the treatment arms were found. It is noteworthy that the time course of the symptom reduction over the 12 weeks showed no differences between the active treatment groups. In a yet unpublished 6-week trial showing no efficacy of lamotrigine in mania, lithium was again found to be superior to placebo on several outcome measures.

In all the industry-generated trials reviewed above, benzodiazepine as a rule was used in combination with the drug(s) under study. This should be borne in mind, when effect sizes and response curves from these studies are considered.

Table 7.2 Company-initiated parallel group designed randomized controlled trials designed for drug approval and using lithium as an internal standard to validate assay sensitivity, published in peer-reviewed international journals, listed by year of publication

Authors and year of publication	Result of comparison[a]	n
Bowden et al.[14] 1994	VAL > P	179
	Li > P	
	Li = VAL	
Tohen et al.[46] 2002	Li/VAL + OL > Li/VAL + P[b]	334
Sachs et al.[44] 2002	Li/VAL + RIS > Li/VAL + P[c]	155
	Li/VAL + HAL > Li/VAL + P[c]	
	Li/VAL + RIS = Li/VAL + HAL	
Yatham et al.[43] 2003	Li/VAL/CAR + RIS > Li/VAL/CAR + P[c, d]	117
Yatham et al.[45] 2004	Li/VAL + QTP > Li/VAL + P[e]	370
Bowden et al.[42] 2005	QTP > P	300
	Li > P	
	Li = QTP	

VAL, valproate; P, placebo; Li, lithium; OL, olanzapine; RIS, risperidone; HAL, haloperidol; CAR, carbamazepine; QTP, quetiapine

[a] Any stated difference means a statistically significant difference at least at the 5% level
[b] In the subgroup with psychotic symptoms, no differences were seen
[c] In the subgroup starting the combination treatment at enrolment, no differences were seen
[d] Only superiority on secondary outcome measures; however, superiority was reached on the primary outcome measure when carbamazepine-treated patients were excluded from the analysis
[e] Essentially, this was a pooled analysis of one positive and one negative trial

Combination therapy trials

Several drug companies have tested their atypical antipsychotic in combination with lithium or valproate (Table 7.2). In these studies, lithium or valproate combined with risperidone[43], risperidone or haloperidol[44], quetiapine[45] or olanzapine[46] were modestly more beneficial in controlling manic symptoms than the monotherapy alone. Yet unpublished data on ziprasidone combined with lithium also showed some superiority as compared to lithium monotherapy, but not on the primary outcome measure. However, since the majority of patients in these trials were treated with lithium or valproate for various periods of time prior to randomization, some of them suffering from break-through prophylaxis mania, interpretations are difficult. When the design allowed, and analyses were made separately on those patients who already received lithium or valproate at the time of randomization and those who did not receive lithium or valproate until the start of the trial, it was clear that no benefit could be demonstrated in the latter group[43,44]. Seemingly, there were no differences in the performance of lithium and valproate in these trials. None of these studies compared the combination therapy with an antipsychotic in monotherapy, presumably because this is not required for drug approval.

CLINICAL ASPECTS OTHER THAN EFFICACY

Predictors of antimanic response to lithium

In terms of predicting an antimanic response per se to any of the available drugs in an individual patient, we still have no tools, and the evidence for any differential efficacy among the alternative drugs in subgroups of patients is sparse. However, in addition to using this sparse evidence (reviewed below) when choosing a specific treatment for an individual patient, the clinician can be guided by combining general knowledge of the side-effect profiles of the various drugs with a careful assessment of the physical status and drug preference of the patient. Also, an evaluation of the previous treatment history of the patient, including prior drug intolerance or lack of effect, is of some help.

Only a few studies have addressed whether any factors predict a poorer or better antimanic response to lithium in comparison with other agents. As previously mentioned, Prien et al.[12] found chlorpromazine to be superior to lithium in a subgroup of highly active manic patients, whereas the compounds were comparable in the remaining subgroup of less active manic patients. In a second part of this study, comparing these two drugs in 83 schizomanic patients, chlorpromazine was also more effective than lithium in the highly active patients, whereas the compounds appeared to be equally effective in the mildly active schizomanic patients[11]. Likewise, in an RCT including a subsample with a manic syndrome in the context of psychosis, Braden et al.[47] found

chlorpromazine to be superior to lithium only in the most overactive patients on various measures. These studies indicate that it may be more the degree of agitation than the presence of psychotic symptoms per se that is associated with a poorer response to lithium (compared to a typical antipsychotic). In the study comparing quetiapine with placebo (and lithium)[42], it was reported that quetiapine and lithium did equally well compared to placebo in terms of reduction in the positive and negative syndrome scale (schizophrenia) (PANSS) positive subscale scores. Also, a post-hoc analysis of data from the valproate–lithium–placebo trial by Bowden et al.[14] found similar responses to lithium and valproate in a subgroup of psychotic patients[48]. In addition, from the studies evaluating an atypical antipsychotic combined with lithium or valproate against monotherapy with lithium or valproate, there were no indications that the presence of psychotic symptoms increased the benefit of adding the antipsychotic to the mood stabilizer[43–46]. As discussed previously, some earlier trials have indicated that the combination of lithium and a typical antipsychotic in psychotic mania may be better than each of the drugs given in monotherapy.

In another post-hoc analysis of the data from the valproate–lithium–placebo trial[14], it was shown that the response to valproate was unaffected by the presence of depressive symptoms (mixed mania), whereas the response to lithium in this subgroup of patients was relatively poor[49]. Unfortunately, no information on the course of depressive symptoms during treatment was given. Based on data from the same trial, it was also found that many previous episodes predicted a poorer response to lithium as opposed to the response to valproate not influenced by this factor[50]. However, a substantial proportion of the sample were non-responders to lithium prior to this trial, since they were and it over-represented among the patients with a high number of previous episodes, interpretations can be difficult.

Tolerability of lithium during treatment of mania

Lithium is relatively well tolerated acutely. However, in the study comparing valproate with lithium and placebo, 11% of patients treated with lithium discontinued because of side-effects, as opposed to 6% and 3% in the groups treated with valproate and placebo, respectively[14]. This may be due to the relatively high levels of serum lithium used in that study. It was mostly tremor as well as nausea and occasionally vomiting that were found to be troublesome. In the recent comparison between quetiapine, lithium and placebo, 6.1% of the patients on lithium dropped out because of side-effects, compared to 6.5% and 4.1% of patients on quetiapine and placebo, respectively[42]. Adverse events occurring in more than 10% of patients in the lithium group were tremor (18.4%), insomnia (16.3%) and headache (12.2%), whereas in the quetiapine group they were dry mouth (24.3%), somnolence (19.6%), weight gain (15.0%) and dizziness (12.1%). A slight negative effect on cognitive functions may also occur in acute treatment, especially in elderly patients, which can be difficult to differentiate from symptoms of the disorder itself. Since all these side-effects are dose dependent they may be managed with dose reduction, although the serum lithium should be kept relatively high as discussed below.

Dosing and monitoring

When treating mania with lithium, a dose–response relationship is generally assumed. However, only one RCT on mania was explicitly designed for testing this assumption[51]. Using three dosing levels and placebo in a complex alternating treatment schedule, a

positive relationship between steady-state serum lithium and antimanic response was shown.

Practically, before treatment with lithium, electrolytes, including serum creatinine, should be measured. However, if there is no clinical suspicion of dehydration or renal disease, acute treatment may be initiated before the results are available. Thyroid stimulating hormone (TSH) should be measured as soon as possible in order to obtain a baseline value. If heart disease is suspected, and in elderly patients, an electroencephalogram should be performed.

The acute dosing of lithium for mania must comply with renal clearance, but can generally be initiated with lithium citrate 6-mmol tablets, four tablets daily, or lithium carbonate 8-mmol tablets, three tablets daily (possibly divided into two doses) with measurement of serum lithium after approximately 5 days. Subsequently, the dose should be adjusted to obtain a serum lithium level between 0.8 and 1.2 mmol/l; this must always be accompanied by a close monitoring for toxic symptoms. In hospitalized, closely monitored patients, according to the clinical state, the dose could be further raised until a serum lithium level of 1.5 mmol/l is reached or cognitive side-effects occur[14]. Very fast dosage increases of lithium have been described in small studies[52]. However, this strategy requires very close monitoring.

The clinician must be aware that the optimal 12- (or 24-) hour serum lithium level varies from patient to patient. In addition to inter-individual differences in sensitivity to lithium, this is due to the fact that the ratio between the 12- (or 24-) hour serum lithium level and the average serum lithium level varies from patient to patient, owing to the inter-individual variations in renal clearance[53]. For the same reason, a low 12- (or 24-) hour serum lithium level does not exclude a high average serum lithium level.

There are no studies addressing when, during the treatment course of mania, the dose can safely be reduced. However, when the manic symptoms have resolved, it seems reasonable to lower the serum lithium concentration, at least in the interest of minimizing side-effects and the risk of subsequent intoxication. Also, the state-dependent kinetics of lithium (with higher lithium clearance during mania) should be taken into account.

Sometimes, a so-called break-through lithium prophylaxis mania can be managed simply by increasing the dose of lithium, although this strategy has not been tested in controlled trials. In these cases, the subsequent prophylactic serum lithium level should be kept at a higher level than was used prior to the episode, unless prophylaxis is optimized through other means.

Implications of lithium-induced rebound mania

As mentioned previously, a good reason to initiate an antimanic treatment with lithium is that a prophylactic treatment is thereby initiated as well. However, assuming that abrupt discontinuation of lithium may induce a rebound mania, for which there is fairly good evidence[54], it can be argued that lithium should not be initiated acutely unless it will be used for at least 2 years from that point on, since otherwise the overall risk would increase the overall benefit[55]. This implication would limit the use of lithium for mania considerably, since a patient at that time only rarely can consent reliably to long-term treatment. On the other hand, the discontinuation effects of the other drugs used for mania may be under-recognized. In fact, a large yet unpublished RCT comparing relapse rates on olanzapine with those of placebo in manic patients stabilized on olanzapine suggests that this phenomenon presumably cannot be attributed to lithium alone[54].

TRANSLATING THE EVIDENCE INTO CLINICAL PRACTICE

As reviewed here, the efficacy, i.e. the pharmacological effect per se, of lithium in mania is well established from placebo-controlled comparisons using modern methodology, and, when compared to other available agents in controlled trials, effect sizes are similar. A delayed onset of action of lithium indicated by earlier trials has not been confirmed in more recent trials, probably because lithium was combined with a benzodiazepine in these trials. Also, combining lithium with antipsychotics seems sometimes to be beneficial, e.g. when mania develops despite ongoing treatment with lithium. However, considerable cooperation from patients is required during treatment with lithium, and many patients treated under routine conditions may therefore not benefit from this drug, thereby reducing the effectiveness, as compared to other drugs which are more easily administered. Side-effects emerging during acute treatment can most often be handled by proper dosing adjustments and are rarely the reason for discontinuing the drug (either by doctor or by patient). Lithium should be preferred for patients with non-mixed mania without severe agitation. There is no convincing evidence that psychotic symptoms per se predict a poorer response specifically to lithium as compared to antipsychotics or valproate. Also, the potential benefit of combining lithium with an antipsychotic (preferably an atypical agent) seems not to be increased in manic patients with psychotic symptoms. On the other hand, since the presence of psychotic symptoms often leads to uncooperativeness, lithium may not always be an option in this subgroup of manic patients.

Despite the sparse information from RCTs on antimanic efficacy of lithium in the younger and elder populations, there is no reason to assume that the effect sizes are different from those seen in populations usually included in RCTs. However, in terms of safety, special precautions should be taken in these populations.

Given the potential risk of the emergence of rebound mania on abrupt discontinuation of lithium, as is probably seen with other agents as well, the necessity of continued compliance after remission has been achieved should be communicated carefully to the patient.

OUTLOOK

The antimanic efficacy of lithium has been well established in non-mixed mania with or without psychotic symptoms, making it a first-line treatment. Therefore, goals for future clinical studies addressing this indication could include answering the question of what role lithium might have in cases resistant to other antimanic treatments. Also, randomized comparisons with other agents addressing the potential phenomenon of rebound mania when the treatment is stopped could be highly useful.

REFERENCES

1. Svendsen SW. Secular trends in first-ever admission rates of affective disorders in Denmark, 1971–93. Nord J Psychiatry 1997; 51: 119–25

2. Royal Australian and New Zealand College of Psychiatrists Clinical Practice Guidelines Team for Bipolar Disorders. Australian and New Zealand clinical practice guidelines for the treatment of bipolar disorder. Aust NZ J Psychiatry 2004; 38: 280–305

3. Licht RW, Vestergaard P, Kessing LV, et al. Psychopharmacological treatment with lithium and antiepileptic drugs: suggested guidelines from the Danish Psychiatric Association and the Child and Adolescent Psychiatric Association in Denmark. Acta Psychiatr Scand 2003; 419 (Suppl): 1–22

4. Grunze H, Kasper S, Goodwin G, et al. The World Federation of Societies of Biological Psychiatry (WFSBP) Guidelines for the Biological Treatment of Bipolar Disorders, Part II: Treatment of Mania. World J Biol Psychiatry 2003; 4: 5–13

5. American Psychiatric Association. Practice guideline for the treatment of patients with bipolar disorder (revision). Am J Psychiatry 2002; 159 (Suppl): 1–50

6. Goodwin GM, Young AH. The British Association for Psychopharmacology guidelines for treatment of bipolar disorder: a summary. J Psychopharmacol 2003; 17 (Suppl): 3–6

7. Licht RW. Limitations in randomised controlled trials evaluating drug effects in mania. Eur Arch Psychiatry Clin Neurosci 2001; 251 (Suppl): II66–71

8. Licht RW, Gouliaev G, Vestergaard P, et al. Treatment of manic episodes in Scandinavia: the use of neuroleptic drugs in a clinical routine setting. J Affect Disord 1994; 32: 179–85

9. Vestergaard P, Licht RW. Fifty years with lithium treatment in affective disorders: present problems and priorities. World J Biol Psychiatry 2001; 2: 18–26

10. Lim PZ, Tunis SL, Edell WS, et al. Medication prescribing patterns for patients with bipolar I disorder in hospital settings: adherence to published practice guidelines. Bipolar Disord 2001; 3: 165–73

11. Prien RF, Caffey EM, Klett CJ. A comparison of lithium carbonate and chlorpromazine in the treatment of excited schizo-affectives. Arch Gen Psychiatry 1972; 27: 182–9

12. Prien RF, Caffey EM Jr, Klett CJ. Comparison of lithium carbonate and chlorpromazine in the treatment of mania. Report of the Veterans Administration and National Institute of Mental Health Collaborative Study Group. Arch Gen Psychiatry 1972; 26: 146–53

13. Licht RW. Experience with benzodiazepines in the treatment of mania. In Modigh K, Robak OH, Vestergaard P, eds. Anticonvulsants in psychiatry. Petersfield: Wrightson Biomedical Publishing, 1994: 37–55

14. Bowden CL, Brugger AM, Swann AC, et al. Efficacy of divalproex vs lithium and placebo in

the treatment of mania. JAMA 1994; 271: 918–24

15. Licht RW. Drug treatment of mania: a critical review. Acta Psychiatr Scand 1998; 97: 387–97

16. Cade JFJ. Lithium salts in the treatment of psychotic excitement. Med J Aust 1949; 36: 349–52

17. Goodwin FK, Jamison KR. Manic–Depressive Illness. New York: Oxford University Press, 1990

18. Johnson G, Gershon S, Burdock EI, et al. Comparative effects of lithium and chlorpromazine in the treatment of acute manic states. Br J Psychiatry 1971; 119: 267–76

19. Platman SR. A comparison of lithium carbonate and chlorpromazine in mania. Am J Psychiatry 1970; 127: 351–3

20. Shopsin B, Gershon S, Thompson H, Collins P. Psychoactive drugs in mania. A controlled comparison of lithium carbonate, chlorpromazine, and haloperidol. Arch Gen Psychiatry 1975; 32: 34–42

21. Spring G, Schweid D, Gray C, et al. A double-blind comparison of lithium and chlorpromazine in the treatment of manic states. Am J Psychiatry 1970; 126: 1306–10

22. Takahashi R, Sakuma A, Itoh K, et al. Comparison of efficacy of lithium carbonate and chlorpromazine in mania. Report of collaborative study group on treatment of mania in Japan. Arch Gen Psychiatry 1975; 32: 1310–18

23. Garfinkel PE, Stancer HC, Persad E. A comparison of haloperidol, lithium carbonate and their combination in the treatment of mania. J Affect Disord 1980; 2: 279–88

24. Lenzi A, Lazzerini F, Grossi E, et al. Use of carbamazepine in acute psychosis: a controlled study. J Int Med Res 1986; 14: 78–84

25. Lerer B, Moore N, Meyendorff E, et al. Carbamazepine versus lithium in mania: a double-blind study. J Clin Psychiatry 1987; 48: 89–93

26. Lusznat RM, Murphy DP, Nunn CMH. Carbamazepine vs. lithium in the treatment and prophylaxis of mania. Br J Psychiatry 1988; 153: 198–204

27. Small JG, Klapper MH, Milstein V, et al. Carbamazepine compared with lithium in the treatment of mania. Arch Gen Psychiatry 1991; 48: 915–21

28. Okuma T, Yamashita I, Takahashi R, et al. Comparison of the antimanic efficacy of carbamazapine and lithium carbonate by double-blind controlled study. Pharmacopsychiatry 1990; 23: 143–50

29. Freeman TW, Clothier JL, Pazzaglia P, et al. A double-blinded comparison of valproate and lithium in the treatment of acute mania. Am J Psychiatry 1992; 149: 108–11

30. Segal J, Berk M, Brook S. Risperidone compared with both lithium and haloperidol in mania: a double-blind randomized controlled trial. Clin Neuropharmacol 1998; 21: 176–80

31. Berk M, Ichim L, Brook S. Olanzapine compared to lithium in mania: a double-blind randomized controlled trial. Int Clin Psychopharmacol 1999; 14: 339–43

32. Walton SA, Berk M, Brook S. Superiority of lithium over verapamil in mania: a randomized, controlled, single-blind trial. J Clin Psychiatry 1996; 57: 543–6

33. Garza-Treviño ES, Overall JE, Hollister LE. Verapamil versus lithium in acute mania. Am J Psychiatry 1992; 149: 121–2

34. Clark HM, Berk M, Brook S. A randomized controlled single blind study of the efficacy of clonazepam and lithium in the tratment of acute mania. Hum Psychopharmacol 1997; 12: 325–8

35. Lenox RH, Newhouse PA, Creelman WL, Whitaker TM. Adjunctive treatment of manic agitation with lorazepam versus haloperidol: a double-blind study. J Clin Psychiatry 1992; 53: 47–52

36. Gouliaev G, Licht RW, Vestergaard P, et al. Treatment of manic episodes: zuclopenthixol and clonazepam versus lithium and clonazepam. Acta Psychiatr Scand 1996; 93: 119–24

37. Biederman J, Lerner Y, Belmaker RH. Combination of lithium carbonate and haloperidol in schizo-affective disorder: a controlled study. Arch Gen Psychiatry 1979; 36: 327–33

38. Johnstone EC, Crow TJ, Frith CD, Owens DGC. The Northwick park 'functional' psychosis study: diagnosis and treatment response. Lancet 1988; 2: 119–25

39. Chou JC, Czobor P, Charles O, et al. Acute mania: haloperidol dose and augmentation

with lithium or lorazepam. J Clin Psychopharmacol 1999; 19: 500–5

40. Kowatch RA, Suppes T, Carmody TJ, et al. Effect size of lithium, divalproex sodium, and carbamazepine in children and adolescents with bipolar disorder. J Am Acad Child Adolesc Psychiatry 2000; 39: 713–20

41. Emrich HM. Experience with oxcarbazepine in acute mania. In Modigh K, Robak OH, Vestergaard P, eds. Anticonvulsant in Psychiatry. Petersfield: Wrightson Biomedical Publishing, 1994: 29–36

42. Bowden CL, Grunze H, Mullen J, et al. A randomized, double-blind, placebo-controlled efficacy and safety study of quetiapine or lithium as monotherapy for mania in bipolar disorder. J Clin Psychiatry 2005; 66: 111–21

43. Yatham LN, Grossman F, Augustyns I, et al. Mood stabilisers plus risperidone or placebo in the treatment of acute mania. International, double-blind, randomised controlled trial. Br J Psychiatry 2003; 182: 141–7

44. Sachs GS, Grossman F, Ghaemi SN, et al. Combination of a mood stabilizer with risperidone or haloperidol for treatment of acute mania: a double-blind, placebo-controlled comparison of efficacy and safety. Am J Psychiatry 2002; 159: 1146–54

45. Yatham LN, Paulsson B, Mullen J, Vagero AM. Quetiapine versus placebo in combination with lithium or divalproex for the treatment of bipolar mania. J Clin Psychopharmacol 2004; 24: 599–606

46. Tohen M, Chengappa KN, Suppes T, et al. Efficacy of olanzapine in combination with valproate or lithium in the treatment of mania in patients partially nonresponsive to valproate or

lithium monotherapy. Arch Gen Psychiatry 2002; 59: 62–9

47. Braden W, Fink EB, Qualls CB, et al. Lithium and chlorpromazine in psychotic inpatients. Psychiatry Res 1982; 7: 69–81

48. Swann AC, Bowden CL, Calabrese JR, et al. Pattern of response to divalproex, lithium, or placebo in four naturalistic subtypes of mania. Neuropsychopharmacology 2002; 26: 530–6.

49. Swann AC, Bowden CL, Morris D, et al. Depression during mania. Treatment response to lithium or divalproex. Arch Gen Psychiatry 1997; 54: 37–42

50. Swann AC, Bowden CL, Calabrese JR, et al. Differential effect of number of previous episodes of affective disorder on response to lithium or divalproex in acute mania. Am J Psychiatry 1999; 156: 1264–6

51. Stokes PE, Kocsis JH, Orestes JA. Relationship of lithium chloride dose to treatment response in acute mania. Arch Gen Psychiatry 1976; 33: 1080–4

52. Keck PE Jr, Strakowski SM, Hawkins JM, et al. A pilot study of rapid lithium administration in the treatment of acute mania. Bipolar Disord 2001; 3: 68–72

53. Amdisen A. Lithium neurotoxicity – the reliability of serum lithium measurements. Hum Psychopharmacol 1990; 5: 281–5

54. Franks MA, Macritchie KAN, Young AH. The consequences of suddenly stopping psychotropic medication in bipolar disorder. Clin Approach Bipolar Disord 2005; 4: 11–17

55. Goodwin GM. Recurrence of mania after lithium withdrawal. Implications for the use of lithium in the treatment of bipolar affective disorder. Br J Psychiatry 1994; 164: 149–52

8 Maintenance treatment with lithium in bipolar disorder

John R Geddes, Guy M Goodwin

Contents   Introduction • Evidence for long-term lithium therapy in bipolar disorder • Dose and lithium levels • The clinical management of long-term lithium therapy • Conclusions

INTRODUCTION

Lithium has long been accepted as the first-line therapy for relapse prevention in bipolar disorder. Early skepticism[1] was at least partly dispelled by a clearer documentation of the usually adverse course of the illness and by randomized clinical trials, exemplified by the seminal Veterans Administration–National Institute of Mental Health (VA-NIMH) trials conducted by Robert Prien and his colleagues[2]. However, uncertainty about the effectiveness of lithium in real-life practice continued. This was fueled in the 1990s by retrospective attacks on the validity of the pivotal efficacy trials conducted in the 1970s[3], concern about toxicity and the increased risk of relapse on withdrawal[4,5], and the introduction and marketing of potential alternative drug treatments, particularly valproate semisodium (Depakote®). Most recently, and a little unexpectedly, new long-term evidence has emerged from large trials conducted primarily to investigate the efficacy of newer agents compared with placebo, but which also included a lithium arm as an active comparator[6]. In this chapter, we summarize the randomized evidence for the long-term efficacy of lithium in the prevention of relapse in bipolar disorder, suggest a method for the clinical application of the randomized evidence to the individual patient and provide a regimen for baseline assessment and monitoring for patients taking long-term lithium therapy.

EVIDENCE FOR LONG-TERM LITHIUM THERAPY IN BIPOLAR DISORDER

We have previously reported a systematic review of the available randomized trials comparing lithium with placebo in the maintenance treatment of bipolar disorder with at least 3 months' follow-up[7,8]. The search for these reviews has been repeated and updated and here we present the updated results of this review.

Selection of trials

Search strategy

(1) *Electronic databases* The Cochrane Collaboration Depression, Anxiety and Neurosis Controlled Trials Register (CCDANCTR) and The Cochrane Controlled Clinical Trials Register (CCTR) were searched using the following search terms: LITHIUM OR CAMCOL-IT OR CARBOLITH OR DUROLITH OR ESKALITH OR LICARBIUM OR LISKONUM OR LITAREX OR LITHANE OR LITHOCARB OR LITHIZINE OR LITHONATE OR LITHOTABS OR MANIALITH OR PHASAL OR PRIADEL OR QUILONORM OR QUILONUM OR LI-LIQUID.

(2) *Reference checking* The reference lists of all identified randomized controlled trials, other relevant papers and major textbooks on mood disorder were checked.

(3) *Hand searching* The journals *Lithium* (1990–1994) and *Lithium Therapy Monographs* (1987–1991) were hand-searched.

(4) *Personal communication* The authors of randomized controlled trials included in the review and other recognized experts in the field were contacted and asked whether they had knowledge of any other studies, published or unpublished, relevant to the review. Pharmaceutical companies marketing lithium products were requested to provide relevant published and unpublished data. Following the publication of the first version of this review, we kept in contact with identified active trialists and companies to identify any emerging trials.

Inclusion criteria

We included randomized trials with at least 3 months of follow-up that compared lithium with placebo in patients with bipolar disorder. We excluded trials that randomized patients who had been stable on long-term lithium either on continuation or sudden discontinuation of the drug because the treatment effect observed in such trials might be inflated by the lithium withdrawal[3]. The primary outcome was relapse of mood disorder with subanalysis of manic and depressive relapse rates. Withdrawal was used as an overall measure of acceptability and the risk of specific adverse events was estimated. Study quality was assessed by appraisal of method of randomization, concealment of allocation, blinding and handling of withdrawals.

Data were meta-analyzed using the METAN routine in STATA. For binary efficacy outcomes, pooled risk ratios (with 95% confidence intervals) were calculated. Statistical heterogeneity was investigated by performing a χ^2 test across the trial-specific results. When statistically significant heterogeneity was identified, possible causes were explored[7]. Fixed effects relative risks were estimated except when significant heterogeneity was detected, in which case estimates of random effects were also used. Intention-to-treat data were used where possible; otherwise endpoint data for trial completers were used. For uncommon adverse events, the Peto odds ratio was used to pool data – this has been found to perform well in such situations and avoids the need to add a continuity correction[9].

We identified five randomized trials comparing lithium with placebo in bipolar patients (770 participants) (Table 8.1)[2, 10–13]. No further trials had been published since the last update of the review. One trial had a factorial design in which participants were randomized to imipramine vs. placebo and separately to

Table 8.1 Characteristics of included trials

Trial	Methods	Participants (n)	Interventions	Definition of relapse	Quality	Previous lithium use
Prien 1973[2]	Randomized trial 2 year follow-up	205 patients with manic depressive disorder, manic type	Lithium (0.5 to 1.4 mEq/l) Placebo	Post-randomization emergent manic or depressive attack measured on Global Affective Scale requiring hospitalization (severe relapse) or supplementary drugs (moderate relapse). Combined moderate or severe relapse rates used	Allocation concealment unclear Participant and clinical raters masked to treatment allocation Treating physician unmasked	All participants stabilized on lithium prior to randomization
Kane 1982[10]	Randomized trial factorial Up to 2 year follow-up	22 patients with bipolar II disorder	Lithium (0.8–1.2 mEq/l) Imipramine (100–150 mg/d) Lithium (0.8–1.2 mEq/l) + imipramine (100–150 mg/d) Placebo	Post-randomization emergent mood episode meeting RDC criteria for major depressive disorder for 1 week, minor depressive disorder for 4 weeks, manic episode for any duration, or hypomanic episode for 1 week	Allocation concealment unclear Masking of patients, clinicians and outcome assessors	6 months' continuation treatment with lithium prior to randomization
Bowden 2000[11]	Randomized trial 1 year follow-up Primary aim of trial was to assess efficacy of divalproex	372 patients with bipolar I disorder High suicide risk excluded	Lithium (0.8–1.2 mmol/l) Divalproex (71–125 µg/ml) Placebo	Post-randomization emergent mood episode – manic if MRS score was 16 or more, or required hospitalization; depressive episode if required antidepressant use or premature study withdrawal	Allocation concealment unclear Masking of patients, clinicians and outcome assessors	1/3 participants on open lithium treatment Lithium discontinued over 2 weeks

continued

Table 8.1 *continued* Characteristics of included trials

Trial	Methods	Participants (n)	Interventions	Definition of relapse	Quality	Previous lithium use
Bowden 2001[12]	Randomized trial 1 year follow-up Primary aim of trial was to assess efficacy of lamotrigine	175 patients with bipolar I disorder recently recovered from a manic episode	Lithium (0.8–1.1 mEq/l) Placebo Lamotrigine 50 mg/200 mg/400 mg	Post-randomization intervention (addition of pharmacotherapy or ECT) for any mood episode. Secondary outcomes subdivided by type of mood episode (manic/hypomanic/mixed or depressive)	Allocation concealment unclear Masking unknown	21% used lithium during run-in phase; prior use of lithium in 63%
Bowden 2002[13]	Randomized trial 1 year follow-up Primary aim of trial was to assess efficacy of lamotrigine	463 patients with bipolar I disorder recently recovered from a depressive episode	Lithium (0.8–1.1 mEq/l) Placebo Lamotrigine 100–400 mg	Post-randomization intervention (addition of pharmacotherapy or ECT) for any mood episode. Secondary outcomes subdivided by type of mood episode (manic/hypomanic/mixed or depressive)	Allocation concealment unclear Masking unknown	25% used lithium during run-in phase; prior use of lithium in 69%

lithium vs. placebo. The lithium vs. placebo comparison was included (ignoring the imipramine vs. placebo comparison). The trials followed participants either until relapse, or for maximum periods of between 11 months and 4 years. Lithium levels were reported in five trials, and were between 0.5 and 1.4 mmol/l.

Lamotrigine trials

Following our first systematic review and meta-analysis[14], two large new trials were published. These trials were sponsored by GlaxoSmithKline and were primarily designed to investigate the efficacy of lamotrigine compared to placebo in the prevention of relapse in bipolar disorder, but each included a lithium comparator arm[12,13]. Both of these trials shared a common design in which patients initially entered an 8–16-week open active run-in phase during which lamotrigine was initiated and other psychotropics were discontinued. Patients were enrolled in the randomized, double-blind phase of the illness if they had a Clinical Global Impression (CGI) score of ≥3 for 4 consecutive weeks, had received medication other than lamotrigine for >1 week (>2 weeks since discontinuing anticonvulsants and mono-oxidase inhibitors; >4 weeks since discontinuing fluoxetine). The design of these trials probably underestimated the relative treatment effect of lithium because the patient sample was not enriched for those who responded or at least could tolerate lithium in the short term. With the exception of the Depakote trial[11], these are the only placebo-controlled studies in which abrupt withdrawal induced relapse on placebo was avoided by tapering the lithium dosage before randomization.

Patients who remained well and who could tolerate lamotrigine were randomized to lamotrigine, lithium or placebo. This design therefore selected patients who could tolerate lamotrigine in the short term.

Prevention of relapse

The meta-analysis found that lithium was more effective than placebo in preventing all new episodes of mood disturbance (fixed effects relative risk 0.66, 95% CI 0.57–0.77; random effects RR 0.65, 95% CI 0.50–0.84; $p = 0.001$, χ^2 for heterogeneity 10.08, df = 4, $p = 0.04$) (Figure 8.1). The statistically significant heterogeneity observed was judged to be quantitative rather than qualitative because all the trials found a benefit for lithium over placebo, although this was not always statistically significant. The average risk of relapse in the placebo group was 61% compared to 40% on lithium. This means that one patient would avoid relapse for every five patients who were treated for a year or two with lithium[15].

Prevention of manic relapse

Lithium was superior to placebo in the prevention of manic episodes (fixed effects RR 0.61; 95% CI 0.39–0.95, $p = 0.008$, χ^2 for heterogeneity 3.89, df = 3, $p = 0.27$) (Figure 8.2). The average risk of relapse in the placebo group was 24% compared to 14% on lithium. This means that one patient would avoid relapse for every ten patients who were treated for a year or two with lithium.

Prevention of depressive relapse

The effect on depressive relapses appeared smaller and just failed to reach statistical significance (fixed effects RR 0.78 95% CI 0.60–1.01, $p = 0.06$, χ^2 for heterogeneity 4.67, df = 3, $p = 0.2$; random effects RR 0.72, 95% 0.49–1.08) (Figure 8.3). The average risk of relapse in the placebo group was 32% compared to 25% on lithium. This means that one patient

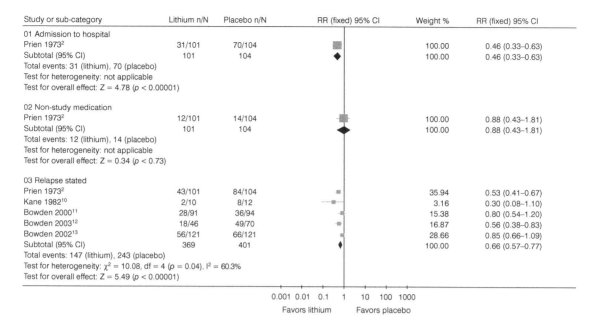

Figure 8.1   Forest plot of meta-analysis of lithium vs. placebo in prevention of relapse in mood disorder: all relapses

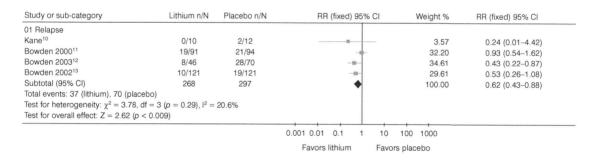

Figure 8.2   Forest plot of meta-analysis of lithium vs. placebo in prevention of relapse in mood disorder: manic relapses

would avoid relapse for 14 patients who were treated for a year or two with lithium.

Prevention of suicide

Goodwin et al.[16] conducted a large obser-vational study of 20 638 members of a US health maintenance organization who were aged ≥14

years, had at least one outpatient diagnosis of bipolar disorder and at least one filled prescription for lithium, divalproex, or carba-mazepine between 1 January 1994 and 31 December 2001. The authors compared the rates of attempted suicide (deliberate self-harm) and completed suicide in the groups of patients prescribed each medicine, and reported that,

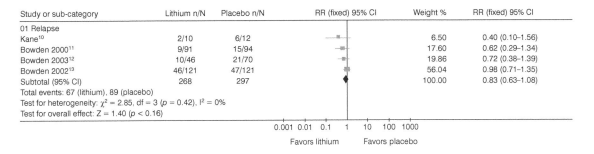

Study or sub-category	Lithium n/N	Placebo n/N	RR (fixed) 95% CI	Weight %	RR (fixed) 95% CI
01 Relapse					
Kane[10]	2/10	6/12		6.50	0.40 (0.10–1.56)
Bowden 2000[11]	9/91	15/94		17.60	0.62 (0.29–1.34)
Bowden 2003[12]	10/46	21/70		19.86	0.72 (0.38–1.39)
Bowden 2002[13]	46/121	47/121		56.04	0.98 (0.71–1.35)
Subtotal (95% CI)	268	297		100.00	0.83 (0.63–1.08)
Total events: 67 (lithium), 89 (placebo)					
Test for heterogeneity: $\chi^2 = 2.85$, df = 3 ($p = 0.42$), $I^2 = 0\%$					
Test for overall effect: Z = 1.40 ($p < 0.16$)					

0.001 0.01   0.1   1   10   100 1000

Favors lithium   Favors placebo

Figure 8.3 Forest plot of meta-analysis of lithium vs. placebo in prevention of relapse in mood disorder: depressive relapse

after adjustment for age, sex, health plan, year of diagnosis, co-morbid medical and psychiatric conditions, and concomitant use of other psychotropic drugs, the risk of suicide was 2.7 times higher (95% CI, 1.1–6.3; $p = 0.03$) during treatment with divalproex than during treatment with lithium. These findings extend and confirm the results of previous combined analyses of observational studies and randomized trials[17–20]. Although these findings suggest that lithium is potently anti-suicidal, the lack of randomization means that the results may be explained by other systematic differences between patients taking lithium and those taking valproate. For example, choice of treatment may be influenced by baseline clinical characteristics of the patient – confounding by indication[21]. Patients who were considered to be suicidal at the time of initiation of treatment might be preferentially prescribed valproate because it is less toxic in overdose.

However, a recent meta-analysis restricted to randomized trials – which exclude the possibility of confounding – and in which original authors were contacted for further details about trial deaths, suggests that the lithium preventative effect is real[22]. In this meta-analysis, patients allocated to lithium were less likely to die by suicide (seven trials; two vs.

11, OR 0.26; 95% CI 0.09–0.77; $p = 0.02$) – indicating a 74% reduction in the risk of suicide in patients allocated to lithium. The composite measure of suicide plus deliberate self harm was also lower in patients allocated to lithium (OR 0.29; 95% CI, 0.13–0.63; $p = 0.002$). There were fewer deaths overall in patients allocated to lithium (12 trials; nine vs. 22, OR 0.42; $p = 0.019$; 95% CI 0.21–0.87). Even when combining all the available studies, the total numbers of suicides and deaths were very low and there was substantial clinical heterogeneity between the trials. Nonetheless, the consistency between these findings and the large-scale observational evidence suggests that the anti-suicidal effect of lithium is real.

Adverse effects

Lithium produces a variety of adverse effects which reduce the quality of life of those who take it. These predictably include thirst and tremor, and in the long term, probably, weight gain. Thus, adverse effects were more common in the lithium-treated participants in clinical trials than those treated with placebo (random effects OR 2.35, 95% CI 1.57–3.53; Peto OR 2.32 95% Cl 1.57–3.43). Only two participants (one in each treatment group) are reported to have dropped out of the studies because of side-effects, although it is likely that the reporting of this outcome was suboptimal in these early trials. Seven of 158 participants on lithium (5%) developed hypothyroidism compared with none of 152 participants on placebo (random effects OR 5.09, 95% CI 0.85–30.51; Peto OR 7.19, 95% Cl 1.6–32.32).

DOSE AND LITHIUM LEVELS

It is usually recommended that patients on long-term lithium therapy should be maintained at serum levels between 0.4 and 1.0 mmol/l. Within this range, there remains uncertainty about the relative efficacy of higher (0.8–1.0 mmol/l) and lower (0.4–0.8 mmol/l). The average level in the early Prien trial was 0.7 mmol/l. More recently, the lamotrigine trials used 0.8–1.1 mmol/l. There is no evidence from the overall meta-analysis that higher levels produce better outcomes than lower levels and there are few directly randomized comparisons. In one randomized controlled trial (RCT)[23], 94 patients who were stable on lithium were randomized to 0.8–1.0 mmol/l or 0.4–0.6 mmol/l. Over 182 weeks, patients in the lower level group were more likely to relapse than those in the high level group. It is possible that these results are explained by the high rates of relapse in patients who were on high levels at baseline, but were randomized to lower levels and were therefore exposed to sudden withdrawal[24]. Further, the higher level patients were more likely to drop out from treatment than those on lower doses and so any potential advantages in efficacy for the higher levels have to be balanced against increased adverse effects and poorer compliance. This finding is consistent with another RCT directly comparing lower and higher levels of lithium[25]. In this open trial, 91 patients with DSM-III unipolar or bipolar (n = 57) disorder were randomly allocated to either high (serum lithium 0.8–1.0 mmol/l) or low (serum lithium 0.5–0.8 mmol/l) levels of lithium. The proportion of patients relapsing was the same in both high and low groups (20%) and the results were the same when repeated excluding the unipolar subgroup.

In general, therefore, the patient should be maintained at the highest well-tolerated level between 0.5 and 1.0 mmol/l[26]. Persevering with high doses or levels in the face of obvious adverse effects is inadvisable in the long term because of the obvious likelihood of discontinuation.

THE CLINICAL MANAGEMENT OF LONG-TERM LITHIUM THERAPY

Initiation of long-term therapy

Previously, long-term treatment was reserved for patients who had already suffered from multiple relapses. Recent guidelines, however, recommend that long-term therapy for relapse prevention should be considered following a single severe manic episode because of the high risk of negative outcomes if the patient suffers from multiple severe episodes before commencing long-term treatment[26,27]. However, adherence with lithium is often poor[28–30] and it can often be difficult to explain the need for lengthy – or even lifelong – treatment to a young patient. Poor treatment adherence will clearly reduce the effectiveness of lithium but the initiation of long-term therapy coupled with poor adherence may worsen outcome because of the increased risk of relapse following sudden cessation of lithium[4,5]. It has been estimated that lithium needs to be taken for a minimum of 2 years to offset the risks of early discontinuation. For this reason, it is essential that the patient understands both the risks of the untreated illness and the effects of long-term lithium therapy *before commencing long-term therapy.* Each patient, therefore, needs an assessment of their own specific baseline risk of relapse plus an estimation of the potential benefits and adverse effects of lithium to allow fully informed decision making. An informed decision implies a high degree of patient education, sometimes called 'psychoeducation', which is a critical requirement for effective disease management.

Three key parameters are required:

(1) *An estimate of the average likely treatment effect (source: RCTs)* The average treatment effects from a meta-analysis provide the best estimate of the likely treatment effect. The average patient might therefore expect a 35% reduction in risk of relapse overall and, more specifically, a 39% reduction in the risk of manic relapse and possibly a 22% reduction in the risk of depressive relapse.

(2) *An estimate of the individual patient's risk of relapse* Accurate estimates of prognosis for individual patients with bipolar disorder are still unavailable. For this reason, most guidelines default to assuming the worst prognosis for all patients. Quantitative estimates of relapse can be derived from inception cohort studies, although extrapolation is required to other settings. The McLean–Harvard First-Episode Mania Study[31] was a prospective 2–4 year follow-up study of 160 patients with bipolar disorder following their first admission to the McLean Hospital. In this study, 34.4% of patients who recovered from a first episode of mania and who remained well for 8 weeks experienced a further mood episode (mania, depression or mixed episode) in the subsequent 2 years. The risk for both depression and mania was 20.1%. This was a treated cohort although long-term treatment appeared to be suboptimal (perhaps reflecting poor compliance) and so this is likely to be an underestimate of the real risk. The McLean–Harvard First-Episode Mania Study is probably the most reliable evidence on prognosis but clinical application in other settings – and to non-hospitalized groups – needs to be cautious. However, the findings are reasonably consistent with routinely collected data from Denmark, which suggest a 2-year readmission risk of 30–40% in patients following first admission with bipolar disorder[31,32].

(3) *An estimate of the risk of specific treatment-emergent adverse events* The best estimate of treatment-emergent adverse events is the systematic review of randomized trials above. Clinically, however, we prefer a trial treatment period for each patient anticipating long-term therapy. Only patients who can tolerate adverse effects at therapeutic doses would be selected for long-term therapy.

On average, therefore, lithium can be expected to reduce the risk of a mood episode by 35% – i.e. for the typical McLean patient from 34.4% to approximately 22.4%. This is an absolute risk reduction (ARR) of 12%. The number needed to treat (NNT) is 100/ARR = 8 for all mood episodes. This size of NNT is normally considered to be at the borderline of those usually considered to be worth the inconvenience, costs and adverse effects of medication. Guidelines are therefore pushing to the limit of what is on average reasonable by promoting earlier treatment. Individual patients will be at different risks and differ in their view of the average level of risk and treatment benefit. Severe illness, a medically orientated acceptance of the fact of the illness and strong family history tend to reinforce the strategy of early long-term treatment.

At higher levels of risk – for example in a patient who has already had two or more severe manic episodes[32], the relative treatment benefit remains constant but the absolute benefit increases and the NNT decreases. The benefits of treatment are much clearer in this situation. This accords with the traditional approach to long-term treatment, which allowed the illness course to emerge before initiating lithium.

Average effects are helpful, but not all patients appear to show a good outcome despite compliance with lithium treatment. Maj *et al.*[33] showed that, in a large lithium clinic, only 25% of patients had good 5-year outcomes. Targeting lithium treatment on likely responders remains an inexact strategy but, with the development of pharmacogenomics, it may become more important in the future. For the present, some aspects of the phenotype such as classical euphoric mania, clear episodes of illness and usual recurrence to the manic pole of the illness may predict lithium responsiveness on the basis of retrospective analysis of data from some of the clinical trials[34].

Realizing the potential benefits of lithium therapy in the real world

There is increasing recognition that adherence must be optimized to realize the potential benefit of long-term lithium therapy. In the past, clinicians tended to expect a passive acceptance (compliance) with prescribed treatment. It is now understood that more sophisticated models of patient–physician collaboration are required to achieve optimal outcomes. Von Korff and colleagues[35] proposed an influential collaborative practice model for chronic medical illness based on social learning and self-regulation theories which contained four main elements:

(1) Collaborative definition of problems;

(2) Joint goal-setting and planning;

(3) Continuum of self-management;
      support

(4) Active and sustained follow-up.

The application of this concept of collaborative chronic disease management is intuitively appealing when applied to bipolar disorder, a disorder in which *self-management* has become popular with patients, and is probably essential for the early detection of relapse. It is a potentially powerful way of improving adherence to long-term lithium therapy – a treatment that is able to confer substantial benefit when used optimally but substantial harm when used suboptimally. The average use of lithium appears to be suboptimal[36] and so the capacity to benefit from the improvements brought by structured collaborative approaches may be considerable. Randomized evidence is now emerging that they can improve outcomes. Bauer[37] has elaborated a collaborative practice model for bipolar disorder which is now being evaluated in a Veterans Administration randomized trial[38].

In a trial of collaborative disease management, Simon and co-workers[39] randomly allocated 441 patients with bipolar disorder to continued usual care or usual care plus a systematic care management program which included:

• Initial assessment and care planning;

• Monthly telephone monitoring (including symptom assessment and medication monitoring);

• Feedback to and coordination with the mental health treatment team;

• A structured group psychoeducational program.

All these components were provided by a nurse care manager. Patients allocated to the intervention group suffered from fewer manic symptoms across the 12-month follow-up period and approximately one-third less time in a hypomanic or manic episode. There was no significant difference in mean depression ratings across the follow-up period, but the intervention group showed a greater decline in depression ratings over time.

The specific objectives in psychosocial interventions all include education about the illness, self monitoring and the development of an action plan in the face of relapse. Modest but worthwhile effects on rates of relapse have been described both for individuals[40] and for young people offered family psychoeducation[41]. Part of the mechanism of action of these interventions is by improved adherence to medicines. The other assumed effects are via changes in lifestyle – especially drug or alcohol misuse and more regular daily activities.

CONCLUSIONS

It is perhaps surprising that lithium, an agent discovered over 50 years ago to be effective in acute mania, should remain the benchmark for maintenance treatment of bipolar disorder. The challenge of providing effective long-term treatment remains the most difficult we face and lithium continues to play a central part. This is because it has proven efficacy in preventing relapse and, probably, reducing the risk of suicide. The modest average benefits of lithium appear to be more substantial in individual cases – an important observation that we are yet fully to understand. Whether modest effects as monotherapy can be amplified by treatment in combination with other agents is a pressing current question. Thus far, the alternatives to lithium remain just that: the newer medicines have not decisively out-performed lithium. Accordingly, lithium will continue for the foreseeable future to set the standards against which we should measure improvements in pharmacological practice.

REFERENCES

1. Blackwell B, Shepherd M. Prophylactic lithium: another therapeutic myth? An examination of the evidence to date. Lancet 1968; 1: 968–71
2. Prien RF, Caffey EM Jr, Klett CJ. Prophylactic efficacy of lithium carbonate in manic-depressive illness. Report of the Veterans Administration and National Institute of Mental Health collaborative study group. Arch Gen Psychiatry 1973; 28: 337–41
3. Moncrieff J. Lithium: evidence reconsidered. Br J Psychiatry 1997; 171: 113–19
4. Suppes T, Baldessarini RJ, Faedda GL, Tohen M. Risk of recurrence following discontinuation of lithium treatment in bipolar disorder. Arch Gen Psychiatry 1991; 48: 1082–8
5. Goodwin GM. Recurrence of mania after lithium withdrawal. Implications for the use of lithium in the treatment of bipolar affective disorder [Editorial]. Br J Psychiatry 1994; 164: 149–52
6. Goodwin GM, Geddes JR. Latest maintenance data on lithium in bipolar disorder. Eur Neuropsychopharmacol 2003; 13: S51–S55
7. Geddes JR, Burgess S, Hawton K, et al. Long-term lithium therapy for bipolar disorder: systematic review and meta-analysis of randomized controlled trials. Am J Psychiatry 2004; 161: 217–22
8. Burgess S, Geddes J, Hawton K, et al. Lithium for maintenance treatment of mood disorders. Cochrane Database Syst Rev CD003013 2001
9. Sweeting MJ, Sutton AJ, Lambert PC. What to add to nothing? Use and avoidance of continuity corrections in meta-analysis of sparse data. Stat Med 2004; 23: 1351–75
10. Kane JM, Quitkin FM, Rifkin A, et al. Lithium carbonate and imipramine in the prophylaxis of unipolar and bipolar II illness: a prospective, placebo-controlled comparison. Arch Gen Psychiatry 1982; 39: 1065–9
11. Bowden CL, Calabrese JR, McElroy SL, et al. A randomized, placebo-controlled 12-month trial of divalproex and lithium in treatment of outpatients with bipolar I disorder. Divalproex

Maintenance Study Group [see comments]. Arch Gen Psychiatry 2000; 57: 481–9

12. Bowden CL, Calabrese JR, Sachs G, et al. A placebo-controlled 18-month trial of lamotrigine and lithium maintenance treatment in recently manic or hypomanic patients with bipolar I disorder. Arch Gen Psychiatry 2003; 60: 392–400

13. Calabrese JR, Bowden CL, Sachs G, et al. A placebo-controlled 18-month trial of lamotrigine and lithium maintenance treatment in recently depressed patients with bipolar I disorder. J Clin Psychiatry 2003; 64: 1013–24

14. Burgess S, Geddes JR, Townsend E, et al. Lithium for preventing relapse in affective disorder [protocol]. Cochrane Library 2000

15. Laupacis A, Sackett DL, Roberts RS. An assessment of clinically useful measures of the consequences of treatment. N Engl J Med 1988; 318: 1728–33

16. Goodwin FK, Fireman B, Simon GE, et al. Suicide risk in bipolar disorder during treatment with lithium and divalproex. JAMA 2003; 290: 1467–73

17. Schou M, The effect of prophylactic lithium treatment on mortality and suicidal behaviour: a review for clinicians. J Affect Disord 1998; 50: 253–9

18. Tondo L, Jamison KR, Baldessarini RJ. Effect of lithium maintenance on suicidal behavior in major mood disorders [Review]. Ann NY Acad Sci 1997; 836: 339–51

19. Tondo L, Hennen J, Baldessarini RJ. Lower suicide risk with long-term lithium treatment in major affective illness: a meta-analysis. Acta Psychiatr Scand 2001; 104: 163–72

20. Müller-Oerlinghausen B, Berghöfer A, Ahrens B. The antisuicidal and mortality-reducing effect of lithium prophylaxis: consequences for guidelines in clinical psychiatry. Can J Psychiatry 2003; 48: 433–9

21. Walker AM. Confounding by indication. Epidemiology 1996; 7: 335–6

22. Cipriani A, Pretty H, Hawton K, Geddes JR. Lithium in the prevention of suicidal behaviour and all-cause mortality in patients with mood disorders: a systematic review of randomised trials. Am J Psychiatry 2005; 162: 1805–19

23. Gelenberg AJ, Kane JM, Keller MB, et al. Comparison of standard and low serum levels of lithium for maintenance treatment of bipolar disorder. N Engl J Med 1989; 321: 1489–93

24. Perlis RH, Sachs GS, Lafer B, et al. Effect of abrupt change from standard to low serum levels of lithium: a reanalysis of double-blind lithium maintenance data. Am J Psychiatry 2002; 159: 1155–9

25. Vestergaard P, Licht RW, Brodersen A, et al. Outcome of lithium prophylaxis: a prospective follow-up of affective disorder patients assigned to high and low serum lithium levels. Acta Psychiatr Scand 1998; 98: 310–15

26. Goodwin GM. Evidence-based guidelines for treating bipolar disorder: recommendations from the British Association for Psychopharmacology. J Psychopharmacol 2003; 17: 149–73

27. American Psychiatric Association. Practice guideline for the treatment of patients with bipolar disorder (revision). Am J Psychiatry 2002; 159: 1–50

28. Gitlin MJ, Cochran SD, Jamison KR. Maintenance lithium treatment: side effects and compliance [see comments]. J Clin Psychiatry 1989; 50: 127–31

29. Jamison KR, Akiskal HS. Medication compliance in patients with bipolar disorder. Psychiatr Clin North Am 1983; 6: 175–92

30. Lee S, Wing YK, Wong KC. Knowledge and compliance towards lithium therapy among Chinese psychiatric patients in Hong Kong. Aust NZ J Psychiatry 1992; 26: 444–9

31. Tohen M, Zarate CAJ, Hennen J, et al. The McLean–Harvard First-Episode Mania Study: prediction of recovery and first recurrence. Am J Psychiatry 2003; 160: 2099–107

32. Kessing LV, Hansen MG, Andersen PK. Course of illness in depressive and bipolar disorders: Naturalistic study, 1994–1999. Br J Psychiatry 2004; 185: 372–7

33. Maj M, Pirozzi R, Magliano L, Bartoli L. Long-term outcome of lithium prophylaxis in bipolar disorder: a 5-year prospective study of 402 patients at a lithium clinic. Am J Psychiatry 1998; 155: 30–35

34. Kleindienst N, Greil W. Differential efficacy of lithium and carbamazepine in the prophylaxis of bipolar disorder: results of the MAP study. Neuropsychobiology 2000; 42 (Suppl): 2–10

35. Von Korff M, Gruman J, Schaefer J, et al. Collaborative management of chronic illness. Ann Int Med 1997; 127: 1097–102

36. Johnson RE, McFarland BH. Lithium use and discontinuation in a health maintenance organization. Am J Psychiatry 1996; 153: 993–1000

37. Bauer MS. The collaborative practice model for bipolar disorder: design and implementation in a multi-site randomized controlled trial. Bipolar Disorders 2001; 3: 233–44

38. Bauer MS, Williford WO, Dawson EE, et al. Principles of effectiveness trials and their implementation in VA Cooperative Study #430: 'Reducing the Efficacy-Effectiveness Gap in Bipolar Disorder'. J Affect Disord 2001; 67: 61–78

39. Simon GE, Ludman EJ, Unutzer J, et al. Randomized trial of a population-based care program for people with bipolar disorder. Psychol Med 2005; 35: 13–24

40. Colom F, Vieta E, Martinez-Aran A, et al. A randomized trial on the efficacy of group psychoeducation in the prophylaxis of recurrences in bipolar patients whose disease is in remission. Arch Gen Psychiatry. 2003; 60: 402–7

41. Miklowitz DJ, George EL, Richards JA, et al. A randomized study of family-focused psychoeducation and pharmacotherapy in the outpatient management of bipolar disorder. Arch Gen Psychiatry 2003; 60: 904–12

9 Effectiveness of lithium in naturalistic settings

Mario Maj

Contents   Introduction • Overall effectiveness of lithium prophylaxis • Effectiveness of lithium prophylaxis in special groups • Persistence of the effectiveness of lithium prophylaxis • Effects of lithium discontinuation • Conclusions

INTRODUCTION

The efficacy of lithium prophylaxis in bipolar disorder has been convincingly documented by several double-blind randomized placebo-controlled trials (see reference 1 for a systematic review). However, there are several reasons why the evidence provided by controlled trials can be usefully complemented by the information collected through well-designed observational studies carried out in ordinary clinical conditions.

First, the patient samples recruited for lithium controlled trials are likely not to be representative of the broad population of people with bipolar disorder, for the following reasons:

(1)   The exclusion criteria adopted in these trials (e.g. exclusion of patients with other concomitant mental or general medical disorders, of those with alcohol or drug abuse, or of those with rapid cycling);

(2)   The inclusion criteria used in some of these trials (e.g. a minimum number of episodes of affective disorder during the last few years, or a period of euthymia of a specified minimum duration before the start of lithium treatment);

(3)   The requirement of patients' informed consent to an experimental procedure involving the use of placebo.

Indeed, it has been reported[2] that 77% of a clinical sample of bipolar patients would have been excluded from the lithium controlled trials of the 1970s. Furthermore, the only placebo-controlled prophylactic lithium trial conducted in the past 25 years[3] has reportedly overincluded the more mildly ill bipolar patients (many participants had not been hospitalized or even treated pharmacologically for the index episode) exactly due to the adopted exclusion and inclusion criteria and the requirement for informed consent[1].

Second, the gap between efficacy (i.e. the impact on the target disorder in controlled conditions) and effectiveness (i.e. the impact on the target disorder in ordinary clinical conditions) has been well documented for several drugs outside the field of psychiatry[4]. Two of the main factors contributing to that gap (patients' inadequate adherence to treatment and physicians' inadequate adherence to good clinical practice in the initiation and supervision of treatment) are likely to be particularly powerful in the specific case of lithium prophylaxis of bipolar disorder. Several lithium controlled trials excluded from the analysis those patients who were not compliant to treatment (as shown by their low plasma lithium levels) and/or did not include those patients who did not tolerate lithium during an initial stabilization phase of open treatment with the drug. Estimates of cost savings related to lithium prophylaxis of bipolar disorder may be more reliably based on effectiveness than efficacy data.

Third, almost all lithium controlled trials have had a duration of no more than 2 years, and it is very unlikely that controlled trials exceeding that duration will be carried out in the future. A longer observation period may be needed to explore the different patterns of response to lithium prophylaxis, a possible decline of the prophylactic effect with time, rebound phenomena after discontinuation, as well as the impact of treatment on crucial variables such as the risk for suicide.

For all the above reasons, observational studies carried out in ordinary clinical conditions may usefully complement lithium controlled trials. However, the biases inherent in the lack of randomization and the absence of a controlled group should always be kept in mind when interpreting the results of naturalistic studies. For example, the comparison of patients who receive lithium prophylaxis versus those who do not receive it in ordinary clinical conditions may be misleading, since the subgroup of patients with the milder forms of the disorder, who are less likely to receive long-term pharmacological treatment, may be over-represented in the non-lithium-treated sample (so that the two groups may have a similar outcome, but this may not reflect a lack of effectiveness of lithium treatment). Equally misleading may be the focus on patients who have completed a minimum period of prophylaxis (e.g. 1 year), because the permanence of these patients on the prophylactic regimen may have been a consequence as well as a determinant of their favorable response (in other terms, they may represent a self-selected group with a better than average response to treatment). Furthermore, even if a 'mirror design' is adopted (i.e. a period of lithium treatment is compared with a period of the same duration preceding the index episode and the start of prophylaxis, so that each patient represents his/her own control), several sources of bias cannot be avoided. For example, if the pre-treatment period is reconstructed retrospectively and the treatment period is observed prospectively, the probability that minor recurrences will be missed may be higher during the pre-treatment period, thus creating a bias in favor of the treatment. On the other hand, the natural course of bipolar disorder is often capricious or may worsen with time; this may create a bias in favor of prophylactic treatment (e.g. if episodes cluster in the period immediately before the start of treatment) or against prophylaxis (e.g. if the natural recurrence rate increases during the treatment period, thus counteracting the effect of prophylaxis).

Finally, the expression 'naturalistic studies' or 'studies carried out in ordinary clinical practice' encompasses investigations conducted in very different contexts and using very different designs. These differences should be recognized, in order to avoid inappropriate generalizations and misleading conclusions. Moreover, the reader should be alert to some crucial variables which make an observational study more or less valid: the reliable continuous documentation of psychopathology in individual patients throughout the observation period, the regular recording of all treatments received by the patients (including non-pharmacological ones) and the monitoring of patients' adherence to treatment (by the regular measurement of plasma lithium levels).

OVERALL EFFECTIVENESS OF LITHIUM PROPHYLAXIS

The most frequently quoted naturalistic studies of the effectiveness of lithium prophylaxis in bipolar disorder can be classified into two groups, very different in their methodology and results. These two groups of studies have led, not surprisingly, to different conclusions, but their clinical implications can be regarded as complementary (Table 9.1).

The first group includes studies conducted in a sample of bipolar patients discharged from hospital after an episode of affective disorder, and followed up after a specified period of time. Patients receiving lithium during that period are compared to those not receiving the drug. The most frequently quoted studies of this group are those published by Markar and Mander[5] and Harrow et al.[6].

The second group includes studies carried out in a lithium clinic or a clinic specializing in the treatment of mood disorders. They evaluate all patients who started lithium prophylaxis in the clinic during a specified period of time, or all those who completed a minimum period of lithium prophylaxis. The lithium treatment period is usually compared with a period of the

Table 9.1 Selected studies exploring the overall effectiveness of lithium prophylaxis in bipolar disorder

Study	Design	Main findings
Markar and Mander[5]	Follow-up of 83 patients from the point when they had been well for 6 months up to readmission or up to 6 years	No significant difference between lithium and control group on number of admissions and mean period spent in hospital per year
Harrow et al.[6]	Follow-up after an average of 1.7 years of 73 patients discharged from hospital after a manic episode	Patients who had been prescribed lithium throughout the year before follow-up did not differ from the others on post-hospital adjustment
Maj et al.[8]	Prospective follow-up of 402 patients who started lithium prophylaxis at a lithium clinic. Evaluation after 5 years	During treatment, 52% of patients had a reduction of at least 50% in the mean annual time spent in hospital; 23.4% had no affective episode
Tondo et al.[12]	Retrospective study of 360 patients who continued lithium prophylaxis for at least 1 year (average 6 years)	During treatment, 64.4% of patients had a reduction of at least 50% in the percentage of time ill; 28.9% had no affective episode

same duration preceding the index episode and the start of prophylaxis. The most frequently quoted studies of this group are those published by Maj *et al.*[7–9] and Baldessarini and co-workers[10–12].

Studies in patients discharged after an episode and followed up after a specified period of time

Markar and Mander[5] studied 83 patients with a DSM-III diagnosis of bipolar disorder who had had at least two admissions in 2 years or three admissions in 5 years. All patients were followed up starting from the point when they had been well for 6 months following the index episode until the occurrence of a readmission or up to 6 years. Forty-one patients took lithium continuously for at least 6 months after the index episode and had a mean serum lithium level higher than 0.4 mmol/l during that 6-month period (lithium group); 42 patients did not receive lithium prophylaxis (control group). The two groups did not differ significantly with respect to the mean duration of the index episode and to several demographic variables (except the mean age at index episode, which was significantly higher in the control group). Lithium treatment was monitored by general practitioners in the majority of cases. The mean number of admissions and the mean period spent in hospital per year of follow-up were found to be not significantly different in the two groups. The conclusion of the authors was that the benefits conferred by the prescription of lithium in clinical practice are modest compared with the results of clinical trials. The authors recognized, however, that patients of the lithium group might have discontinued the drug after the first 6 months of follow-up and may have had withdrawal relapses.

Harrow *et al.*[6] studied 73 patients discharged from hospital after an episode fulfilling DSM-III criteria for mania. They evaluated these patients an average of 1.7 years after discharge. During that period, 63% of them had been treated by a psychiatrist and 23% had received no form of treatment. The 25 patients who had been prescribed lithium throughout the year before follow-up evaluation did not differ from the others with respect to overall post-hospital adjustment, as evaluated by the LKP scale. Moreover, full manic syndromes occurred among 40% of the patients who had been prescribed lithium throughout the year before follow-up evaluation, and 42% of those who had not been prescribed lithium at all during that period (this comparison was carried out in the 38 patients who received a complete standardized clinical interview at follow-up). The conclusion of the authors was that the outcome of lithium prophylaxis in routine clinical practice is not as positive as suggested by the studies carried out under controlled conditions. The authors recognized, however, that they had no data on patients' treatment compliance, and that probably some patients did not follow their treatment plan and stopped taking lithium.

The main implication of the above two studies is that pointed out by Schou[13]. 'Ordinary clinical conditions' are often not good enough for long-term lithium prophylaxis. Patients are given lithium treatment 'under conditions of insufficient information, support and supervision'. The solution to the problem 'is not to use lithium less, but to use it better'. Hospital physicians and general practitioners should be provided with guidelines about minimum requirements for the monitoring of lithium treatment. Training courses may be useful. 'It is not lithium alone but the mode of service delivery which confers the benefits'[4]. Obviously, both main factors contributing to the gap between efficacy and effectiveness of any drug are at work in this context: patients' inadequate adherence to treatment and physicians' inadequate surveillance of treatment.

Prospective and retrospective studies carried out in specialized units

Maj et al.[8] studied prospectively all patients fulfilling Research Diagnostic Criteria for bipolar I disorder who started lithium prophylaxis at a lithium clinic throughout a period of more than 15 years. Patients with other concomitant mental disorders, alcohol or drug abuse, or rapid cycling, as well as patients with concomitant physical diseases (except those in which lithium treatment is contraindicated), were not excluded. Patients were evaluated bimonthly with standardized instruments for as long as they took lithium. Treatment surveillance conformed to internationally accepted guidelines. Five years after starting prophylaxis, each patient was contacted for a follow-up interview. Of the 402 enrolled patients, 10.7% were not available at follow-up; 27.9% were not taking lithium at follow-up; 9.5% were taking lithium and had had at least one affective episode during the treatment period, without a reduction of at least 50% in the mean annual time spent in hospital (compared to a reference pre-treatment period); 28.6% were taking lithium and had had at least one recurrence, with a reduction of at least 50% in the mean annual time spent in hospital; and 23.4% were taking lithium and had had no affective episode during the treatment period. Of the interviewed patients who were not taking lithium at follow-up, 84.8% had interrupted prophylaxis on their own initiative. The most frequent alleged reasons for interruption were perceived inefficacy, trouble related to side-effects, the conviction to be cured and to need no more drugs, and the annoyance of taking medicines. Among patients who were taking lithium at follow-up, the percentage of those who had had psychotic symptoms during the index episode was significantly lower than in the group of patients who had interrupted lithium. The main conclusions of the authors

were that: (1) 'information, support and supervision' are not sufficient to counteract the tendency of bipolar patients receiving long-term lithium treatment to drop out; and (2) lithium, if taken regularly for several years, has a substantial impact on the course of illness in most bipolar patients. The authors warned, however, against the bias of self-selection in patients who remain on lithium for several years (i.e. the permanence on lithium prophylaxis may be a consequence as well as a determinant of the favorable response).

Baldessarini and co-workers[11,12] studied 360 patients fulfilling DSM-IV criteria for bipolar I ($n = 218$) or bipolar II ($n = 142$) disorder, who started lithium prophylaxis from 1970 and continued it for at least 1 year (average 6 years). They excluded patients misusing drugs or alcohol during treatment and those considered non-compliant with treatment recommendations (because of repeated interruptions or self-reduction of dosage). Of the studied patients, 28.9% had no new episodes during treatment; 35.5% had at least one new episode, but with a reduction of at least 50% of the percentage of time ill during lithium treatment versus a pre-treatment period; and 35.6% had at least one new episode, without a reduction of at least 50% of the percentage of time ill (with 21.4% showing no improvement). The conclusion of the authors was that long-term lithium treatment produces substantial levels of improvement in compliant patients with bipolar disorder without co-morbid substance abuse.

Overall, the above two studies carried out in lithium clinics suggest that a drastic reduction of affective morbidity is almost the rule in bipolar patients who keep on taking lithium for several years, although a complete suppression of morbidity occurs only in less than one-third of them. However, bipolar patients who remain on a lithium regimen for several years represent a self-selected population, in which some subgroups at high risk of poor outcome (for example, psychotic patients and those with concomitant substance abuse) may be under-represented.

EFFECTIVENESS OF LITHIUM PROPHYLAXIS IN SPECIAL GROUPS

Observational studies carried out in ordinary clinical conditions have allowed the collection of information about the impact of lithium prophylaxis on some varieties of bipolar disorder which have usually been excluded from controlled trials (e.g. bipolar disorder with rapid cycling or with mood-incongruent psychotic features) or which have not been evaluated separately in those trials (e.g. bipolar II disorder) (Table 9.2).

Within the above-mentioned study carried out in a lithium clinic[11,12], Baldessarini et al.[14] compared response to lithium in bipolar patients with and without rapid cycling (defined as the occurrence of at least four DSM-IV depressive, manic or mixed episodes within any year before intake). Among the 56 rapid cyclers, the percentage of those presenting no recurrences during the treatment period was significantly lower than among the 304 non-rapid cyclers (17.9% vs. 31.6%, $p = 0.04$), but the proportion of those presenting a reduction of at least 50% of the time ill during treatment (compared with a pre-treatment period) was not different (66.1% vs. 60.5%), nor was the percentage of those who showed no improvement (16.1% vs. 25.4%). The percentage of improvement during versus before lithium treatment was very similar between the two groups on all variables (reduction in recurrence rates or in the proportion of time ill for all episodes, manic episodes and depressive episodes). The time to 50% recurrence risk during lithium treatment was also not significantly different. The conclusion of the authors was that rapid cycling is not associated with a poorer response to lithium prophylaxis in bipolar patients.

Within the above-mentioned study carried out in a lithium clinic[8], Maj et al.[15] compared

Table 9.2 Selected studies exploring the effectiveness of lithium prophylaxis in some varieties of bipolar disorder

Study	Variety of bipolar disorder	Main findings
Baldessarini et al.[14]	Rapid cycling	The proportion of patients presenting a reduction of at least 50% of time ill during treatment and the percentage of those who showed no improvement did not differ in rapid vs. non-rapid cyclers
Maj et al.[15]	With mood-incongruent psychotic features	Significant reduction of the time to 50% risk of readmission during treatment in both psychotic patients ($p < 0.004$) and non-psychotic controls ($p < 0.001$)
Tondo et al.[10]	Bipolar II disorder	The time to 50% recurrence during lithium treatment was 5.9-fold longer in bipolar II than in bipolar I patients

the response to lithium in bipolar patients with and without mood-incongruent psychotic features (as defined by the DSM-III). Out of 58 recruited patients, 53 with mood-incongruent psychotic features and 54 without mood-incongruent psychotic features could be interviewed 5 years after the start of lithium prophylaxis. Thirty (56.6%) of the psychotic patients and 42 (77.8%) of the controls were still on lithium at follow-up ($p < 0.02$). Among the psychotic patients who were still on lithium, 23.3% had had no recurrence during the treatment period, and 56.7% had had a reduction of at least 50% of the time spent in hospital during that period compared to a pre-treatment period. The corresponding figures for the non-psychotic patients were 35.7% and 78.6% ($p = 0.26$ and $p < 0.05$, respectively). The time to 50% risk of readmission was 10 months before lithium treatment and 20 months during treatment in the psychotic patients ($p < 0.004$), and 17 vs. 39 months in non-psychotic controls ($p < 0.001$). The conclusion of the authors was that lithium prophylaxis does exert an impact on the course of bipolar disorder with mood-incongruent psychotic features, although this impact is less pronounced than in bipolar disorder without those features.

Within the above-mentioned study carried out in a lithium clinic[11,12], Tondo et al.[10] compared response to lithium in bipolar II versus bipolar I patients. Survival analyses indicated that bipolar II patients ($n = 129$) and bipolar I patients ($n = 188$) had the same time to 50% recurrence before lithium treatment (8.0 months). However, the time to 50% recurrence during lithium treatment was 5.9-fold longer in bipolar II patients (100.0 vs. 17.0 months). Furthermore, the ratio of computed time to 50% risk of a first recurrence during lithium treatment versus before lithium treatment (a measure of benefit of lithium treatment) was 5.9 times greater in bipolar II patients (12.50 vs. 2.12 months). The authors' conclusion was that the

benefit of lithium prophylaxis may be somewhat greater in bipolar II than in bipolar I patients.

PERSISTENCE OF THE EFFECTIVENESS OF LITHIUM PROPHYLAXIS

Observational studies carried out in ordinary clinical conditions allow a systematic assessment to be made of the persistence of lithium prophylactic effect over time. This assessment is important, because it has been maintained that lithium exerts its prophylactic activity on relapses but not on recurrences of bipolar disorder, so that its effect does not persist after the first year of recovery from the index episode[16], and that about one-third of lithium non-responders show a pattern of gradual loss of efficacy of the drug, suggesting the development of tolerance[17].

Berghöfer et al.[18] studied 86 patients with an ICD-9 diagnosis of mood or schizoaffective disorder (55 of whom were bipolar) who received lithium treatment at a lithium clinic for at least 3 years (mean 8.2 years). Of the 36 patients receiving lithium for more than 10 years, 30 had at least one recurrence during the treatment period. The number and severity of the manic episodes decreased during the second treatment period (years 6–10) compared with the first one (years 1–5), whereas the number and severity of the depressive episodes did not change significantly. The morbidity index was lower in the first year of treatment, but subsequently did not change over time. The conclusion of the authors was that the effect of regular lithium prophylaxis remains constant over a period of up to 10 years.

In an extension of the above-mentioned study carried out in a lithium clinic[8], Maj[9] studied 161 bipolar I patients who were still on lithium prophylaxis at a 10-year follow-up interview. In these patients, the number of episodes per year was not significantly different in the second 5-year treatment period compared with the first one (0.82 ± 1.10 vs. 0.88 ± 0.95). No significant difference was observed between the two periods with respect to the time spent by the patients in hospital per year (1.39 ± 2.16 vs. 1.44 ± 2.04). However, of the 77 patients who had had no affective episode during the first 5-year period, ten (13%) had at least two episodes during the second period, without a reduction of at least 50% of the mean annual time spent in hospital during that period compared with the pre-treatment reference period. The conclusion of the authors was that, in bipolar patients who remain on lithium for many years, the effect of prophylaxis does not usually decrease over time. However, a minority of patients who had had no episode for several years may have multiple recurrences subsequently. Whether the latter finding indicates a loss of efficacy of the drug over time in individual patients, or simply reflects the irregular natural course of the disorder, remains unclear.

EFFECTS OF LITHIUM DISCONTINUATION

Observational studies carried out in ordinary clinical conditions allow one to approach the issue of whether the discontinuation of lithium prophylaxis is followed by rebound phenomena. This is a question of great clinical relevance: if the drop-out rate in patients receiving lithium in ordinary clinical practice is high, as seems to have been shown[8], and discontinuation of lithium treatment is usually followed by a period of increased risk of recurrence, then the prophylactic impact of the drug may be counterbalanced, and the overall net effect of initiating lithium treatment in a population of bipolar patients may be null or even negative[19].

Baldessarini et al.[20] studied 227 bipolar patients (136 with bipolar I and 91 with bipolar II disorder) who discontinued lithium prophylaxis in a non-experimental fashion (i.e. the interruption of treatment was not required by an experimental protocol). Discontinuation was rapid (over 1–14 days) in 112 patients, gradual (over 15–30 days) in 84 patients, and uncertain in 31 patients. The time to 50% risk of recurrence was 6 months in the first group, 24 months in the second and 18 months in the third ($p < 0.0001$). Following rapid discontinuation, the time to 50% risk of recurrence was three times shorter than the average spontaneous cycling interval in the same subjects before they started lithium prophylaxis (6 vs. 18 months).

Davis et al.[21] noticed that much of the evidence concerning the consequences of lithium discontinuation came from studies published after 1990, which 'may reflect something about this time period'. In fact, both Schou[22] and Grof[23], who failed to find any increase of recurrence rate in the first few months following lithium discontinuation, have submitted the opinion that the rebound phenomenon does not occur in typical manic-depressive patients, whereas it may be observed in atypical (e.g. schizoaffective) cases, the percentage of which may have increased in recent studies using DSM-III or DSM-IV criteria for the diagnosis of bipolar disorder. This, however, is not supported at the moment by convincing research evidence.

Baldessarini and co-workers have also repeatedly approached the question of whether re-treatment after lithium discontinuation is associated, at least in some cases, with a loss of the prophylactic effect of lithium, as has been suggested by several authors[24–27]. In a sample of 86 bipolar patients[28], Tondo et al. found that affective morbidity was similar during a second versus a first period of lithium prophylaxis, but that the use of an adjunctive antipsychotic or antidepressant for acute symptoms was significantly more frequent ($p = 0.002$) during the second period. In a further report concerning 106 patients[29], this group described a significant increase (by 38%) of the percentage of time ill during a second versus a first lithium maintenance period. In a third report concerning 130 patients[20], they found a non-significant increase of affective morbidity during the second lithium treatment period ($p = 0.09$), but a significant increase of the time in depression during that period compared with the first one ($p = 0.02$). In a fourth report regarding 85 patients[12], they found only minor and non-significant increases in annual rates of recurrence or in the proportion of time ill in the second treatment period compared with the first.

The issue has also been addressed by Coryell et al.[30] in a sample of 28 bipolar patients. In those patients, the recurrence rate at 2 years was not significantly different during two subsequent periods of lithium prophylaxis, but the recurrence rate at 1 year was about 10% during the first treatment period and about 30% during the second (a difference that is not discussed in the paper, but is likely to be significant). This seems to support the notion of a reversible discontinuation effect.

Further long-term prospective studies of large patient samples are obviously needed in order to clarify the effect of treatment discontinuation on response to lithium prophylaxis.

CONCLUSIONS

Well-designed observational studies carried out in ordinary clinical conditions add useful information to the evidence provided by lithium controlled trials. However, the biases inherent in the lack of randomization and the absence of a control group should always be kept in mind when interpreting the results of these naturalistic studies. Moreover, the differences in the designs of these studies and in the contexts in which they are carried out should always be acknowledged when reporting and interpreting their results.

Overall, studies carried out in ordinary clinical conditions confirm that lithium, if taken regularly for several years, has a significant impact on the course of the illness in most bipolar patients. However, patients receiving long-term lithium treatment have a high tendency to drop out. This tendency is more pronounced if they are not provided with sufficient information, support and supervision, but is remarkable even if treatment surveillance is adequate. Adjunctive psychoeducational interventions may improve patients' acceptance of lithium prophylaxis, but their ability to reduce the impact of factors such as perceived inefficacy of treatment or trouble related to side-effects remains to be documented.

Well-designed observational studies carried out in ordinary clinical practice suggest that lithium prophylaxis is effective also in bipolar disorder with mood-incongruent psychotic features or with rapid cycling. Although the larger study focusing on the impact of lithium prophylaxis in bipolar II versus bipolar I patients suggests a greater efficacy in the former group, this finding requires independent confirmation.

Naturalistic studies suggest that the effect of lithium prophylaxis does not decrease over time in the vast majority of bipolar patients, and that abrupt discontinuation of lithium treatment is followed by a period of increased risk of recurrence. The effect of treatment discontinuation on response to lithium prophylaxis requires further investigation.

REFERENCES

1. Burgess S, Geddes J, Hawton K, et al. Lithium for maintenance treatment of mood disorders. Cochrane Database Syst Rev 2001; (3): CD003013

2. Sachs GS, Lafer B, Truman CJ, et al. Lithium monotherapy: miracle, myth and misunderstanding. Psychiatr Ann 1994; 24: 299–306

3. Bowden CL. Efficacy of lithium in mania and maintenance therapy of bipolar disorder. J Clin Psychiatry 2000; 61 (Suppl 9): 35–40

4. Guscott R, Taylor L. Lithium prophylaxis in recurrent affective illness. Efficacy, effectiveness and efficiency. Br J Psychiatry 1994; 164: 741–6

5. Markar HR, Mander AJ. Efficacy of lithium prophylaxis in clinical practice. Br J Psychiatry 1989; 155: 496–500

6. Harrow M, Goldberg JF, Grossman LS, Meltzer HY. Outcome in manic disorders: a naturalistic follow-up study. Arch Gen Psychiatry 1990; 47: 665–71

7. Maj M, Pirozzi R, Kemali D. Long-term outcome of lithium prophylaxis in patients initially classified as complete responders. Psychopharmacology 1989; 98: 535–8

8. Maj M, Pirozzi R, Magliano L, Bartoli L. Long-term outcome of lithium prophylaxis in bipolar disorder: a 5-year prospective study of 402 patients at a lithium clinic. Am J Psychiatry 1998; 155: 30–5

9. Maj M. Long-term impact of lithium prophylaxis on the course of bipolar disorder. In Christodoulou G, Lecic-Tosevski D, Kontaxakis VP, eds. Issues in Preventive Psychiatry. Basel: Karger, 1999: 79–82

10. Tondo L, Baldessarini RJ, Hennen J, Floris G. Lithium maintenance treatment of depression and mania in bipolar I and bipolar II disorder. Am J Psychiatry 1998; 155: 638–45

11. Baldessarini RJ, Tondo L. Does lithium treatment still work? Evidence of stable responses over three decades. Arch Gen Psychiatry 2000; 57: 187–90

12. Tondo L, Baldessarini RJ, Floris G. Long-term clinical effectiveness of lithium maintenance treatment in types I and II bipolar disorders. Br J Psychiatry 2001; 178 (Suppl 41): S184–S190

13. Schou M. Lithium prophylaxis: 'about naturalistic' or 'clinical practice' studies. Lithium 1993; 4: 77–81

14. Baldessarini RJ, Tondo L, Floris G, Hennen J. Effects of rapid cycling on response to lithium maintenance treatment in 360 bipolar I and II disorder patients. J Affect Disord 2000; 61: 13–22

15. Maj M, Pirozzi R, Bartoli L, Magliano L. Long-term outcome of lithium prophylaxis in bipolar disorder with mood-incongruent psychotic features: a prospective study. J Affect Disord 2002; 71: 195–8

16. Coryell W, Winokur G, Solomon D, et al. Lithium and recurrence in a long-term follow-up of bipolar affective disorder. Psychol Med 1997; 27: 281–9

17. Post RM, Leverich GS, Pazzaglia PJ, et al. Lithium tolerance and discontinuation as pathways to refractoriness. In Birch NJ, Padgham C, Hughes MS, eds. Lithium in Medicine and Biology. Carnforth: Marius Press, 1993: 71–84

18. Berghöfer A, Kossman B, Müller-Oerlinghausen B. Course of illness and pattern of recurrences in patients with affective disorders during long-term lithium prophylaxis: a retrospective analysis over 15 years. Acta Psychiatr Scand 1996; 93: 349–54

19. Goodwin G. Recurrence of mania after lithium withdrawal. Implications for the use of lithium in the treatment of bipolar affective disorder. Br J Psychiatry 1994; 164: 149–52

20. Baldessarini RJ, Tondo L, Viguera AC. Discontinuing lithium maintenance treatment in bipolar disorders: risks and implications. Bipolar Disord 1999; 1: 17–24

21. Davis JM, Janicak PG, Hogan DM. Mood stabilizers in the prevention of recurrent affective disorders: a meta-analysis. Acta Psychiatr Scand 1999; 100: 406–17

22. Schou M. Perspectives on lithium treatment of bipolar disorder: action, efficacy, effect on suicidal behavior. Bipolar Disord 1999; 1: 5–10

23. Grof P. Has the effectiveness of lithium changed? Impact of the variety of lithium's effects. Neuropsychopharmacology 1998; 19: 183–8

24. Koukopoulos A, Reginaldi D, Minnai G, et al. The long term prophylaxis of affective disorders. Adv Biochem Psychopharmacol 1995; 49: 127–47

25. Post RM, Leverich GS, Altshuler L, Mikalauskas K. Lithium-discontinuation-induced refractoriness: preliminary observations. Am J Psychiatry 1992; 149: 1727–9

26. Bauer M. Refractoriness induced by lithium discontinuation despite adequate serum lithium levels. Am J Psychiatry 1994; 151: 1522

27. Maj M, Pirozzi R, Magliano L. Non-response to reinstituted lithium prophylaxis in previously responsive bipolar patients: prevalence and predictors. Am J Psychiatry 1995; 152: 1810–11

28. Tondo L, Baldessarini RJ, Floris G, Rudas N. Effectiveness of restarting lithium treatment after its discontinuation in bipolar I and bipolar II disorders. Am J Psychiatry 1997; 154: 548–50

29. Suppes T, Baldessarini RJ, Motohashi N, et al. Special treatment issues: maintaining and discontinuing psychotropic medications. In Rush AJ, ed. Mood Disorders. Systematic Medication Management. Basel: Karger, 1997: 235–54

30. Coryell W, Solomon D, Leon AC, et al. Lithium discontinuation and subsequent effectiveness. Am J Psychiatry 1998; 155: 895–8

10 Lithium maintenance of unipolar depression

John M Davis

Contents   Introduction • Method • Results • Discussion

INTRODUCTION

I will examine the evidence that prophylactic lithium is effective in unipolar depression. Presented elsewhere in this volume is the discussion of the use of lithium for the treatment of acute depression. My view is that there are a small number of controlled studies showing that lithium may have some efficacy in acute depression and has clear efficacy as augmentation for acute depression. I review here the large body of information on maintenance lithium for prophylaxis in unipolar depression, based on both double-blind, random-assignment studies and case-controlled studies, generally carried out in the 1950s, 1960s and 1970s. Although antidepressants are now considered the standard treatment for preventing the recurrence of depression and are recommended by various guidelines, there may still be a role for lithium in selected cases. Depressed patients currently would have received antidepressants for their acute episode, so continued treatment with a drug that is effective for the acute episode would be the first choice for maintenance treatment. There are more data on the preventive properties of lithium for unipolar depression than there are for the prophylactic properties of many of the anticonvulsants used for bipolar illness. I have identified the controlled studies of maintenance lithium for unipolar depression and present in this chapter a new meta-analysis of the efficacy of lithium for unipolar depression. I compare the prophylactic efficacy of lithium in unipolar disease to that of lithium in bipolar disease, as an active comparator. The efficacy of lithium for this purpose has been questioned by many authors (for example in references 1 and 2, the possibility that withdrawal of lithium induces abrupt relapse). We move beyond rhetoric to examine what the data show about the efficacy of lithium from approximately 400 unipolar patients and 2000 bipolar patients, for comparison, in controlled clinical trials, with an emphasis on methodological rigor.

Many texts of evidence-based medicine present a hierarchy of methodological rigor, starting with the random-assignment, double-blind, placebo-controlled trial as the most precise evidence, followed by a various hierarchy of less rigorously controlled studies, such as randomized open studies, and various types of case-controlled studies, because blind evaluation and random assignment prevents bias known and also bias unknown to the investigator. Nothing can replace it for its methodological rigor. This noted, many important discoveries in clinical medicine and epidemiology that yield valid time-tested results were based on case-control studies (classes 2 and 3, above). There are a substantial number of case-controlled studies on the efficacy of lithium in unipolar depression. These methodologies are seldom used for most psychotropic drugs, and I feel that this type of control study has certain advantages for treatment evaluation. For this reason, I review them as well. Mirror-image studies are critically important because they do not involve the possible withdrawal-induced relapse that is central to Moncrieff's critiques[1,2]. Randomized open studies do have the protection of randomization to ensure that groups are reasonably comparable, but they are subject to many important systematic biases. Case-controlled studies have potential biases as well. Both randomized open and case-controlled designs have the following problems: (1) the suggestive effect in the patient of having received a medication, the well-known placebo effect; (2) patients may expect to get better if they received the medication; (3) the physicians may expect them to get better; (4) raters may try hard to find improvements since they know which patient is receiving medication; and (5) it is possible that a physician wishing a favorable outcome may place the most severe patients on medication or conversely be unwilling not to use medication in the severe cases. This said, some case-control designs do have marked advantages. The before-drug after-drug design holds the patient constant. There is substantial variation patient-to-patient and, since the patient is the same, this variation is substantially reduced. There is a large body of litera-

ture showing that only selected patients are entered in double-blind, placebo-controlled studies. This selected population is not necessarily representative of the wide variety of patients with a given disorder. Being much easier to do, case-controlled studies may much better reflect the wider variety of patients in the real world. I feel that the case-control methodology is often underutilized. Case-controlled studies do not control for time-dependent bias. Insofar as the case-control design has biases, the biases roughly should (in my view) be similar for both unipolar and bipolar forms of the disorder. If anything, they would more likely show a bias against unipolar depression, as lithium is used more widely for bipolar patients, and this use is and was better accepted, even in the early days. Since the prophylactic effect of lithium has been repeatedly demonstrated, and if lithium has an equal effect in unipolar depression in the same studies, the bipolar arm of the study serves as a positive control. It is impossible to classify studies rigidly as to quality, because opinion differs on this issue. In my opinion, even blinded randomized studies can be invalid. For example, some studies continue to collect data on patients assigned to a new drug or comparator even though the patients are switched to another drug or stop taking medication entirely. Discarding studies from a meta-analysis can create substantial bias as well. I followed our hierarchy (see Method) exactly, including all studies in each category, and feel that they are all valid studies, but with some complementary limitations, with strengths and weaknesses.

In recent years, pharmaceutical company-sponsored evaluation has become more commercialized. Many studies, particularly in unipolar depression, are based on symptomatic volunteers as opposed to patients seeking help from physicians. Furthermore, patients can be entered in one trial and as soon as that is finished entered in another trial. These are often chronic, treatment-resistant patients and they may not necessarily be in an episode, only sick enough to meet the entrance criteria. The patients are often evaluated by trained (or sometimes only partially trained) raters, and sometimes the endpoint is not an actual relapse but a surrogate endpoint, such as worsening on a rating scale. In contrast, the early studies were done in real patients who sought help in the hospital or clinic for an acute severe episode, or who had a severe, recurrent form of the disease and real relapses versus no relapse were determined. The early mirror-image studies were often evaluated as to whether the patient was rehospitalized or not. The earlier studies were often done by the authors of the paper themselves rather than having them outsourced to clinical trial organizations where they were rated by trained raters. If lithium were not efficacious or less efficacious in unipolar patients, then it should be less efficacious in unipolar than bipolar patients. Comparison of unipolars with bipolars as an active control group has certain analogies to including an active comparator in a study comparing a new drug to an old comparator, and to placebo.

METHOD

I searched the world literature (all languages) on the use of lithium to prevent future episodes of affective disorders, using Medline and other computer databases, and meticulously traced the references of each paper to other papers. Since much of this literature was published in the 1950s, 1960s and 1970s, hand searching was mandatory. I classified these studies into four design classes, because the studies differ in methodological rigor (ranked 1 as the most rigorous and 4 the least):

1.   Random-assignment, double-blind, placebo-control clinical trials

2.   Prospective case-control matched-subject studies;

3.   Case-control 'before and after' mirror-image studies;

4.   Placebo-controlled discontinuation studies.

When the results were available just in a graph or a diagrammatic life chart, I evaluated the graph and digitized these data. Most random-assignment, double-blind, matched-design and placebo-controlled discontinuation studies base their results primarily on the number of patients who relapsed or who did not relapse, i.e. dichotomous data. As a result, I used the Mantel-Haenszel[3] and the Peto methods[4]. These methods employ raw data from each individual patient. These methods underestimate the lithium efficacy. Psychotropic-treated subjects have fewer relapses, and will be at risk for relapse for a longer period of time. Case-controlled mirror-image studies compare the number and the length of episodes (or length of hospitalization) in a comparable time period prior to administration of lithium versus the lithium treatment period. Some mirror-image studies use two or more indices of improvement; therefore, insofar as was possible I made two compilations of data, one on frequency of relapse and the other on duration or severity of relapse. I used our recent modification[5] of the method of Hedges and Olkin[6] for use with paired data for our meta-analysis of the mirror-image studies (using n, mean and standard deviation (SD)). (If no pooled SD was available but individual SDs were, since the correlation between pre-lithium and lithium values was close to zero in all studies, I averaged individual group SDs. In one case, I used the SD reported in a preliminary publication of a partial sample, or calculated effect size using T, F, or p value.) Since almost all the case-controlled studies did not involve a design for patients who were suddenly discontinued from lithium but rather patients who had never received it previously, this methodology is not influenced by the possibility that abrupt lithium withdrawal can precipitate an episode of unipolar or bipolar affective illness. I initially carried out a systematic meta-analysis of antipsychotic and antidepressant lithium in the prevention of schizophrenia or recurrent bipolar and unipolar illness published in 1975–1976[7,8], the first meta-analysis done in psychiatry or behavioral science, before the term was coined, and re-examined lithium prophylaxis in 1999[9].

RESULTS

Efficacy of lithium

Nine double-blind, random-assignment, controlled trials of lithium prophylaxis in 229 unipolar depressed patients found that lithium was highly effective (Table 10.1). Seventy-five per cent of patients had a recurrence on placebo versus 36% on maintenance lithium, a 39% decrease in relapses, which is a highly significant difference ($\chi^2 = 37$; df = 1, $p = 10^{-9}$). This is roughly similar to bipolar disease: placebo relapse = 64%, lithium relapse = 32% (i.e. 32% decrease in relapses, $\chi^2 = 111$, df = 1, $p = 10^{-28}$)[10–24]. For all 1402 patients, 66% relapsed on placebo and 33% on lithium ($\chi^2 = 159$, df = 1, $p = 10^{-36}$, Peto odds ratio = 0.24). Excluding placebo-controlled discontinuation studies (class 4) and using just class 1, the results for all subtypes (unipolar, bipolar and atypical) were significant ($\chi^2 = 111$, df = 1, $p = 10^{-28}$). For bipolar disorder classes 1 and 2 studies only, the reduction of relapse was highly significant: $\chi^2 = 126$; df = 1, $p = 10^{-29}$. The magnitude of the reduction of relapse by lithium of unipolar patients was similar to that of bipolar patients. The results of just the class 1 studies are similar to those of all studies.

Mirror-image studies

A meta-analysis comparing the frequency of relapse before lithium and after lithium treatment (Table 10.2) found that lithium reduced the frequency of relapse by 69% (effect size = 0.72, 95% CI = 0.56–0.88, z = 8.7, $p < 10^{-17}$) in unipolar patients, by 50% (effect size = 0.68, 95% CI = 0.57–0.75, z = 17, $p < 10^{-41}$) in bipolar patients, and for all patients, including atypical bipolars, yielded an effect size = 0.67, 95% CI = 0.60–0.74, z = 18.2, $p < 10^{-91}$). The fact that as many did not relapse on lithium could be due to the existence of the proposed lithium-withdrawal syndrome, which is not applicable in these studies because the control group consisted of the same patients before any treatment with lithium.

I combined the data for all controlled studies, including a few that did not provide overall data to fit with the above analysis, and tested the significance of the reduction by lithium of affective episodes, with the result of $p < 10^{-1}$ for all affective patients. Data on continuous lithium prophylaxis on 79 patients nonrelapsed after 2 years[25] showed 35 still nonrelapsed at 7 years. Page et al.[26] found 41% completely remitted without episodes, and 41% partially remitted in a 13–17-year follow-up of 59 patients. Many patients (41%) had not relapsed at all.

Review of evidence on the lithium-withdrawal relapse

Suppes et al.[24] have suggested that sudden withdrawal of psychotropics may produce a widespread biological withdrawal phenomenon opposite in direction to that of the drug's beneficial effect, and that this may lead to relapse. This is an interesting idea. Since most maintenance trials switch patients from lithium to placebo, a lithium–placebo difference hypothetically might be inflated by a lithium-withdrawal-induced relapse. Clinically, I feel we should assume that the syndrome could exist. Lithium should be discontinued gradually. If a withdrawal syndrome existed, it might explain why many patients relapse while on lithium: that is, because inadvertent abrupt non-compliance for a few days due to forgetfulness, accidental, or other reasons consequently may result in relapse. I do not feel that relapse withdrawal has been proven, and even if it were, its effect would be too small to account for the prophylactic effect of lithium. I respectfully disagree with the hypothesis. Suppes and co-workers[24] very carefully compiled data from a wide variety of anecdotal information, chart review, and retrospective evaluations in support of the hypothesis to

Table 10.1 Prophylactic effiicacy of lithium in unipolar depression

Author	Year	Study type	n	Relapsed on lithium (%)	Relapsed on placebo (%)	Difference, reduction of relapse (%)
Kane et al.[39]	1982	u	13	29	100	71
Prien et al.[40]	1973	u	53	63	92	29
Glen et al.[41]	1984	u	20	45	89	44
Baastrup et al.[32]	1970	u	34	0	53	53
Coppen et al.[31]	1971	u	26	9	80	71
Fieve et al.[42]	1976	u	28	57	64	7
Persson[18]	1972	cr	42	29	67	38
Melia[43]	1970	u	3	0	100	100
Cundall et al.[13] and Christodoulou et al.[44]	1972 1982	d	10	40	40	0
Summary			229	36	75	39

$\chi^2 = 37$, df = 1, $p = 0.000000001$, odds ratio = 0.18
u, uncrossed (parallel group); cr, crossed; d, discontinuation studies

Table 10.2 Mirror image studies of lithium prophylaxis in unipolar depression

Study	Year	n	Baseline before lithium	Lithium	Decrease frequency relapse (%)	Baseline	Lithium	Decrease duration illness (%)
Persson[18]	1972	21	1.7	0.3	82	6.2	0.7	89
Holinger[14]	1979	9	4.11	1.69	59	4.11	1.69	59
Bouman[12]	1986	20	3.1	2	35	1.4	0.3	79
Lepkifker[45]	1985	33	0.86	0.15	83	0.87	0.06	93
Angst et al.[10]	1970	58	1.19	0.33	72	0.59	0.17	71
Melia[17]	1967	4	37.8	21.3	44	37.8	21.3	44
Baastrup[11]	1967	22	1.56	0.4	74	3.88	0.27	93
Cundall[13]	1972	5	3.8	1.36	64	3.8	1.36	64
Stancer[46]	1970	21	4.48	1.76	61	4.48	1.76	61
Kukopulos[15]	1973	2	1	0.25	75	4.5	1	78
Total		195			69			78

provide some evidence. Because I found this an interesting hypothesis, I analyzed the empirical data to see whether I could support it or refute it. My analysis refuted the hypothesis. I have critiqued this evidence in detail elsewhere[9] and will not repeat the discussion here, other than the above statements. Specifically, I question the assertion of a cause–effect relationship, that a relapse must surely be a withdrawal relapse, for the relapse could be caused by unchecked disease. Anecdotal and/or retrospective case reports from a practitioner's experience are no more precise than a practitioner's experience with patients in a clinical trial. Extensive statistical analysis might quantitate a real finding or an artifactual finding.

While I respectfully disagree with some of the evidence that supports this hypothesis, I would hasten to add that, because one can criticize the evidence or the hypothesis, it does not mean the hypothesis is false. Assorted defects in study design and problems with anecdotal information, plus a variety of arguments against the hypothesis, do not disprove the withdrawal hypothesis, and, by the same token, do not disprove that lithium has prophylactic activity. I feel that there is a major fallacy in the assumption that if something can be criticized the opposite is true, although there are some who act as if that were the case. In the first place, the criticisms may be wrong. Secondly, the hypothesis may be true even if the methodological criticisms are correct, or if the evidence for the hypothesis is much weaker than was initially assumed. The hypothesis could be true even if the methodology in support of the evidence is completely wrong. Reports of individual patients relapsing after abruptly discontinuing lithium certainly do exist. I would suggest that one of the reasons for this is that the patients may have been undergoing a relapse and, because of the denial of illness surfacing, may have stopped taking the lithium and relapsed, not because of the abrupt withdrawal of lithi-

um, but rather because they had already started to relapse. In addition, the natural course of this illness may worsen over time. Clinicians working with a drug-free research protocol are justifiably concerned that patients might suffer a destructive relapse and may be very vigilant for any symptoms suggesting a relapse. Even day-to-day fluctuations in mood may be falsely identified as a relapse. Faedda et al.[27] compared relapse in patients who abruptly discontinued lithium versus gradual discontinuation and found more relapses in the former group. Suppes et al.'s composite survival curves[24] are drawn in part from open clinical experience, such as that of Faedda and co-workers[27], and not exclusively from controlled trials, and thus the many uncontrolled variables make the interpretation problematical. There are plausible alternate explanations of all the data on the withdrawal hypothesis.

There is substantial evidence against the withdrawal hypothesis. Neither Baastrup and Schou[11] nor Goodnick et al.[28] reported worsening in the week following abrupt lithium discontinuation. I plotted the time course of data from Schou et al.[29], Grof et al.[30] and others (data not shown) as a rate, and could not find any increase in the rate of relapse in the first month or so in comparison with later months (3, 4, 5, 6, etc.). Inspection of the pooled data of Suppes et al.[24] fails to show more relapses during this time in comparison with several weeks later (e.g. weeks 3 to 4). Schou et al.[29] plotted the data as a semi-log plot and also failed to find evidence of an increase in relapse rate immediately after discontinuation. They (Baastrup and Schou)[11] were the first to examine the question in 25 cases in which lithium administration was stopped because the patients had been relapse free for a long time. The average time to relapse was 3.2 months, a time identical to the time to relapse before initial lithium treatment. Schou et al.[29] reviewed the evidence for withdrawal relapses and concluded that there was some limited evidence in favor of withdrawal relapses but some important evidence against. I agree. Particularly important are the Persson[18] results, and the mirror-image study is free of such an artifact because he studied patients on lithium compared with a group of matched patients who were never on lithium. I would give the Scottish verdict of 'not proven', but keep an open mind that it might be a real phenomenon.

DISCUSSION

There is a large body of data in support of the prophylactic properties of lithium against recurrent unipolar depression. A further strength is that these studies were conducted with somewhat different designs, in different countries, with different clinical settings, but all class 1 studies were random-assignment, double-blind studies that differ in other design features. Some studies followed patients to first relapse (e.g. patients drop out when they have relapsed), others (Coppen et al.[31]) used a set time period and allowed other concurrent treatments, a design closer to clinical practice, and some (Baastrup et al.[32]) used stabilized patients, whereas others (e.g. Prien et al.[19]), studied patients immediately following an acute episode. Since a great variety of controlled trials are available for lithium, and since many of these methodologies have been seldom used or not used at all for many of the other psychotropic drugs, the methodological advantages and disadvantages are discussed in considerable detail below. These early studies were performed at a time when there were substantially fewer alternative treatments than there are today, so there is a much greater likelihood that patients with severe, uncomplicated disease would be included in the trial, and not symptomatic volunteers. The case–control studies have much strength: (1) each patient is his own control (each is very well matched), and (2) they

often reflect real-world settings. Insofar as objective indices of outcome are used, bias is avoided. A variety of time-dependent changes could confound the results. Lithium withdrawal effects are avoided since patients were not on lithium 'before'. This design complements the random-assignment studies, in which lithium withdrawal effects could be a factor.

One persistent problem in meta-analysis is 'the file drawer problem', i.e. studies that are not published but filed away, or put in the file drawer. There is systematic evidence that negative studies may tend not to be published and that the pharmaceutical industry does not publish some of its trials when the results of the sponsored drug are completely negative or lackluster. Another variant of the file drawer problem is that the meta-analysis excludes studies that do not fit with the author's preconception of what the results should be. Exclusion for all these reasons does produce systematic bias. Even though it is reasonable to restrict meta-analysis to randomized controlled trials with double-blind evaluation, I feel that other controlled studies yield important data as well. I carried out an exhaustive search for trials and have included every trial I could find. I examined methodological rigor as a variable and analyzed the less rigorous trials separately. The results of all trials are consistent.

Consistency of results

I evaluated whether the effect size of the superiority of lithium was constant in the 26-strata Mantel–Haenszel controlled clinical trials meta-analysis and found it to be roughly consistent and constant. Overall, 70% of patients relapsed on placebo, and 28% on lithium. The effect was homogeneous in that the test of variability between studies was not significant. Lithium reduced relapse by a factor of 2.5. Studies using substantially different methods found lithium superior to placebo to a roughly similar degree. The mirror-image studies also showed a similar degree of efficacy for lithium. Here, it reduced relapse by a factor of three. Taking into account that patients in mirror-image studies can have more than one relapse, I would expect the magnitude of the efficacy of lithium to be larger than that seen in randomized studies.

Most medical practice is based on clinical opinion. Rarely do we have such good data as exist for lithium. Moncrieff[1] argues that lithium's prophylactic properties are a myth. If so, this myth is (1) shared by different investigators, (2) in different countries, (3) using different methods, (4) a myth that obeys the dose–response curve[9,33–38], and (5) a myth where less efficacious studies and the better-controlled studies had the same efficacy.

At the time these studies were done, the concept of bipolar II and the variants of bipolar disease were not well understood. (This is much better understood now and is reviewed in this book.) It is quite possible that some patients labeled 'unipolar' in the 1950s and 1960s may have had some variant of bipolar II disorder. The entrance criteria of many of the early studies required the occurrence of two or three episodes in the past 2 years. This said, the distinction between unipolar and bipolar was well understood at this time. At the present time, since patients with unipolar depression will most likely have been treated with antidepressants, the natural choice for preventive treatment would be to continue the antidepressants on which they were doing well. Unfortunately, there are many treatment-resistant patients, with recurrent episodes. Many alternative therapies exist, e.g. maintenance electroconvulsive therapy and various drug combinations, strategies often with very little evidence supporting them. Candidates for maintenance included patients who were on the borderline between unipolar depression and the bipolar II variant of the disorder, and patients

who responded only to antidepressants augmented with lithium. Indeed, an important role of meta-analysis and evidence-based medicine is to identify where there is evidence (or no evidence). The latter empowers clinicians to trust their intuition and patients to follow their experience and preferences. It is relevant to know that prophylactic lithium produces statistically significant and clinically important benefits. The data for this are unusual and have many of the advantages in depth, breadth and generalizability. Most clinical decisions are made based on clinical wisdom, not on controlled clinical trials. For this particular indication of prophylactic lithium as a second-line treatment for recurrent unipolar depression, we do have a substantial body of evidence that lithium is efficacious. It should be considered for selected patients. The stakes are high for our patients and their families, and hence the clinician needs to give these data careful consideration.

REFERENCES

1. Moncrieff J. Lithium revisited. A re-examination of the placebo-controlled trials of lithium prophylaxis in manic-depressive disorder [see comment]. Br J Psychiatry 1995; 167: 569–73; discussion 573–64
2. Moncrieff J. Forty years of lithium treatment.[see comment]. Arch Gen Psychiatry 1998; 55: 92–3
3. Mantel N, Haenszel W. Statistical aspects of the analysis of data from retrospective studies of disease. J Natl Cancer Inst 1959; 22: 719–48
4. Peto R, Pike MC, Armitage P, et al. Design and analysis of randomized clinical trials requiring prolonged observation of each patient. II. Analysis and examples. Br J Cancer 1977; 35: 1–39
5. Gibbons RD. Estimation of effect size from a series of experiments involving paired comparisons. J Ed Stat 1993; 18: 271–9

6. Hedges LV, Olkin I. Statistical Methods for Meta-Analysis. Orlando, FL: Academic Press, 1985

7. Davis JM. Overview: maintenance therapy in psychiatry: I. Schizophrenia. Am J Psychiatry 1975; 132: 1237–45

8. Davis JM. Overview: maintenance therapy in psychiatry: II. Affective disorders. Am J Psychiatry 1976; 133: 1–13

9. Davis JM, Janicak PG, Hogan DM. Mood stabilizers in the prevention of recurrent affective disorders: a meta-analysis. Acta Psychiatr Scand 1999; 100: 406–17

10. Angst J, Weis P, Grof P, et al. Lithium prophylaxis in recurrent affective disorders. Br J Psychiatry 1970; 116: 604–14

11. Baastrup PC, Schou M. Lithium as a prophylactic agents. Its effect against recurrent depressions and manic-depressive psychosis. Arch Gen Psychiatry 1967; 16: 162–72

12. Bouman TK, Niemantsverdriet-van Kampen JG, Ormel J, Slooff CJ. The effectiveness of lithium prophylaxis in bipolar and unipolar depressions and schizo-affective disorders. J Affect Disord 1986; 11: 275–80

13. Cundall RL, Brooks PW, Murray LG. A controlled evaluation of lithium prophylaxis in affective disorders. Psychol Med 1972; 2: 308–11

14. Holinger PC, Wolpert EA. A ten year follow-up of lithium use. Illinois Med J 1979; 156: 99–104

15. Kukopulos A, Reginaldi D. Does lithium prevent depressions by suppressing manias? Int Pharmacopsychiatry 1973; 8: 152–8

16. Maj M, Pirozzi R, Starace F. Previous pattern of course of the illness as a predictor of response to lithium prophylaxis in bipolar patients. J Affect Disord 1989; 17: 237–41

17. Melia PI. A pilot trial of lithium carbonate in recurrent affective disorders. J Ir Med Assoc 1967; 60: 160–70

18. Persson G. Lithium prophylaxis in affective disorders: an open trial with matched controls. Acta Psychiatr Scand 1972; 48: 462–79

19. Prien RF, Caffey EM Jr, Klett CJ. Prophylactic efficacy of lithium carbonate in manic-depressive illness. Report of the Veterans Administration and National Institute of Mental Health collaborative study group. Arch Gen Psychiatry 1973; 28: 337–41

20. Bowden CL, Calabrese JR, McElroy SL, et al. A randomized, placebo-controlled 12-month trial of divalproex and lithium in treatment of outpatients with bipolar I disorder. Divalproex Maintenance Study Group [see comment]. Arch Gen Psychiatry 2000; 57: 481–9

21. Bowden CL, Calabrese JR, Sachs G, et al, Lamictal 606 Study G. A placebo-controlled 18-month trial of lamotrigine and lithium maintenance treatment in recently manic or hypomanic patients with bipolar I disorder. [erratum appears in Arch Gen Psychiatry 2004; 61: 680]. Arch Gen Psychiatry 2003; 60: 392–400

22. Calabrese JR, Bowden CL, Sachs G, et al, Lamictal 605 Study G. A placebo-controlled 18-month trial of lamotrigine and lithium maintenance treatment in recently depressed patients with bipolar I disorder. [see comment]. J Clin Psychiatry 2003; 64: 1013–24

23. Goodwin GM, Bowden CL, Calabrese JR, Grunze H, Kasper S, White R, Greene P, Leadbetter R. A pooled analysis of 2 placebo-controlled 18-month trials of lamotrigine and lithium maintenance in bipolar I disorder. J Clin Psychiatry 2004; 65: 432–41

24. Suppes T, Baldessarini RJ, Faedda GL, Tohen M. Risk of recurrence following discontinuation of lithium treatment in bipolar disorder. Arch Gen Psychiatry 1991; 48: 1082–8

25. Maj M, Pirozzi R, Kemali D. Long-term outcome of lithium prophylaxis in patients initially classified as complete responders. Psychopharmacology 1989; 98: 535–8

26. Page C, Benaim S, Lappin F. A long-term retrospective follow-up study of patients treated with prophylactic lithium carbonate. Br J Psychiatry 1987; 150: 175–9

27. Faedda GL, Tondo L, Baldessarini RJ, et al. Outcome after rapid vs gradual discontinuation of lithium treatment in bipolar disorders. Arch Gen Psychiatry 1993; 50: 448–55

28. Goodnick PJ. Clinical and laboratory effects of discontinuation of lithium prophylaxis. Acta Psychiatr Scand 1985; 71: 608–14

29. Schou M, Thomsen K, Baastrup PC. Studies on the course of recurrent endogenous affective

disorders. In Pharmacopsychiatry 1970; 5: 100–6

30. Grof P, Cakuls P, Dostal T. Lithium drop outs, a follow-up study of patients who discontinued prophylatic lithium in recurrent affective disorders. Int Pharmacopsychiatry 1970; 5: 162–9

31. Coppen A, Noguera R, Bailey J, et al. Prophylactic lithium in affective disorders. Controlled trial. Lancet 1971; 2: 275–9

32. Baastrup PC, Poulsen JC, Schou M, et al. Prophylactic lithium: double blind discontinuation in manic-depressive and recurrent-depressive disorders. Lancet 1970; 2: 326–30

33. Gelenberg AJ, Kane JM, Keller MB, et al. Comparison of standard and low serum levels of lithium for maintenance treatment of bipolar disorder. N Engl J Med 1989; 321: 1489–93

34. Hullin RP, McDonald R, Allsopp MN. Prophylactic lithium in recurrent affective disorders. Lancet 1972; 1: 1044–6

35. Hullin RP, McDonald R, Allsopp MN. Further report on prophylatic lithium in recurrent affective disorders. Br J Psychiatry 1975; 126: 281–4

36. Jerram TC, McDonald R. Plasma lithium control with particular reference to minimum effective levels. In: Johnson FN, Johnson S, eds. Lithium in Medical Practice. Baltimore, MD: University Park Press, 1978

37. Maj M, Starace F, Nolfe G, Kemali D. Minimum plasma lithium levels required for effective prophylaxis in DSM III bipolar disorder: a prospective study. Pharmacopsychiatry 1986; 19: 420–3

38. Waters B, Lapierre Y, Gagnon A, et al. Determination of the optimal concentration of lithium for the prophylaxis of manic-depressive disorder. Biol Psychiatry 1982; 17: 1323–9

39. Kane JM, Quitkin FM, Rifkin A, et al. Lithium carbonate and imipramine in the prophylaxis of unipolar and bipolar II illness: a prospective, placebo-controlled comparison. Arch Gen Psychiatry 1982; 39: 1065–9

40. Prien RF, Klett CJ, Caffey EM Jr. Lithium carbonate and imipramine in prevention of affective episodes. A comparison in recurrent affective illness. Arch Gen Psychiatry 1973; 29: 420–5

41. Glen AI, Johnson AL, Shepherd M. Continuation therapy with lithium and amitriptyline in unipolar depressive illness: a randomized, double-blind, controlled trial. Psychol Med 1984; 14: 37-50

42. Fieve RR, Kumbaraci T, Dunner DL. Lithium prophylaxis of depression in bipolar I, bipolar II, and unipolar patients. Am J Psychiatry 1976; 133: 925–9

43. Melia PI. Prophylactic lithium: a double-blind trial in recurrent affective disorders. Br J Psychiatry 1970; 116: 621–4

44. Christodoulou GN, Lykouras EP. Abrupt lithium discontinuation in manic depressive patients. Acta Psychiatr Scand 1982; 65: 310–14

45. Lepkifker E, Horesh N, Floru S. Long-term lithium prophylaxis in recurrent unipolar depression. A controversial indication? Acta Psychiatr Belg 1985; 85: 434–43

46. Stancer HC, Furlong FW, Godse DD. A longitudinal investigation of lithium as a prophylactic agent for recurrent depressions. Can Psychiatr Assoc J 1970; 15: 29–40

11 The acute antidepressive effects of lithium: from monotherapy to augmentation therapy in major depression

Michael Bauer, Nicolas Andres Crossley, Sonja Gerber, Tom Bschor

Contents   Introduction • Acute depression: monotherapy studies with lithium • Acceleration therapy • Augmentation therapy • Mechanisms of lithium augmentation: neurobiological basis • Practical aspects of the use of lithium in major depressive episodes

INTRODUCTION

Lithium has been considered mainly as a prophylactic treatment for mood disorders and in the acute treatment of mania, but it is also of potential value for acute depressive episodes. In this chapter, its uses as a monotherapy and as an acceleration and augmentation therapy will be reviewed, as well as the neurobiological mechanisms thought to underlie its action.

ACUTE DEPRESSION: MONOTHERAPY STUDIES WITH LITHIUM

Although the majority of open and controlled studies have delivered clear evidence for lithium's antidepressive effect, clinicians still hesitate to use it as an antidepressive drug. It is known as a medication of first choice in the prophylactic treatment of mood disorders and in the management of acute mania[1–3]. For unipolar depressive patients, studies have confirmed a comparable prophylactic effect and have established lithium as a first-line prophylactic agent for these patients (see Chapter 10). Despite these findings, however, practitioners are reticent to use lithium to treat acute and prophylactic depressive disorders. This might be due to its relatively narrow therapeutic range of application and the necessity with lithium treatment to monitor lithium serum levels regularly.

The antidepressive effect of lithium was first tested with disappointing results in 1949 in a small group of depressive patients[4]. Since then several clinical trials have tested lithium as a monotherapy in depressive disorders.

Clinical trials

As early as in the 1960s and 1970s the antidepressant effect of lithium was verified by numerous studies. In 1976 Mendels[5] reviewed nine uncontrolled studies[4,6–13], six of which showed antidepressant effects. Of the three negative reports reviewed[4,6,7], two were early trials with small numbers of patients (reviewed in 14).

In 1968 Fieve *et al.* reported that imipramine showed more antidepressant effect than did lithium[15], and Stokes *et al.* found no significant difference between lithium and placebo[16].

However, even though some of these studies used control groups of some sort, they did not meet today's criteria for controlled clinical trials[17]. The duration of lithium administration was very short (10 days in the Stokes study) and blood levels were presumably too low to show any antidepressant effect[5] (Table 11.1).

Randomized double-blind trials

In 1991, Souza and Goodwin[18] published a first meta-analysis confirming the efficacy of lithium in the treatment of acute unipolar depression. It encompassed six of the studies shown in Table 11.2 (all studies except that of Linder et al.[19]) with a wide range of serum lithium levels (0.4–1.5 mmol/l).

As shown in Table 11.2, lithium was at least as effective as conventional tricyclic

Table 11.1 Uncontrolled studies of lithium as an antidepressant

Study	Number of patients	Patients' characteristics	Lithium outcome
Cade 1949[4]	3	Chronic depressive psychosis	No effect
Noack and Trautner 1951[6]	n.a.	—	No effect
Vojtěchovský 1957[8]	14	Depression, ECT failure	8 improved
Andreani et al. 1958[9]	24	Severe depression	10 improved
Dyson and Mendels 1968[10]	31	Heterogeneous group of depressed patients	19 improved, especially those with bipolar and cyclothymic disorder
Van der Velde 1970[7]	n.a.	Mixed affective disorder (BP and UP), relapsing BP	No effect after 14 days of treatment
Náhunek et al. 1970[11]	98	UP	55 improved
Goodwin et al. 1972[24]	24	UP, inpatients	8 improved, 4 did not
Noyes et al. 1971[12]	5	BP (n = 3), UP (n = 2)	4 improved: 2 relapsed with placebo
Noyes et al. 1974[25]	23	UP	9 improved, 7 did not
Baron et al. 1975[26]	36	UP (n = 20), BP (n = 16)	UP: 7 improved, 3 did not, BP: 1 improved, 7 did not
Bennie 1975[13]	14	Depression, no response to ECT and/or tricyclics	14 improved
Mendels 1976[5]	34	UP (n = 12), BP (n = 22)	UP: 4 improved with lithium, 4 did not, BP: 4 improved, 9 did not

n.a., information not available; BP, bipolar disorder, UP, unipolar disorder; ECT, electroconvulsive therapy

Table 11.2 Randomized double-blind trials of lithium as monotherapy in the treatment of acute depression

Study	Comparator treatment	Number of patients	Duration (weeks)	Outcome
Mendels et al. 1972[107]	Desipramine	24	3	Lithium = desipramine
Watanabe et al. 1975[23]	Imipramine	45	3	Lithium = imipramine
Worrall et al. 1979[20]	Imipramine	29	3	Lithium > imipramine
Khan 1981[22]	Amitriptyline	25	3	Lithium = amitriptyline
Arieli and Lepkifker 1981[21]	Clomipramine, placebo	33	3	Lithium = clomipramine > placebo
Khan et al. 1987[108]	Placebo	31	6	Lithium > placebo
Linder et al. 1989[19]	Clomipramine	22	4	Lithium = clomipramine

=, comparable efficacy; >, higher efficacy

antidepressants and proved superior to the placebo. Worral and colleagues[20] even found lithium to be more effective than imipramine. In 1981, Arieli and Lepkifker[21] found a comparable effectiveness of lithium and clomipramine. In the latter trial, serum levels and lithium dosage were extremely high (0.8–2.95 mmol/l and 1500–2500 mg/day) and induced severe side-effects in all patients. Lithium was found particularly effective for depression and anxiety, while clomipramine exhibited earlier onset than lithium. Khan[22] and Linder et al.[19], showed that lithium's antidepressant effect was comparable to that of tricyclic antidepressants. In the study by Linder et al.[19] time until symptom reduction did not differ between both groups, but the rate of side-effects was lower in the lithium than in the clomipramine group. Watanabe et al.[23] tested lithium and desipramine and reported a comparable overall efficacy for both drugs.

Predictors of outcome

Psychopathological and biological characteristics as well as patient history were examined to identify predictors for a favorable outcome in the treatment of acute depression with lithium. Most studies found it particularly effective in patients with bipolar disorder[17,21,24–26].

Predictors of good outcome in unipolar depressed patients were a family history of bipolar disorder, mood fluctuation and light hypomania, cyclothymic personality, an 'endogenous' type of depression, early onset of illness and postnatal depression[17,27]. One possible conclusion might be to classify these patients as 'pseudo-unipolar', i.e. having genotypical factors for bipolar disorder with a unipolar phenotype[16].

Regarding biological factors, Mendels and Frazer[28] found a higher red blood cell (RBC) lithium : plasma lithium concentration ratio in depressed responders during lithium treatment. They also reported a higher RBC lithium : plasma lithium ratio when the sodium baseline was higher. Carman and colleagues[29] discovered a positive correlation of high baseline calcium : magnesium ratio in plasma and an antidepressant effect of lithium as well as an initial increase in plasma calcium and magnesium concentration. Furthermore, a reduced accumulation of 5-hydroxyindoleacetic acid in the lumbar spinal fluid was observed[30]. Other research studies focused on neurophysiological parameters as well as on the activity of enzymes involved in the metabolism of neurotransmitters (e.g. catecholamine-O-methyltransferase (COMT)) and metabolites of depression-relevant neurotransmitters, e.g. (methoxyhydroxyphenylglycole (MHPG) and 5-hydroxy-indoleacetic acid[17,31,32], but results were inconsistent or negative. In summary, none of these biological parameters could serve as a reliable predictor for the outcome of lithium treatment in acute depression.

ACCELERATION THERAPY

The delayed onset of response to antidepressants remains a major clinical dilemma. To date, no antidepressant has yielded any apparent benefit before the second or third week of treatment. Reducing this latency time would markedly reduce the morbidity and impairment associated with depression. Following an open report of the 2-week response of three subjects being treated simultaneously from the beginning with a combination of lithium and a tricyclic antidepressant[33], several studies have tried to find an acceleration effect of lithium. However, as noted by Altshuler et al.[34], a study of an acceleration drug with sufficient power to detect meaningful clinical differences would require far more subjects than are typically included in studies.

The authors systematically reviewed the evidence for an acceleration effect of lithium in randomized placebo-controlled trials. Studies comparing lithium in combination with other antidepressants versus antidepressant plus placebo in previously untreated bipolar or unipolar patients were retrieved by a Medline computer database search (from 1966 to June 2005). The characteristics of six studies reviewed are shown in Table 11.3.

Table 11.3 Randomized placebo-controlled lithium acceleration studies

Study	Subjects	Intervention	Depression scale and/or response criteria	Quality	Results
Lingjaerde et al. 1974[35]	37 UP, 8 BP 35 F, 10 M only inpatients Mean age 48 years (lithium group) and 50 (placebo group)	Any tricyclic antidepressant (225 mg/day) plus lithium carbonate (BM 0.8–1.3 mEq/l)	HAM-D Clinical global assessment (+ to +++)	Randomized No analysis by ITT Double blind Placebo group > duration of current episode; lithium group > number of previous episodes LFUP 40%	No difference between the two groups in the first 3 weeks
Nick et al. 1976[40]	20 UP, 10 BP 22 F, 8 M only inpatients Mean age 53 years	Clomipramine i.v. for 15 days on average (range 50–125 mg) plus lithium carbonate (range of serum concentration 0.35–1.1 mEq/l)	BPRS	Randomized No analysis by ITT Double blind Prognostic factors of groups not given LFUP not reported	No difference in BPRS scores at day 15

continued over

Table 11.3 *continued*   Randomized placebo-controlled lithium acceleration studies

Study	Subjects	Intervention	Depression scale and/or response criteria	Quality	Results
Januel *et al.* 1994[36]	6 UP 3 F, 3 M Hospitalization status not represented Age range 21–51 years	Clomipramine, maprotiline or tianeptine (minimum 150 mg clomipramine-equivalent) plus lithium carbonate (700 mg/day)	MADRS	Randomized No analysis by ITT Double blind Prognostic factors of groups not given LFUP 17%	Mean MADRS score at day 10 dropped significantly more ($p < 0.05$) in patients treated with lithium
Ebert *et al.* 1995[37]	40 BP 0 F, 40 M only inpatients Age range 30–45 years	Amitriptyline (225 mg/day) plus lithium carbonate (900 mg/day)	HAM-D CGI improved or much improved	Semi-randomized (half of the sample paired) No analysis by ITT Double blind Groups comparable LFUP not reported	No difference in the reduction of depressive symptoms at weeks 1 or 2
Bloch *et al.* 1997[38]	29 UP, 2 BP 17 F, 14 M only outpatients Mean age 46 (lithium group) and 49 years (placebo group)	Desipramine (150 mg at day 7) plus lithium carbonate (BM 0.7–1 mmol/l)	HAM-D 50% reduction with final score less than 16	Randomized (separate for bipolar group) Analysis by ITT Double blind Groups comparable LFUP 13%	No difference in time to respond between groups
Januel *et al.* 2003[39]	149 UP 92 F, 57 M only inpatients Mean age 44 years	Clomipramine (150 mg at day 4) plus lithium carbonate (750 mg/day)	MADRS 50% reduction	Randomized Analysis by ITT Double blind LFUP 30%	Mean percentage reduction of MADRS score was lower for lithium after 11 days ($p = 0.07$)

UP, unipolar; BP, bipolar; F, female; M, male; BM, blood monitored; ITT, intention to treat; LFUP, lost to follow-up; HAM-D, Hamilton Depression Rating Scale[24]; BPRS, Brief Psychiatric Rating Scale; CGI, Clinical Global Impression; MADRS, Montgomery Asberg Depression Rating Scale

As can be seen in Table 11.3, the original articles reviewed are of varying quality. Some report a non-significant difference between the two groups but a perceptible trend supporting an effect of lithium. For an initial pooling, data from five studies[35–39] were available at the time of writing. The study by Nick *et al.*[40] was not included because it reported only significance levels. The depressive scores of 231 patients at 7–14 days of treatment were pooled and in congruence with the original articles; a positive trend was found in favor of lithium ($p < 0.10$) (Crossley and Bauer, unpublished data).

AUGMENTATION THERAPY

Although there are many drugs available for the treatment of major depression, the overall treatment outcome of depressed patients is usually far from optimal. Regardless of the initial choice of antidepressant, about 30–50% of patients with a major depressive episode will not respond sufficiently to adequately performed first-line treatment and will not return to pre-morbid levels of functioning[41]. Various treatment strategies have been proposed for patients only partially or not at all responding to a monotherapy trial with an antidepressant. Some authors have argued for choosing augmentation strategies because they eliminate the period of transition between one antidepressant to another and build on the partial response without losing the benefit gained by the initial treatment.

Lithium salts have been used to augment the efficacy of antidepressant medications for more than 20 years. The first study to test this hypothesis in patients with major depression was performed by de Montigny and associates in 1981[42]. They reported a dramatic response within 48 hours to the addition of lithium in eight patients who had not responded to at least 3 weeks of treatment with tricyclic antidepressants. The efficacy of the combination and rapidity of response have led many clinical research groups to pursue study of this treatment intervention.

Subsequent randomized controlled trials have confirmed de Montigny's initial findings from 1981. The recent unpublished update of a previous meta-analysis[43] addressing the question pooled ten randomized, double-blind, placebo-controlled trials[44–53] and included 269 patients. Lithium dosage, duration of treatment and other characteristics of the studies are detailed in Table 11.4. Figure 11.1 shows the odds ratio for subjects responding to the treatment in each study and by publication year and data pooling.

As can be seen in Figure 11.1, lithium has a significant positive effect versus placebo with an odds ratio of 3.11, which corresponds to a number-needed-to-treat (NNT) of 5.

Five of the studies pooled did not show a significant difference. Reasons for these negative findings may be: low power[44–46], use of insufficient lithium doses[47], short duration of treatment[44,46], and concerns about the efficacy of lithium augmentation with noradrenergic antidepressants[48,54]. Previous studies had demonstrated that only doses of lithium carbonate higher than 600 mg/day and a duration of 7 days were useful in augmenting therapies[43].

Since the original publication of this meta-analysis[43], only one article has been published. Most investigators have probably been convinced by the current weight of evidence for lithium's effect. As noted in the original meta-analysis published in 1999[43], a new negative study would have to include more than 2500 patients per group to change the results of this pooling. However, it remains to be examined whether the response to lithium augmentation represents true augmentation resulting from synergistic effects or whether the response is simply due to the antidepressant effect of lithium itself. Experimental studies supporting the former alternative are reviewed below.

From the clinical point of view, arguments for a true augmentation effect derive from a controlled clinical trial showing that the antidepressant effects of lithium addition were significantly higher in depressed patients pretreated with amitriptyline than in those pretreated with placebo, who showed no improvement after a 3-week treatment[55]. Still, a randomized, double-blind study is warranted

Table 11.4 Characteristics of double-blind, placebo-controlled augmentation studies included in a meta-analysis

Study	Subject	Antidepressant	Lithium dosage (serum level) and duration	Response criteria and response rates
Heninger et al. 1983[49]	14 UP, 1 BP 12 F, 3 M Mean age 50 years	Various TCA and tetracyclics	Lithium carbonate 900–1200 mg/day (0.5–1.1 mEq/l); 12 days	Decrease of 2 or more points on SCRS; Lithium: 62.5% Placebo: 0%
Kantor et al. 1986[44]	7 UP Sex nr Mean age nr	Various TCA	Lithium carbonate 900 mg/day; 48 hours	≥40% decrease in HAM-D score; Lithium: 25% Placebo: 0%
Zusky et al. 1988[45]	16 UP 13 F, 3 M Mean age 45 years	Various TCA and MAOI	Lithium carbonate 300 mg/day first week, 900 mg/day second week; 14 days	Final HAM-D ≤7; Lithium: 38% Placebo: 25%
Schöpf et al. 1989[50]	18 UP, 9 BP 19 F, 8 M Mean age 54 years	Various antidepressants	Lithium carbonate 600–800 mg/day (0.6–0.8 mEq/l); 14 days	≥50% decrease in HAM-D; Lithium: 50% Placebo: 0%
Browne et al. 1990[46]	14 UP, 3 BP 10 F, 7 M Mean age 42 years	Various TCA and tetracyclics	Lithium carbonate 900 mg/day; 48 hours	≥50% decrease in HAM-D; Lithium: 43% Placebo: 20%
Stein and Bernadt 1993[47]	34 UP 27 F, 7 M Mean age 47 years	Various TCA	Lithium carbonate 250 mg/day or 750 mg/day; 21 days	≥50% decrease in HAM-D; Lithium (250 mg): 18% Lithium (750 mg): 44% Placebo: 22%
Joffe et al. 1993[51]	33 UP 18 F, 15 M Mean age 37 years	Various TCA	Lithium carbonate 900 mg/day (>0.55 mEq/l); 14 days	≥50% decrease in HAM-D; Lithium: 52% Placebo: 18.7%

continued over

Table 11.4 *continued* Characteristics of double-blind, placebo-controlled augmentation studies included in a meta-analysis

Study	Subject	Antidepressant	Lithium dosage (serum level) and duration	Response criteria and response rates
Katona et al. 1995[52]	61, polarity nr 35 F, 26 M Mean age 40 years	SSRI and TCA	Lithium carbonate 800 mg/day; (0.6–1 mmol/l) 42 days	≥50% decrease in HAM-D; Lithium: 53% Placebo: 25%
Baumann et al. 1996[53]	23 UP, 1 BP 17 F, 7 M Mean age 41 years	Citalopram	Lithium carbonate 800 mg/day; (0.5–0.8 mmol/l) 14 days	≥50% decrease in HAM-D; Lithium: 58% Placebo: 14%
Nierenberg et al. 2003[48]	35 UP 16 F, 19 M Mean age 38 years	Nortriptyline	Lithium carbonate 900 mg/day; 42 days	≥50% decrease in HAM-D; Lithium: 12.5% Placebo: 20%

UP, unipolar; BP, bipolar; F, female; M, male; nr, not reported; MAOI, monoamine oxidase inhibitor; TCA, tricyclic antidepressant; SSRI, selective serotonin reuptake inhibitor; HAM-D, Hamilton Depression Rating Scale; SCRS, Short Clinical Rating Scale

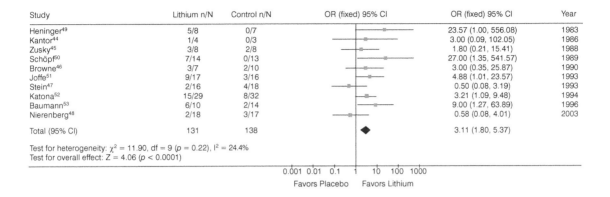

Study	Lithium n/N	Control n/N	OR (fixed) 95% CI	OR (fixed) 95% CI	Year
Heninger[49]	5/8	0/7		23.57 (1.00, 556.08)	1983
Kantor[44]	1/4	0/3		3.00 (0.09, 102.05)	1986
Zusky[45]	3/8	2/8		1.80 (0.21, 15.41)	1988
Schöpf[50]	7/14	0/13		27.00 (1.35, 541.57)	1989
Browne[46]	3/7	2/10		3.00 (0.35, 25.87)	1990
Joffe[51]	9/17	3/16		4.88 (1.01, 23.57)	1993
Stein[47]	2/16	4/18		0.50 (0.08, 3.19)	1993
Katona[52]	15/29	8/32		3.21 (1.09, 9.48)	1994
Baumann[53]	6/10	2/14		9.00 (1.27, 63.89)	1996
Nierenberg[48]	2/18	3/17		0.58 (0.08, 4.01)	2003
Total (95% CI)	131	138		3.11 (1.80, 5.37)	

Test for heterogeneity: $\chi^2 = 11.90$, df = 9 ($p = 0.22$), $I^2 = 24.4\%$
Test for overall effect: $Z = 4.06$ ($p < 0.0001$)

0.001 0.01   0.1   1   10   100 1000
Favors Placebo   Favors Lithium

Figure 11.1 Forest plot of meta-analysis of lithium augmentation vs. placebo in major depression. Number of patients responding (*n*) of total patients treated (*N*) in each group. Odds ratios are pooled using the Mantel–Haenszel test

which describes the effects of lithium alone and compares them with the effects of lithium in combination with an antidepressant.

Lithium augmentation versus other strategies for treatment-refractory depression

Several randomized controlled studies comparing lithium augmentation to other strategies have been published, the other strategies being: electroconvulsive therapy[56], a monoamine oxidase-inhibitor (MAOI)[57], thyroid hormone[58], carbamazepine supplementation[59] and high-dose selective serotonin reuptake inhibitor (SSRI) or tricyclic augmentation in SSRI users[60]. The last study has recently been repeated by the same group with a larger sample[61]. Details of these six studies are shown in Table 11.5.

These studies have shown no difference between lithium augmentation and any other strategy, but the varying quality of the studies – for example, problems with trial duration[58], use

of sub-therapeutic doses of lithium and desipramine[60–62], and low power – precludes drawing any definite conclusions.

Predictors of response to lithium augmentation

Although lithium has been shown to be an effective augmenting therapy, approximately 50% of the treated patients do not respond sufficiently. Efforts have therefore been made to identify clinical and biological variables that allow outcome to be predicted on lithium augmentation.

Several studies have investigated clinical variables in lithium augmentation trials[50,55,63–67]. In none of these has age or gender been found to be associated with response. Some have found that bipolar patients respond better than unipolar patients[63], but this has not been confirmed by all[64]. The severity of the depressive episode has been one of the variables most intensively probed, with some studies reporting better outcomes in less depressed

Table 11.5 Characteristics of studies comparing lithium augmentation to other strategies for treatment-refractory depression

Study	Subjects	Lithium group	Group 2	Group 3	Results
Dinan and Barry 1989[56]	22 UP, 8 BP, 20 F, 10 M Mean age 55 years	Lithium carbonate (600–800 mg/day) plus amitriptyline or other antidepressant (mean dose 175 mg/day)	Bilateral ECT (6 treatments in 3 weeks)	—	Responses (HAM-D <10 at 3 weeks): Li 67%, ECT 73% No significant difference
Joffe et al. 1993[58]	50 UP 30 F, 20 M Mean age 37 years	Lithium carbonate (900–1200 mg/day) plus desipramine or imipramine (>2.5 mg/kg/day)	Liothyronine sodium (37.5 µg/day) plus desipramine or imipramine (>2.5mg/kg/day)	Placebo plus desipramine or imipramine (>2.5 mg/kg/day)	Responders (50% reduction HAM-D and less than 10 at 2 weeks): Li 53%, liothyronine 59%, placebo 19% No difference between thyroid supplementation and lithium. Both groups performed significantly better than placebo
Hoencamp et al. 1994[57]	46 UP, 3 dysthymia, 2 psychotic 32F, 19M Mean age 39 years	Lithium (BM 0.6–1.0 mmol/l) plus maprotiline (BM 75–150 ng/ml)	Brofaromine (150 mg/day at 3rd week)	—	Responses (reduction >50% HAM-D): Li = 30%, brofaromine = 24%. No significant difference
Fava et al. 1994[60]	41 UP 25 F, 16 M Mean age 40 years	Lithium carbonate (300–600 mg/day) plus fluoxetine (20 mg/day)	Desipramine (25–50 mg/day) plus fluoxetine (20 mg/day)	Fluoxetine (40–60 mg/day)	Responses (reduction >50% of HAM-D and score >10 at 4 weeks): Li 29%, high fluoxetine 53%, desipramine 25%; no significant differences between the two groups
Rybakowski et al. 1999[59]	41 UP, 18 BP 49 F, 10 M Mean age 49 years	Lithium carbonate (mean dose 965 mg/day, adjusted to plasma level of 0.5–0.8 mmol/l) plus various antidepressants (SSRIs, TCAs, MAOIs)	Carbamazepine (400 mg/day adjusted to maintain plasma concentration of 4–8 µg/ml) plus various antidepressants (SSRIs, TCAs, MAOIs)	None	Responders (>50% HAM-D) at 4 weeks: Li 68%, CBZ 57% No significant difference between the two groups
Fava et al. 2002[61]	101 UP 49 F, 52 M Mean age 42 years	Lithium carbonate (300–600 mg/day) plus fluoxetine (20 mg/day)	Desipramine (25–50 mg/day) plus fluoxetine (20 mg/day)	Fluoxetine (40–60 mg/day)	Response at 4 weeks (<7 points in HAM-D): Li 24%, TCA 29%, fluoxetine 60 mg 42% No significant difference between the three groups

UP, unipolar; BP, bipolar; F, female; M, male; nr, not reported; BM, blood monitored; MAOI, monoamine oxidase inhibitor; TCA, tricyclic antidepressant; SSRI, selective serotonin reuptake inhibitor; Li, Lithium; CBZ, carbamazepine; ECT, electroconvulsive therapy; HAM-D, Hamilton Depression Rating Scale patients[63,65,66] and others not finding this correlation[50,55,64]. A recent retrospective analysis of 71 depressed patients refractory to a treatment trial with a tricyclic antidepressant demonstrated that patients with a more severe depressive syndrome were more likely to respond to lithium augmentation[67]. This result is in line with studies on treatment with antidepressants in which more severely depressed patients showed a greater response[68].

Findings regarding the type of antidepressant used and the response to lithium augmentation have been contradictory. Concerns have been raised after the negative findings of a recent study which used an antidepressive agent without a marked serotonergic profile[48,54]. To the authors' knowledge, no study has used lithium augmentation with a selective norepinephrine antidepressant, but such a study would be of great theoretical and clinical interest.

Another area of interest has been the study of the hypothalamo–pituitary–adrenocortical (HPA) system. In one study[69], HPA system status was analyzed with regard to its predictive value. Non-responders to lithium augmentation showed a cortisol/adrenocorticotropic hormone (ACTH) peak ratio in the combined dexamethasone/corticotropin releasing hormone (DEX/CRH) test which was statistically significantly higher than that of responders. This ratio is considered to be indicative of the sensitivity of the adrenal cortex to ACTH[70]. The higher ratio in non-responders could point to a more chronic course of the depression with more marked biological changes, since chronic depression was found to result in an enlargement of the adrenal gland and increased sensitivity to ACTH[71,72].

In depressed patients treated with antidepressants, a high cortisol response in the combined DEX/CRH test at admission to hospital has been demonstrated to be significantly associated with a depressive relapse in the continuation treatment phase[73,74]. No correlation between the DEX/CRH test results and a depressive relapse were detected in a follow-up study after lithium augmentation. The follow-up interval had a mean of 18 months (range 12–28). Only 48% of the 23 patients studied had a favorable course, defined as no occurrence of a major depressive syndrome. A favorable or unfavorable course did not correlate with any demographic, clinical or therapeutic variable (Bschor et al., unpublished observation).

Lithium augmentation: continuation treatment and discontinuation studies

A randomized controlled trial has inquired into the efficacy of lithium augmentation in the continuation treatment of unipolar major depressive disorder[75]. Twenty-nine patients with a refractory major depressive episode who had responded to acute lithium augmentation therapy during an open 6-week study were randomized after a 2–4-week stabilization period to a double-blind continuation treatment for another 4 months with either lithium ($n = 14$) or placebo ($n = 15$). The antidepressant was continued at the same dosage throughout the study[75] (Figure 11.2).

Seven of the 15 patients on placebo suffered a relapse (five depressive and two manic) in the double-blind study phase, while no patients from the lithium group relapsed. Even more patients relapsed during the subsequent open 6-month phase after lithium was withdrawn in the group previously receiving lithium[76]. It was concluded that patients who respond to lithium augmentation should be maintained on lithium augmentation for a minimum of 12 months[76].

Another randomized study pursued the effects of a gradual discontinuation of lithium augmentation therapy in elderly depressed patients. Hardy et al. conducted a placebo-controlled discontinuation study in 12 geriatric

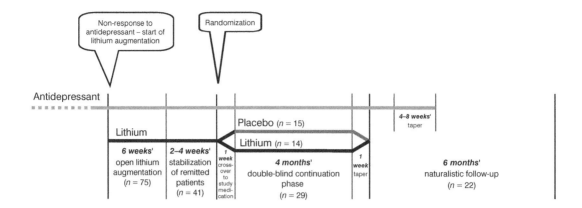

Figure 11.2 Design of a double-blind, placebo-controlled trial of lithium augmentation continuation treatment in patients with major depressive disorder

patients who had responded to lithium augmentation during their most recent refractory unipolar depressive episode[77]. Patients were randomized to receive continued lithium augmentation or matching placebo; two of six patients in the lithium maintenance group had a recurrence of depression at 61 and 96 weeks, respectively, immediately after a stressful life event. Similarly, two of six patients had a recurrence in the placebo group at 7 and 92 weeks, respectively, without any apparent changes in life stresses. In a second, naturalistic discontinuation study in an elderly cohort of patients with major depressive disorder, approximately half of the patients relapsed following discontinuation of lithium augmentation[78].

MECHANISMS OF LITHIUM AUGMENTATION: NEUROBIOLOGICAL BASIS

Treatment strategies for major depression that show well-documented effects on the outcome of patients have heuristic value for the investigation of the pathophysiology of the disorder. There is strong evidence that the serotonergic

(5-hydroxytryptamine (5-HT)) system plays a key role in mood regulation[79,80], and studies have indicated that lithium has a net enhancing effect on serotonin function[81,82]. Neurochemical and neuroendocrine research has provided hypotheses for the mechanisms involved in lithium augmentation therapy based on studies in animals and humans. Arguments for a true augmentation effect derive from animal studies showing that a potentiation of antidepressant treatment by lithium might be mediated through an enhancement of serotonin neurotransmission, and from neuroendocrine studies in humans that also demonstrate that lithium augments the function of the serotonergic system. These two lines of experimental evidence are outlined here.

The serotonin system in animal studies

There is consistent evidence from animal studies that lithium enhances serotonergic responsiveness by acting on turnover and release[83–85]. Grahame-Smith and Green reported that an increase in 5-HT transmission, produced by enhancing the function of 5-HT neurons, was demonstrated behaviorally by the appearance of '5-HT syndrome' in rats following short-term application of lithium[86]. The combination of lithium and MAOIs produced a behavioral overactivity syndrome in rats that was indistinguishable from that evoked by MAOIs and tryptophan; this lithium-induced overactivity syndrome was blocked by prior administration of an inhibitor of serotonin synthesis[86]. Lithium administration has also been shown to augment 5-HT release in the rat dorsal hippocampus[87] and to enhance 5-HT synthesis[88]. Furthermore, short-term administration of lithium augments the efficacy of electrically stimulating the ascending 5-HT pathway, which suppresses the firing of postsynaptic neurons in the dorsal hippocampus of rats[81].

Subsequently, and as already mentioned, it was postulated that a pharmacodynamic action mediated via the serotonergic systems may account for the synergistic effect of lithium when added to a tricyclic antidepressant (TCA)[55]. The development of this hypothesis was based on several observations of the neurobiological effects of tricyclic antidepressant drugs in combination with lithium's effects on the serotonin system. De Montigny and Aghajanian[89] demonstrated that long-term TCA treatment induced a selective increase in the responsiveness to serotonin in rat dorsal hippocampus which has since been shown to be mediated by post-synaptic 5-HT$_{1A}$ receptors[90]. If this is also true for humans, it would mean that, in patients who fail to respond to an antidepressant, chronic TCA usage may induce post-synaptic sensitization to 5-HT, as seen in animals. Second, if lithium has similar effects on 5-HT turnover in humans, lithium augmentation of antidepressant therapy may alter 5-HT neurotransmission[55,91].

Further evidence for a true augmentation effect derived from animal studies showed that, in contrast to lithium alone, the addition of lithium to antidepressant treatment with the SSRI citalopram potentiated presynaptic serotonergic function in rats[92]. Using microdialysis techniques, addition of subchronic lithium to chronic citalopram therapy further elevated basal levels of 5-HT in the rat ventral hippocampus[93].

Neuroendocrine studies

Human neuroendocrine challenge tests have repeatedly been studied in depressed patients during lithium augmentation therapy. The pharmacologic challenge test used most frequently to assess central 5-HT function is the prolactin response to intravenous L-tryptophan[84]. Cowen et al. found that the administration of lithium increased the prolactin response to L-tryptophan in patients receiving TCAs after both 4 days and 4 weeks of treatment[94]. These results provide evidence that lithium might facilitate 5-HT neurotransmission. However, the magnitude of the prolactin increase did not correlate with the clinical outcome. Some lithium augmentation responders showed little increase in prolactin release while others had a more pronounced prolactin response[94]. Similar results were obtained by McCance-Katz et al., who reported that primary antidepressant medication did not increase the prolactin response, but lithium augmentation increased it significantly as compared to both placebo pre-treatment and antidepressant alone[95]. Furthermore, neither depression severity nor response status to lithium augmentation correlated with the increase in the prolactin response[95].

Another endocrine system that has been studied during lithium augmentation is the HPA system[96,97]. The combined DEX/CRH test is a sensitive neuroendocrinological challenge test to investigate HPA system function[98]. A significant proportion of patients with major depression show an overstimulation in the DEX/CRH test[98].

In 30 unipolar depressed subjects who had not responded to a treatment trial with an antidepressant of at least 4 weeks, the combined DEX/CRH test was performed directly before and (depending on the response status) 2–4 weeks after the initiation of lithium augmentation therapy (n = 24 for the second test). In contrast to results from studies in depressed patients treated with tricyclic antidepressants[98], where a decline was found, the cortisol and ACTH response to CRH stimulation after dexamethasone pre-treatment displayed a significant rise under lithium augmentation compared to the baseline[99,100]. Eleven patients responded according to the criteria applied (based on weekly ratings with the Hamilton Depression Rating Scale) and it is noteworthy that both responders and non-responders demonstrated that increase. This led to the assumption that the stimulation of the HPA system might be a direct effect of the lithium ion, probably mediated by the serotonergic actions of the pharmacon[99]. In a recent study in patients with a major depressive episode, treatment with lithium monotherapy also led to a (for most parameters significant) increase in the HPA axis activity[101].

Early studies in patients[102,103], animals and cell cultures[104–106] demonstrated a stimulating effect of lithium on cortisol or ACTH production. These results contradict the established decline of HPA system activity during treatment with tricyclic antidepressants and therefore throw into question the paradigm in major depression that the normalization of HPA system overstimulation in the combined DEX/CRH test is a necessary prerequisite for recovery[98]. To elucidate the effects of lithium on the HPA system, studies are needed to investigate the effects of lithium monotherapy on the HPA system in healthy controls.

PRACTICAL ASPECTS OF THE USE OF LITHIUM IN MAJOR DEPRESSIVE EPISODES

Lithium monotherapy may be considered when treating a depressive episode in a bipolar patient at high risk of switching to a manic phase with the use of other antidepressants. If a rapid response is desired for a depressive episode, lithium added to an antidepressant treatment should be considered as an initial therapy, especially in patients for whom long-term prophylactic lithium therapy is indicated.

Finally, following the same line of previously published guidelines[41] (see Chapter 5), the evidence reviewed here supports the recommendation of lithium augmentation as a first-line therapy for non-responding and refractory depressed patients. Lithium carbonate should be started with a dose of 800–1200 mg (equivalent to approximately 24–36 mmol/day), which should achieve serum levels of 0.6–0.8 mmol/l and be administered for 2–4 weeks to allow assessment of the patient's response. In depressed patients who respond to lithium augmentation, effective lithium doses should be continued in combination with the antidepressant for at least 12 months after remission.

REFERENCES

1. Schou M. Lithium in psychiatric therapy and prophylaxis. J Psychiatr Res 1968; 6: 67–95
2. Goodwin FK, Jamison KR. Manic-depressive illness. Oxford: Oxford University Press, 1990
3. Bauer M, Ahrens B. Bipolar disorder. A practical guide to drug treatment. CNS Drugs 1996; 6: 35–52
4. Cade JFJ. Lithium salts in the treatment of psychotic excitement. Med J Aust 1949; 36: 349–52
5. Mendels J. Lithium in the treatment of depression. Am J Psychiatrry 1976; 133: 373–8

6. Noack CH, Trautner EM. The lithium treatment of maniacal psychosis. Med J Aust 1951; 38: 219–22

7. Van der Velde CD. Effectiveness of lithium carbonate in the treatment of manic-depressive illness. Am J Psychiatry 1970; 127: 345–51

8. Vojtěchovský M, Zkuśenosti s lecbou solemi lithia. In Problémy psychiatrie v praxi a ve vyskumu. Prague, 1957

9. Andreani G, Caselli G, Martelli G. Clinical and electroencephalographic changes during treatment with lithium salts in mental disorders. G Psichiatr Neuropathol 1958; 86: 273–328

10. Dyson WL, Mendels J. Lithium and depression. Curr Ther Res 1968; 10: 601–8

11. Náhunek K, Svestka J, Rodová A. Zur Stellung des Lithiums in der Gruppe der Antidepressiva in der Behandlung von akuten endogenen und Involutions depressionen. Int Pharmacopsychiatry 1970; 5: 249–57

12. Noyes R Jr, Ringdahl IC, Andreasen NJC. Effect of lithium citrate on adrenocortical activity in manic-depressive illness. Compr Psychiatry 1971; 12: 337–47

13. Bennie EH. Lithium in depression [Letter]. Lancet 1975; 1: 216

14. Hansen CJ, Retboll K, Schou M. Lithium in psychiatry: a review. J Psychiatr Res 1968; 6: 67–95

15. Fieve RR, Platman SR, Plutchick RR. The use of lithium in affective disorders: I. Acute endogenous depression. Am J Psychiatry 1968; 125: 487–98

16. Stokes PE, Shamonian CA, Stoll PM, Patton MJ. Efficacy of lithium as acute treatment of manic-depressive illness. Lancet 1971; 1: 1319–25

17. Adli M, Bschor T, Canata B, et al. Lithium in der Behandlung der akuten Depression. Fortschr Neurol Psychiatr 1998; 66: 435–41

18. Souza FGM, Goodwin GM. Lithium treatment and prophylaxis in unipolar depression – a meta-analysis. Br J Psychiatry 1991; 158: 666–75

19. Linder J, Fyrö B, Petterson U, Werner S. Acute antidepressant effect of lithium is associated with fluctuation of calcium and magnesium in plasma. Acta Psychiatr Scand 1989; 80: 27–36

20. Worral E, Moody JP, Peet M, et al. Controlled studies of the acute antidepressant effects of lithium. Br J Psychiatry 1979; 135: 255–62

21. Arieli A, Lepkifker E. The antidepressant effect of lithium. Curr Dev Psychopharmacol 1981; 6: 165–90

22. Khan MC. Lithium carbonate in the treatment of acute depressive illness. Bibl Psychiatr 1981; 161: 244–8

23. Watanabe S, Ishino H, Otsuki S. Double-blind comparison of lithium carbonate and imipramine in the treatment of depression. Arch Gen Psychiatry 1975; 32: 659–68

24. Goodwin FK, Murphy DL, Dunner DL, Bunney WE Jr. Lithium response in unipolar versus bipolar depression. Am J Psychiatry 1972; 129: 44–7

25. Noyes R Jr, Dempsey GM, Blum A, Chavanaugh GL. Lithium treatment of depression. Compr Psychiatry 1974; 15: 187–93

26. Baron M, Gershon ES, Rudy V, et al. Lithium carbonate response in depression: prediction by unipolar/bipolar illness, average evoked response, catechol-O-methyl transferase, and family history. Arch Gen Psychiatry 1975; 32: 1107–11

27. Kupfer DJ, Pickar D, Himmelhoch JM, Detre TP. Are there two types of unipolar depression? Arch Gen Psychiatry 1975; 32: 866–71

28. Mendels J, Frazer A. Intracellular lithium concentration and clinical response: towards a membrane theory of depression. J Psychiatr Res 1973; 10: 9–18

29. Carman JS, Post RM, Teplitz TA, Goodwin FK. Divalent cations in predicting antidepressant response to lithium [Letter]. Lancet 1974; 2: 1454

30. Goodwin FK, Post RM. Brain serotonin, affective illness, and antidepressant drugs: cerebrospinal fluid studies with probenecid. In Costa E, Gessa Gl, Sander M, eds. Serotonin – New Vistas: Histochemistry and Pharmacology, Advances in Biochemical Psychopharmacology. New York: Raven Press, 1974; 10: 341–55

31. Marini JL. Predicting lithium responders and nonresponders: physiological indicators. In

Johnson FN, ed. Handbook for Lithium Therapy. Lancaster: MTP Press, 1980: 118–25

32. Mendlewicz J. Responders and non-responders to lithium therapy: some potential biological indicators. Bibl Psychiat 1981; 161: 63–8

33. Austin LS, Arana GW, Ballenger JC. Rapid response of patients simultaneously treated with lithium and nortriptyline. J Clin Psychiatry 1990; 51: 124–5

34. Altshuler LL, Frye MA, Gitlin MJ. Acceleration and augmentation strategies for treating bipolar depression. Biol Psychiatry 2003; 53: 691–700

35. Lingjaerde O, Edlund AH, Gormsen CA, et al. The effects of lithium carbonate in combination with tricyclic antidepressants in endogenous depression. A double-blind, multicenter trial. Acta Psychiatr Scand 1974; 50: 233–42

36. Januel D, Galinowski A, Poirier MF, et al. Prospective study of antidepressants combined with lithium in unipolar depression: preliminary results. Lithium 1994; 5: 253–7

37. Ebert D, Jaspert A, Murata H, Kaschka WP. Initial lithium augmentation improves the antidepressant effects of standard TCA treatment in non-resistant depressed patients. Psychopharmacology (Berl) 1995; 118: 223–5

38. Bloch M, Schwartzman Y, Bonne O, Lerer B. Concurrent treatment of nonresistant major depression with desipramine and lithium: a double-blind, placebo-controlled study. J Clin Psychopharmacol 1997; 17: 44–8

39. Januel D, Poirier MF, D'alche-Biree F, et al. Multicenter double-blind randomized parallel-group clinical trial of efficacy of the combination clomipramine (150 mg/day) plus lithium carbonate (750 mg/day) versus clomipramine (150 mg/day) plus placebo in the treatment of unipolar major depression. J Affect Disord 2003; 76: 191–200

40. Nick J, Luaute JP, Des Lauriers A, et al. The clomipramine–lithium combination: controlled trial. Encephale 1976; 2: 5–16

41. Bauer M, Whybrow PC, Angst J, et al. World Federation of Societies of Biological Psychiatry (WFSBP) Guidelines for Biological Treatment of Unipolar Depressive Disorders, Part 1: Acute and continuation treatment of major depressive disorder. World J Biol Psychiatry 2002; 3: 5–43

42. De Montigny C, Grunberg F, Mayer A, Deschenes JP. Lithium induces rapid relief of depression in tricyclic antidepressant drug non-responders. Br J Psychiatry 1981; 138: 252–6

43. Bauer M, Döpfmer S. Lithium augmentation in treatment-resistant depression: meta-analysis of placebo-controlled studies. J Clin Psychopharmacol 1999; 19: 427–34

44. Kantor D, McNevin S, Leichner P, et al. The benefit of lithium carbonate adjunct in refractory depression – fact or fiction? Can J Psychiatry 1986; 31: 416–18

45. Zusky PM, Biederman J, Rosenbaum JF, et al. Adjunct low dose lithium carbonate in treatment-resistant depression: a placebo-controlled study. J Clin Psychopharmacol 1988; 8: 120–4

46. Browne M, Lapierre YD, Hrdina PD, Horn E. Lithium as an adjunct in the treatment of major depression. Int Clin Psychopharmacol 1990; 5: 103–10

47. Stein G, Bernadt M. Lithium augmentation therapy in tricyclic-resistant depression. A controlled trial using lithium in low and normal doses. Br J Psychiatry 1993; 162: 634–40

48. Nierenberg AA, Papakostas GI, Petersen T, et al. Lithium augmentation of nortriptyline for subjects resistant to multiple antidepressants. J Clin Psychopharmacol 2003; 23: 92–5

49. Heninger GR, Charney DS, Sternberg DE. Lithium carbonate augmentation of antidepressant treatment. An effective prescription for treatment-refractory depression. Arch Gen Psychiatry 1983; 40: 1335–42

50. Schöpf J, Baumann P, Lemarchand T, Rey M. Treatment of endogenous depressions resistant to tricyclic antidepressants or related drugs by lithium addition. Results of a placebo-controlled double-blind study. Pharmacopsychiatry 1989; 22: 183–7

51. Joffe RT, Singer W, Levitt AJ, MacDonald C. A placebo-controlled comparison of lithium and triiodothyronine augmentation of tricyclic antidepressants in unipolar refractory depression. Arch Gen Psychiatry 1993; 50: 387–93

52. Katona CL, Abou-Saleh MT, Harrison DA, et al. Placebo-controlled trial of lithium augmen-

tation of fluoxetine and lofepramine. Br J Psychiatry 1995; 166: 80–6

53. Baumann P, Nil R, Souche A, et al. A double-blind, placebo-controlled study of citalopram with and without lithium in the treatment of therapy-resistant depressive patients: a clinical, pharmacokinetic, and pharmacogenetic investigation. J Clin Psychopharmacol 1996; 16: 307–14

54. Bschor T, Bauer M. Is successful lithium augmentation limited to serotonergic anti-depressants? J Clin Psychopharmacol 2004; 24: 240–1

55. de Montigny C, Cournoyer G, Morissette R, et al. Lithium carbonate addition in tricyclic antidepressant-resistant unipolar depression. Correlations with the neurobiologic actions of tricyclic antidepressant drugs and lithium ion on the serotonin system. Arch Gen Psychiatry 1983; 40: 1327–34

56. Dinan TG, Barry S. A comparison of electro-convulsive therapy with a combined lithium and tricyclic combination among depressed tricyclic nonresponders. Acta Psychiatr Scand 1989; 80: 97–100

57. Hoencamp E, Haffmans PM, Dijken WA, et al. Brofaromine versus lithium addition to maprotiline. A double-blind study in maproti-line refractory depressed outpatients. J Affect Disord 1994; 30: 219–27

58. Joffe RT, Singer W, Levitt AJ, MacDonald C. A placebo-controlled comparison of lithium and triiodothyronine augmentation of tricyclic antidepressants in unipolar refractory depression. Arch Gen Psychiatry 1993; 50: 387–93

59. Rybakowski JK, Suwalska A, Chlopocka-Wozniak M. Potentiation of antidepressants with lithium or carbamazepine in treatment-resistant depression. Neuropsychobiology 1999; 40: 134–9

60. Fava M, Rosenbaum JF, McGrath PJ, et al. Lithium and tricyclic augmentation of fluoxetine treatment for resistant major depression: a double-blind, controlled study. Am J Psychiatry 1994; 151: 1372–4

61. Fava M, Alpert J, Nierenberg A, et al. Double-blind study of high-dose fluoxetine versus lithium or desipramine augmentation of fluox-etine in partial responders and nonresponders to fluoxetine. J Clin Psychopharmacol 2002; 22: 379–87

62. Nelson JC, Price LH. Lithium or desipramine augmentation of fluoxetine treatment. Am J Psychiatry 1995; 152: 1538–9

63. Rybakowski J, Matkowski K. Adding lithium to antidepressant therapy: factors related to therapeutic potentiation. Eur Neuro-psychopharmacol 1992; 2: 161–5

64. Price LH, Charney DS, Heninger GR. Variability of response to lithium augmentation in refractory depression. Am J Psychiatry 1986; 143: 1387–92

65. Joffe RT, Levitt AJ, Bagby RM, et al. Predictors of response to lithium and triiodothyronine augmentation of antidepressants in tricyclic non-responders. Br J Psychiatry 1993; 163: 574–8

66. Alvarez E, Perez-Sola V, Perez-Blanco J, et al. Predicting outcome of lithium added to anti-depressants in resistant depression. J Affect Disord 1997; 42: 179–86

67. Bschor T, Canata B, Müller-Oerlinghausen B, Bauer M. Predictors of response to lithium aug-mentation in tricyclic antidepressant-resistant depression. J Affect Disord 2001; 64: 261–5

68. Müller HJ, Fischer G, Zerssen VD. Prediction of therapeutic response in acute treatment with antidepressants. Results of an empirical study involving 159 endogenous depressive patients. Eur Arch Psychiatr Neurol Sci 1987; 236: 349–57

69. Bschor T, Baethge C, Adli M, et al. Association between response to lithium augmentation and the combined DEX/CRH test in major depressive disorder. J Psychiatr Res 2003; 37: 135–43

70. Holsboer F, Lauer CJ, Schreiber W, Krieg JC. Altered hypothalamic–pituitary–adrenocortical regulation in healthy subjects at high familial risk for affective disorders. Neuroendocrinology 1995; 62: 340–7

71. Amsterdam JD, Winokur A, Abelman E, et al. Cosyntropin (ACTH alpha 1-24) stimulation test in depressed patients and healthy subjects. Am J Psychiatry 1983; 140: 907–9

72. Barden N, Reul JM, Holsboer F. Do antidepressants stabilize mood through actions on the hypothalamic–pituitary–adrenocortical system? Trends Neurosci 1995; 18: 6–11

73. Zobel AW, Yassouridis A, Frieboes RM, Holsboer F. Prediction of medium-term outcome by cortisol response to the combined dexamethasone-CRH test in patients with remitted depression. Am J Psychiatry 1999; 156: 949–51

74. Zobel AW, Nickel T, Sonntag A, et al. Cortisol response in the combined dexamethasone/CRH test as predictor of relapse in patients with remitted depression. a prospective study. J Psychiatr Res 2001; 35: 83–94

75. Bauer M, Bschor T, Kunz D, et al. Double-blind, placebo-controlled trial of the use of lithium to augment antidepressant medication in continuation treatment of unipolar major depression. Am J Psychiatry 2000; 157: 1429–35

76. Bschor T, Berghöfer A, Ströhle A, et al. How long should the lithium augmentation strategy be maintained? A 1-year follow-up of a placebo-controlled study in unipolar refractory major depression. J Clin Psychopharmacol 2002; 22: 427–30

77. Hardy BG, Shulman KI, Zucchero C. Gradual discontinuation of lithium augmentation in elderly patients with unipolar depression. J Clin Psychopharmacol 1997; 17: 22–6

78. Fahy S, Lawlor BA. Discontinuation of lithium augmentation in an elderly cohort. Int J Geriatr Psychiatry 2001; 16: 1004–9

79. Maes M, Meltzer HY. The serotonin hypotheses of major depression. In Bloom FE, Kupfer DJ, eds. Psychopharmacology: The Fourth Generation of Progress. New York: Raven Press, 1995: 933–44

80. Schatzberg AF, Garlow SJ, Nemeroff CB. Molecular and cellular mechanisms in depression. In Davis KL, Charney D, Coyle JT, Nemeroff C, eds. Neuropsychopharmacology: The Fifth Generation of Progress. American College of Neuropsychopharmacology. Philadelphia, PA: Lippincott Williams and Wilkins, 2002: 1039–50

81. Blier P, De Montigny C. Short-term lithium administration enhances serotonergic neurotransmission: electrophysiological evidence in the rat CNS. Eur J Pharmacol 1985; 113: 69–77

82. Price LH, Charney DS, Delgado PL, Heninger GR. Lithium and serotonin function: implications for the serotonin hypothesis of depression. Psychopharmacology (Berl) 1990; 100: 3–12

83. Müller-Oerlinghausen B. Lithium long-term treatment – does it act via serotonin? Pharmacopsychiatry 1985; 18: 214–17

84. Price LH, Charney DS, Delgado PL, et al. Clinical studies of 5-HT function using i.v. L-tryptophan. Prog Neuropsychopharmacol Biol Psychiatry 1990; 14: 459–72

85. de Montigny C. Lithium addition in treatment-resistant depression. Int Clin Psychopharmacol 1994; 9 (Suppl 2): 31–5

86. Grahame-Smith DG, Green AR. The role of brain 5-hydroxytryptamine in the hyperactivity produced in rats by lithium and monoamine oxidase inhibition. Br J Pharmacol 1974; 52: 19–26

87. Treiser SL, Cascio CS, O'Donohue TL, et al. Lithium increases serotonin release and decreases serotonin receptors in the hippocampus. Science 1981; 213: 1529–31

88. Broderick P, Lynch V. Behavioral and biochemical changes induced by lithium and L-tryptophan in muricidal rats. Neuropharmacology 1982; 21: 671–9

89. de Montigny C, Aghajanian GK. Tricyclic antidepressants: long-term treatment increases responsivity of rat forebrain neurons to serotonin. Science 1978; 202: 1303–6

90. Chaput Y, de Montigny C, Blier P. Presynaptic and postsynaptic modifications of the serotonin system by long-term administration of antidepressant treatments. An in vivo electrophysiologic study in the rat. Neuropsychopharmacology 1991; 5: 219–29

91. De Montigny C. Lithium addition in treatment-resistant depression: evidence for the involvement of the serotonin system. In Racagni G, Brunello N, Fukuda T, eds. Biological Psychiatry. Amsterdam: Elsevier Science Publishers, 1991; 1: 243–4

92. Okamoto Y, Motohasi N, Hayakawa H, et al. Addition of lithium to chronic antidepressant treatment potentiates presynaptic serotonergic

function without changes in serotonergic receptors in the rat cerebral cortex. Neuropsychobiology 1996; 33: 17–20

93. Wegener G, Bandpey Z, Heiberg IL, et al. Increased extracellular serotonin level in rat hippocampus induced by chronic citalopram is augmented by subchronic lithium: neurochemical and behavioural studies in the rat. Psychopharmacology (Berl) 2003; 166: 188–94

94. Cowen PJ, McCance SL, Ware CJ, et al. Lithium in tricyclic-resistant depression. Correlation of increased brain 5-HT function with clinical outcome. Br J Psychiatry 1991; 159: 341–6

95. McCance-Katz E, Price LH, Charney DS, Heninger GR. Serotonergic function during lithium augmentation of refractory depression. Psychopharmacology (Berl) 1992; 108: 93–7

96. Dinan TG. Psychoneuroendocrinology of mood disorders. Curr Opin Psychiatry 2001; 14: 51–5

97. Steckler T, Holsboer F, Reul JM. Glucocorticoids and depression. Baillières Best Pract Res Clin Endocrinol Metab 1999; 13: 597–614

98. Holsboer F. The corticosteroid receptor hypothesis of depression. Neuropsychopharmacology 2000; 23: 477–501

99. Bschor T, Adli M, Baethge C, et al. Lithium augmentation increases the ACTH and cortisol response in the combined DEX/CRH test in unipolar major depression. Neuropsychopharmacology 2002; 27: 470–8

100. Bschor T, Baethge C, Adli M, et al. Lithium augmentation increases post-dexamethasone cortisol in the dexamethasone suppression test in unipolar major depression. Depress Anxiety 2003; 17: 43–8

101. Bschor T, Ritter D, Lewitzka U, et al. Effects of lithium on the HPA axis in patients with unipolar major depression [Abst]. Pharmacopsychiatry 2005; 38: 233

102. Platman SR, Fieve RR. Lithium carbonate and plasma cortisol response in the affective disorders. Arch Gen Psychiatry 1968; 18: 591–4

103. Platman SR, Hilton JG, Koss MC, Kelly WG. Production of cortisol in patients with manic-depressive psychosis treated with lithium carbonate. Dis Nerv Syst 1971; 32: 542–4

104. Sugawara M, Hashimoto K, Hattori T, et al. Effects of lithium on the hypothalamo–pituitary–adrenal axis. Endocrinol Jpn 1988; 35: 655–63

105. Zatz M, Reisine TD. Lithium induces corticotropin secretion and desensitization in cultured anterior pituitary cells. Proc Natl Acad Sci USA 1985; 82: 1286–90

106. Reisine T, Zatz M. Interactions among lithium, calcium, diacylglycerides, and phorbol esters in the regulation of adrenocorticotropin hormone release from AtT-20 cells. J Neurochem 1987; 49: 884–9

107. Mendels J, Secunda SK, Dyson WL. A controlled study of the antidepressant effects of lithium. Arch Gen Psychiatry 1972; 26: 154–7

108. Khan MC, Wickham EA, Reed JV. Lithium versus placebo in acute depression: a clinical trial. Int Clin Psychopharmacology 1987; 2: 47–54

12 Lithium in schizoaffective disorder and schizophrenia

Christopher Baethge, Christian Simhandl

Contents Introduction • Schizoaffective disorder – diagnostic issues • Lithium for the long-term treatment of schizoaffective disorders • Randomized controlled trials • Other lithium studies • Lithium in the long-term treatment of schizoaffective disorder – conclusions • Lithium for the treatment of acute schizoaffective episodes • Combinations in acute treatment of schizoaffective disorder • Lithium in schizophrenia

INTRODUCTION

In addition to the host of studies on its efficacy in bipolar disorders and unipolar depression, lithium has also been examined as a medication for other psychotic disorders. Its well-established mood-stabilizing properties suggested lithium as a treatment for schizo-affective disorder (SAD), but lithium has also been used in schizophrenia, in particular for treatment-resistant patients.

In this chapter the evidence for using lithium in SAD and in schizophrenia is reviewed. In the first part, diagnostic issues pertaining to SAD are briefly described in order to explain the most important problems of almost all studies in this group of patients. These limitations have to be kept in mind when the available evidence is presented. The focus is

on long-term treatment, because this is the most important indication for lithium in this recurrent psychosis[1]. However, the data regarding lithium as an anti-schizomanic agent is touched upon as well. In the second part of this chapter, the studies on lithium in schizophrenia are reviewed. The bulk of these data stem from studies dealing with the addition of lithium to ongoing antipsychotic treatment.

SCHIZOAFFECTIVE DISORDER – DIAGNOSTIC ISSUES

Patients suffering from SAD constitute a considerable subgroup in general psychiatric settings. With regard to outpatients, Müller–Oerlinghausen et al.[2] reported that between 7% and 30% of all cases in mood disorder clinics were diagnosed with SAD.

Even though there is no doubt that SAD is very important in everyday clinical practice, the main problem in the field is the accuracy of the diagnosis. The concept of SAD has undergone many diagnostic refinements since the term was introduced by Kasanin in 1933[3,4]. The first diagnostic criteria that were generally accepted and widely used were the DSM-III-R criteria of 1987[5]. To date, the criteria of DSM-IV[6] and ICD-10[7] differ considerably: the DSM requires a time-span of 2 weeks of delusions or hallucinations and absent prominent mood symptoms.

As a result of this diagnostic confusion, study samples differ according to the diagnostic system used[4]. A case in point is the important study by Greil and coworkers[8]. Of 90 patients who were schizoaffective according to ICD-9, 74 were included on the basis of a Research Diagnostic Criteria (RDC) diagnosis of SAD. Of those, the authors reported, only 17 fulfilled DSM-III-R criteria for SAD. In a similar vein, Maj and co-workers[9] reported that only 33 out of 48 ICD-9 schizoaffective patients maintained that diagnosis when RDC were applied. Moreover, the inter-rater reliability of the diagnosis seems to be unsatisfactorily low[10], with a Cohen's kappa for the DSM-IV-diagnosis of, in one study, 0.2[9].

Given the status of SAD as a borderline category between schizophrenia and bipolar disorder, it is not surprising that study samples also differ, depending on the centers where the investigations were carried out. Williams and McGlashan[11] reported that, in their group of chronic hospitalized study participants at Chestnut Lodge, the schizoaffective patients resembled their schizophrenic patients. On the other hand, Rosenthal et al.[12], using RDC in a lithium clinic, found their patients very similar to their bipolar patients with regard to treatment outcome. Referring to this sampling bias, Angst and Preisig[1] commented in their follow-up study: 'The high similarity between our affective and schizoaffective samples is likely to be attributable to our sampling strategy. We studied the schizoaffective patient group within a large sample of initial affective patients.'

Against the backdrop of the diagnostic difficulties described above, the studies in this overview are divided into those carried out before standardized diagnostic instruments came into use and studies using modern diagnostic criteria, i.e. from RDC on. In a literature search (restricted to German and English articles and using Medline, Embase and the Cochrane Controlled Trials Register) the terms 'schizoaffective' and 'lithium' were used. In addition, the bibliographies of the retrieved references and of handbook articles were searched. All publications reporting on five or fewer patients were excluded, as were studies reporting on mixed samples (e.g. bipolar and schizoaffective patients) without presenting the results for the schizoaffective study participants in particular. The results presented in this chapter are updated from an earlier study[4].

LITHIUM FOR THE LONG-TERM TREATMENT OF SCHIZOAFFECTIVE DISORDERS

We found 25 studies on lithium in the long-term treatment of schizoaffective disorders (Table 12.1). Eight studies[8,12–19] used modern diagnostic criteria (Table 12.2), 17[20–36] did not, many of which were carried out from the late 1960s until the early 1980s (Table 12.3). In total, the studies included 607 patients (170 in modern studies), and the average follow-up amounted to approximately 3.0 years (range: 0.9–6.8 years). Only five of 25 studies were prospective and controlled, and only three were randomized controlled trials (RCT) (see Tables 12.2 and 12.3). Another RCT, Prien and co-workers[26],

Table 12.1 General characteristics of studies on lithium long-term treatment in schizoaffective disorder

	Number
Number of studies	25
No modern diagnostic criteria	17
Modern diagnostic criteria	8
Prospective and controlled	5
Randomized	3
Number of patients	607
Average follow-up	3.0 years (0.9–6.8)

was not randomized with regard to the SAD sub group in the sample (only one patient in the placebo group).

The studies do not lend themselves to a quantitative meta-analytic approach because the methodology and the outcome measures are too different. Therefore, we will describe the most important studies in detail and, if necessary, summarize the studies in a qualitative way.

RANDOMIZED CONTROLLED TRIALS

The earliest of the randomized trials[14] compared lithium with fluphenazine in a group of 14 'mainly schizophrenic' schizoaffective patients diagnosed according to RDC. In this double-blind, 1-year follow-up study, six of seven patients who received lithium relapsed as opposed to only two out of five study completers in the fluphenazine group. Unfortunately, the authors did not document the success of their randomization with regard to illness severity, a critical issue in a small study.

The two other RCTs compared lithium with carbamazepine. Bellaire and co-workers[36] included 17 patients on the diagnostic basis of DSM-III (no formal criteria). After 1 year of observation five of nine lithium patients and three of eight patients taking carbamazepine

had a recurrence, a statistically non-significant difference. Both groups benefited from the treatment when the follow-up period was compared with the time prior to the study.

In the largest RCT in this field to date, the open study of Greil and co-workers[8], the authors treated 43 patients with lithium and 47 patients with carbamazepine for a period of 2.5 years. The patients had been diagnosed according to ICD-9 (no formal criteria). With respect to this group there were no statistically significant differences between the two treatments. Seventy-four patients of the sample were diagnosed as schizoaffective according to RDC (62 mainly affective, 12 mainly schizophrenic). Among the 35 RDC-schizodepressive patients carbamazepine turned out to be statistically superior to lithium in preventing recurrences whereas among the 39 RDC-schizomanic patients no differences between the treatments were observed. Also, in an intention-to-treat analysis of the whole group there were no differences between lithium (five drop-outs) and carbamazepine (15 drop-outs). Subjectively the patients felt more satisfied with carbamazepine than they did with lithium. Unfortunately, the authors did not present data on the course of the illness prior to the study. Thus, there is no evidence in this study that lithium and carbamazepine work better than no treatment in this group of patients.

Table 12.2 Long-term treatment of schizoaffective disorder (SAD) with lithium: studies using modern diagnostic criteria ($n = 8$) (adapted from reference 4)

Author (first)	Year	Diagnostic criteria	Design	Medication	SAD (n)	Follow-up (years)	Results, comments
Rosenthal[12]	1980	RDC	Open, prospective	Li	15	2	RDC-positive vs. RDC-negative. SAD: 49% remaining well (bipolar disorder, 55%), no before and after comparison
Sarantidis[13]	1981	RDC mirror image	Retrospective, mirror image	Li	9	>2	Six of patients, no recurrences; two of nine significantly fewer days in hospital; patient had to be on Li for 2 years to be included. Negative predictor: number of episodes prior to Li. Follow-up not stated for SAD (SAD + bipolar disorder, 4.2 years)
Mattes[14]	1984	RDC	Double blind, controlled randomized	Li vs. fluphenazine	14	≤ 1	Six of seven Li patients and one of five fluphenazine patients relapsed. Sample mainly schizophrenic; no before and after comparison
Maj[15]	1988	RDC	Open, prospective, mirror image	Li	33	2	18 of 33 labeled as responders (no relapse though high risk for relapse). Significant decrease in number of episodes, mainly schizophrenic SAD <mainly affective SAD; 62 SAD according to ICD-9
Minnai[16]	1990	RDC	Open, retrospective, mirror image	Li	22	5	SAD manic type (RDC), 86% decrease in time spent in hospital
Grossman[17,18]	1991 1984	RDC	Open, prospective, controlled	Li vs. AP vs. no medication	41	4–5	Li or AP either alone or in combination; no detailed information on medication; no differences in outcome between groups; patients taking AP showed non-significantly more functional impairment
Greil[8]	1997	RDC	Open, prospective, controlled, randomized	Li vs. Cbz	74	2.5	Cbz >Li among schizodepressive SAD; no differences among schizomanic SAD; 90 ICD-9 SAD, 19 DSM-III-R SAD; Cbz appeared to be better tolerated; no before and after comparison
Baethge[19]	2004	ICD-10, DSM-IV	Open, retrospective	Li, Cbz	49	6.8	Li, $n = 41$, Cbz: $n = 8$, predictor study of long-term mood stabilizer treatment; no predictors found; 85% decrease in days spent in hospital; no different results for the 34 DSM-IV SAD patients

Cbz, carbamazepine; Li, lithium; AP, antipsychotics ; '>' and '<', 'more' and 'less' effective

Table 12.3 Long-term treatment of schizoaffective disorder (SAD) with lithium: studies without modern diagnostic criteria (n = 17) (adapted from reference 4)

Author (first)	Year	Diagnostic criteria	Design	Medication	SAD (n)	Follow-up (years)	Results, comments
Baastrup[20]	1967	Author's ('atypical')	Open, prospective	Li	15	2.5	Li effective in reducing no. of episodes and hospitalizations, less among BD and UD, no effect on paranoid delusions
Angst[21]	1969	ICD	Open, controlled, prospective, mirror image	Li vs. imipramine	Li: 24 I: 11	Li: 0.9 I: 1.4	Li: 76% reduction of episodes; imipramine: 56% increase of episodes; Li better in SAD than in BD and UD
Angst[22]	1970	ICD	Open, prospective, mirror image	Li	72	2.3	Episode reduction by 39%, in 49% of SAD patients episodes reduced, 35% no difference, 16% deteriorated; Li better in BD and UD than in SAD; negative predictor: number of episodes
Hofmann[23]	1970	Author's	Open	Li	19	>0.5	In 6 (32%) patients no recurrences, in 4 (21%) only moderate symptoms, SAD <BD, UD; follow-up not stated for SAD as a group, for the whole sample about 1.5 years
Aronoff[24]	1970	Author's	Open, prospective	Li	6	<3	In 5 patients only mild symptoms recurred, 1 patient treated with Li + fluphenazine
Egli[25]	1971	Author's	Retrospective	Li	25	2	No. of episodes reduced by 60% and in 64% of patients, episode duration reduced by 67%
Prien[26]	1974	DSM-II	(Double blind, randomized)	Li (vs. placebo)	6	<2	3 of 5 lithium patients relapsed, study not controlled and randomized with respect to SAD since only 1 patient in placebo group
Smulevitch[27]	1974	Author's	Open, controlled, mirror image	Li vs. no medication	49	1	In 32 (65%) fewer or no recurrences, in 9 episode duration shortened, in 8 deterioration; study was controlled but results for SAD were not stated in particular
Tress[28]	1979	Author's	Open, retrospective	Li	22	2.4	Reduction of episodes by 73%, SAD > cyclothymia
Perris[29]	1983	Author's: CP (cycloid psychoses), SAD	Open, prospective, mirror image	Li, Li (+AP)	56	1–16	CP (n = 41): significant reduction of episodes and time spent in hospital, 8 patients + depot AP. SAD (n = 15): no significant change; 7 patients + depot AP, SAD similar to chronic S

continued over

Table 12.3 *continued* Long-term treatment of schizoaffective disorder (SAD) with lithium: studies without modern diagnostic criteria (*n* = 17) (adapted from reference 4)

Author (first)	Year	Diagnostic criteria	Design	Medication	SAD (n)	Follow-up (years)	Results, comments
Küfferle[30]	1983	ICD-9	Open, retrospective, mirror image	Li	68	5.1	Reduction of episodes by 48%, Li not effective in patients with schizophrenic thought disturbance and blunted affect, only 36 diagnosed SAD longitudinally, sample biased towards affective symptomatology
Emrich[31]	1985	ICD-9	Open	Li + Val	6	3.9	Significant extension of phase interval from 1 to 3 years, Li+Val in affective disorders >SAD
Romeo[32]	1985	DSM-III	Open, prospective	Li	6	(2)	All patients received co-medication, only small prophylactic effect due to author's rating system SAD <BD, follow-up not stated for SAD group
Bouman[33]	1986	Kendell	Retrospective	Li	28	3.3	Significant improvement in no. of episodes and hospitalizations compared to time prior Li, Li better in SAD and BD than in UD
Koufen[34]	1989	ICD-9	Open, retrospective	Li	17	> 8	Inclusion criterion: ≥8 years on Li, physician's ratings: 78% improved, in 12% no relapses
Hayes[35]	1989	Not stated	Retrospective	Val, Val + Li	14	1.3	Only 4 patients Val monotherapy, 11 of 14 improved in GAS and due to author's rating system ('global response'), very moderate degree of improvement
Bellaire[36]	1990	DSM-III	Open, prospective, controlled randomized, mirror image	Li vs. Cbz	17	1	Li: 4 of 9 no relapse, Cbz: 5 of 8 no relapse (no significant difference), Cbz in whole sample (n = 109) better tolerated, Cbz in SAD better than in BD (5/8 vs. 10/24)

AP, antipsychotic; BD, bipolar disorder; Cbz, carbamazepine; CP, cycloid psychosis; GAS, Global Assessment Scale; Li, lithium not relapsed: S, schizophrenia; UD, unipolar disorder; VAL, valproate; '>' and '<', 'move' and 'less' effective;

OTHER LITHIUM STUDIES

Given the lack of placebo-controlled studies in this field, only mirror-image studies provide evidence regarding the basic question whether lithium is effective in the prophylaxis of SAD at all. In one of the classical early lithium studies[22], the illness course of 72 SAD patients from three study centers during 2.3 years of follow-up was compared with the illness course in the time before lithium had been started. Outcome parameters in this open and uncontrolled study were number of episodes and number of hospitalizations. Forty-nine per cent of the patients showed an improved course, in 35 no change was observed and 16 patients deteriorated. Overall, the number of episodes decreased during lithium therapy by 39%. In another mirror image study[21], lithium was associated with a reduction of the number of episodes among SAD patients ($n = 35$) by 76% after approximately 1 year of follow-up, and it performed better than imipramine (56% increase of episodes).

One study compared lithium in an open design with no treatment in a large group of patients, 49 of whom had a diagnosis of schizoaffective disorder (according to author's criteria)[27]. Although lithium significantly improved the illness course of the group as a whole, the results were unfortunately not broken down for the subgroup of SAD patients.

Maj[15] included 33 schizoaffective patients (RDC) in a prospective and naturalistic study dividing the sample into ten 'mainly schizophrenic', 14 'mainly affective' and nine patients who could not be allocated to either group. Over 2 years of follow-up, the number of episodes and length of illness significantly improved when the illness course was compared to the period prior to treatment. Interestingly, nine of the 'mainly affective' (9/14) and only three of the 'mainly schizophrenic' (3/10) patients responded. When the patients in this study were diagnosed with regard to their affective course, that is, schizodepressive versus schizobipolar, lithium appeared to be very effective in the group of schizobipolar patients ($n = 14$). No improvement, however, could be shown among the 19 patients suffering from a schizodepressive illness.

Baethge and co-workers[19] reported on an observational study at the Berlin Lithium Clinic. Forty-nine schizoaffective patients were followed up for 6.8 years and the illness course was compared to the period before long-term treatment was started. Of the patients, 41 were treated with lithium and eight with carbamazepine. All 49 patients had been diagnosed as schizoaffective according to ICD-10, 34 of whom were also schizoaffective in the terms of DSM-IV. The main purpose of this project was to find predictors of long-term mood stabilizer treatment success or failure. In this sample, however, polarity of schizoaffective disorder (schizobipolar versus schizoaffective) was not associated with treatment outcome and neither were time between onset of the disorder and start of mood stabilizer long-term treatment (latency), severity of illness (as measured in days spent in hospital per year), sex, age at illness onset, family history, or type of treatment (lithium or carbamazepine). However, the study documented successful long-term treatment in a group of patients diagnosed with modern diagnostic criteria over a very long follow-up period: the illness course improved dramatically (number of hospitalized days declined from 71 to 11 days per year). Küfferle and Lenz[30], in another observational study, found formal thought disturbances and schizophrenic symptoms to be associated with a worse outcome in a group of patients with schizoaffective disorder according to ICD-9.

LITHIUM IN THE LONG-TERM TREATMENT OF SCHIZOAFFECTIVE DISORDER – CONCLUSIONS

One of the most important findings of this overview is that there are no placebo-controlled studies with lithium in schizoaffective patients. Unfortunately, the lack of placebo studies applies also to other mood stabilizers and to antipsychotics[4].

Therefore, the evidence that lithium works at all in SAD is derived from six prospective mirror-image studies involving 242 lithium patients with an average follow-up time of 1.4 years (range 0.9–2.3). Only one study ($n = 33$) used modern diagnostic criteria; the remaining were carried out before operationalized criteria came into use. In addition, ten further studies ($n = 321$), most of them retrospective, compared the time span of lithium treatment with the period of no treatment and found evidence for lithium's efficacy in this group of patients. Three of those studies employed RDC, ICD-10, or DSM-IV. In the vast majority of the studies lithium was administered as the sole medication. The authors are not aware of studies using the mirror image methodology or any other kind of before and after comparison that yielded negative results concerning lithium's efficacy or effectiveness in SAD long-term treatment.

Most of the studies reported on SAD patients as part of a larger study sample also comprised bipolar disorder patients. In eight studies, the outcome of SAD patients was compared to that of the bipolar patients; five studies showed that lithium worked better in bipolar patients, whereas three reported the opposite result.

There is evidence from three studies[14,15,30] that lithium does not work well in SAD patients with predominant schizophrenic symptoms.

The only study, albeit small, that compared lithium with an antipsychotic showed lithium to be inferior in this subgroup[14]. However, the data from the mirror image studies in predominantly affective patient samples indicate that a comparison between lithium and an antipsychotic could yield different results in a sample balanced with regard to schizophrenic and affective psychopathology.

Also, two studies[8,15] indicated that lithium works better in preventing schizomania than in preventing schizodepression. One study[19], however, could not corroborate this finding. Other studies have shown that schizodepressive patients constitute a subgroup that is particularly difficult to treat[4]. Therefore, the results of Greil and co-workers merit particular attention; they found that, in schizodepressives, carbamazepine appeared to be superior to lithium. As regards the comparison of lithium[8] and carbamazepine, the results of the two controlled studies[8,36] indicate that they have similar efficacy in SAD in general. In contrast, the available data are not sufficient to recommend valproate for SAD long-term treatment because, to the knowledge of the authors, there are only four schizoaffective patients in the English and German literature, who underwent valproate monotherapy[35]. However, in this study, the clinical course of those patients is not documented in detail.

In conclusion, in terms of evidence-based medicine, there is level 2b and 2c evidence of lithium's efficacy in the long-term treatment of SAD (as defined by the Oxford Centre for Evidence-Based Medicine). On the other hand, with 16 studies indicating efficacy or effectiveness of lithium among predominantly affective SAD patients, many clinicians would consider it unethical to perform a placebo-controlled study with lithium in SAD patients. What is clearly warranted, however, is a comparison of lithium, and perhaps also carbamazepine, with an antipsychotic in a sample of SAD patients that is balanced in terms of 'mainly affective' and 'mainly schizophrenic' participants.

It seems justified from the data at hand to use lithium as a first-line long-term treatment in predominantly affective schizoaffective patients. This applies particularly to patients with a mainly schizomanic course. In patients with a mainly schizodepressive course of the illness, a trial with carbamazepine appears reasonable. For mainly schizophrenic SAD patients, lithium is not a first-line option. Here, antipsychotics are the long-term treatment of choice.

LITHIUM FOR THE TREATMENT OF ACUTE SCHIZOAFFECTIVE EPISODES

Most of the trials on the acute treatment of SAD were conducted before the diagnostic criteria mentioned above had been published (Table 12.4). The only placebo-controlled study[39] showed that lithium was superior to placebo in mainly schizoaffective patients. In the first – and smallest – of three studies comparing lithium with chlorpromazine in SAD patients, Johnson et al.[37] found that among 'excited schizoaffective' (today likely to be considered schizomanic patients), lithium was inferior to chlorpromazine with regard to Brief Psychiatric Rating Scale (BPRS) and Clinical Global Impression (CGI) ratings after 3 weeks. However, larger studies by Prien and co-workers[40] and by Brockington and co-workers[38] came to a different conclusion. Prien and co-workers[40] compared lithium and chlorpromazine in a group of 83 excited schizoaffective patients according to the authors' diagnoses. The authors divided the sample with regard to their excitation into a 'highly active' group and a 'mildly active' group. Owing to a high rate of drop-outs of lithium patients in the 'highly active' group, chlorpromazine was superior after 3 weeks of treatment (regarding several ratings, e.g. the BPRS). On the other hand, both compounds were similarly effective in the mildly affected subsample. Most of the treatment-related drop-outs in the lithium group occurred during the first 10 days of therapy. This observation points to the lag time between administering lithium and the onset of its effect. Braden and co-workers[41], in a 4-week RDC-based study of 31 SAD patients, also found similar effectiveness of lithium and CPZ, except for highly active partients; the latter responded better to CPZ. In summary, lithium appears to be a treatment option in acute SAD as long as the patients are not too excited.

Table 12.4 Acute treatment of schizoaffective disorder (SAD) with lithium

	No. of patients	Methods	Medications	Result
Johnson et al. 1971[37]	13	db RCT	Li vs. CPZ	Chlorpromazine superior
Prien et al. 1972	83	sb RCT	Li vs. CPZ	CPZ superior in highly active SAD patients (high rate of lithium drop-outs in this group); both compounds similar with regard to mildly active SAD patients
Brockington et al. 1978[38]	19	sb RCT	Li vs. CPZ	Both treatments equally effective
Alexander et al. 1979[39]	8	db	Li vs. placebo	Lithium superior

Db, double blind; RCT, randomized controlled trial; sb, single blind; Li, lithium; CPZ, chlorpromazine

Apart from the impression that lithium seems to be far more useful in mainly affective schizoaffectives, in particular in mainly affective schizomanic patients, we do not know much about predictors of lithium treatment success in SAD. Nevertheless, it might prove clinically valuable to treat particularly mainly affective SAD patients with a family history of bipolar disorder and an episodic (as opposed to a chronic) illness course. However, it has to be kept in mind that this is an analogy to bipolar disorder[42]. Among other clinical characteristics that suggest a consideration of lithium, suicidality should be particularly mentioned[43,44].

With regard to atypical antipsychotics, probably the group of substances most frequently used today in SAD treatment, there are no comparisons with lithium. The same applies to anticonvulsants. In fact, there are only few data supporting the common use of anticonvulsants in this area. Data for valproate are naturalistic[45,46]. For a long time, lamotrigine has been reported to be possibly helpful, for example in three schizoaffective patients documented by Erfurth et al.[47]. An interesting finding from a family study has been published, indicating that bipolar lamotrigine responders had relatives who were schizoaffective significantly more often than were bipolar lithium responders[42]. However, no controlled study has been published to date.

COMBINATIONS IN ACUTE TREATMENT OF SCHIZOAFFECTIVE DISORDER

As for the combination of lithium and antipsychotics, the results are unequivocal: Biederman and co-workers[48] as well as Carman and co-workers[49] found evidence for the superiority of the combination as compared to antipsychotics alone. Both groups had diagnosed their patients

using RDC. It is noteworthy that in Biederman's study both the mainly affective SAD patients and the predominantly schizophrenic SAD patients responded as defined by the BPRS score. However, in the latter group, comprising only 13 participants, the result did not quite reach statistical significance ($p = 0.06$). In a more recent RCT, lithium (or placebo) was combined with clozapine in ten schizophrenic and ten SAD patients. The combination proved to be very well tolerated and, in the SAD subgroup, the lithium patients improved on the CGI, on the Positive and Negative Syndrome Scale (PANSS) total, on negative symptom scales, and on various cognitive measures. A study by Small and co-workers[50] added further support to these findings. The authors found that, among schizoaffective patients ($n = 10$) who were treated with lithium and clozapine as compared with a clozapine–placebo combination, the schizophrenic patients ($n = 10$) did not benefit from the combination.

The observations cited above are in keeping with a recent Cochrane review by Leucht et al.[51], who reported that there is 'inconsistent evidence' that lithium augmentation to ongoing antipsychotic treatment is superior to antipsychotic treatment alone among patients with schizoaffective disorders. However, this study revealed also that more patients dropped out in the combination groups. This highlights the fact that benefits and side-effects of a combination must be carefully pondered before treatment, and closely monitored during an add-on trial.

To the knowledge of the authors, there are no convincing data indicating that lithium is a powerful monotherapy in acute schizo-depression, notably one of the most difficult to treat conditions in psychiatry[4,52,53]. It seems plausible to use antidepressants in combination with antipsychotics. However, in the schizo-depressive patients of the study by Brockington et al.[38] mentioned above, amitriptyline plus chlorpromazine was not superior to placebo plus chlorpromazine. Also, in another study of 58 depressed patients meeting RDC criteria for schizoaffective disorder, haloperidol plus placebo was superior to the combination of the antipsychotic with either amitriptyline or desipramine. Müller-Siecheneder et al.[54] found no superiority of haloperidol plus amitriptyline over risperidone monotherapy in 46 patients diagnosed with SAD, of the depressed type.

There are preliminary data from one RCT that adding lithium to antipsychotics might be of benefit for depressed mainly schizophrenic depressed SAD patients[55]. Preliminary data regarding olanzapine indicated that this drug might be of benefit for schizodepressed patients when compared to haloperidol[56].

In summary, most of the data on lithium as monotherapy in schizomanic patients indicate that lithium is as effective as chlorpromazine except in the group of highly excited patients. In this group of patients the time until lithium becomes effective is probably too long to keep the patients in treatment. Therefore, patients in this subgroup should not be treated with lithium as a monotherapy. In moderately excited patients lithium is a considerable treatment option, in particular because, in mainly affective SAD patients, it is also a powerful long-term treatment. Therefore, even in highly excited mainly affective SAD patients lithium should be considered as an add-on medication. In the light of the limited data at hand for predominantly schizophrenic SAD patients the first-line treatments are antipsychotics, alone or in combination with lithium.

The treatment of schizoaffective disorder is remarkably poorly studied, in particular compared with schizophrenia and with bipolar disorder. Randomized controlled trials are lacking, in particular studies that test antipsychotics versus mood stabilizers, the most promising of which being lithium so far. Also, given the difficulties with reliably diagnosing SAD and the wide spectrum of SAD sympto-matology it will be of great importance to describe the psychopathology of the study participants in the most accurate way. In the absence of those studies the acute and long-term treatment of schizoaffective patients is very challenging for the psychiatrist. It is important to determine whether the schizoaffective disorder is mainly affective or mainly schizo-phrenic. Also, the often variable course of the patients has to be monitored closely without changing the prophylactic treatment too quickly.

LITHIUM IN SCHIZOPHRENIA

The following overview is based on a Medline (1966 to July 2005) search using the terms 'schizophrenia' and 'lithium'. Owing to the lack of double-blind, placebo-controlled mono-therapy trials, other articles were also taken into account – for example, those on randomized add-on treatment with lithium and consecutive studies (Table 12.5)[39,51,55,57–67].

As one of the first reports, in 1967 Gjessing published on lithium as a therapy for a patient with periodic catatonia[68]. He posited that a periodic catatonic course or prominent affective symptoms were indications for the use of lithium in schizophrenic patients. In keeping with this opinion, Weizsäcker et al.[59] reported on the successful treatment of two patients with periodic catatonia. Prakash[60] published two cases of patients suffering from paranoid schizophrenia, chronic subtype (DSM III), who improved during lithium treatment and experienced a relapse when lithium was with-drawn. The authors proposed that paraphrenia, a diagnostic subtype of the Leonhard's criteria, might help to differentiate lithium responders from non-responders because of the sensitivity of these patients to lithium.

Lithium monotherapy for DSM II schizo-phrenic patients was investigated by Alexander

Table 12.5 Acute treatment of schizophrenia with lithium

	Methods	Treatment	n	Remarks
Alexander et al., 1979[39]	db 3 weeks	13/7 Li	13	Positive
Delva et al., 1982[57]	Li withdrawal		6	2 of 6 relapsed
Delva et al., 1982[58]	Rev			Positive in some
Weizsäcker et al., 1984[59]	Case reports		2	Periodic catatonia
Prakash, 1985[60]	On/off		2	Positive, Leonhard criteria
Lerner et al., 1988[55]	db 8 weeks add-on	Hal + Li/PLC	36	Positive in baseline more depressed
Atre-Vaidya, 1989[61]	Rev			Positive in some
Collins, 1991[62]	sb 4 weeks add-on	Severe	44	No improvement; 21 finished
Schulz et al., 1999[63]	db 8 weeks + ol	Depot + Li/PLC	41	Negative for poorly responsive patient
Wilson, 1993[64]	db 8 weeks add-on	Hal + Li/PLC	21	Negative in non-responsive patient
Schexnayder et al., 1995[65]	Consecutive	Sch + schform	66	Predictors of response
Terao et al., 1995[66]	db 8 weeks add-on		21	Positive, SANS no improvement
Simhandl et al., 1996[67]	db 8 weeks add-on	Li/CBZ/PLC	42	13 on Li, improvement on CGI
Leucht et al., 2004[51]	Meta-analysis		611	Positive in some add-on

db, double blind; ol, open label; li, lithium; hal, haloperidol; PLC, placebo; sch + schform, schizophrenia and schizophreniform; sb, single blind; CBZ, carbamazepine; SANS, Scale for the Assessment of Negative Symptoms

and co-workers[39] in a double-blind setting. Eight of 13 patients had an RDC diagnosis of a schizoaffective disorder (see above). Seven out of 13 improved and four of the seven patients relapsed after lithium withdrawal. There were no predictors for treatment success except for response in the first week.

Schexnayder et al.[65] carried out a therapeutic trial in 66 patients with schizophrenia and schizophreniform disorder (DSM III, RDC) with lithium alone. The authors applied various response criteria after 10 and 14 days of treatment, respectively. Ten patients were considered as responders, as shown in an improvement of negative symptoms. It is noteworthy that among the responders, there was no family history of schizophrenic spectrum disorder. Collins and co-workers[62] found no improvement after adding lithium to neuroleptic medication in their 4-week single-blind, randomized, placebo-controlled trial in 44

severely psychotic patients (DSM-III-R schizophrenia). In a similar vein, Wilson[64] reported on an 8-week double-blind, placebo-controlled study in patients with chronic schizophrenia (DSM-III-R). The addition of lithium (0.98 ± 0.13 mEq/l) to stable haloperidol (13.6 ± 8.1 mg/day) was not superior to haloperidol monotherapy. A somewhat different result was found in a study by Terao and co-authors[66]: The authors studied the effect of adding lithium to antipsychotic treatment using a randomized, double-blind, placebo-controlled, cross-over design over 8 weeks in 21 chronic schizophrenic patients with constant additional medication. Among 18 patients who completed the trial a significant improvement in the BPRS anxiety–depression subscore was observed.

Lerner[55], already mentioned above with regard to schizoaffective disorder, treated patients with schizophrenia and mainly schizophrenic schizoaffective disorder (RDC) with haloperidol. After 2 weeks, lithium was added under randomized placebo-controlled conditions for the duration of 6 weeks. When DSM-III criteria were applied to the same patient group, 28 patients out of the 36 who entered the trial met the diagnosis of schizophrenia. The group with the higher BPRS depression–anxiety baseline score needed higher haloperidol doses and responded to lithium.

Simhandl et al.[67] reported on a double-blind, controlled study with treatment-resistant chronic schizophrenic patients receiving neuroleptic medication. Lithium, carbamazepine or placebo was administered over 6 weeks. BPRS scores improved in all three groups. Regarding the CGI severity score, patients taking lithium or carbamazepine showed a significant improvement compared with those on placebo. Schulz et al.[63] investigated 41 patients (schizophrenic, 31 and schizoaffective, ten) in a double-blind augmentation trial (to ongoing neuroleptic treatment). Results were presented only for the whole group. The study revealed no effects of lithium on BPRS and HAM-D scores. In an open-label trial in addition following the double-blind phase, the patients showed no improvement.

A review by Delva and Letemendia[58] summarized their findings thus: 'a surprisingly high proportion (40–55%) of those diagnosed as schizophrenic without affective overlay or excitement also respond to lithium'. Delva and Letemendia concluded that lithium can be used safely at usual serum levels at least for short-term treatment. The same authors reported on a lithium withdrawal trial in six schizophrenic patients who, in addition to antipsychotics, were treated with lithium for at least 2 years. Two patients displayed a relapse within 2 weeks. The remaining four patients had no relapse after 1 year of follow-up[57].

In another review, Atre-Vaidya and Taylor[61] found seven controlled short-term studies in the literature: three studies compared lithium and placebo alone, two studies compared lithium with chlorpromazine and two augmentation studies were of neuroleptic treatment. They also emphasized diagnostic problems and that fulfilling diagnostic criteria for schizophrenia alone did not predict a response or give justification for the use of lithium. Affective symptoms, previous affective episodes and a family history of affective disorder may predict a favorable response to lithium even if the diagnosis of schizophrenia is fulfilled and there is no full affective syndrome. A recent meta-analysis by Leucht and co-authors[51] summarizing 20 controlled studies used the following main outcome parameters: a clinically significant response and the number of patients leaving the study early. Studies covering 611 patients were included and showed insufficient evidence for lithium as an effective monotherapy for the acute treatment of schizophrenia. It was concluded from augmentation trials that more patients with lithium augmentation were classified as responders than those with neuroleptic treatment alone. However, when patients with affective symptoms were excluded from the analysis, lithium augmentation was not significantly related to a positive outcome ($p = 0.07$).

In summary, the data published to date indicate that lithium monotherapy is not well supported for schizophrenic patients. Regarding the use of lithium as an augmentation to antipsychotic treatment the study results are inconsistent. Several studies – and, in part, consequently one meta-analysis – revealed that about one-third of the patients might benefit from lithium augmentation to ongoing neuroleptic treatment. A positive family history of affective disorder, absence of positive family history of schizophrenic spectrum disorders, current affective symptomatology as well as previous affective episodes or higher depression scores might identify patients who would respond to lithium augmentation. All data refer to a relatively short period of time: from 2 to 8 weeks. There are no data available for long-term use in schizophrenia.

REFERENCES

1. Angst J, Preisig M. Outcome of a clinical cohort of unipolar, bipolar and schizoaffective patients. Results of a prospective study from 1959 to 1985. Schweiz Arch Neurol Psychiatrie 1995; 146: 17–23

2. Müller-Oerlinghausen B, Ahrens B, Grof E, et al. The effect of long-term lithium treatment on the mortality of patients with manic–depressive and schizoaffective illness. Acta Psychiatr Scand 1992; 86: 218–22

3. Kasanin J. The acute schizo-affective psychoses. Am J Psychiatry 1933; 57: 41–8

4. Baethge C. The long-term treatment of schizoaffective disorder: review and recommendations. Pharmacopsychiatry 2003; 36: 45–56

5. American Psychiatric Association. Diagnostic and Statistical Manual of S, 3rd edn., revised (DSM-III-R). Washington, DC: APA, 1987

6. American Psychiatric Association. Diagnostic and Statistical Manual of Mental Disorders, 4th edn. (DSM-IV). Washington, DC: APA, 1994

7. World Health Organization. The ICD-10 Classification of Mental and Behavioural Disorders. Clinical Descriptions and Diagnostic Guidelines. Geneva: WHO, 1992

8. Greil W, Ludwig-Mayerhofer W, Erazo N, et al. Lithium vs carbamazepine in the maintenance treatment of schizoaffective disorder: a randomised study. Eur Arch Psychiatry Clin Neurosci 1997; 247: 42–50

9. Maj M, Pirozzi R, Formicula RM, et al. Reliability and validity of the DSM-IV diagnostic category of schizoaffective disorder: Preliminary data. J Affect Disord 2000; 57: 95–8

10. Faraone SV, Blehar M, Pepple J, et al. Diagnostic accuracy and confusability analyses: an application to the Diagnostic Interview for Genetic Studies. Psychol Med 1996; 26: 401–10

11. Williams PV, McGlashan TH. Schizoaffective psychosis. I. Comparative long-term outcome. Arch Gen Psychiatry 1987; 44: 130–7

12. Rosenthal NE, Rosenthal LN, Stallone F, et al. Toward the validation of RDC schizoaffective disorder. Arch Gen Psychiatry 1980; 37: 804–10

13. Sarantidis D, Waters B. Predictors of lithium prophylaxis effectiveness. Prog Neuro-psychopharmacol 1981; 5: 507–10

14. Mattes JA, Nayak D. Lithium versus fluphenazine for prophylaxis in mainly schizophrenic schizo-affectives. Biol Psychiatry 1984; 19: 445–9

15. Maj M. Lithium prophylaxis of schizoaffective disorders: a propspective study. J Affect Disord 1988; 14: 129–35

16. Minnai GP, Tundo A. Effects of lithium on the course and symptoms of schizo-affective disorder. Lithium 1990; 1: 191–3

17. Grossman LS, Harrow M, Goldberg JF, Fichtner CG. Outcome of schizoaffective disorder at two long-term follow-ups: comparison with outcome of schizophrenia and affective disorders. Am J Psychiatry 1991; 148: 1359–65

18. Grossman L, Harrow M, Lechert F, Meltzer HY. The longitudinal course of schizoaffective disorders. J Nerv Ment Dis 1984; 172: 140–9

19. Baethge C, Gruschka P, Berghöfer A, et al. Prophylaxis of schizoaffective disorder with lithium or carbamazepine: outcome after long-term follow-up. J Affect Disord 2004; 79: 43–50

20. Baastrup PC, Schou M. Lithium as a prophylactic agent. Arch Gen Psychiatry 1967; 16: 162–72

21. Angst J, Dittrich A, Grof P. Course of endogenous affective psychoses and its modification by prophylactic administration of imipramine and lithium. Int Pharmacopsychiatry 1969; 2: 1–11

22. Angst J, Weis P, Grof P, et al. Lithium prophylaxis in recurrent affective disorders. Br J Psychiatry 1970; 116: 604–13

23. Hofmann G, Kremser M, Katschnig H, Schreiber V. Prophylaktische Lithiumtherapie bei manisch-depressivem Krankheitsgeschehen und bei Legierungspsychosen. Int Pharmacopsychiat 1970; 4: 187–93

24. Aronoff MS, Epstein RS. Factors associated with poor response to lithium carbonate: a clinical study. Am J Psychiatry 1970; 127: 472–480

25. Egli H. Erfahrungen mit der Lithium-prophylaxe phasischer affektiver Erkrankungen in einer psychiatrischen Poliklinik. Schweiz Med Wochenschr 1971; 101: 157–64

26. Prien RF, Caffey EM, Klett J. Factors associated with treatment success in lithium carbonate prophylaxis. Arch Gen Psychiatry 1974; 31: 189–92

27. Smulevitch AB, Zavidovskaya GI, Igonin AL, Mikhailova NM. The effectiveness of lithium in affective psychoses. Br J Psychiatry 1974; 125: 65–72

28. Tress W, Haag H. Vergleichende Erfahrungen mit der rezidivprophylaktischen Lithium-Langzeitmedikation bei schizoaffektiven Psychosen. Nervenarzt 1979; 50: 524–6

29. Perris C, Smigan L. The use of lithium in the long term morbidity suppressive treatment of cycloid and schizoaffective psychoses. 7th World Congress of Psychiatry. Pharmaco-psychiatry 1983; 3: 375–80

30. Küfferle B, Lenz G. Classification and course of schizo-affective psychoses. Psychiatr Clin 1983; 16: 169–77

31. Emrich HM, Dose M, von Zerssen D. The use of sodium valproate, carbamazeoine and oxcarbazepine in patients with affective disorders. J Affect Disord 1985; 8: 243–50

32. Romeo R, Bastianello S, Janiri L, et al. Slow-release lithium in the treatment of schizo-affective syndromes. Int J Clin Pharm Res 1985; 5: 205–11

33. Bouman TK, Niemantsverdriet-van Kampen JK, Ormel J, Sloof CJ. The effectiveness of lithium prophylaxis in bipolar and unipolar depressions and schizo-affective disorders. J Affect Disord 1986; 11: 275–80

34. Koufen H, Consbruch U. Langzeitkatamnese zur Frage von Nutzen und Nebenwirkungen der Lithiumprophylaxe der phasischen Psychosen. Fortschr Neurol Psychiat 1989; 57: 374–82

35. Hayes SG. Long-term use of valproate in primary psychiatric disorders. J Clin Psychiatry 1989; 50 (Suppl 3): 35–9

36. Bellaire W, Demisch K, Stoll KD. Carbamazepin vs. lithium. Münch Med Wochenschr 1990; 132 (Suppl 1): S82–S86

37. Johnson G, Gershon S, Burdock EI, et al. Comparative effects of lithium and chlor-promazine in the treatment of acute manic states. Br J Psychiatry 1971; 119: 267–76

38. Brockington IF, Kendell RE, Kellet JM, et al. Trials of lithium, chlorpromazine and amitriptyline in schizoaffective patients. Br J Psychiatry 1978; 133: 162–8

39. Alexander PE, van Kammen DP, Bunney WE. Antipsychotic effects of lithium in schizophrenia. Am J Psychiatry 1979; 136: 283–7

40. Prien RF, Caffey EM Jr, Klett CJ. A comparison of lithium carbonate and chlorpromazine in the treatment of excited schizo-affectives. Arch Gen Psychiatry 1972; 27: 182–9

41. Braden W, Fink EB, Quals CB, et al. Lithium and chlorpromazine in psychotic inpatients. Psychiatry Res 1982; 7: 69–81

42. Passmore MJ, Garnham J, Duffy A, et al. Phenotypic spectra of bipolar disorder in responders to lithium versus lamotrigin. Bipolar Disord 2003; 5: 110–14

43. Baldessarini RJ, Tondo L, Hennen J. Lithium treatment and suicide risk in major affective disorders: update and new findings. J Clin Psychiatry 2003; 64 (Suppl 5): 44–52

44. Müller-Oerlinghausen B, Felber W, Berghöfer A, et al. The impact of lithium long-term medication on suicidal behavior and mortality of bipolar patients. Arch Suicide Res 2005; 9: 307–19

45. Bogan AM, Brown ES, Suppes T. Efficacy of divalproex therapy for schizoaffective disorder. J Clin Psychopharmacol 2000; 20: 520–2

46. Basan A, Leucht S. Valproate for schizophrenia. Cochrane Database Syst Rev 2004; 1: CD004028

47. Erfurth A, Walden J, Grunze H. Lamotrigine in the treatment of schizoaffective disorder. Neuropsychobiology 1988; 38: 204–5

48. Biederman J, Lerner Y, Belmaker R. Combination of lithium carbonate and haloperidol in schizoaffective disorder. A controlled study. Arch Gen Psychiatry 1979; 36: 327–33

49. Carman JS, Bigelow LB, Wyatt RJ. Lithium combined with neuroleptics in chronic schizophrenic and schizoaffective patients. J Clin Psychiatry 1981; 42: 124–8

50. Small JG, Klapper MH, Malloy FW, Steadman TM. Tolerability and efficacy of clozapine combined with lithium in schizophrenia and schizoaffective disorder. J Clin Psychopharmacol 2003; 23: 223–8

51. Leucht S, Kissling W, McGrath J. Lithium for schozophrenia revisited: a systematic review and meta-analysis of randomized controlled trials. J Clin Psychiatry 2004; 65: 2: 177–86

52. McElroy SL, Keck PE, Strakowski SM. An overview of the treatment of schizoaffective disorder. J Clin Psychiatry 1999; 60 (Suppl 5): 16–21

53. Levinson DF, Umapathy C, Musthaq M. Treatment of schizoaffective disorder and schizophrenia with mood symptoms. Am J Psychiatry 1999; 156: 1138–48

54. Müller-Siecheneder F, Müller MJ, Hillert A, et al. Risperidone versus haloperidol and amitriptyline in the treatment of patients with a combined psychotic and depressive syndrome. J Clin Psychopharmacol 1998; 18: 111–20

55. Lerner Y, Mintzer Y. Lithium combined with haloperidol in schizophrenia patients. Br J Psychiatry 1988; 153: 359–62

56. Tran PV, Tollefson GD, Sanger TM, et al. Olanzapine versus haloperidol in the treatment of schizoaffective disorder. Br J Psychiatry 1999; 4: 15–22

57. Delva NJ, Letemendia FJJ, Prowse AW. Lithium withdrawal trial in chronic schizophrenia. Br J Psychiatry 1982; 141: 401–6

58. Delva NJ, Letemendia FJJ. Lithium treatment in schizophrenia and schizo-affective disorder. Br J Psychiatry 1982; 141: 387–400

59. Weizsäcker M, Wöller W, Tegeler J. Lithium in der Behandlung periodisch auftretender katatoner Erregungszustände bei Schizophrenien. Nervenarzt 1984; 55: 382–4

60. Prakash R. Lithium-responsive schizophrenia: case reports. J Clin Psychiatry 1985; 46: 141–2

61. Atre-Vaidya N, Taylor MA. Effectiveness of lithium in schizophrenia: do we really have an answer? J Clin Psychiatry 1989; 50: 170–3

62. Collins PJ, Larkin EP, Shubsachs APW. Lithium carbonate in chronic schizophrenia – a brief trial of lithium carbonate added to neuroleptics for treatment of resistant schizophrenic patients. Acta Psychiatr Scand 1991; 84: 150–4

63. Schulz SC, Thompson PA, Jacobs M, et al. Lithium augmentation fails to reduce symptoms in poorly responsive schizophrenic outpatients. J Clin Psychiatry 1999; 60: 366–72

64. Wilson WH. Addition of lithium to haloperidol in non-affective, antipsychotic non-responsive schizophrenia: a double blind, placebo controlled, parallel design clinical trial. Psychopharmacology 1993; 111: 359–66

65. Schexnayder LW, Hirschowitz J, Sautter FJ, Garver DL. Predictors of response to lithium in patients with psychoses. Am J Psychiatry 1995; 152: 1511–13

66. Terao T, Oga T, Nozaki S, et al. Lithium addition to neuroleptic treatment in chronic schizophrenia: a randomized, double-blind, placebo-controlled, cross-over study. Acta Psychiatr Scand 1995; 92: 220–4

67. Simhandl C, Meszaros K, Denk E, et al. Adjunctive carbamazepine or lithium carbonate in therapy-resistant chronic schizophrenia. Can J Psychiatry 1996; 41: 317

68. Gjessing LR. Lithium citrate loading of a patient with periodic catatonia. Acta Psychiatr Scand 1967; 43: 372–5

13 Lithium in rapid cycling bipolar disorder

David J Muzina, Michael Bauer, Joseph R Calabrese

Contents Introduction • Historical background for rapid cycling and lithium • Lithium in rapid cycling bipolar disorder • Conclusion

INTRODUCTION

The objective of this chapter is to review the available literature on the use of lithium in the treatment of rapid cycling bipolar disorder with an emphasis on evidence from long-term, randomized controlled trials. Early studies are reviewed that suggested poor response to lithium among rapid cyclers, some characteristics thought to be associated with rapid cycling and potential resistance to treatment, including endocrine and immune factors, and newer evidence supporting an equitable role for lithium in rapid cycling treatment.

HISTORICAL BACKGROUND FOR RAPID CYCLING AND LITHIUM

Early descriptions, definitions and criteria

The first descriptions of a rapid cycling phenomenon, although not termed as such, were originally made by Falret in 1854[1] and by Emil Kraepelin[2]. In his treatise on 'manic-depressive insanity' Kraepelin distinguished manic-depressive illness from the degenerative course of schizophrenia by its periodic cycling and noted that cycling occurred with remarkable frequency (in excess of four per year) in a subgroup of patients with bipolar disorder. It was this observation of various manic-depressive illness courses as forms of a single disease process that led Kraepelin further to describe patients who had only very brief periods of remission between episodes and associated them with poorer prognosis.

Dunner and Fieve[3] first used the term 'rapid cycling' in 1974 in their landmark paper describing clinical factors associated with lithium prophylaxis failure in bipolar disorder: 'patients who had frequent episodes of mania and depression immediately prior to their acceptance into the clinic were termed "rapid cyclers" if they had four or more affective episodes per year.' They reported lithium prophylaxis failure in 18 of 44 (41%) of patients without rapid cycling but a disproportionately higher rate of lithium prophylaxis failure in nine of 11 (82%) rapid cyclers. In a subsequent paper, Dunner *et al.* further detailed their definition of rapid cycling as somewhat arbitrary yet included at least two episodes of mania and two depressions per year[4]. Kukopulos *et al.*[5] replicated and extended their findings through longitudinal study of 434 patients with bipolar disorder, noting lithium prophylaxis failure in 82% of rapid cyclers.

As a result, these early reports and investigations led not only to the recognition and first definitions of 'rapid cycling', but also to the longstanding belief that lithium was ineffective in the treatment of rapid cycling bipolar disorder.

Modern definition and criteria – the DSM

The validity of a rapid cycling course as a distinct modifier for bipolar disorder was first demonstrated only in 1994. This was accomplished as a result of a meta-analysis performed by Bauer and colleagues[6], with differences noted in gender, prospectively assessed outcome and perhaps social class between rapid cycling patients and others. This multi-site data reanalysis showed a relationship of gender to episode frequency that supported the DSM-IV[7] cutoff of four or more episodes that had been discussed in the literature and used in earlier studies[6].

According to DSM-IV-TR, the course specifier of rapid cycling applies to 'at least four episodes of a mood disturbance in the previous 12 months that meet criteria for a Major Depressive, Manic, Mixed, or Hypomanic Episode'[8]. The episodes must be 'demarcated either by partial or full remission for at least 2 months or a switch to an episode of opposite polarity'[8]. Per DSM-IV criteria, many patients with very rapid alteration (over days) between manic symptoms and depressive symptoms who do not meet minimal duration criteria for a

manic episode or a major depressive episode are classified as 'Bipolar Disorder Not Otherwise Specified'. Early studies often employed alternative rapid cycling definitions, suggesting that the DSM-IV and DSM-IV-TR criteria cover only part of a spectrum of rapid cycling conditions[9].

Prevalence of and factors associated with rapid cycling

The percentage of the rapid cycling variant of bipolar disorder has been estimated at 14–53% of patients who have bipolar disorder[3,5,10,11]. Women have consistently been reported to be disproportionately more affected by rapid cycling than men, although a careful meta-analysis of ten studies by Tondo and colleagues suggested that rapid cycling was only moderately more common in bipolar women than men; rapid cycling occurred in 29.6% of women and 16.5% of men[11]. The prevalence of rapid cycling appears to be as low as 4% in bipolar I disorder and as high as 31% in bipolar II disorder[11], although elsewhere an equal frequency in bipolar I and bipolar II disorder has been reported[12,13]. Hypothyroid states may increase both the risk for rapid cycle development in bipolar disorder as well as prophylactic treatment resistance[14].

Tricyclic antidepressants (TCA), and perhaps other drugs that affect monoaminergic neurotransmitter systems, have been implicated in triggering rapid mood cycling[15]. Wehr and colleagues[16] noted that continued administration of antidepressant drugs was responsible for rapid cycling in approximately 50% of 51 bipolar patients. Kukopulos and colleagues[5] demonstrated that antidepressant use caused an acceleration in the cycle frequency from 0.8 per year prior to treatment to 6.5 episodes per year following administration of these drugs. Others have estimated that 20% of all cases of rapid cycling are caused by antidepressant treatment and that 95% of spontaneous rapid cycling patients may worsen with antidepressants, mainly tricyclics[6]. There is some evidence that the newer, more selective antidepressants have a lowered risk of inducing cycling acceleration[17,18].

LITHIUM IN RAPID CYCLING BIPOLAR DISORDER

Early observations led to the conclusion that lithium was ineffective in the treatment of rapid cycling bipolar disorder. Some clinicians and investigators still argue that lithium has poor efficacy in treating rapid cycling bipolar disorder, even with adjunctive treatment with antidepressants or neuroleptics[19,20]. However, other reports have supported lithium efficacy in the treatment of rapid cycling bipolar disorder[21–23] or at least equivalent efficacy with other mood stabilizers[24]. Here we review the evidence regarding the use of lithium in this difficult, often refractory, form of bipolar disorder.

The early work of Dunner, Fieve and colleagues (1974–77)

In an attempt to clarify factors associated with the failure of lithium prophylaxis in all types of bipolar disorder, Dunner and Fieve[3] carried out a placebo-controlled, double-blind maintenance study in a general cohort of 55 patients, of whom 20% were rapid cyclers. Lithium failure was defined in this study as hospitalization for or treatment of mania or depression during lithium therapy or mood symptoms. A disproportionate number of rapid cyclers were represented in the lithium failure group, with 82% (nine of 11) of rapid cyclers failing lithium therapy compared with 41% (18 of 44) of those not experiencing rapid cycling. This led to the conclusion that 'a beneficial effect of lithium

carbonate in rapid cyclers is difficult to demonstrate' and served as the foundation for the clinical belief that lithium is ineffective in rapid cycling bipolar disorder, although it was based on data that included only 11 rapid cyclers.

However, although the majority of patients with rapid cycling continued to be ill after more than 2 years of lithium therapy, the percentage of time spent in remission tended to be greater during periods of lithium treatment than during placebo periods in each patient. A report on the prophylactic effect of lithium in bipolar II disorder in a double-blind placebo-controlled study of 40 outpatients included a small number of rapid cyclers who were noted to stay in the study longer and had fewer hypomanic episodes (but more depressive episodes) than did those who received placebo[25]. A subsequent retrospective chart review of 390 patients seen in this same lithium clinic identified 40 rapid cyclers and observed that most patients treated with lithium experienced a reduction in frequency of mood episodes compared to the frequency at baseline periods[26].

Kukopulos et al., 1980

Kukopulos replicated the findings of Dunner and Fieve in a study of the longitudinal clinical course of 434 bipolar patients[5]. Fifty of these patients were rapid cyclers on continuous lithium therapy for more than 1 year, with poor response in 72% and good-to-partial prophylaxis in only 28%. However, the allowance of concomitant antidepressant medications for intervening depressive episodes may have confounded these results. Indeed, the authors reported that they later 'persuaded 21 of these patients to endure their depressions without the help of antidepressants' with 15 patients reaching stabilization immediately after the untreated depression and only two patients staying unchanged. This effect of slowing or stopping rapid cycling simply through discontinuation of antidepressant medication in bipolar patients has been reported by other investigators, including a 51% stabilization response through antidepressant discontinuation in one study of 51 bipolar rapid cyclers[16].

Okuma, 1993

This retrospective study of 215 bipolar disorder patients treated for more than 2 years with lithium or carbamazepine in Japan examined the characteristics of responders and non-responders to prophylactic monotherapy with either agent and included 91 DSM-III-R-defined rapid cyclers[27]. Patients with current or lifetime history of rapid cycling did worse relative to patients not rapid cycling regardless of assignment to carbamazepine or lithium. This study supports the notion that rapid cycling confers a negative prognostic impact on the course of bipolar illness whatever the treatment offered.

Maj et al., 1998

Maj and colleagues[28] published a 5-year prospective study of lithium therapy in a general cohort of 402 patients with bipolar disorder and noted the absence of rapid cycling in good responders to lithium but an incidence rate of 26% in non-responders to lithium. This study cohort of patients included those with co-morbid disorders (psychiatric, substance use, medical) and permitted concomitant use of other psychotropic drugs, including anti-convulsants. In these complex bipolar patients, those who remained on lithium for several years experienced a remarkable reduction in hospitalization. Although the presence of rapid cycling predicted poor prophylaxis, the authors noted that this variable predicted poor outcome independently of treatment and was not necessarily a true predictor of lithium failure in and of itself.

Tondo et al., 1998

The effects of long-term lithium treatment for bipolar I and bipolar II disorders, including rapid cycling, were compared by Tondo et al. during the time prior to lithium initiation (mean 8.38 years) and the period on lithium maintenance (mean 6.35 years) in 317 patients with DSM-IV-defined bipolar disorder[11]. Of this cohort, 15% demonstrated rapid cycling, which was observed to be 6 times more common in bipolar II than bipolar I disorder. Overall, 50% of all lithium-treated bipolar patients relapsed within 3 years, although the median survival was significantly longer in bipolar II compared to bipolar I patients (8.3 years vs. 1.5 years). The authors concluded that lithium maintenance therapy led to notable reduction of morbidity due to relapsing mood episodes. A more robust effect was observed in bipolar II patients. Potential limitations to this study include sample enrichment, since long-term outcome was assessed in patients known to be responsive to lithium. Despite these limitations this study also offers additional evidence that lithium treatment is not ineffective in rapid cycling bipolar disorder, particularly for type II disorder and when initiated earlier rather than later in the course of illness.

Baldessarini et al., 2000

In a cohort of 360 subjects with DSM-IV bipolar I ($n = 218$) or II ($n = 142$) disorder followed over an average of 13.3 years, bivariate and multivariate techniques were utilized to evaluate factors associated with rapid cycling status and response to lithium maintenance treatment[29]. Women represented 64% of the total population studied. Although the risk for rapid cycling in this overall sample was 15.6%, the risk was 5.1 times greater in subjects with bipolar II versus bipolar I disorder (30.3% vs. 6.0%). A slightly higher rate was observed in women versus men (17.9% vs. 11.5%). The two groups did not differ significantly regarding the time to 50% recurrence risk during treatment and the proportion of subjects showing no improvement in the percentage of time ill during versus before lithium maintenance. Limitations of this study include its naturalistic design, lack of random assignment or blind assessment, and the exclusion of any patient given maintenance treatments other than lithium at any time. Nonetheless, these findings suggest beneficial effects from lithium during the maintenance treatment of even rapid cycling bipolar disorder.

Swann et al., 2000

Previous depressive and manic episodes may have a differential effect on response to treatment with lithium[30]. A total of 372 stabilized patients were randomized to three groups: divalproex, lithium, or placebo. Observations from this study led to the conclusion that a history of at least four previous depressive or 12 previous manic episodes is associated with reduced antimanic response to lithium. Response to lithium, but not to divalproex or placebo, worsened with increased depressive or manic episodes. Having more than 11 manic or four depressive episodes was associated with response to lithium that did not differ from that to placebo. Effects of previous depressive and manic episodes appeared independent and could not be accounted for by increased rapid cycling or mixed states. Although subjects with many episodes had a high incidence of rapid cycling, only one subject with more than 11 manic episodes randomized to lithium had rapid cycling. Therefore, the reduced response to lithium occurred among subjects who were not rapid cyclers, and current rapid cycling did not account for the reduced response to lithium in patients with many previous episodes of

mania or of depression. This cross-sectional dataset cannot distinguish whether this phenomenon represents progressive development of lithium resistance with repeated episodes or indicates that those patients who had frequent episodes were also lithium resistant from the start. The reported increased episodes could be associated with increased incidents of lithium discontinuation, which may have led to neurophysiologic changes adversely affecting response to lithium but not to divalproex. However, a previous favorable response to lithium in the present study predicted a favorable response in the index episode, arguing against loss of lithium response with repeated episodes of treatment. Furthermore, most patients had similar responsiveness to lithium before and after lithium discontinuation.

Kupka et al., 2003 (meta-analysis)

Kupka and colleagues systematically analyzed all studies that made direct comparisons between bipolar disorder that included rapid cycling and bipolar disorder that did not, and utilized clear descriptions of patient characteristics, diagnostic criteria, stated lifetime or current history of rapid cycling, and addressed one or more factors associated with the course of this illness[31]. This meta-analysis was composed of 20 studies including 3709 subjects from five different countries. The prevalence of rapid cycling was approximately 16% and was found to be slightly more common in women and in bipolar type II disorder. Lithium prophylaxis was associated with beneficial effects in rapid cyclers when severity and duration of subsequent episodes were taken into account, with 59% of lithium-treated patients achieving at least 50% improvement. Again, the role of antidepressants must be considered, because in 38% of cases rapid cycling was preceded by their use.

Tondo *et al.*, 2003 (meta-analysis)

Data obtained by Tondo and colleagues[32] from 16 studies involving 1856 bipolar patients (905 rapid cycling, 951 not rapid cycling) were analyzed for effects of rapid cycling and treatment type on clinical outcome. Although only lithium and carbamazepine could be directly compared meta-analytically in rapid cyclers, pooled recurrence rates and non-improvement rates did not suggest any best or superior treatment. Overall, rapid cycling was associated with lower effectiveness of all treatments evaluated.

Calabrese *et al.,* 2005

Calabrese and colleagues[24] aimed to test the hypothesis that divalproex was moderately more effective than lithium in the long-term treatment of rapid cycling bipolar disorder based on a preliminary study[33]. A total of 254 DSM-IV-defined rapid cycling bipolar outpatients without major health problems or drug or alcohol dependence in the prior 6 months were openly prescribed the combination of lithium ($\geq 0.8\,mEq/l$) and divalproex ($\geq 50\,\mu g/ml$) during the initial pre-randomization stabilization phase. Of the patients treated with the combination, 24% stabilized and these responders were entered into the double-blind phase of the trial stratifying for bipolar I and II disorder and lasting 20 months. These stabilized patients met rigorous definitions for response. Randomized patients received either lithium or divalproex monotherapy.

The rate of relapse was 51% on divalproex and 56% on lithium. In both groups, 22% of patients relapsed into manic/mixed states. No statistically significant differences were observed between treatment groups in terms of premature discontinuation due to side-effects, median time to treat emerging symptoms, or

median survival in the study. Neither the time to treatment for a depressive episode (Figure 13.1) nor the time to treatment for a manic, hypomanic, or mixed episode (Figure 13.2) significantly differed between rapid cycling patients treated with lithium or divalproex. A greater number of completers was observed in the divalproex group as significantly more lithium-treated patients experienced tremor, polyuria and polydipsia, which may have led to discontinuation from the study.

The results suggest that both divalproex and lithium are equally efficacious in the long-term management of rapid cycling bipolar disorder. Lithium was not found to be inferior to divalproex, although divalproex exhibited a marginally preferential safety profile, which may make it more effective in some patients based solely on this tolerability advantage.

Hormonal factors associated with rapid cycling and lithium

Thyroid axis abnormalities in rapid cycling bipolar disorder

There is a long debate whether thyroid axis abnormalities may contribute to the development of rapid mood shifts in bipolar patients. Several studies have found an association among indices of low thyroid function and/or clinical hypothyroidism and rapid cycling bipolar disorder[34], while other studies refute this association (for example, reference 35). However, the conclusions to be drawn from these studies are often limited by their retrospective design and frequently the lack of a healthy control comparison group. Most importantly, many of these studies included patients with rapid cycling bipolar disorder who were receiving prophylactic long-term lithium treatment. Cross-sectional studies of unmedicated rapid cycling bipolar patients, on the other hand, found no abnormalities in basal

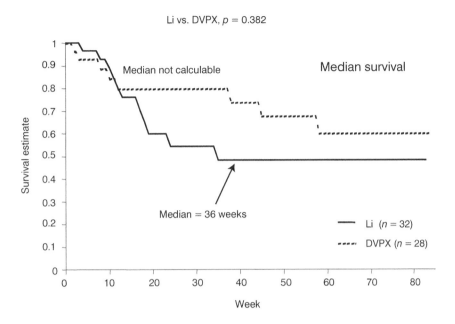

Figure 13.1 Time to treatment for a depressive episode in patients with rapid cycling bipolar disorder treated with lithium (Li) or divalproex (DVPX) (Kaplan–Meier survival curves) (from reference 24, with permission)

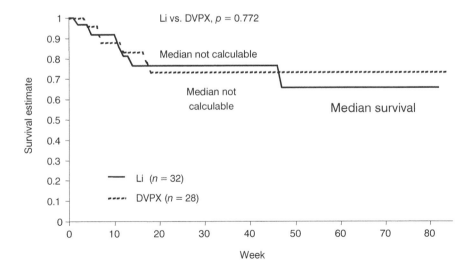

Figure 13.2 Time to treatment for a manic, hypomanic, or mixed episode in patients with rapid cycling bipolar disorder treated with lithium (Li) versus divalproex (DVPX) (Kaplan–Meier survival curves) (from reference 24, with permission)

thyroid stimulating hormone (TSH) and thyroxine levels in this patient population[12,13]. Bauer and colleagues postulated that patients with rapid cycling may manifest no thyroid abnormalities until physiologically challenged by 'antithyroid' stressors. Such stressors may include spontaneously occurring thyroid disease or goiterogenic drugs such as lithium[36] (See Chapter 22).

Consistent with these physiological 'anti-thyroid' actions of lithium, a recent controlled study indicated that short-term treatment with lithium led to diminished thyroid function in rapid cycling bipolar disorder. When previously unmedicated patients were challenged with therapeutic doses of lithium, they were found to have a significantly higher delta TSH level after thyrotropin releasing hormone stimulation than did age- and gender-matched healthy controls who were also treated with lithium[34]. This finding of thyroid hypofunction unmasked by short-term lithium treatment provides a pathophysiologic model that may explain the potential role of the thyroid axis in precipitating the rapid cycling phenotype of bipolar disorder. Under this model, a dysfunction in the hypothalamic-pituitary-thyroid (HPT) system is latent until the axis is challenged by the thyroprivic effect of lithium. These studies again support that changes in the thyroid economy may play a modulating role in affective illness, and specifically in the development of the rapid cycling pattern of bipolar disorder.

Thyroid hormones in lithium-treated patients with mood disorders

Efforts to employ thyroid hormones alone as therapeutic agents in mood disorder, or in other psychiatric disability, have rarely been successful. Nonetheless, a series of open and controlled clinical trials have confirmed the adjunctive therapeutic value of thyroid hormones in refractory mood disorders. Specifically, in a series of open-label studies, adjunctive treatment with supraphysiological doses of L-thyroxine have proven effective and well tolerated in the maintenance treatment of patients suffering the malignant phenotype of rapid cycling and in otherwise prophylaxis-resistant bipolar disorders[13,37,38]. The evidence that high doses of L-thyroxine, when added to the established treatment regimen of patients with rapid cycling bipolar disorder who are refractory to lithium and other psychotropic drugs, can reverse the rapid cycling pattern further, and supports the hypothesis of thyroid metabolism as modulator in affective illness.

CONCLUSION

The summed body of evidence (Table 13.1) does not readily or convincingly support the common clinical assumption that lithium is ineffective or less effective than other agents for rapid cycling bipolar patients. Serious consideration of lithium as a potential first-line prophylactic treatment for rapid cycling bipolar disorder must be made as either monotherapy or more likely combination therapy with other mood stabilizers, particularly emphasizing cautious use versus discontinuation of anti-depressants. Furthermore, given the putative role of the HPT axis in the initiation and/or modulation of affective states along with the knowledge that lithium itself may perturb the axis through induction of relative hypothyroidism, clinicians may consider early co-prescription of thyroid hormone with lithium for the management of rapid cycling bipolar disorder.

In some patients with rapid cycling, simply discontinuing antidepressant drugs may allow lithium to act as a more effective anti-cycling mood-stabilizing agent[16]. The addition of an

Table 13.1 Summary of reports and studies examining lithium in rapid cycling (RC) bipolar disorder (RCBD)

Author(s)	Study	Outcome
Dunner and Fieve, 1974[3]	n = 55 (only 11 with RC) Double-blind, placebo controlled	Although 9 of 11 (82%) rapid cycling patients relapsed on lithium, overall per cent time spent ill was reduced while on lithium compared to placebo
Dunner et al., 1977[26]	n = 390 (40 with RC) Retrospective chart review	Most patients treated with lithium had fewer and less severe mood episodes while on lithium
Kukopulos et al., 1980[5]	n = 434 (50 with RC) Longitudinal follow-up	Although only 28% of RC patients had good/partial prophylaxis on lithium, when antidepressants stopped most stabilized
Okuma, 1993[27]	n = 215 (91 with RC) Retrospective chart review	RC patients had poorer outcomes than non-RC counterparts, whether on lithium or carbamazepine
Maj et al., 1998[28]	n = 402 Prospective study of lithium therapy in a cohort of patients with bipolar disorder	RC absent in bipolar patients deemed good responders to lithium, but observed in 26% of those with poor response. RC predicted poor outcome independent of treatment
Tondo et al., 1998[11]	n = 317 (47 with RC) Comparison of mood state prior to lithium initiation versus time on lithium maintenance	Lithium maintenance reduced morbidity due to relapse in all bipolar patients, although there were more robust effects against mania and hypomania than depression
Baldessarini et al., 2000[29]	n = 360 patients with bipolar I or II disorder followed on average for more than 13 years	Similar morbidity was observed while on lithium in both RC and non-RC cases, arguing against the idea that lithium is less effective in RCBD
Swann et al., 2000[30]	n = 372 stabilized bipolar patients randomized to divalproex, lithium, or placebo	Although response to lithium decreased in patients with increased numbers of past depressive or manic episodes, only one subject randomized to lithium had RCBD
Kupka et al., 2003[31]	n = 3709 (RC prevalence approximately 16%) Meta-analysis of 20 studies that made direct comparisons between RC and non-RCBD	59% of all lithium-treated rapid cyclers achieved at least 50% improvement. A significant association between current RC and hypothyroidism was noted
Tondo et al., 2003[32]	n = 1856 (905 with RC) Meta-analysis	Overall RC was associated with lower effectiveness of all treatments evaluated, not specific to lithium
Calabrese et al., 2005[24]	n = 254 (all with RC) Randomized, 20-month, double-blind, parallel group comparison of divalproex (DVPX) versus lithium (Li)	24% responded to combined lithium and divalproex and entered into double-blind maintenance phase on either DVPX or Li. Although DVPX was better tolerated than Li, rates of relapse were not significantly different in RC patients

anticonvulsant to lithium is a common clinical strategy that has been shown to have benefits for rapid cycling bipolar patients[24,39,40]. In the management of rapid cycling bipolar disorder, lithium should have equal footing with all other available treatments to date, since it appears most likely that this phase of bipolar illness itself is the most significant factor in any treatment's failure, and not a particular therapy such as lithium. This more difficult phase or variant of bipolar disorder most commonly requires clinical pharmacologic management consisting of combinations of medications. The ease and relative safety with which lithium can be added to other drugs such as anticonvulsants makes lithium a valued option for patients with rapid cycling bipolar disorder. Close monitoring for response, side-effects and toxicity is required, with particular attention paid to any disturbance in thyroid functioning. Stabilization of thyroid balance may also contribute to improved mood stability in many rapid cycling patients, especially those on lithium.

REFERENCES

1. Sedler MJ. Falret's discovery: the origin of the concept of bipolar affective illness. Translated by MJ Sedler and Eric C Dessain. Am J Psychiatry 1983; 140: 1127–33
2. Kraepelin E. Psychiatrie III, Klinische Psychiatrie II. Leipzig: Verlag von Johann Ambrosius Barth, 1913
3. Dunner DL, Fieve RR. Clinical factors in lithium carbonate prophylaxis failure. Arch Gen Psychiatry 1974; 30: 229–33
4. Dunner DL, Murphy D, Stallone F, Fieve RR. Episode frequency prior to lithium treatment in bipolar manic–depressive patients. Compr Psychiatry 1979; 20: 511–15
5. Kukopulos A, Reginaldi D, Laddomada P, et al. Course of the manic-depressive cycle and changes caused by treatment. Pharmakopsychiatr Neuropsychopharmakol 1980; 13: 156–67
6. Bauer MS, Calabrese JR, Dunner DL, et al. Multisite data reanalysis of the validity of rapid cycling as a course modifier for bipolar disorder in DSM-IV. Am J Psychiatry 1994; 151: 506–15
7. American Psychiatric Association. Diagnostic and Statistical Manual of Mental Disorders, 4th edn. Washington, DC: American Psychiatric Association, 1994
8. American Psychiatric Association. Diagnostic and Statistical Manual of Mental Disorders, 4th edn. Text Revision. Washington, DC: American Psychiatric Association, 2000
9. Maj M, Pirozzi R, Formicola AM, Tortorella A. Reliability and validity of four alternative definitions of rapid-cycling bipolar disorder. Am J Psychiatry 1999; 156: 1421–4
10. Maj M, Magliano L, Pirozzi R, et al. Validity of rapid cycling as a course specifier for bipolar disorder. Am J Psychiatry 1994; 151: 1015–19
11. Tondo L, Baldessarini RJ, Hennen J, Floris G. Lithium maintenance treatment of depression and mania in bipolar I and bipolar II disorders. Am J Psychiatry 1998; 155: 638–45
12. Bauer MS, Whybrow PC, Winokur A. Rapid cycling bipolar affective disorder. I. Association with grade I hypothyroidism. Arch Gen Psychiatry 1990; 47: 427–32
13. Bauer MS, Whybrow PC. Rapid cycling bipolar affective disorders. II. Treatment of refractory rapid cycling with high-dose levothyroxine: a preliminary study. Arch Gen Psychiatry 1990; 47: 435–40
14. Whybrow PC, Bauer MS, Gyulai L. Thyroid axis considerations in patients with rapid cycling affective disorder. Clin Neuropharmacol 1992; 15 (Suppl 1): 391A–2A
15. Altshuler LL, Post RM, Leverich GS, et al. Antidepressant-induced mania and cycle acceleration: a controversy revisited. Am J Psychiatry 1995; 152: 1130–8
16. Wehr TA, Sack DA, Rosenthal NE, Cowdry RW. Rapid cycling affective disorder: contributing factors and treatment responses in 51 patients. Am J Psychiatry 1988; 145: 179–84
17. Peet M. Induction of mania with selective serotonin re-uptake inhibitors and tricyclic antidepressants. Br J Psychiatry 1994; 164: 549–50

18. Bauer M, Rasgon N, Grof P, et al. Mood changes related to antidepressants: a longitudinal study of patients with bipolar disorder in a naturalistic setting. Psychiatry Res 2005; 133: 73–80

19. Bowden CL. Clinical correlates of therapeutic response in bipolar disorder. J Affect Disord 2001; 67: 257–65

20. Post RM, Frye MA, Denicoff KD, et al. Emerging trends in the treatment of rapid cycling bipolar disorder: a selected review. Bipolar Disord 2000; 2: 305–15

21. Baldessarini RJ, Tondo L, Hennen J, Viguera AC. Is lithium still worth using? An update of selected recent research. Harvard Rev Psychiatry 2002; 10: 59–75

22. Tondo L, Baldessarini RJ, Floris G. Long-term clinical effectiveness of lithium maintenance treatment in types I and II bipolar disorders. Br J Psychiatry 2001; 178: S184–90

23. Viguera AC, Baldessarini RJ, Tondo L. Response to lithium maintenance treatment in bipolar disorders: comparison of women and men. Bipolar Disord 2001; 3: 245–52

24. Calabrese JR, Rapport DJ, Youngstrom EA, et al. New data on the use of lithium, divalproate, and lamotrigine in rapid cycling bipolar disorder. Eur Psychiatry 2005; 20: 92–5

25. Dunner DL, Stallone F, Fieve RR. Lithium carbonate and affective disorders. V: A double-blind study of prophylaxis of depression in bipolar illness. Arch Gen Psychiatry 1976; 33: 117–20

26. Dunner DL, Patrick V, Fieve RR. Rapid cycling manic depressive patients. Compr Psychiatry 1977; 18: 561–6

27. Okuma T. Effects of carbamazepine and lithium on affective disorders. Neuropsychobiology 1993; 27: 138–45

28. Maj M, Pirozzi R, Magliano L, Batoli L. Long-term outcome of lithium prophylaxis in bipolar disorder: a 5-year prospective study of 402 patients at a lithium clinic. Am J Psychiatry 1998; 155: 30–5

29. Baldessarini RJ, Tondo L, Floris G, Hennen J. Effects of rapid cycling on response to lithium maintenance treatment in 360 bipolar I and II disorder patients. J Affect Disord 2000; 61: 13–22

30. Swann AC, Bowden CL, Calabrese JR, et al. Mania: differential effects of previous depressive and manic episodes on response to treatment. Acta Psychiatr Scand 2000; 101: 444–51

31. Kupka RW, Luckenbaugh DA, Post RM, et al. Rapid and non-rapid cycling bipolar disorder: a meta-analysis of clinical studies. J Clin Psychiatry 2003; 64: 1483–94

32. Tondo L, Hennen J, Baldessarini RJ. Rapid-cycling bipolar disorder: effects of long-term treatments. Acta Psychiatr Scand 2003; 108: 4–14

33. Calabrese JR, Delucchi GA. Spectrum of efficacy of valproate in 55 patients with rapid-cycling bipolar disorder. Am J Psychiatry 1990; 147: 431–4

34. Gyulai L, Bauer M, Bauer MS, et al. Thyroid hypofunction in patients with rapid cycling bipolar disorder after lithium challenge. Biol Psychiatr 2003; 53: 899–905

35. Kupka RW, Nolen WA, Post RM, et al. High rate of autoimmune thyroiditis in bipolar disorder: lack of association with lithium exposure. Biol Psychiatr 2002; 51: 305–11

36. Lazarus JH. The effects of lithium therapy on thyroid and thyrotropin-releasing hormone. Thyroid 1998; 8: 909–13

37. Stancer HC, Persad E. Treatment of intractable rapid-cycling manic-depressive disorder with levothyroxine. Arch Gen Psychiatr 1982; 39: 311–12

38. Bauer M, Berghöfer A, Bschor T, et al. Supraphysiological doses of L-thyroxine in the maintenance treatment of prophylaxis-resistant affective disorders. Neuropsychopharmacology 2002; 27: 620–8

39. Denicoff KD, Smith-Jackson EE, Disney ER, et al. Comparative prophylactic efficacy of lithium, carbamazepine, and the combination in bipolar disorder. J Clin Psychiatry 1997; 58: 470–8

40. Bowden CL, Calabrese JR, McElroy SL, et al. The efficacy of lamotrigine in rapid cycling and non-rapid cycling patients with bipolar disorder. Biol Psychiatry 1999; 45: 953–8

14 Responders to long-term lithium treatment

Paul Grof

Contents   Introduction • Initial challenges • Gathering lithium responders • The importance of clinical profile • Clinical profile: course of illness • Clinical profile: family history • Clinical profile: symptom presentation • Clinical profile: co-morbidity • Childhood recollections • Neurobiological findings • Case histories of lithium responders and non-responders • Selectivity, stability, mortality and side-effects • Children of lithium responders • Misconceptions about lithium and response • Conclusions

INTRODUCTION

Since this book is written primarily for practicing psychiatrists, the emphasis in this chapter is on identifying lithium-responsive patients clinically, differentiating them from patients with other mood disorders, and on providing some background needed for understanding how the response characteristics can be applied in practice.

The chapter focuses exclusively on the response of patients with recurrent mood disorders to long-term lithium treatment. Lithium may provide psychiatric patients with a variety of benefits: stabilization (prophylaxis), antimanic, antidepressive, anti-suicidal, anti-aggressive and antipsychotic action, and augmentation of antidepressants[1]. However, the stabilization by lithium is not only the clinically most important, but also the most striking and relatively specific effect.

Earlier studies attempting to forecast lithium response struggled with obstacles such as spontaneous changes of clinical course, low predictability and huge variability of recurrences, patients' fluctuating compliance with long-term treatment and psychiatrists' changing habits when they diagnose bipolar disorders. Until now stabilization has been the only sufficiently predictable aspect of lithium treatment[2].

Several lessons can be learned from investigating patients who had been markedly ill with a recurrent mood disorder and became stabilized during long-term lithium treatment. For clinical practice it is important to know the clinical profile of patients who should receive lithium prophylaxis as the treatment of choice.

Once this profile is recognized, the response to lithium stabilization becomes so predictable that we have been confidently giving patients with a pronounced profile a 'written guarantee'. Such a guarantee improves the patients' compliance and they report an increased feeling of security.

For research it is important that bipolar patients who demonstrate excellent lithium response are a relatively homogeneous group[3], in contrast to the marked heterogeneity of groups selected simply on the basis of diagnostic criteria. Investigating such a core group of bipolar patients is likely to generate more replicable findings than has usually been obtained from bipolar research. This uniformity of lithium responders is also reflected in the clustering of the response in families[4] and in the observations on the patients' offspring[5,6].

INITIAL CHALLENGES

Many earlier studies investigated the prediction of lithium response but struggled with the task for two main reasons: they overestimated the potential of a primarily laboratory approach to the problem and underestimated the methodological complexities. Biologically oriented psychiatry expanded quickly after 1970, stimulated in particular by the discovery of the stabilizing effect of lithium in mood disorders. The fact that a simple ion could stabilize mood nourished the fantasy that the striking response reflected some underlying biological abnormality that could be picked up by newer laboratory methods, flourishing particularly in neurochemistry and neurophysiology. The resulting studies yielded a number of promising, but not replicable, biological differences between lithium responders and non-responders.

To identify individuals who are unequivocally well because of lithium also turned out to

be an unexpectedly challenging task. In practice we are satisfied if a patient who has been prescribed lithium functions much better. We consider it a poor response if a patient continues having recurrences. Much research into lithium response has been carried out in a similar way, by dividing all lithium-treated patients into responders and non-responders and comparing the two groups. This approach did not succeed because, unfortunately, the reality is more complex. For example, a patient on lithium may fare well because the initial episodes may have had strong reactive triggers and the subsequent long stability is spontaneous, unrelated to lithium treatment. Or, despite having a lithium-responsive illness, the patient may do poorly because of poor compliance with lithium.

It was also not appreciated in earlier studies that there are important methodological differences between assessing the recurrence risk in a large group of patients and in a single individual. In a clinical trial, a sufficiently large group of patients will usually have a sufficiently high average number of previous episodes. It then becomes possible to estimate with reasonable accuracy how many episodes on the average the group would experience during the coming years, if no effective treatment had been given[7,8]. Because the course of untreated illness is extremely variable, the forecast of the expected recurrences in each bipolar patient is much more problematic, particularly after only a few episodes, for example in the early stage of illness.

An individual patient must first experience multiple or frequent episodes before one can count on a significant recurrence risk[9–12]. After only one or two episodes, the risk of another recurrence is highly variable. In some patients a setback will follow shortly. In other patients recurrences will take time to appear. Many years may elapse before a second or third recurrence develops, and such patients remain well even without treatment. This high variability in bipolar course, particularly early in the illness, may lead to misleading interpretations. If, for example, a patient recovers from his first manic episode after treatment with lithium and is then recurrence-free on lithium for 3 years, the clinician often concludes that the patient has responded to lithium. If a patient then suffers a recurrence on lithium, the clinician may assume that lithium is losing its efficacy and will add another medication. Yet, this 3-year-long remission may have been spontaneous and a comprehensive clinical assessment of the patient could show that he has a non-responsive profile and may require a different treatment.

Useful statistical predictions can be made about the average course of bipolar illness in a population of relapsing patients; an individual course is a different matter. The prediction is particularly difficult at the early stage at which physicians now usually intervene. Furthermore, very few clinicians now have the opportunity to see the unfolding of an untreated bipolar illness, and they overestimate their ability to assess the recurrence risk. The capriciousness of bipolar illness often leads to incorrect assumptions about the treatment benefits.

The methodology of research on lithium response must be commensurate with the complexity of the issue. To identify the markers of lithium response, each patient's recurrence risk and treatment adequacy must be carefully evaluated and the data about the clinical profile must be analyzed by multivariate techniques.

GATHERING LITHIUM RESPONDERS

Response and non-response

When we started treating patients with recurrent mood disorders in 1959, the prevailing opinion was that recurrences of mood disorders could not be stopped by any medication. The studies with antidepressants and neuroleptics supported these views[13,14]. It then came as a big surprise that lithium prophylaxis could keep many patients completely well. Equally perplexing was that many patients whose symptoms appeared similar to those of lithium responders failed to stabilize on long-term treatment. These observations raised intriguing questions about the markers of response. To attempt to answer them, we needed to study, prospectively, large samples of lithium responders and non-responders, and we have been accumulating them ever since.

Defining responders

This chapter summarizes long-term, prospective observations of 296 patients who, despite a history of frequently recurring bipolar and unipolar disorders of marked severity, remained well on lithium for many years. The task has been to identify with a high probability those patients who would have been repeatedly ill if untreated but remain well because of lithium. The responder to long-term treatment was therefore defined as a patient who, despite frequent recurrences, remained fully stabilized during adequate lithium treatment. (For research criteria see Table 14.1.) Three years was considered the minimum duration of observation on adequate lithium treatment, but the average duration of treatment in the sample of excellent lithium responders is now approaching 20 years.

The critical elements in defining a responder have been a high risk of further recurrences, given by the patient's history prior to lithium treatment, and a lengthy period of full stability during lithium monotherapy. Supportive evidence may come from therapeutic serum lithium levels during the period of stability, from low serum lithium levels preceding a relapse and from a recurrence within a

Table 14.1   Retrospective criteria of lithium response in research subjects

The criterion A is used to determine an association between clinical improvement and lithium treatment. The criteria B establish whether there is a causal relationship between the improvement and the treatment.

A: Rate the degree of response (activity of the illness while on adequate lithium treatment) on a 10-point scale.

10   complete response, no episodes, no residual symptoms

9   very good response, no major episodes, there may be residual minimal mood or anxiety symptoms (not requiring any intervention)

1–8   incomplete response, but episodes of abnormal moods less frequent compared to the pre-treatment period; rate as a relative decrease in episode frequency

0   no change or increase in episode frequency

B: Rate the degree of confidence about the response – subtract 0, 1 or 2 points for each of the following items:

B1:   *Number of episodes before lithium*
0   4 or more
1   2 or 3 episodes
2   1 episode

B2:   *Frequency of episodes before lithium*
0   average to high, including rapid cycling
1   low, spontaneous remissions of 3 or more years on average
2   1 episode only, risk of recurrence cannot be established

B3:   *Duration of lithium treatment*
0   2 or more years
1   1–2 years
2   less than 1 year

B4:   *Compliance during period(s) of stability*
0   excellent, documented by lithium levels in the therapeutic range
1   good, more than 80% levels in the therapeutic range
2   poor, repeated periods of more than 1 week off lithium, fewer than 80% levels in the therapeutic range

B5:   *Use of additional medication during the period of stability*
0   None except infrequent sleep medication (1 dose per week or less); no other mood stabilizers, antidepressants or antipsychotics for control of mood disorder
1   low-dose antidepressants or antipsychotics as an 'insurance' or prolonged use of sleep medication
2   systematic use of antidepressant or antipsychotic medications or additional mood stabilizers

C: Diagnosis of a mood disorder

Note: This scale should be applied to the period of treatment closest to optimal, i.e. adequate dosage and least use of medications interfering with effect of lithium.

reasonable period of time after lithium discontinuation.

Canadian lithium responders

We collected data on lithium responders, and compared them with non-responders in the Affective Disorders Program at McMaster University in 1968–1988[15–17]. We continued the collection in Ottawa in 1988–2004. All patients in our programs who were suffering from recurrent mood disorders were first treated systematically with monotherapy. For research purposes partial responders and non-compliant patients were carefully excluded. The patient samples collected were otherwise unselected but, owing to the referral pattern, the collection has had an overrepresentation of more severe and possibly fewer responsive patients.

All lithium responders included in family studies met the DSM-IV diagnostic criteria for a major mood disorder. They were interviewed according to the SADS-L format[18] (lifetime version) and the course of illness preceding treatment was described from information obtained from all available sources. Family history was obtained from two or more first-degree relatives in each family, with the aid of SADS-FH[18] (family history version).

European lithium responders

The second half of the cohort was gathered over several years in the European IGSLI centers (IGSLI, International Group for the Study of Lithium-treated patients, see Preface). The goal was to create a large, relatively homogeneous sample suitable particularly for systematic molecular genetic studies, coordinated by Dr. Martin Alda[19–23]. In all IGSLI centers the patients were selected according to the same criteria (Table 14.1). The details of selection and findings have been reported elsewhere (see also Chapter 35)

In Canadian IGSLI centers the response to lithium monotherapy was one of our main research tasks. In the European IGSLI centers the issue of lithium response was not necessarily their long-term preoccupation, and the researchers often had more difficulty with finding patients who met the stringent criteria, mainly because of problems with additional medications. To ensure the uniformity of the Canadian and European patients, I have re-interviewed and tested all English-, German-, Czech- and French-speaking patients. I have also reviewed clinical and research documentation of Swedish-, Danish- and Polish-speaking patients, together with their psychiatrists.

The initial purpose of the IGSLI collection was molecular genetic studies of bipolar disorders. However, since the group of excellent lithium responders is relatively homogeneous, presumably with a uniform set of biological abnormalities underlying the illness, we proceeded to explore their neurochemical and neuropsychological features also in other studies[24,25].

Limitations

In a single patient one can never determine the response with certainty. The analyses of untreated clinical course indicated that over 95% of the patients whom we identified as lithium responders according to the mentioned criteria remained well because of lithium treatment.

Subtypes of lithium responders

In addition to a striking response to lithium prophylaxis, excellent responders share other clinical characteristics, such as complete remission, but they may be less uniform in other characteristics, for instance, acute symptoms.

According to their psychopathology they can be divided into three subgroups:

(1) Bipolar disorder, classic type: the vast majority of our sample;

(2) Bipolar disorder, cycloid type. Over a quarter could be best characterized as suffering from a cycloid type of bipolar illness[26–28];

(3) Pseudounipolar mood disorder: 'hidden bipolar', 'unipolar with hypomanias' not recognized[29].

A group of patients diagnosed according to DSM criteria as suffering from recurrent unipolar disorder and in whom hypomania was missed prior to lithium treatment, or who met the broader criteria for hypomania[29], were included only in some Canadian studies but the group may turn out to be much larger in the future, given the results of recent epidemiological studies[30].

THE IMPORTANCE OF CLINICAL PROFILE

Fewer studies of lithium response focused on clinical than on laboratory variables, but they have been more fruitful. Agreement has been achieved that patients with an episodic, fully remitting course of illness, a family history of manic-depressive illness in first-degree relatives, classical symptoms of mania and freedom from personality disorder respond best to lithium[15,31–37]. Although the hope for a simple laboratory predictor persists, the patient selection and treatment decisions are best based on clinical evaluation. However, to identify a patient who has a very high probability of responding to long-term lithium treatment, it is important to consider the full clinical profile, especially the variables of clinical course and family history. Each of the elements of a clinical profile is important, but none by itself is sufficient to identify the responder.

CLINICAL PROFILE: COURSE OF ILLNESS

Most useful information about lithium responders usually comes from the clinical course of the illness. Various aspects of the course, such as an episodicity, complete remissions free of any psychopathology and polarities starting with mania[2,34,36–40], have all been associated with the response to lithium treatment.

Remission

The most important of all clinical characteristics of lithium responders turned out to be the quality of the remission (interepisodic interval). In the multivariate analyses contrasting excellent lithium responders and clear non-responders, the quality of remission explained most of the variance and was the strongest predictor. Surprisingly, the acute psychopathology on which we ordinarily base our psychiatric diagnosis carried much less weight.

It is difficult to assess the quality of remission in patients whose course became destabilized into continuous or rapid cycling by antidepressants. In such situations the clinician may have to utilize the information prior to the use of antidepressants, or must re-evaluate the patient after discontinuation of the antidepressant.

The completeness of remission is expressed qualitatively in a clinical interview and can be supported quantitatively by psychological testing, with a Minnesota Multiphasic Personality Inventory (MMPI) profile. In a clinical interview carried out outside of the acute episodes, the future lithium responder is free of all psychopathology, affective as well as non-affective, and views the previous episodes of illness as ego-dystonic. However unusual or atypical the acute symptoms, in remission the patients are clear that these were the manifestations of their illness. If they had some psychotic symptoms during episodes, when a psychiatrist interviews them in remission, the psychiatrist does not find them in some way still reflected in the patient's thinking.

It is helpful to support the qualitative clinical evaluation by a quantitative psychological testing. The MMPI profile has been found particularly useful for this purpose[2,15,41]. However, it is important to perform the psychological testing at, or close to, the patient's optimum functioning. In practice one should wait at least a month after the clinical recovery from any acute episode. Otherwise some symptoms tend to 'spill over' from the acute state into the MMPI profile. The clinician may need to follow a patient during remission for a period of time, in order correctly to select the time for the psychological testing and distinguish good responders with a complete remission from patients who experience a functional remission but have persisting or fleeting residual symptoms. In contrast to MMPI profiles which, during acute illness, may change in the same patient every few days, the MMPI profiles obtained at the optimum functioning have been found to be individually reproducible for up to 10 years.

The normal psychological profile (i.e. all MMPI scales having T score less than 70) may be viewed simply as a quantitative confirmation that the patient is in a complete remission, free of any significant residual symptoms. The profile was within normal limits in 96% of tested responders. The 4% of profiles that deviated from the norm may perhaps belong to patients with a very irregular course who, during much longer follow-up, may prove not to be lithium responsive or whose profile may be contaminated by unrelated medical or psychological problems.

Daily subjective ratings of mood, anxiety, energy and sleep may also be helpful when the completeness of free interval is assessed.

The importance of the quality of remission may explain why so many earlier studies failed to find reproducible features of responders. They usually focused either on acute symptoms or on biological variables but left out the critical characteristics of the clinical course.

Unfortunately, psychiatrists are neither trained nor accustomed to evaluate the degree of remission. Many find it therefore difficult to identify potential lithium responders. Training of psychiatrists focuses on acute symptoms in identifying and managing mood disorders; little attention is paid to assessing the quality of remission. When psychiatrists then move to practice, they naturally continue with the same approach. They focus intensely on acutely ill patients but, once these markedly improve, the psychiatrist's attention moves to other clients. However, the information about the quality of the remission is particularly valuable for choosing the medication that will work in long-term stabilization.

Age at onset of the disorder

In our cohort of lithium responders the first identified episode of illness took place when the patients were on average 28 years old (Figure 14.1). This is earlier than we found in our previous studies[42–44], but much later than the findings in recent studies on bipolar spectrum disorders with high co-morbidity[45,46]. The criteria of lithium responders skewed the selection to more severe cases with several frequent previous recurrences and consequently an earlier age of onset.

Age at onset has always been considered one of the important clinical characteristics. Earlier long-term follow-ups of manic-depressive

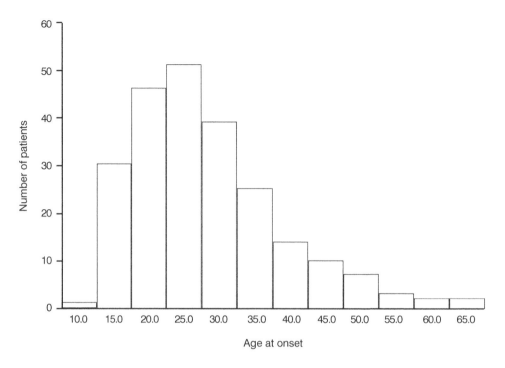

Figure 14.1 Excellent lithium responders. The age of onset at the first diagnosable episode (*n* = 296, mean 28.2 years, SD 10.2)

illness – the predecessor of bipolar disorder – found generally that the average age at onset of the disorder was higher than 30 years. The expanded concept of the bipolar spectrum added many patients with co-morbid conditions and with a much earlier onset, even in their teens.

Pre-lithium patterns of recurrence and polarity

Patterns and polarity of recurrences also add some characteristic features. If the course has already evolved into several recurrences, lithium responders usually experience a predominance of depressions over overactive episodes. The sequence of manic and depressive

phases within the same episode can also be helpful when one evaluates the likelihood of lithium response. Biphasic and multiphasic episodes of lithium responders start more often with mania than with depression[40,47].

However, clinicians must often start lithium treatment before a longer pattern of recurrences is established: the history of patterns and sequences of polarities is rarely documented well enough to be useful in treatment decisions.

Frequency of episodes before lithium treatment

Most lithium responders have experienced two or fewer episodes per year. Rapid or continuous cycling is less common in lithium responders, but a number of patients with rapid cycling responded well to lithium, particularly if rapid cycling was earlier induced by the administration of antidepressants.

This point needs to be stressed, because it has been incorrectly presented in the literature. Antiepileptics are usually recommended as a better treatment than lithium[48], but this conclusion has been drawn when antiepileptics were given to rapid cyclers who failed to respond to lithium. A recent study randomized the rapid cyclers and found lithium and lamotrigine similarly effective[49].

CLINICAL PROFILE: FAMILY HISTORY

To stress the assessment of family history in choosing an effective long-term treatment is not new. Over the years a number of studies recognized the importance of inheritance for lithium response[20,32,33,50-56]. The existence of bipolar disorders among the first-degree relatives is predictive of good response to lithium prophylaxis. Other psychiatric disorders with an episodic course such as, for example, episodic unipolar depression, may also be increased among the relatives of responders. Furthermore, the response to long-term lithium clusters in families[4].

Only lithium responders have been observed to have a significant excess of bipolar illness in the families. In this respect they differ from patients responding to alternative long-term treatment. The first-degree relatives of bipolar patients responding to lamotrigine have an overabundance of anxiety disorders, panic attacks, substance abuse and alcohol addictions, while families of those benefiting from neuroleptics lack bipolar or anxiety disorders but do have chronic psychiatric (e.g. personality disorders) or psychotic illnesses among relatives[34,57,58].

Patients with the cycloid type of bipolar disorder often have no ill family members, or at times have a relative with episodically running psychotic disorder.

CLINICAL PROFILE: SYMPTOM PRESENTATION

In clinical practice we are accustomed to assess primarily the patient's symptoms during episodes of depression or mania. When we evaluate a patient with recurrent mood disorder for long-term treatment, the acute presentation is also important but it is not sufficient for selecting an effective treatment. Unfortunately, this point is often not appreciated. By themselves the symptoms are not enough to identify which medication will stabilize the patient.

Prior to treatment, lithium responders most often have depressions and manic episodes of the classical type. Depressive syndromes are dominated by mood abnormalities. The emphasis is on sadness and hopelessness rather than inability to think clearly and/or low motivation. The depressed mood, with sadness and hopelessness, persists for weeks and months and changes mainly in intensity. If patients complete daily mood ratings, they have no difficulty in characterizing each day by a particular number, because the abnormal mood remains similar over a period of time. Changes in mood are usually positively correlated with low energy and negatively with anxiety. Manic episodes are often euphoric, elated and expansive rather than dysphoric and irritable.

In lithium non-responders the symptoms are often quite different. Sadness and hopelessness are often fleeting, frustration and anger are common and mood is changeable from day to day, or even changing several times within the same day ('ultrarapid cycling').

These presentations during acute episodes are characteristic of the majority but not of all responders to long-term lithium treatment. In the cycloid lithium responders, for example, non-classical symptoms may appear in particular during mania. Low mood may be described in a variety of ways and may cycle faster. Psychotic symptoms, hallucinations and delusions can be mood incongruent, but the course of the illness is fully remitting and, in hindsight, the patient views the past episodes as ego-dystonic. When long-term treatment is considered, it is therefore important to look at the overall clinical profile, not just at symptom presentation.

CLINICAL PROFILE: CO-MORBIDITY

Bipolar spectrum disorders have been described as having much co-morbidity with other psychiatric disorders, particularly anxiety and panic disorders, alcoholism and addictions. That is not so for lithium-responsive bipolar disorders. Twelve per cent abused alcohol, but the prevalence of other psychiatric disorders among lithium responders is similar to that of the general population and markedly lower than in bipolar spectrum disorders and in bipolar responders to atypical neuroleptics or lamotrigine[34,58,59].

CHILDHOOD RECOLLECTIONS

All responders from Ontario were interviewed in detail about their developmental issues. As adults, lithium responders characteristically recalled normal childhood and described predominantly positive, pleasant experiences stretching from their earliest memories to adolescence. They denied any psychiatric symptoms in childhood, such as anxiety, panic, phobias, nightmares, recurrent insomnia, depressions or manic experiences. The patients were, of course, intimately familiar with many

of these symptoms because they encountered them later in life. If they had a major loss (e.g. a death of a family member) or major stresses in childhood, they reacted with a short-lived grief or adjustment reaction.

These reports are markedly different from those of adults suffering from other types of bipolar illness, for example, from lamotrigine or neuroleptic responders who often describe emotional problems and adverse experiences since early childhood. To some extent, these reports also deviate from what Duffy[5,6] (see also Chapter 16) observed when she and her team followed prospectively the offspring of adult lithium responders. Followed because they were at high risk of mood disorders, some children of responders experienced emotional problems: sleep disorders, anxiety, panic, phobias and later mood disorders. The episodic course of these childhood problems, and in some adolescents also their response to lithium, indicate that these manifestations probably reflect the same mood dysregulation as that of their parents. Yet, as adults the parents do not report childhood precursors of the mood disorder.

Further follow-up of the children of responders will hopefully clarify this discrepancy. Perhaps the adult responders had such symptoms in childhood but their memory rewrites the past in the service of the present. Alternatively, our interviews might not be sophisticated enough to retrieve such memories. As some epidemiological studies suggest, the recent generation has a higher prevalence of emotional problems, with an earlier onset.

NEUROBIOLOGICAL FINDINGS

In the late 1960s and 1970s biologically oriented psychiatry was expanding quickly and researchers were hoping that the striking lithium response in bipolar patients would shed light on some underlying biological abnormality identifiable by the newer laboratory methods. The scientists focused on neurochemical, neurophysiological and psychological tests. Many promising differences between responders and non-responders were reported, but eventually not replicated. The deviations often turned out to reflect incomplete understanding of multivariate influences on the investigated biological function. Unfortunately, only a very few studies have been carried out in the way that could give some answers: comparing excellent lithium responders with indisputable lithium non-responders.

There is a wealth of literature on neurobiological findings, and a few examples are quoted here. Some of the domains of intense research have been lithium transport in red blood cells[60], the red blood cell/plasma lithium ratio[61], urinary lithium excretion[62], platelet monoaminase activity[63], urinary MHPG and other expressions of central amine metabolism[64,65], serum calcium and magnesium[66], average evoked potentials[67,68], human leukocyte antigens (HLA)[69,70] and psychological indicators[71].

We reported characteristic neuroendocrine responses in lithium responders[72,73]. While these responses were indistinguishable between healthy controls and lithium responders off lithium at the time of testing, the differences were unmasked after 3 weeks of lithium treatment. The neuroendocrine responses can be best explained by a serotonergic or endorphin dysregulation in these patients. The tests are unfortunately too cumbersome to use in clinical practice.

Lithium responders also had characteristic abnormalities in the MNS blood groups[74]. The NN groups were found only in 6% of patients, compared to 24% in other psychiatric and healthy controls.

Finally, a number of important genetic studies of lithium responders have now been completed. The studies of transmission mode supported autosomal recessive transmission as probably the most common mode for this group[75,76]. While the initial genome scan implicated particularly the chromosomal regions 15q14 and 7q11[77,78], detailed mapping of these regions has not as yet identified specific genes. The gene for phospholipase C[79] has shown a significant association with this group of patients, but the increased risk in the presence of this gene is limited. Another series of molecular genetic studies on excellent lithium responders has been performed by Rybakowski *et al.*[80,81] (for details see Chapter 36).

The lack of success is surprising. Those with classical manic-depressive illness, and lithium responders in particular, undoubtedly have a strong genetic contribution to their illness, probably the strongest of all psychiatric disorders, but to date no specific genes have been identified in lithium responders.

While the search for a predictive laboratory test still goes on, there is not yet a laboratory test that can be clinically useful in predicting lithium response. The patient selection and treatment decisions are best based on a comprehensive clinical evaluation and careful judgment.

CASE HISTORIES OF LITHIUM RESPONDERS AND NON-RESPONDERS

Most good and poor responders to lithium prophylaxis can be identified beforehand by their differing clinical profiles. One of the best ways to illustrate the differences is by their characteristic case histories. The responders have typically an episodic course of illness, full remissions free of residual symptoms, no rapid cycling, no psychiatric co-morbidity and often also a positive bipolar family history and classic manic and depressive symptoms. Lithium non-responders lack these features and differ in clinical profile.

For clinical practice perhaps the most revealing may be the clinical vignettes of distinct, characteristic clinical profiles.

Case history: bipolar type 1 disorder, classical presentation

Forty-nine-year-old male, divorced, with two children

Course

Became ill at age 19 with mania followed by depression. Subsequently frequent severe depressions bringing him to a hospital for several months and interspersed with the occasional manic episode. Tended to discontinue psychotropic medication after discharge and remained completely well and fully functional during remissions. After 14 recurrences, mostly biphasic episodes, he was placed on lithium. Remained stable for 14 months, then discontinued lithium and after 5 months experienced another recurrence of depression and hypomania. Since then he has been completely stable on lithium for 14 years.

Family history

Mother and one of her three sisters suffered from bipolar illness, and so does his daughter. One aunt on his mother's side suffered from frequently recurrent depressions and stabilized well on lithium.

Symptoms

During his depressions he was intensely sad, crying uncontrollably, had insomnia with early morning awakening, suffered marked weight loss and suicidal impulses and attempts, frequently found it very difficult to make decisions, was unable to concentrate. When manic, he was elated, spoke with pressure of speech, and expressed grandiose ideas. Slept only 2–4 hours but didn't miss the sleep. Increased sexual drive, involved in extramarital affairs that were accompanied by expenses he could not afford.

No psychiatric co-morbidity, but abuse of alcohol during hypomanic and manic episodes.

Development

Happy memories of his childhood years, excelled academically, no emotional problems until the age of 19 when he became ill.

Case history: bipolar type 2 disorder, classical presentation

Forty-five-year-old married man, with three daughters.

Course

Episodes of mild depression since age 25, manifesting primarily as dissatisfaction with his job. Psychiatrically treated episodes started at age 30, with onsets in December 1991, October 1992, November 1993 and October 1994. Treated with tricyclic antidepressants, selective serotonin reuptake inhibitors (SSRIs) and psychotherapy, with no clear benefit and continuing recurrences. Short-lived hypomanic episodes often followed depressions. MMPI profile taken in remission was within normal limits. Past 11 years on 1200 mg of lithium carbonate, fully stabilized.

Family history

Father suffered from bipolar disorder. A nephew suffers from depressions which worsen during winter.

Symptoms

During depressions sad, worried excessively about everything, multiple fears. Became unusually quiet, no longer extroverted, afraid to talk to people, was afraid that they would find out how incompetent he was. He was worried that he had picked the wrong career. When hypomanic had marital strifes, kept falling in love with other women and behaved inappropriately.

Development

Very good memories of early childhood. Was very outgoing, extroverted. Was in the gifted class and was receiving straight A marks. Played a number of sports competitively, particularly tennis. Successful student and athlete both in the USA and Canada. The only negatively charged childhood memories are those of his father's drinking behavior: father became drunk, exposed himself in public and was arrested. Patient felt very close to his mother.

Case history: pseudounipolar disorder

Thirty-year-old woman, living common-law, no children

Course

Started experiencing depressions at age 13. Initially the episodes were 2–3 weeks long, once a year, gradually increasing in length and frequency. Treated by her family physician with SSRIs, venlafaxin, quetiapine and tri-iodthyronine augmentation, all without clear benefit and with no stabilization. Because of her lack of response to antidepressants, between the ages of 18 and 21 the patient saw several adolescent and adult psychiatrists in consultations. Her striking family history was noted and the possibility of bipolar illness considered. Therefore, she was placed on 900 mg of lithium carbonate, along with 300 mg of venlafaxin but continued having very lengthy recurrences of depression.

At age 24, referred by her family physician for a comprehensive consultation to a mood disorders center, because of a history of recurrent depressions that did not respond to treatment. Her hypomanias were identified, her diagnosis was changed from recurrent depression to bipolar type II disorder, lithium responsive (previous course was viewed as a pseudounipolar disorder). The lithium kinetics test indicated that she excreted lithium rapidly and the lithium had a rather short half-life. She was placed on lithium carbonate 1350 mg at bedtime, giving her serum lithium levels around 0.8 mEq/l. For the past 6 years she has remained fully stabilized on lithium alone.

Family history

Patient's mother was treated for depressions and a hypomania. Mother's mother was taking medication 'for her nerves'. An aunt on her mother's side was depressed and hospitalized. No history of psychiatric problems on her father's side.

Symptoms

When depressed, crying, pervasive feelings of sadness, hopelessness, pessimistic thoughts, low self-esteem. Unable to work or function at home. The patient and her parents reported that, following a few of her depressions, she experienced energy, and activity increased uncharacteristically for her.

No psychiatric co-morbidity. Tried smoking marihuana once with her schoolmates.

Development

Very happy memories of her childhood, no psychiatric symptoms at that time. Family functioning was healthy. Graduated from high school and has been working for an embroidery company.

Case history: bipolar disorder, cycloid type

Forty-three-year-old male, divorced, no children.

Course

Became ill at age 14, experienced a total of seven major episodes, three exclusively overactive, one predominantly overactive and two episodes of low mood. On one occasion, after he spontaneously reduced his dosage of lithium, he became acutely overactive within 3 weeks. Otherwise, he has been well on lithium for 15 years.

Family history

No positive family history identified when interviewing all his first-degree and several second-degree relatives.

Symptoms

During the overactive episodes, he was agitated; his mood was elevated, at times with rapid changes, pressure of speech and excessive spending. He felt an increased drive, was restless, could not sleep and complained bitterly about his insomnia. His thinking ranged from overvalued ideas to Messianic delusions, with a need to convince others about the veracity of his beliefs. At times, he felt ecstatic happiness, spending much energy writing letters to various celebrities and to the prime minister. Other times during his mania he felt insecure. He was very angry at his wife and had to fight impulses to harm her, although he had no obvious reason for his rage.

During the periods of a low mood, he felt depressed, desperate, hopeless, had a very low drive; had guilt feelings, feelings of insufficiency, early morning awakening and anxiety.

Co-morbidity

He abused alcohol and cannabis.

Development

No psychological problems in childhood identified.

Case history: non-responder to lithium; subsequently lamotrigine responder

Seventy-one-year-old man, married, with four adult children.

Course

A man with a pre-existing anxiety disorder, for which he was not treated, developed in his early fifties intense depressive and hypomanic episodes requiring hospitalizations. In between episodes both clinical interview and an MMPI profile confirmed florid anxiety disorder. Over 10 years his recurrences were unresponsive to lithium, carbamazepine, divalproex and antidepressants but for the past 9 years he has been completely free of mood problems on 200 mg of lamotrigine, with an adequate therapeutic level.

Family history

His son struggles with alcoholism and his aunt has been ill with an anxiety disorder.

Symptoms

While depressed, he complains of emotional emptiness, apathy, indifference, occasional sadness and crying, with great difficulty to motivate himself. While he is hypomanic, it is his wife who complains about his excessive activation, rather than euphoria.

Co-morbidity

Anxiety disorder, stuttering. Did not, however, go for any help until he became depressed in his early fifties.

Development

Since childhood, throughout his life he has been 'nervous, tense', stuttering.

Case history: lithium non-responder, subsequently clozapine responder

Forty-four-year-old woman, divorced three times, living common law, no children.

Course

Became ill at age 19 with a protracted period of low mood. During the next 12 years had 25 hospitalizations because of manias with psychotic features.

Failed to respond to lithium in a high dosage, to fluphenazine and haloperidol both given first orally and then in long-acting injections, and to divalproex alone and in combination. The past 8 years fully stabilized on 400 mg of clozapine at night.

Family history

One sister suffering from chronic problems with anger or uncontrollable rage, one aunt abroad treated for some form of psychotic illness. No evidence of any bipolar disorder in the family.

Symptoms

During manic episodes irritable and expansive mood, feverishly writing songs, stories and a novel. Pressure of speech, flight of ideas, when challenged hostile or physically aggressive, promiscuity and sexual indiscretions. During low periods feels empty, unmotivated, with diminished pleasure, insomnia and fatigue.

Co-morbidity

Intermittent periods of addiction to street drugs that virtually stopped on clozapine.

Development

No emotional problems reported by the patient before the age of 19, corroborated by her family.

Note: Some personal details of the case histories were adjusted in order to protect the patients' privacy.

SELECTIVITY, STABILITY, MORTALITY AND SIDE-EFFECTS

There is a growing body of observations indicating that the response to long-term lithium is, by and large, stable over time and selective vis-à-vis treatment alternatives. Patients with recurrent mood disorders who benefit from long-term lithium monotherapy often fail miserably on the alternative therapies and vice versa[82–86]. These observations of selective response do not support the often stated clinical impression that most, if not all, bipolar patients benefit only when treated with combinations.

There are more and more clinical data on bipolar patients systematically treated with long-term lithium, who have remained successfully stabilized for years or decades[87–92]. This is particularly true for patients with the classical type of bipolar disorder who constitute the majority in these long-term studies. It is not yet clear whether the same stability of response exists in the cycloid bipolar disorder.

The patients on long-term lithium show a striking normalization of mortality and markedly decreased suicidal behavior[93,94]. In addition, lithium responders show fewer subjective and objectively measured side-effects than do non-responders[95,96].

CHILDREN OF LITHIUM RESPONDERS

Duffy has carried out systematic prospective studies of offspring of lithium responders and non-responders[6,97]. Her major findings include the observation that, despite a genetic risk for bipolar disorder, these offspring manifest a broad range of psychopathology. Furthermore, the type of clinical course breeds true from parent to offspring. The investigators showed that children of adult lithium responders present, like their parents, with a recurrent, completely remitting course. After a normal or gifted early development, the offspring of lithium-responsive patients develop an episodic illness with a variety of psychopathologies. The

offspring of lithium non-responsive parents also developed a broad range of disorders including mood disorders, but more often starting as anxiety and sleep disorders and unfolding without full remissions. Duffy *et al.* have also made observations supporting a selective response to long-term mood stabilizers among the affected offspring. This topic is further explored in Chapter 16.

These findings that parents and their children who suffer from the same brain dysfunction have the same course of illness but strikingly divergent symptoms challenge the long-held, strongly embedded belief that we can diagnose psychiatric entities and select effective long-term treatment primarily on clinical symptoms.

MISCONCEPTIONS ABOUT LITHIUM AND RESPONSE

Unfortunately, particularly in some countries, several misconceptions prevail about lithium response: the response to lithium was seen only in the 1960s and 1970s; lithium responders are now rare; it takes too much time to find out whether a patient will respond to lithium treatment; lithium treatment has many side-effects and is usually poorly tolerated.

However, lithium responders exist now as much as they existed in the 1970s and they represent a sizeable proportion of bipolar patients. When diagnosed according to DSM-IV, the percentage could be estimated at 35% of bipolar patients[98]. When, in addition to the bipolar diagnosis, the psychiatrist includes the patient's clinical profile, the great majority of selected patients respond. Furthermore, if one considers that up to 40–50% of patients with recurrent unipolar disorders have unrecognized hypomanias[29], the number of likely lithium responders increases dramatically.

The prediction of lithium response takes time. It requires comprehensive assessment; a simple accounting of DSM symptoms is not enough, but once a patient is stabilized, the savings of time are large. The identification of future responders requires skill: learning about the untreated course of mood disorders, learning about recurrence risk and family history and, above all, learning to evaluate the quality of remission. This is a task that is not taught in medical schools or during residency. Psychiatrists who want to identify future lithium responders will have to learn this skill.

Excellent responders seem ubiquitous: they have been observed in many hospitals and clinics. Yet, there are a number of psychiatrists who treat mood disorders and report that they have never seen a lithium responder. The problem is that they do not know how to look for them. Many recent graduates from psychiatric residency in North America have never used lithium during their extensive training. They may not be comfortable with lithium; they may not know how to use it properly; they may be afraid of it and of its potential side-effects. For bipolar patients they may use only combinations and may maintain their patients on a particular combination that was helpful in acute treatment. As a result, these psychiatrists will never see an excellent responder to lithium monotherapy.

Despite contrary statements in the literature, most good lithium responders tolerate lithium well and have few side-effects, if maintained at a correct serum lithium level.

CONCLUSIONS

To identify a patient who has a high probability of responding to long-term lithium treatment, it is important to consider not just symptom presentation but also the broad clinical profile, including the clinical course, family history, co-morbidity and early development. The essential features are the diagnosis of recurrent mood disorder and an episodic course of illness with a complete, symptom-free remission. Supporting features identifiable prior to lithium treatment are a predominance of depressions over manias/hypomanias, the absence of rapid cycling, a family history of episodic bipolar disorder, no co-morbid psychiatric illness and a classical presentation of depressive and over-active episodes. While complete remissions appear essential for an excellent response, each of the elements of a clinical profile is important and none by itself is sufficient to identify the responder. One needs to consider the whole clinical profile.

There may be challenges in the decision-making process. When a patient arrives for the initial assessment not all information may be available by the time long-term treatment needs to be instituted. There are situations when sufficient information, for example about clinical course or family history, is missing, incomplete or contradictory. Such patients will have to be initially treated with a combination of stabilizers, and the clinician will have to revert to combinations if individual stabilizers do not succeed.

If the clinical profile is not sufficiently known and information for a rational decision is not available, such patients should be carefully considered for both lithium and the alternatives. If such patients are placed on a lithium trial, this trial should be time-limited and the patients should be closely monitored. If the patients continue to relapse and show no striking improvement, despite an adequate lithium dosage and sufficient serum levels, they should be carefully reassessed and alternatives to lithium considered.

On the other hand, if a patient improves quickly and remains well for a longer period of time, a thorough reassessment with additional information is needed, to see whether the patient does or does not have a lithium-responsive profile. The patient may be a true lithium responder and require long-term maintenance, or the reassessment may suggest that the patient's well-being may have nothing to do with the lithium treatment. For instance, the patient's mood may have been destabilized by antidepressants that preceded lithium. Gradual discontinuation of lithium may be considered.

Finally, lithium responders represent an important population for psychiatric research because of their relative homogeneity. Genetic and other biological investigations need to be performed on fairly uniform groups of patients, and lithium responders as a group are good candidates for such tasks. Comparing lithium responders with lithium non-responders may be the best way to discover the mechanism of lithium action. This may lead to the development of new substances that are effective in maintenance treatment and are better tolerated than lithium.

REFERENCES

1. Grof P. Has the effectiveness of lithium changed? Impact of the variety of lithium's effects. Neuropsychopharmacology 1998; 19: 183–8

2. Grof P, Alda M, Grof E, et al. The challenge of predicting response to stabilising lithium treatment. The importance of patient selection. Br J Psychiatry 1993; (Suppl 21): 16–19

3. Duffy A, Grof P. Psychiatric diagnoses in the context of genetic studies of bipolar disorder. Bipolar Disord 2001; 3: 270–5

4. Grof P, Duffy A, Cavazzoni P, et al. Is response to prophylactic lithium a familial trait? J Clin Psychiatry 2002; 63: 942–7

5. Duffy A, Alda M, Kutcher S, et al. A prospective study of the offspring of bipolar parents responsive and nonresponsive to lithium treatment. J Clin Psychiatry 2002; 63: 1171–8

6. Duffy A, Alda M, Kutcher S, et al. Psychiatric symptoms and syndromes among adolescent children of parents with lithium-responsive or lithium-nonresponsive bipolar disorder. Am J Psychiatry 1998; 155: 431–3

7. Isaksson A, Ottosson JO, Perris C. Methodologische Aspekte der forschung unber prophylaktische Behandlung bei affektiven Psychosen. In Hippius H, Selbach H, eds. Das Depressive Syndrom. Munich: Urban & Schwarzenberg, 1969: 561–74

8. Grof P. Designing long-term clinical trials in affective disorders. J Affect Disord 1994; 30: 243–55

9. Angst J, Grof P. Selection of patients with recurrent affective illness for a long-term study: testing research criteria on prospective follow-up data. In Cooper TN, Gershon S, Kline N, et al., eds. Lithium: Controversies and Unresolved Issues. Amsterdam: Excerpta Medica, 1979: 355–69

10. Grof P, Angst J, Karasek M, Keitner G. Patient selection for long-term lithium treatment in clinical practice. Arch Gen Psychiatry 1979; 36: 894–7

11. Zis AP, Grof P, Goodwin FK. The natural course of affective disorders: implications for lithium prophylaxis. In Cooper TB, Gershon ES, Kline N, et al., eds. Lithium: Controversies and Unresolved Issues. Amsterdam: Excerpta Medica, 1979: 381–97

12. Coryell W, Endicott J, Maser JD, et al. The likelihood of recurrence in bipolar affective disorder: the importance of episode recency. J Affect Disord 1995; 33: 201–6

13. Grof P, Vinar O. Maintenance and prophylactic imipramine doses in recurrent depressions. Activ Nerv Sup (Prague) 1966; 8: 383–5

14. Grof P, Vinar O. Verlaufsrhytmus and prophylaktische beeinflussunsmoeglichkeiten der affectiven psychosen. In Hippius H, Selbach H, eds. Das Depressive Syndrom. Munich: Urban and Schwarzenberg, 1969: 101–4

15. Grof P, Lane J, MacCrimmon D, et al. Clinical and laboratory correlates of the response to

long-term lithium treatment. In Stromgren E, Schoua M, eds. Origin, Prevention and Treatment of Affective Disorders. London: Academic Press, 1979: 27–40

16. Grof P, Hux M, Grof E, Arato M. Prediction of response to stabilizing lithium treatment. Pharmacopsychiatry 1983; 16: 195–200

17. Grof P. Response to long-term lithium treatment: research studies and clinical implications. In Davis JM, Mass JW, eds. Affective Disorders. Washington: American Press, 1983: 357–66

18. Endicott J, Spitzer RL. A diagnostic interview: the schedule for affective disorders and schizophrenia. Arch Gen Psychiatry 1978; 35: 837–44

19. Alda M. Pharmacogenetics of lithium response in bipolar disorder. J Psychiatry Neurosci 1999; 24: 154–8

20. Alda M, Cavazzoni P, Grof P. Treatment response to prophylactic lithium and family history of psychiatric disorders. Biol Psychiatry 1999; 45: 1078

21. Alda M, Turecki G, Grof P, et al. Association and linkage studies of CRH and PENK genes in bipolar disorder: a collaborative IGSLI study. Am J Med Genet 2000; 96: 178–81

22. Alda M. Genetic factors and treatment of mood disorders. Bipolar Disord 2001; 3: 318–24

23. Alda M. Pharmacogenetic aspects of bipolar disorder. Pharmacogenomics 2003; 4: 35–40

24. Alda M, Keller D, Grof E, et al. Is lithium response related to $G_s\alpha$ levels in transformed lymphoblasts from subjects with bipolar disorder? J Affect Disord 2001; 65: 117–22

25. MacQueen GM, Hajek T, Alda M. The phenotypes of bipolar disorder: relevance for genetic investigations. Mol Psychiatry 2005 Sep; 10 (9) : 811–26

26. Perris C. Morbidity suppressive effect of lithium carbonate in cycloid psychosis. Arch Gen Psychiatry 1978; 35: 328–31

27. Perris P, Smigan L. The use of lithium in the long term morbidity suppressing treatment of cycloid and schizoaffective psychoses. In Pichot P, Berner P, Wolf R, Thau K, eds. Psychiatry: The State of the Art. New York: Plenum, 1985: 375–80

28. Perris C. The concept of cycloid psychotic disorder. Psychiatr Dev 1988; 1: 37–56

29. Angst J, Gamma A, Benazzi F, et al. Diagnostic issues in bipolar disorder. Eur Neuropsychopharmacol 2004; 13 (Suppl 2): S43–S50

30. Angst J, Gamma A. Prevalence of bipolar disorders: traditional and novel approaches. Clin Appr Bipol Disord 2002; 1: 10–14

31. Prien R, Kupfer DJ, Mansky PA, et al. Drug therapy in the prevention of recurrences in unipolar and bipolar affective disorders: report of the NIMH collaborative study group comparing lithium carbonate, imipramine, and a lithium carbonate–imipramine combination. Arch Gen Psychiatry 1984; 41: 1096–104

32. Maj M, Del Vecchio M, Starace F, et al. Prediction of affective psychoses response to lithium prophylaxis: the role of socio-demographic, clinical, psychological and biological variables. Acta Psychiatr Scand 1984; 69: 37–44

33. Maj M. Clinical prediction of response to lithium prophylaxis in bipolar patients: a critical update. Lithium 1992; 3: 15–21

34. Grof P. Selecting effective treatments for bipolar disorders. J Clin Psychiatry 2003; 64 (Suppl 5): 53–61

35. Tyrer SP. Lithium in the treatment of mania. J Affect Disord 1985; 8: 251–7

36. Abou-Saleh MT. Predictors of response to prophylactic lithium. In Birch NJ, ed. Lithium: Inorganic Pharmacology and Psychiatric Use. Washington DC: IRL Press 1987: 143–4

37. Abou-Saleh MT. Who responds to prophylactic lithium therapy? Br J Psychiatry 1993; 21 (Suppl): 20–26

38. Deshauer D, Duffy A, Alda M, et al. The cortisol awakening response in bipolar illness: a pilot study. Can J Psychiatry 2003; 48: 462–6

39. Kukopoulos A, Reginaldi D. Recurrences of manic depressive episodes during lithium treatment. In: Johnson FN, ed. Handbook of lithium therapy. Lancaster: MTP Press, 1980

40. Haag M, Heidorn A, Haag H, Greil W. Response to stabilizing lithium therapy and sequence of affective polarity. Prog Neuropsychopharmacol Biol Psychiatry 1987; 11: 205–8

41. Lane J, Grof P, Daigle L, Varma R. The Minnesota multiphasic personality inventory in the prediction of response to lithium stabilization. In Dufour H, et al., eds. The Prediction of Lithium Response. University of Marseille, 1983: 215–20

42. Angst J, Baastrup PC, Grof P, et al. Clinical course of affective disorders. Psychiatry 1973; 76: 489–500

43. Angst J, Grof P. The course of monopolar depressions and bipolar psychoses. Lithium in Psychiatry, a Synopsis. Quebec City: Université de Laval Press, 1976: 93–104

44. Angst J. The course of affective disorders. Psychopathology 1986; 19 (Suppl): 47–52

45. Keller MB. Differential diagnosis, natural course, and epidemiology of bipolar disorders. Psychiatry Update: The American Psychiatric Association Annual Review. Washington, DC: American Psychiatric Press, 1987: 10–31

46. Akiskal HS, Bourgeois ML, Angst J, et al. Re-evaluating the prevalence of and diagnostic composition within the broad clinical spectrum of bipolar disorders. J Affect Disord 2000; 59: S5–S30

47. Grof E, Haag M, Grof P, Haag H. Lithium response and the sequence of episode polarities: preliminary report on a Hamilton sample. Prog Neuropschopharmacol Biol Psychiatry 1987; 2: 199–203

48. Post RM, Ketter TA, Pazzaglia PJ, et al. Rational polypharmacy in the bipolar affective disorders. Epilepsy Res 1996; (Suppl 11): 153–80

49. Calabrese JR, Rapport DJ, Youngstrom EA, et al. New data on the use of lithium, divalproate, and lamotrigine in rapid cycling bipolar disorder. Eur Psychiatry 2005; 20: 92–5

50. Zvolsky P, Vinarova E, Dostal T, Soucek K. Family history of manic-depressive and endogeneous depressive patients and clinical effect of treatment with lithium. Activ Nerv Sup (Prague) 1974; 16: 194–5

51. Mendlewicz J, Fieve RR, Stallone F, Fleiss JL. Genetic history as a predictor of lithium response in manic-depressive illness. Lancet 1973; 1: 599–600

52. Mendlewicz J, Fieve RR, Stallone F. Relationship between the effectiveness of lithium therapy and family history. Am J Psychiatry 1973; 130: 1011–13

53. Alda M, Grof P. Genetics and lithium response in bipolar disorders. In Soares JC, Gershon S, eds. Basic Mechanisms and Therapeutic Implications of Bipolar Disorder. New York: Marcel Dekker, 2000

54. Alda M. Bipolar disorder: from families to genes. Can J Psychiatry 1997; 42: 378–7

55. Coryell W, Endicott J, Reich T, et al. A family study of bipolar II disorder. Br J Psychiatry 1984; 145:49-54

56. Coryell W, Winokur G. Predicting lithium responders and nonresponders: familial indicators. In Johnson FN, ed. Handbook of Lithium Therapy. Lancaster: MTP Press, 2005: 137–42

57. Passmore MJ, Garnham J, Duffy A, et al. Phenotypic spectra of bipolar disorder in responders to lithium versus lamotrigine. Bipolar Disord 2003; 5: 110–14

58. Alda M. The phenotypic spectra of bipolar disorder. Eur Neuropsychopharmacol 2004; 14 (Suppl 2): S94–S99

59. Passmore MJ, Garnham J, Duffy A, et al. Phenotypic spectra of bipolar disorder in lithium responders vs. lamotrigine. Bipolar Disord 2004; 5: 110–14

60. Upadhyaya AK, Varma VK, Sankarana-yanaran A. Lithium in prophylactic therapy of manic–depressive illness: biochemical correlates of response. Biol Psychiatry 1985; 20: 202–5

61. Mendels J, Fraser A, Baron J. Intraerythrocyte lithium ion concentration and longterm maintenance treatment. Lancet 1976; 7966: 966

62. Serry M. Lithium retention and response. Lancet 1969; 7608: 1267–68

63. Sullivan JL, Cavenar JO, Maltbie A. Platelet-monoaminooxidase activity predicts response to lithium in manic–depressive illness. Lancet 1977; 2: 1325–7

64. Carroll BJ. Prediction of treatment outcome with lithium. In Cooper TN, Gershon S, Kline N, et al., eds. Lithium, Controversies and Uunresolved Issues. World Congress Lecture Series. Amsterdam: Excerpta Medica, 1979: 171–97

65. Goodwin FK, Post R, Dunner DL, Gordon EK. Cerebrospinal amine metabolites in affective illness. Am J Psychiatry 1973; 130: 73–9

66. Carman JS, Post RH, Teplitz TA, Goodwin FK. Divalent cations in predicting antidepressant response to lithium. Lancet 1974; 2: 1454

67. Baron M, Gershon ES, Rudy V, et al. Lithium carbonate response in depression. Arch Gen Psychiatry 1975; 32: 1107–11

68. Buchsbaum M, Goodwin F, Murphy D. AER in affective disorders. Am J Psychiatry 1971; 128: 19–25

69. Maj M. The impact of lithium prophylaxis on the course of bipolar disorder: a review of the research evidence. Bipolar Disord 2000; 2: 93–101

70. Maj M, Arena F, Loverno N, et al. Factors associated with response to lithium prophylaxis in DSM III major depression and bipolar disorder. Pharmacopsychiatry 1985; 18: 309–13

71. Johnson FN. Predicting lithium responders and nonresponders. In Johnson FN, ed. Handbook of Lithium Therapy. Lancaster: MTP Press, 1980: 126–32

72. Grof E, Grof P, Brown GM, Downie S. Lithium effects on neuroendocrine function. Prog Neuropsychopharmacol Biol Psychiatry 1984; 8: 541–6

73. Grof E, Grof P, Brown GM. Investigations of lithium effects on neuroendocrine function in man. In Birch NJ, ed. Lithium: Inorganic Pharmacology and Psychiatric Use. Washington: IRL Press, 1987: 177

74. Alda M, Grof P, Grof E. MN blood groups and bipolar disorder: evidence of genotypic association and Hardy–Weinberg disequilibrium. Biol Psychiatry 1998; 44: 361–3

75. Alda M, Grof E, Cavazzoni P, et al. Autosomal recessive inheritance of affective disorders in families of responders to lithium prophylaxis? J Affect Disord 1997; 44: 153–7

76. Alda M, Grof P, Grof E, et al. Mode of inheritance in families of patients with lithium-responsive affective disorders. Acta Psychiatr Scand 1994; 90: 304–10

77. Alda M, Turecki G, Grof E, et al. Genome scan of bipolar disorder using a pharmacogenetic strategy. Mol Psychiatry 1999; 4 (Suppl 1): 16 (Abstr)

78. Turecki G, Grof P, Grof E, et al. Mapping susceptibility genes for bipolar disorder: a pharmacogenetic approach based on excellent response to lithium. Mol Psychiatry 2001; 6: 570–8

79. Turecki G, Grof P, Cavazzoni P, et al. Evidence for a role of phospholipase C-gamma1 in the pathogenesis of bipolar disorder. Mol Psychiatry 1998; 3: 534–8

80. Rybakowski JK, Suwalska A, Skibinska M, et al. Prophylactic lithium response and polymorphism of the brain-derived neurotrophic factor gene. Pharmacopsychiatry 2005; 38: 166–70

81. Rybakowski JK, Suwalska A, Czerski PM, et al. Prophylactic effect of lithium in bipolar affective illness may be related to serotonin transporter genotype. Pharmacol Rep 2005; 57: 124–7

82. Grof P. Lithium update: selected issues. In Ayd F, Taylor JT, Taylor BT, eds. Affective Disorders Reassessed. Baltimore: Ayd Medical Publications, 1983

83. Greil W, Ludwig-Mayerhofer W, Erazo N, et al. Lithium versus carbamazepine in the maintenance treatment of bipolar disorders – a randomized study. J Affect Disord 1997; 43: 151–61

84. Greil W, Kleindienst N, Erazo N, Muller-Oerlinghausen B. Differential response to lithium and carbamazepine in the prophylaxis of bipolar disorder. J Clin Psychopharmacol 1998; 18: 455–60

85. Bowden CL. Predictors of response to divalproex and lithium [Review]. J Clin Psychiatry 1995; 56 (Suppl 3): 25–30

86. Tohen M, Chengappa K, Suppes T, et al. Efficacy of olanzapine in combination with valproate or lithium in the treatment of mania in patients partially nonresponsive to valproate or lithium monotherapy. Arch Gen Psychiatry 2002; 59: 62–9

87. Berghofer A, Mueller-Oerlinghausen B. No loss of efficacy after discontinuation and

reinstitution of long-term lithium treatment? In Gallicchio VS, Birch MJ, eds. Lithium. Biochemical and Clinical Advances. Cheshire, CT: Weidner Publishing Group, 1996: 39–46

88. Maj M, Pirozzi R, Kemali D. Long-term outcome of lithium prophylaxis in patients initially classified as complete responders. Psychopharmacology 1989; 98: 535–8

89. Tondo L, Baldessarini RJ, Hennen J, et al. Lithium maintenance treatment of depression and mania in bipolar I and bipolar II disorders. Am J Psychiatry 1998; 155: 638–45

90. Grof P. Excellent lithium responders: people whose lives have been changed by lithium prophylaxis. In Birch NJ, Gallicchio VS, Becker RW, eds. Lithium: 50 years of Psychopharmacology. Cheshire, CT: Weidner Publishing Group, 1999: 36–51

91. Baldessarini RJ, Tondo L. Does lithium treatment still work? Evidence of stable responses over three decades. Arch Gen Psychiatry 2000; 57: 187–90

92. Baldessarini RJ, Tondo L, Hennen J, et al. Is lithium still worth using? An update of selected recent research. Harvard Rev Psychiatry 2002; 10: 59–75

93. Mueller-Oerlinghausen B, Wolf T, Ahrens B, et al. Mortality during initial and during later lithium treatment: a collaborative study by the International Group for the Study of Lithium treated Patients (IGSLi). Acta Psychiatr Scan 1994; 90: 295–7

94. Coppen A, Standish-Barry H, Bailey J, et al. Does lithium reduce the mortality of recurrent mood disorders? J Affect Disord 1991; 23: 1–7

95. Grof P, O'Sullivan K. Somatic side effects of long-term lithium treatment. In Stancer H, Persad E, eds. Guidelines for the Use of Psychotropic Drugs. New York: Spectrum, 1984: 105–18

96. Grof P, Grof E, Hux M. Side effects of responders and nonresponders to longterm stabilization. Proceedings, 33rd Annual Meeting of the CPA, Banff, Alberta, 1983; 96

97. Duffy A, Alda M, Kutcher S, et al. A prospective study of the offspring of bipolar parents responsive and non-responsive to lithium treatment. J Clin Psychiatry 2002; 63: 1171–8

98. Garnham JS, Munro A, Teehan A, et al. Naturalistic study of outcome of mood stabilizing treatment in bipolar disorder. Eur Neuropsychopharmacol 2003; 13 (Suppl 4): S201

15 The suicide-preventive and mortality-reducing effect of lithium

Bruno Müller-Oerlinghausen, Bernd Ahrens, Werner Felber

Contents Introduction • Can adequate lithium prophylaxis change the suicide risk and mortality of patients with affective disorders? • Is the anti-suicidal and mortality-reducing effect of lithium specific? • The efficacy of lithium prophylaxis expressed as number of saved lives • Integrating mortality findings into therapeutic algorithms

INTRODUCTION

Suicidal behavior is frequent in affective disorders, including bipolar disorders. The relevant data have recently been reviewed by Oquendo *et al.*[1].

It is generally assumed that antidepressant treatment reduces the suicide risk. However, in spite of some positive epidemiologic findings[2,3], the evidence for this is shockingly scarce. This sceptical statement refers particularly to the effect of long-term medication[1,4]. The assumption might explain the fact that, to date, drug regulatory agencies have not considered changes of the death rate as an essential endpoint criterion for approval of new anti-depressants or 'mood stabilizers'. The present debate on the suicidality-inducing effects of selective serotonin reuptake inhibitors (SSRIs) and other antidepressants adds another question mark as to the net effects of long-term

antidepressive treatment in terms of suicide prevention[5]. The recent re-analysis of data from the Zurich cohort by Angst *et al.* is one notable exception, suggesting a mortality-reducing effect of antidepressants, as well as neuroleptics and lithium[6,7].

Apart from antidepressant drugs, mood stabilizers and antipsychotics are used for symptomatic treatment in mood-disordered patients. Surprisingly, lithium is the only compound for which increasing evidence of a suicide preventive effect has been accumulated during the past 15 years. It is disturbing that it took so long for the knowledge of this special feature of lithium salts to be perceived by the majority of psychiatrists, particularly in the USA[8–11]. Maj[11] gave four reasons for the denial of existing data and the decreased use of lithium in psychiatric practice during the past decade: (1) problems with patients' compliance; (2) the increased attention to atypical and complicated forms of bipolar disorder that seemed to be less sensitive to lithium than classical bipolar disorder; (3) the introduction and vigorous marketing of other mood stabilizers; and (4) the appearance of reports underscoring the methodological limitations of the placebo-controlled trials of lithium treatment published in the 1970s, and the consequent doubts about the efficacy of the drug.

In this context it appears remarkable that the recent guideline of the World Federation of Societies of Biological Psychiatry[12,13] provides valid, updated information about lithium (see Chapter 5).

We here outline briefly the history and development of the international research on the suicide-preventive effect of lithium. Many of the large studies in this area have included patients with affective disorders, among them mostly a large percentage of those with bipolar disorder. We then discuss the potential specificity of the anti-suicidal effect, focusing on the important question of whether, first, the suicide- and mortality-reducing effect of lithium is shared by other psychotropics; and second, whether this effect might be independent of the episode-suppressing effect.

Finally, we present an estimate of how many lives could be saved annually by lithium and what the consequences should be for modern guidelines and therapeutic algorithms in psychiatric practice.

CAN ADEQUATE LITHIUM PROPHYLAXIS CHANGE THE SUICIDE RISK AND MORTALITY OF PATIENTS WITH AFFECTIVE DISORDERS?

Patients with affective disorders exhibit a 2–3 times increased mortality when compared to the general population[14–17]. This excess mortality is caused primarily by the possibly 30–70-fold higher suicide-related mortality[18], which is particularly high in patients with a history of suicide attempts[19,20]. The meta-analysis by Guze and Robins from 1970[21] calculated the lifetime suicide risk as 15% for affective disorders, whereas 20 years later Goodwin and Jamison, on the basis of more recent literature, reported an overall risk of 19%[22].

According to Harris and Barraclough[23], the suicide-related standardized mortality rate (SMR[24]) is 21.24 in major depression, and 11.73 in bipolar disorder, with, however, large confidence intervals. Although some studies found a somewhat lower suicide rate in bipolar as compared to unipolar patients[25,26], others found higher rates in bipolar patients[5,27,28], particularly in bipolar II patients.

The intriguing question of whether long-term medication with lithium salts can improve the course of the manic-depressive disease or of affective disorders altogether in terms of suicide prevention was given little attention until the 1980s (Table 15.1)[29–42].

Barraclough[29] was one of the first investigators postulating a potential association between long-term lithium medication and suicide prevention. Based on a detailed analysis of the charts of 100 suicide victims he concluded that about 20% of the suicides could have been prevented by adequate lithium medication. The first systematic retrospective study demonstrating a highly significant reduction of suicide attempts in a sample of 64 high-risk patients during long-term lithium treatment was published by Müller-Oerlinghausen et al. in 1992[30]. The authors emphasized that suicides and suicide attempts occurred nearly exclusively in a group of 13 patients who had taken lithium irregularly or had stopped the medication.

Felber's group in Dresden analyzing suicide attempts during accumulated periods on and off

Table 15.1 Anti-suicidal effect of lithium: history

	References
Anecdotal reports and findings from follow-ups in the 1970s and 1980s on possible reduction of suicidal behavior in lithium-treated patients	Barraclough 1972[29] and others
First systematic follow-ups of high-risk patients during long-term lithium treatment	
Berlin study: 2 suicides, 4 suicide attempts in 55 patients with regular lithium treatment; 4 suicides, 7 suicide attempts in 13 patients having discontinued lithium	Müller-Oerlinghausen *et al.* 1992[30]
Dresden study: 6 suicide attempts in 36 patients on lithium; 3 suicides, 36 suicide attempts in 36 patients off lithium	Felber, Kyber 1994[31]
Mortality studies	
First Berlin studies on general mortality-reducing effects of lithium	Ahrens, Müller-Oerlinghausen 1990[32]
Coppen shows reduced mortality in mostly unipolar patients on lithium	Coppen *et al.* 1991[33]
The IGSLI-studies on mortality (MORTA I-IV)	Müller-Oerlinghausen *et al.* 1992[34]; Ahrens *et al.* 1995[24]; Wolf *et al.* 1996[35]
First systematic multicenter analysis of 6000 patient-years	
Further studies	
The MAP-study (randomized, prospective, 2.5 years, $n = 285$). No suicidal acts on lithium, 9 suicidal acts on carbamazepine	Thies-Flechtner *et al.* 1996[36]; Greil *et al.* 1997[37]
Two large Swedish studies and one Sardinian study confirm the IGSLI findings	Nilsson 1995[38]; Kallner *et al.* 2000[39];
Tondo and Baldessarini review the existing data	Tondo *et al.* 1997[40]; Baldessarini *et al.* 1999[41]
Risk of suicidal acts 7–8 times higher in bipolar patients off lithium	
Algorithms	
Berghöfer and Müller-Oerlinghausen develop algorithms as a first step to integrate the existing evidence into therapeutic guidelines	Berghöfer *et al.* 2002[42]

Table 15.2 Selection of studies on the course of affective disorders and suicide rates in patients with long-term lithium treatment (modified according to reference 43)

Studies	Study length (years)	Patient-years	Suicides per 1000 patient-years
After discharge from hospital			
Goldacre et al.[48]	1	6050	10.4
No long-term medication			
Lee and Murray[45]	16	1296*	6.9
Kiloh et al.[46]	15	1785*	5.1
Lehmann et al.[47]	11	948*	11.6
Coppen et al.[33]	16	330	9.1
Lithium long-term medication			
Coppen[43]	16	1519	0.7
Nilsson[38]	20	3911	1.5
Müller-Oerlinghausen et al.[44]	7	5603	1.3
Summary of lithium studies			
All patients with long-term lithium medication	7–16	11 033	1.3
All patients without long-term lithium medication	11–16	4359	7.3

* Recalculated according to the values presented by the authors

lithium had similar findings: 90% of the suicide attempts occurred in the off-lithium period[31].

Several studies on the mortality of affective disorders during long-term lithium treatment by Coppen et al.[33] and by the International Group for the Study of Lithium-treated Patients (IGSLI[24,34]) demonstrated that the SMR of patients with affective disorders during adequate lithium medication was normalized down to the level of the general population*. Coppen[43] reviewed the studies existing in the mid-1990s on the suicide rates in patients on lithium versus off lithium and concluded that adequate lithium medication reduced the suicide-related mortality by 82% (Table 15.2)[33,38,44–48].

The IGSLI studies

In the main IGSLI study well-documented data were evaluated from lithium clinics in Austria, Canada, Denmark and Germany on the course of illness of 827 patients with affective disorders who had been treated with lithium for at least 6 months[24,34]. Of these patients, 55% were bipolar,

* In studies investigating potential effects of a therapeutic intervention on suicide rates, a specific methodical difficulty usually has to be dealt with: a reasonable estimate has to be created of how many cases of death are to be expected in a matched, non-treated patient sample. Since mostly it is not possible for ethical reasons to treat a control group of patients suffering from affective disorders with placebo over many years, IGSLI and other research groups used a reference group of the general population. This made it possible to calculate the standardized mortality rate either for any causes of death or for specific causes such as cardiovascular disease, accident or suicide.

Table 15.3 Overall mortality and cause-specific mortality rates (SMR) of the major diagnostic subgroups (from reference 24)

	Unipolar (n = 182) Patient-years = 1252	Bipolar (n = 440) Patient-years = 3167	Schizoaffective (n = 171) Patient-years = 1030	Total (n = 793) Patient-years = 5450
No. of all observed deaths	7	29	8	44
No. of all expected deaths	9.24	23.49	5.13	37.86
Ratio (observed/expected)*	0.76	1.23	1.56	1.16
95% confidence limits	0.25–1.77	0.80–1.82	0.51–3.64	0.75–1.71
No. of observed suicides	0	4	3	7
No. of expected suicides	0.31	0.76	0.23	1.30
Ratio (observed/expected)	—	5.26	13.04	5.38
95% confidence limits	—	1.43–13.48	2.69–38.11	1.75–12.57
No. of observed CVS deaths	2	11	1	14
No. of expected CVS deaths	3.43	9.49	1.93	14.85
Ratio (observed/expected)	0.58	1.16	0.52	0.94
95% confidence limits	0.07–2.11	0.56–2.13	0.01–2.89	0.45–1.73
No. of other observed deaths	5	14	4	23
No. of other expected deaths	5.50	13.24	2.97	21.71
Ratio (observed/expected)	0.91	1.06	1.35	1.06
95% confidence limits	0.30–2.12	0.51–1.94	0.37–3.45	0.65–1.64

CVS, cardiovascular system
*SMR (reference 24)

25% unipolar, 2% unipolar–manic, 16% schizoaffective and 2% had other diagnoses. At onset of the lithium prophylaxis, patients were 41 years old on the average. The mean duration of lithium treatment was 81 months (6–21 years), equaling 5600 patient years.

The ratio of 44 observed and 38 expected cases of death is not statistically different from 1.0, which is the mortality of the general population. Thus, the expected 2–3-fold excess mortality in patients with affective disorders (see above) does no longer apply in this lithium-treated patient sample (Table 15.3).

Unipolar patients do not differ essentially from other diagnostic groups in this respect. Although the specific suicide-related SMR is still higher than in the general population, it can

be clearly shown that it is definitely lower in all diagnostic groups compared to what could be expected in untreated patient samples.

It has been argued on various occasions that patients accepting lithium prophylaxis might generally benefit from a better prognosis. In this case the specific patient selection would have been primarily responsible for the 'normalization' of the SMR.

In a successive analysis of 270 German and Danish patients from the original IGSLI sample, the initial SMR was compared to the SMR after treatment of more than 1 year[44]. During the first year the overall mortality was increased 2-fold, and the suicide-related mortality 17-fold as compared to the general population. The SMR normalized after the first year of treatment, indicating that patients for whom lithium prophylaxis is indicated are in fact patients with a high risk of suicide.

Further mortality studies in bipolar patients

There are very few studies that apparently contradict the findings of the IGSLI. Vestergaard and Aagaard[49] and Brodersen et al.[50] were not able to demonstrate a reduced mortality in cohorts of lithium-treated manic-depressive patients. However, the average duration of the lithium treatment was less than in the IGSLI study, and control of compliance might not have been sufficient, e.g. one-third of the deaths that occurred in their study took place after the patients had discontinued lithium. It was also argued that the reduction of mortality might essentially be due to the optimal care and attention patients receive in specialized lithium clinics. In this context two Swedish studies are of particular interest. In an open field setting Nilsson[38] did not observe a full normalization of the SMR. However, as in other studies, reviewed by Schou[51], she found a rise of the SMR up to the expected level in untreated affective disorders after discontinuation of lithium.

Kallner et al.[39] analyzed a mixed sample of 497 patients including 405 bipolar patients treated with lithium during an observation period of 30 years. Patients were divided into three groups according to the regularity of attending the outpatient clinic. Among bipolar patients the suicide rate was in excess in all three groups. However, the suicide rate increased by 80% when patients stopped taking lithium.

This study deserves special interest because it generally confirms the findings by IGSLI and by Nilsson[38], but it also suggests that the suicide-preventing effect of lithium might be more marked in patients being cared for in specialized lithium clinics. The suicide-related

SMR in patients on lithium was 14.0 when they had regular visits to the clinic, and 21.4 when treated elsewhere. This difference could possibly be explained by the generally higher quality of the treatment regimens and by the closer monitoring of the patients.

Further support for the anti-suicidal effect of lithium in bipolar patients came from studies in a Sardinian patient sample[52]. A meta-analysis on about 17 000 patients demonstrated an 8.6-fold higher mortality from suicide in patients treated without lithium than in patients during long-term lithium treatment[40].

Recently, two large studies have again confirmed the main findings quoted above. A Danish observational cohort study with linkage of registers of all recorded suicides and of all lithium prescriptions in Denmark over a period of 5 years ($n = 13 186$) clearly showed that patients who purchased lithium had a higher rate of suicide than persons who did not purchase lithium. For those persons who had received lithium at a pharmacy at least twice, the rate of suicide was 194 per 100 000 person-years compared to 448 in persons who had received only one lithium prescription. Age and gender did not significantly influence this finding[53]. Bocchetta from Sardinia (Italy) published a short report on a follow-up of 18 154 patient-years ($n = 1394$)[54]. The study shows that controlled treatment with lithium for more than 5 years reduced the standardized mortality to the rates expected for the general population. However, death rates doubled again in patients having dropped out after years of initial adherence to the medication. The author emphasized the impact of specialized lithium clinics in order to improve compliance and thus prevent suicides. The disastrous effects of lithium discontinuation in terms of re-occurring suicidal acts have been reported by Baldessarini et al.[55]. The authors observed 14 times more frequent fatalities after discontinuation of lithium.

IS THE ANTI-SUICIDAL AND MORTALITY-REDUCING EFFECT OF LITHIUM SPECIFIC?

In view of these rather robust and consistent empirical findings, the intriguing question arises of whether the suicide-preventive effect of lithium should be considered a 'specific' effect and what could be the underlying mechanism?

For the sake of clarity we may subdivide the issue of potential specificity into two questions:

(1) Is this effect specific for lithium salts? In other words, is it shared by other drugs, such as other mood stabilizers or antidepressants?

(2) Is this effect strictly related to the episode-preventive effect of lithium prophylaxis or might it act independently?

Do other drugs possess anti-suicidal activity?

The question of whether the anti-suicidal effect is shared by other psychotropic agents was addressed in the German multicentered MAP study, a prospective randomized controlled trial with a treatment time of 2.5 years. A total of 146 bipolar and schizoaffective patients were randomized to lithium, 139 to carbamazepine. No suicidal act was observed in the lithium group, but four suicides and five suicide attempts occurred in the carbamazepine group – a statistically significant difference[36,56].

Recently, a study by Goodwin et al.[57] comparing the suicide risk in lithium- versus valproate-treated patients from the USA attracted much attention and publicity. The authors conducted a retrospective cohort study at two large integrated health plans in California and Washington. In this follow-up of more than 20 000 patients having received lithium, carbamazepine or valproate during 1994 and 2001 the adjusted suicide risk was 2.7 times (95% CI 1.1–6.3; $p = 0.03$) higher in valproate-treated as compared to lithium-treated patients. Hazard ratios for suicide attempts amounted to 1.7–1.8. Also, carbamazepine-treated patients had a significantly higher risk of suicide attempts leading to hospitalization in comparison to patients having been prescribed lithium at least once during the observation period.

Further evidence comes from a study by Modestin and Schwarzenbach[58], who conducted a follow-up of 64 former psychiatric inpatients who committed suicide within 1 year after discharge, and compared them with a carefully matched control group of patients not having committed suicide. A significantly higher proportion of the controls had been receiving various kinds of psychopharmacotherapy including seven patients who had been treated with lithium. However, none of the 64 patients who committed suicide had been receiving lithium at the time of his or her death – the only statistically significant difference between the two groups.

What could be the mechanism of this suicide preventive effect? Although it was postulated by Baldessarini et al.[59] that the reduction of the suicide risk by lithium prophylaxis is primarily caused by its depression-preventive effect, our hypothesis from the very beginning has been that lithium differs from other mood stabilizers and also from most antidepressants by its marked serotonin-agonistic effects, which are related predominantly to its pre-synaptic functions[60,61]. It appears at least an attractive speculation that this serotoninergic action, possibly in connection with other effects, is related to its well-established anti-aggressive effects in animals as well as humans[62] (see Chapter 19), but also to its anti-suicidal effects.

Is the anti-suicidal effect of lithium coupled to its antidepressive effect?

The second and decisive question is whether the antisuicidal effect of lithium would also occur in patients not responding optimally in terms of episode prevention.

This question again implies two different issues:

(1) Do neurobiological concepts and epidemiological data support the description of suicidal behavior as an independent nosological entity?

(2) Does lithium effectively reduce suicidal behavior in patients who do not benefit from lithium treatment in terms of episode reduction?

In fact, some concepts and findings suggest that suicidal behavior might be seen as a particular, possibly anger-related, form of affective dysregulation, also associated with disturbance of the 5-HT-system, and, thus, as an independent nosological syndrome.

Data from the recent large WHO study show that the prevalence of suicidal behavior is not fully related to the existence of ICD psychiatric diagnoses, but that it occurs frequently in symptomatic individuals and in subjects with subthreshold disorders[63]. Many of such individuals, according to WHO data from Germany, are characterized by symptoms of overt or suppressed anger[64], which van Praag[65] considers as one of the core constituents of the stress syndrome, together with anxiety. Van Praag postulated that in certain types of depression – characterized by a 5-HT disturbance – anxiety and aggression regulation are primarily disturbed while mood lowering is a derivative symptom. Consequently, he expected that certain drugs such as L-tryptophan, the azapirones, or lithium might ameliorate anxiety and/or aggression via regulation of the 5-HT

system to exert in addition an overall therapeutic effect in depression.

As to the second aspect, namely whether the anti-suicidal effect of lithium would also occur in patients not responding optimally in terms of episode prevention, part of the IGSLI data do in fact support such a concept. For this sub-analysis Ahrens and Müller-Oerlinghausen[66] selected only patients with at least one suicide attempt in the past before onset of lithium medication (n = 176; 55% bipolar, 18% schizo-affective). The sample was divided into three subgroups according to their response to long-term lithium treatment in terms of reduction of depressive inpatient episodes. In spite of the clearly different overall efficacy of lithium prophylaxis, a statistically significant reduction of suicide attempts occurred in all three groups, even in the poor responders who did not show a significant decrease of the depressive inpatient episodes. In other words, in 50% of the clear-cut non-responders, no further suicide attempt was observed during lithium treatment (Table 15.4). The standardized suicide mortality in the poor responders was 17.0 compared to an expected figure of about 100.

Certainly, these findings can neither prove the suicide-preventive effect of lithium nor its potential specificity. However, the accumulated evidence strongly supports such a hypothesis.

THE EFFICACY OF LITHIUM PROPHYLAXIS EXPRESSED AS NUMBER OF SAVED LIVES

In a recent editorial it was asked 'Does lithium save lives?'[9]. We tried to answer this question in a quantitative way based on data collected within the Epidemiological Catchment Area Study[67] and the epidemiological data of Weeke from Denmark[17] as well as on the assumption that about 60% of all suicides in the population

Table 15.4 Specificity of lithium. Reanalysis of IGSLI data from 176 high-risk patients

	No. of suicide attempts per year before lithium treatment	No. of suicide attempts per year during lithium treatment	p Value
Poor response (n = 41)	0.33	0.10	<0.007
Questionable response (n = 81)	0.27	0.06	<0.0001
Excellent response (n = 45)	0.26	0.02	<0.0001

Table 15.5 Expected rates of death and suicide in the general population and in patients with affective disorders vs. observed death and suicide rates in the 827 patients of the IGSLI sample (see reference 66 and text)

	Males	Females	Total
Expected no. of deaths			
General population	19.69	18.74	38.43
Affective disorders (ECA[67])	42.40	25.69	68.09
Affective disorders (Weeke[17])	39.85	34.35	74.20
Expected no. of suicides			
General population	0.80	0.54	1.34
Affective disorders (ECA[67])	23.50	7.50	31.00
Affective disorders (Weeke[17])	20.96	16.16	37.12
Observed no. of deaths			
Lithium-treated affective disorders (Data from IGSLI)	21	23	44
Observed no. of suicides			
Lithium-treated affective disorders (data from IGSLI)	2	5	7

are committed by patients with affective disorders. We developed a model for the calculation of deaths and suicides to be expected in the general population and in untreated patients with affective disorders[66]. Table 15.5 shows that for a sample of 827 subjects of the general population (matched with the patients of the IGSLI sample) 1.34 suicides had to be expected, whereas in a corresponding sample of patients with affective disorders, on the average 34 (31–37) suicides were predicted. In the lithium-treated IGSLI sample seven suicides were observed, in other words 27 of the predicted suicides did not occur. Thus, we can conclude that five suicides/year per 1000 treated patients can be prevented. This would result in

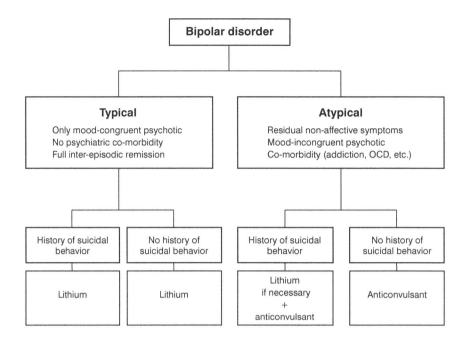

Figure 15.1 Algorithm for the selection of the primary long-term medication in bipolar patients. OCD, obsessive compulsive disorder

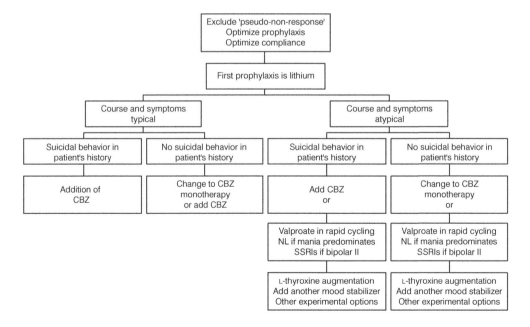

Figure 15.2 Algorithm for a rational procedure in treating patients insufficiently responding to the initial long-term lithium medication. CBZ, carbamazepine; NL, neuroleptics

about 250 suicides per year prevented in Germany. The IGSLI data also showed that the average age of patients having committed suicide was 44. Thus, the gain for the gross national product in Germany would be 3060 working years before individuals had completed the age of 65.

This positive effect adds to the net gain of about 110 million Euro per year in Germany produced by lithium prophylaxis within the National Health Scheme, although the number of lithium-treated patients in Germany appears to be much too low[68]. For further information on the economics of long-term lithium treatment refer to Chapter 42.

INTEGRATING MORTALITY FINDINGS INTO THERAPEUTIC ALGORITHMS

In view of the bewildering variety of compounds studied and propagated today for the long-term treatment of bipolar patients it appears essential to offer a rational, operationalized basis for adequate treatment decisions in psychiatric practice. A psychotropic compound may have been approved in Europe or in the USA for maintenance treatment of bipolar patients, and it may be recommended or listed in independent guidelines following criteria of evidence-based medicine. However, for the selection of the optimal drug in an individual patient the benefit/risk ratio has to be considered (e.g. the risk of obesity and diabetes in the use of olanzapine) as well as the kind of studies having been submitted to the regulatory agencies. Thus, results from maintenance studies using so-called enriched designs can only indicate a potential usefulness of the tested compound in patients having responded favorably to it during an acute episode of the disease. Hardly any prospective trial carried out

with the aim of having a new compound approved for maintenance therapy in bipolar patients provides information on a reduction of suicidality, not to say mortality. In the lamotrigine study of Calabrese et al. in bipolar patients (after a depressive episode) four suicides and 11 suicide attempts occurred during open lamotrigine treatment and one suicide occurred 3 weeks after discontinuation of lamotrigine[69]. One suicide attempt was observed in the placebo group.

To select the appropriate bipolar patient for long-term treatment with lithium the existing findings on lithium's anti-suicidal effect should be taken into account as well as atypical features of the course of the disease. We have worked on suitable algorithms which are depicted in Figures 15.1 and 15.2[42]. Figure 15.1 illustrates the use of the discriminating criterion 'suicidality (suicide attempts in the history of a patient)'. Figure 15.2 suggests an operationalized procedure if the primary lithium medication has not been found successful in terms of episode prevention.

REFERENCES

1. Oquendo MA, Chandbury SR, Manu JJ. Pharmacotherapy of suicidal behaviour in bipolar disorder. Arch Suicide Res 2005; 9: 237–50

2. Isacsson G. Frequency of suicides reduced with 25 percent: Probably by the increased use of antidepressive agents. Lakartidningen 2000; 97: 1644–50

3. Isacsson G, Holmgren P, Druid H, Bergman U. The utilization of antidepressants – a key issue in the prevention of suicide. An analysis of 5281 suicides in Sweden 1992–94. Acta Psychiatr Scand 1997; 96: 94–100

4. Wolfersdorf M, Mauerer C, Franke C. Suizidalität und Antriebssteigerung: Provokation und/oder Prävention von Suizidgefahr durch Psychopharmaka. In

Bronisch T, Felber W, Wolfersdorf M, eds. Neurobiologie suizidalen Verhaltens. S Regensburg: Roderer Verlag, 2001; 303–23

5. Lapierre YD. Suicidality with selective serotonin reuptake inhibitors: valid claim? J Psychiatry Neurosci 2003; 28: 340–47

6. Angst J, Sellaro R, Angst F. Long-term outcome and mortality of treated vs. untreated bipolar and depressed patients: a preliminary report. Int J Psychiatry Clin Pract 1998; 2: 115–19

7. Angst J, Angst F, Gerber-Werder R, Gamma A. Suicide in mood-disorder patients with and without longterm medication: a 40 to 44 years follow-up. Arch Suicide Res 2005; 9: 279–300

8. Fieve RR. Lithium therapy at the millennium: a revolutionary drug used for 50 years faces competing options and possible demise. Bipolar Disord 1999; 1: 67–70

9. Solomon DA, Keller MB, Leon AC, et al. Multiple recurrences of major depressive disorder. Am J Psychiatry 2000; 157: 229–33

10. Joffe RT. Does lithium save lives? J Psychiatry Neurosci 2004; 29: 9

11. Maj M. Lithium – the forgotten drug. Paper presented at the Conference of the European Foundation of Psychiatry. Bipolar Disorder: The Upswing in Research and Treatment. London, 2003

12. Bauer M, Whybrow PC, Angst J, et al. World Federation of Societies of Biological Psychiatry (WFSBP) Guidelines for Biological Treatment of Unipolar Depressive Disorders, Part 1: Acute and continuation treatment of major depressive disorder. World J Biol Psychiatry 2002; 3: 5–43

13. Bauer M, Whybrow PC, Angst A, et al. WFSBP Task Force on Treatment Guidelines for Unipolar Depressive Disorders. World Federation of Societies of Biological Psychiatry (WFSBP) Guidelines for Biological Treatment of Unipolar Depressive Disorders, Part 2: Maintenance treatment of major depressive disorder and treatment of chronic depressive disorders and subthreshold depressions. World J Biol Psychiatry 2002; 3: 67–84

14. Lundquist G. Prognosis and cause of manic depressive psychosis. Acta Psychiatr Neurol Scand 1945; 35: 1–96

15. Kay DWK, Petterson U. Mortality. In Petterson U, ed. Manic depressive illness: a clinical, social and genetic study. Acta Psychiatr Scand 1977; 269 (Suppl): 55–60

16. Tsuang MT, Woolson RF. Excess mortality in schizophrenia and affective disorders. Do suicides and accidental deaths solely account for this excess? Arch Gen Psychiatry 1978; 35: 1181–85

17. Weeke A. Causes of death in manic depressives. In Schou M, Strömgren E, eds. Origin, Prevention and Treatment of Affective Disorders. London: Academic Press, 1979: 289–99

18. Hagnell O, Lanke J, Rorsman B. Suicide rates in the Lundby study: mental illness as a risk factor for suicide. Neuropsychobiology 1981; 7: 248–53

19. Tuckman J, Youngman W. Identifying suicide with groups among attempted suicide. Public Health Rep 1963; 78: 763–6

20. Motto I. Suicide attempts: a longitudinal view. Arch Gen Psychiatry 1965; 13: 516–20

21. Guze SB, Robins E. Suicide in primary affective disorders. Br J Psychiatry 1970; 117: 437–8

22. Goodwin FK, Jamison KR. Manic-depressive Illness. New York: Oxford University Press, 1990

23. Harris EC, Barraclough B. Excess mortality of mental disorder. Br J Psychiatry 1998; 173: 11–53

24. Ahrens B, Müller-Oerlinghausen B, Schou M, et al. Excess cardiovascular and suicide mortality of affective disorders may be reduced by lithium-prophylaxis. J Affect Disord 1995; 33: 67–75

25. Newman S, Bland R. Suicide risk varies by subtype of affective disorder. Acta Psychiatr Scand 1991; 83: 420–6

26. Österby U, Brandt L, Correia N, et al. Excess mortality in bipolar and unipolar disorder in Sweden. Arch Gen Psychiatry 2001; 58: 844–50

27. Lester D. Suicidal behavior in bipolar and unipolar affective disorders: a meta-analysis. J Affect Disord 1993; 27: 117–21

28. Bottlender R, Jager M, Strauss A, Möller HJ. Suicidality in bipolar compared to unipolar depressed inpatients. Eur Arch Psychiatry Clin Neurosci 2000; 250: 257–61

29. Barraclough B. Suicide prevention, recurrent affective disorder and lithium. Br J Psychiatry 1972; 121: 391–2

30. Müller-Oerlinghausen B, Müser-Causemann B, Volk J. Suicides and parasuicides in a high-risk patient group on and off lithium long-term medication. J Affect Disord 1992; 25: 261–70

31. Felber W, Kyber A. Suizide und Parasuizide während und außerhalb einer Lithium-prophylaxe. In Müller-Oerlinghausen B, Berghöfer A, eds. Ziele und Ergebnisse der medikamentösen Prophylaxe affektiver Psychosen. Stuttgart: Georg Thieme Verlag, 1994: 53–9

32. Ahrens B, Müller-Oerlinghausen B. Lithium-prophylaxe und Mortalität bei Langzeit-behandlung: Die Mortalität normalisiert sich bei Langzeitbehandlung. Psycho 1990; 16: 489–95

33. Coppen A, Standish-Barry H, Bailey J, et al. Does lithium reduce the mortality of recurrent mood disorders? J Affect Disord 1991; 23: 1–7

34. Müller-Oerlinghausen B, Ahrens B, Grof E, et al. The effect of long-term lithium treatment on the mortality of patients with manic-depressive and schizo-affective illness. Acta Psychiatr Scand 1992; 86: 218–22

35. Wolf T, Müller-Oerlinghausen B, Ahrens B, et al. How to interpret findings on mortality of long-term lithium treated manic-depressive patients? Critique of different methodological approaches. J Affect Disord 1996; 39: 127–32

36. Thies-Flechtner K, Müller-Oerlinghausen B, Seibert W, et al. Effect of prophylactic treatment on suicide risk in patients with major affective disorders. Data from a randomized prospective trial. Pharmacopsychiatry 1996; 29: 103–7

37. Greil W, Ludwig-Mayerhofer W, Erazo N, et al. Lithium versus carbamazepine in the maintenance treatment of bipolar disorders – a randomised study. J Affect Disord 1997; 43: 151–61

38. Nilsson A. Mortality in recurrent mood disorders during periods on and off lithium. A complete population study in 362 patients. Pharmacopsychiatry 1995; 28: 8–13

39. Kallner G, Lindelius R, Petterson U, et al. Mortality in 497 patients with affective disorders attending a lithium clinic or after having left it. Pharmacopsychiatry 2000; 33: 8–13

40. Tondo L, Jamison KR, Baldessarini RJ. Effect of lithium maintenance on suicidal behavior in major mood disorders. In Stoff DM, Mann JJ, eds. The Neurobiology of Suicide: From the Bench to the Clinic. Ann NY Acad Sci 1997; 836: 339–51

41. Baldessarini KJ, Tondo L, Hennen J. Effect of lithium treatment and its discontinuation on suicidal behaviour in bipolar manic-depressive disorders. J Clin Psychiatry 1999; 60 (Suppl 2): 77–84

42. Berghöfer A, Bauer M, Müller-Oerlinghausen B. Antisuicidal effect of lithium as a criterion for the selection of appropriate long-term medication in bipolar patients. In Kaschka WP, ed. Perspectives in Affective Disorders. Advanced Biological Psychiatry. Basel: Karger, 2002; 21: 1–9

43. Coppen A. Depression as a lethal disease: prevention strategies. J Clin Psychiatry 1994; 55 (Suppl 4): 37–45

44. Müller-Oerlinghausen B, Wolf T, Ahrens B, et al. Mortality during initial and during later lithium treatment: a collaborative study by IGSLI. Acta Psychiatr Scand 1994; 90: 295–7

45. Lee AS, Murray RM. The long-term outcome of Maudsley depressives. Br J Psychiatry 1988; 153: 741–51

46. Kiloh LG, Andrews G, Neilson M. The long-term outcome of depressive illness. Br J Psychiatry 1988; 153: 752–7

47. Lehmann HE, Fenton FR, Deutsch M et al. An 11-year follow-up study of 110 depressed patients. Acta Psychiatr Scand. 1988; 78: 57–65

48. Goldacre M, Seagroatt V, Hawton K. Suicide after discharge from psychiatric inpatient care. Lancet 1993; 342: 283–6

49. Vestergaard P, Aagaard J. Five-year mortality in lithium-treated manic-depressive patients. J Affect Disord 1991; 21: 33–8

50. Brodersen A, Licht RW, Vestergaard P, et al. Sixteen-year mortality in patients with affective disorder commenced on lithium. Br J Psychiatry 2000; 176: 429–33

51. Schou M. The effect of prophylactic lithium treatment on mortality and suicidal behavior: a review for clinicians. J Affect Disord 1998; 50: 253–9

52. Tondo L, Baldessarini RJ, Floris G, et al. Lithium maintenance treatment reduces risk of suicidal behavior in bipolar disorder patients. In: Gallicchio VS, Birch NJ, eds. Lithium: Biochemical and Clinical Advances. Cheshire, CT: Weidner Publishing, 1996: 161–71

53. Kessing LV, Sondergard L, Kvist K, Andersen PK. Suicide risk in patients treated with lithium. Arch Gen Psychiatry 2005; 62: 860–6

54. Bocchetta A. Mortality follow-up of patients since commencing lithium therapy. J Clin Psychopharmacol 2005; 25: 197–9

55. Baldessarini RJ, Tondo L, Hennen J. Effects of lithium treatment and its discontinuation on suicidal behavior in bipolar manic-depressive disorders. J Clin Psychiatry 1999; 60 (Suppl 2): 77–84

56. Goodwin FK. Anticonvulsant therapy and suicide in affective disorders. J Clin Psychiatry 1999; 60 (Suppl 2): 89–93

57. Goodwin FK, Fireman B, Simon GE, et al. Suicide risk in bipolar disorder during treatment with lithium and divalproex. JAMA 2003; 290: 1467–73

58. Modestin J, Schwarzenbach F. Effect of psychopharmacotherapy on suicide risk in discharged psychiatric in-patients. Acta Psychiatr Scand 1992; 85: 173–5

59. Baldessarini RJ, Tondo L, Hennen J. Reduced suicide risk during long-term treatment with lithium. Ann NY Acad Sci 2001; 932: 24–43

60. Müller-Oerlinghausen B. Lithium long-term treatment – does it act via serotonin? Pharmacopsychiatry 1985; 18: 214–17

61. Müller-Oerlinghausen B. Die Wirkung von Lithium auf serotoninerge Funktionen. In Müller-Oerlinghausen B, Greil W, Berghöfer A, eds. Die Lithiumtherapie. Berlin: Springer-Verlag, 1997: 61–8

62. Nilsson A. The anti-aggressive actions of lithium. Rev Comtemp Pharmacother 1993; 4: 269–85

63. Linden M, Zäske H, Ahrens B. Correlates of suicidal ideation in general healthcare patients – results of the WHO collaborative study on psychological problems in general health care (WHO-PPGHC). Int J Psychiatry Clin Pract 2003; 7: 17–25

64. Painuly N, Sharan P, Mattoo SK. Relationship of anger and anger attacks with depression. Eur Arch Psychiatry Clin Neurosci 2005; 255: 215–22

65. Van Praag HM. Anxiety and increased aggression as pacemakers of depression. Acta Psychiatr Scand 1998; 393 (Suppl): 81–8

66. Ahrens B, Müller-Oerlinghausen B. Does lithium exert an independent antisuicidal effect? Pharmacopsychiatry 2001; 34: 132–6

67. Weissman MM, Bruce ML, Leaf PJ, et al. Affective disorders. In Robins LN, Regier DA, eds. Psychiatric Disorders in America. New York: Free Press, 1991

68. Müller-Oerlinghausen B, Lohse MJ. Psychopharmaka. In Schwabe U, Paffrath D, eds. Arzneiverordnungs-Report 2002. Berlin: Springer-Verlag, 2003

69. Calabrese JR, Bowden CL, Sachs G, et al, Lam Study Group. A placebo-controlled 18-month trial of lamotrigine and lithium maintenance treatment in recently depressed patients with bipolar disorder. J Clin Psychiatry 2003; 64: 1013–24

16 Lithium treatment in children and adolescents: a selected review and integration of research findings

Anne Duffy

Contents Introduction • Lithium as an acute treatment for pediatric mania • Lithium as a prophylactic treatment for recurrent mood disorders in children and adolescents • Lithium in the affected offspring of lithium-responsive parents • Other indications for lithium in children and adolescents • Concluding remarks

INTRODUCTION

Relative to the number of studies investigating the various uses of lithium in adult populations, the literature pertaining to the use of lithium in pediatric populations is lacking. In the late 1970s reviews of this topic pointed out the need for the systematic study of lithium in specific pediatric patient populations in which there were some data from case reports to suspect benefit[1,2]. These populations included bipolar youth, psychiatrically ill offspring of lithium-responding parents and some aggressive and behaviorally disordered children. However, over the next two decades, few new systematic studies were completed, and the question is: why?

The answer is complex, and may include a lack of enthusiasm by clinicians, a lack of interest by industry and mediocre results from studies in poorly responsive populations. Further, there was disenchantment with lithium treatment in adult bipolar patients in the 1980s and 1990s which had to do with concerns and myths of reduced effectiveness, poor tolerability, toxicity to the kidney, rebound worsening after abrupt discontinuation and loss of effectiveness over time or after discontinuation[3]. Another factor may be that the pediatric bipolar populations studied have often suffered from complex illnesses with high rates of co-morbidity, chronicity and atypicality which are negative predictors for lithium response in adult bipolar patients[4]. Overriding all of the above issues, there was and still is in many parts of the world a reluctance to use psychotropic medications in children.

The next logical question is: why study lithium in pediatric populations? The answer is relatively straightforward. Essentially, there is convergent information from the adult literature, pediatric case series and some controlled trials in manic adolescents to suggest that lithium may be of benefit for identifiable subgroups of pediatric patients. Further, we have good reason to believe that a proportion of bipolar adolescents can be completely stabilized on long-term lithium monotherapy. Given the morbidity and mortality among untreated youth with mood disorders, the prospect of long-term stability, and for some complete remission, is of critical importance. Furthermore, there are data in bipolar adults supporting the concept of differential treatment response. That is, patients who selectively do well on lithium, do not respond similarly to other mood stabilizers[5]. It is therefore possible that bipolar youth may also have a selective response to a given mood stabilizer. The importance of this line of research is underscored by the current paradox: The popular hypothesis is that long-term polypharmacy will be required in the early-onset bipolar population, yet the clear preference in this population is not to use medication at all and if needed to use the minimum[6].

This chapter provides a selected review of the use of lithium in children and adolescents integrating our own related research findings. The emphasis is on mood disorders, but included is a brief overview of lithium benefits in other pediatric clinical populations. The chapter is divided into the following sections: (1) pediatric mania; (2) recurrent mood disorders in children; (3) affected offspring of lithium-responsive parents; and (4) aggression and other indications.

LITHIUM AS AN ACUTE TREATMENT FOR PEDIATRIC MANIA

There are data from case reports, open studies and randomized double-blind studies supporting the effectiveness of lithium in the treatment of acute mania. The most recent studies are summarized below. For a review of earlier studies, the reader is directed to references 7 and 8.

In a recent well-designed retrospective study of the naturalistic treatment in a series of 133 early-onset patients (mean age 13.1 years) meeting DSM-IV criteria for a manic or mixed index episode (45% with psychotic features and 59% requiring hospitalization), evidence was provided supporting the effectiveness of lithium alone or in combination with antipsychotics for the acute treatment[9]. In this study the majority of patients were drug naive at intake and the vast majority (83%) were started on a single mood stabilizer, usually lithium. All subjects recovered from the acute episode and antipsychotics were added to mood stabilizers in 58% of patients when other mood stabilizers alone proved ineffective in rapidly resolving the episode. The antipsychotic medications were typically tapered by 10–25% every month after remission was achieved. In this study the patients had relatively low rates of co-morbidity: attention-deficit hyperactivity disorder (ADHD) (11%), rapid cycling (28%) and lifetime histories of mixed episodes (30%).

A number of open studies of lithium treatment of manic episodes in adolescents and children have been reported. Specifically, in a novel study by Strober and colleagues[10], the antimanic response to an open 6-week trial of lithium was assessed in two groups of bipolar I adolescents divided on the basis of prepubertal versus adolescent onset (of any psychiatric disturbance). Differences in treatment effectiveness emerged by week 4, at which time over

65% of the adolescent-onset probands met criteria for significant improvement compared to only 33% of the prepubertal onset probands; by week 6 the response rates were 80% compared to 40%, respectively. This study provided evidence of heterogeneity within the early-onset bipolar population; that is, those with prepubertal onset may differ genetically and pharmacologically from those with adolescent onset.

Further evidence of differential treatment response was provided in a subsequent study[11] of a cohort of hospitalized manic patients divided on the basis of presence or absence of childhood ADHD. Improvement in manic symptom scores was evident in both lithium treatment groups as early as the first week; however, the mean change in scores was greater for the manic patients without a childhood history of ADHD. The percentage of patients meeting variable responder criteria at study completion was 33–67% in those with childhood ADHD compared to 67–87% without a history of ADHD. The rate of any use of adjunctive antipsychotic use was comparable in both subgroups (20% vs. 23%, respectively).

However, in a subsequent study the association of a poorer response to acute lithium treatment and early childhood psychopathology was not replicated[12]. In this study the only predictor of non-response to lithium used as an acute manic treatment was the presence of prominent psychotic features. In the sample of manic adolescents studied, the majority of childhood disturbances was broader than in the sample described by Strober and colleagues and included mood and anxiety disorders, as well as ADHD and conduct problems. In addition, the response to lithium in this study was determined after discontinuation of adjunctive antipsychotics, unlike the earlier studies. Therefore, the significance of early childhood psychopathology and effectiveness of lithium anti-manic treatment response remains unclear.

To compare effect sizes for three mood stabilizers – lithium, divalproex sodium and carbamazepine – 42 outpatients in a mixed or hypomanic/manic episode, and ranging in age from 8 to 18, were randomnly assigned to 6 weeks of open treatment[13]. Large and comparable effect sizes using the change in the Young Mania Rating Scale (YMRS) scores from baseline to exit were reported for all three mood stabilizers. Response rates were comparable to those of adult mania studies (42% for lithium and 46% for sodium divalproex). This was a very young study sample with the mean age of onset of bipolar symptoms of 7.1 years and mean age at enrollment of 11.4 years. Of the sample, 71% had a co-morbid diagnosis of ADHD and 79% of the sample had had prior treatment with psychotropic medications.

In the first published placebo-controlled trial of short-term lithium treatment in a heterogeneous group of bipolar youth with secondary substance use disorders, lithium was reported to have benefits in terms of the global assessment of functioning scores and a decrease in substance use[14]. This study suggests that lithium may be effective in a subset of bipolar youth with co-morbid substance dependency. However, interpretation is limited, given that there was a variance in clinical state (nature of the current mood episode, severity of residual symptoms) between subjects at the start of the trial and the short-term nature of the trial (6 weeks of treatment).

While there is evidence to suggest that acute episodes of non-psychotic mania may respond well to lithium monotherapy, episodes of psychotic mania may require an antipsychotic alone or in combination. Specifically, Kafantaris and colleagues[15] reported that 64% of acutely manic adolescents with prominent psychotic features (89% delusions, 71% auditory hallucinations and 21% with formal thought disorder) treated openly with a combination of lithium and an antipsychotic showed significant improvement in 4 weeks. The mean decline in YMRS scores was 81%. When adjunctive antipsychotic medication was discontinued in 14 of 28 of these patients (meeting stabilization criteria), six (43%) experienced a major exacerbation within the first week, which resolved within days of reintroduction of the antipsychotic. Only eight of the 28 adolescents treated openly with a combination of lithium and antipsychotic could be weaned from the antipsychotic and continued on lithium monotherapy for an additional 4 weeks.

The question of whether lithium alone can maintain acute recovery from a severe manic episode was addressed more recently, in a companion study involving 85 acutely manic adolescents[16]. Subjects with psychotic features and/or extreme aggression were less likely to meet lithium response criteria compared to patients without these characteristics (20% response rate vs. 60%, respectively). In this study, 19 of 40 responders to a 4-week trial of lithium monotherapy were randomly assigned to continue lithium and 21 to discontinue lithium for a 2-week trial period. It was reported that ten of the 19 patients continuing on lithium compared to 13 of the 21 placebo-treated patients experienced a clinically significant exacerbation. The high relapse rate in the lithium-treated group was surprising, but may relate to the group of patients studied and to the design. There was insufficient information provided to judge how classical the cases of bipolar disorder were in this sample (age of onset, nature of the clinical course, lifetime psychotic symptoms, previous treatment). However, there was an indication that the vast majority of these adolescents had co-morbid disorders and ten of the 40 had required adjunctive antipsychotic medication prior to randomization for stabilization – although the results did not differ when these subjects were excluded from the analysis. Finally, as pointed out by the authors, the 4-week stabilization period was probably too short to determine response to lithium monotherapy, especially given the severity of illness in these patients.

Summary

There is convergent evidence that lithium is an effective antimanic agent in pediatric patients; however, the data from controlled studies remain relatively sparse. From the available information it appears that lithium is indicated particularly in the treatment of uncomplicated non-psychotic mania. Although from adult and adolescent studies the effectiveness is usually not evident until after the first week of treatment, other pharmacological agents in the short term are indicated[17]. In more severe adolescent manic episodes with prominent psychotic features, the adjunctive use of an antipsychotic medication appears warranted. At this stage it is not clear whether lithium in combination with an antipsychotic provides more benefit than the antipsychotic alone in the acute treatment of severe psychotic mania. We do not have reliable predictors of lithium response in acutely manic children or adolescents, nor do we have a good understanding of the factors contributing to lithium resistance in this population. Finally, it needs to be emphasized that treatment of acute mania is not the same undertaking as selecting efficacious long-term mood-stabilizing treatment for individual patients with recurrent mood disorders.

LITHIUM AS A PROPHYLACTIC TREATMENT FOR RECURRENT MOOD DISORDERS IN CHILDREN AND ADOLESCENTS

While there is substantial evidence of the long-term efficacy of lithium in preventing recurrences of both depressive and manic episodes in bipolar adults, there is no adequate controlled study evidence of the long-term prophylactic efficacy of any mood stabililzer, including lithium, in early-onset bipolar disorder. Given the complexity and chronicity described in some cohorts of bipolar youth, it is hypothesized that early-onset bipolar patients may be resistant to monotherapy and to lithium in particular[18]. However, there are convergent data from small case series, naturalistic and discontinuation studies to suggest that at least a subset of bipolar youth benefit from long-term lithium treatment.

In a review of small case series using lithium in the treatment of bipolar disorder in persons under age 18, Campbell and colleagues[19] concluded that the heterogeneity of the diagnoses and the variable duration of illness and clinical states posed significant interpretation difficulties. Subsequently, Delong and Aldershof[20] reported on a large cohort of lithium-treated youth. Of these, 59 were diagnosed with childhood bipolar disorder, and had started treatment at a mean age of 11 years. Twenty-eight youths were continued on long-term lithium following on average 30 months of treatment and having been identified as clearly benefiting.

The first naturalistic follow-up study evaluating long-term lithium treatment in a cohort of rigorously diagnosed and systematically followed adolescent manic patients who responded to lithium acutely was reported by Strober and colleagues[21]. They found a significantly increased relapse rate in those non-adherent or discontinuing lithium (based on sub-therapeutic plasma levels) over an 18-month follow-up period compared to those compliant with lithium (92% vs. 37.5% rate of relapse, respectively). In both groups (non-completers and completers) relapses clustered in the first year. Strober and colleagues made mention of the fact that the 4-week period on

which to base response may in retrospect have contributed to the high relapse rate early on, and that a longer duration to determine acute treatment response would be helpful.

In a recently reported naturalistic prospective follow-up study of juvenile manic patients advised to continue prophylactic treatment, mostly lithium alone or in combination, a high relapse rate was reported over an average of 52 months[22]. The rate of relapse was 53% for compliant and 100% for non-compliant patients. The authors concluded that lithium prophylaxis delayed the mean time to relapse and reduced the overall number of recurrences.

An extension study following acutely treated hypomanic and manic/mixed children (7–18 years) totaling 24 weeks of prospective treatment examined the effectiveness of combination therapy[18]. Twenty of 35 subjects (58%) required combination treatment and 16 of these subjects (80%) responded to the combination. There were no clinical characteristics that reliably differentiated those successfully continued on monotherapy to those requiring combination. This sample was relatively young, with a mean age of onset of bipolar symptoms at age 7 years, and most had co-morbidity including ADHD (80%), oppositional defiant disorder (38%) and anxiety disorder (17%). Moreover, 80% of this sample had prior psychotropic medication including stimulants for several years.

One often cited clinical concern is that co-morbid conditions may require separate or additional treatment. This hypothesis has not been adequately put to the test. There are observational data to suggest that the use of low-dose stimulant medication in combination with a mood stabilizer in children diagnosed with bipolar disorder and ADHD may be clinically helpful[18,23]. However, there are concerns that stimulants may trigger mania and/or exacerbate psychotic features[24]. Also, there is the concern of rapid cycling or chronicity of course in using adjunctive antidepressants in bipolar youth[25,26]. Furthermore, high-risk studies have shown that children at specific familial risk for bipolar disorder manifest a wide variety of psychopathological conditions in the early course of illness.

Along these lines, one aspect so far not taken into account in long-term treatment studies has been the heterogeneity of the early-onset bipolar population. There is evidence of both etiologic and phenotypic heterogeneity among adults with established bipolar disorder. A three-spectra model has been proposed, differentiating subtypes based on family history, clinical course and treatment response[27]. Furthermore, in our high-risk studies comparing the children of parents with bipolar disorder clearly responsive and clearly non-responsive to long-term lithium monotherapy,

we have found differences in early childhood functioning, psychopathology, clinical course and co-morbidity[28,29].

Briefly, children of lithium responders develop episodic recurrent emotional/psychiatric problems, mostly mood disorders. The mood disorder usually starts with a depressive episode in mid-adolescence following normal or gifted functioning in early childhood. In contrast, children of lithium non-responders develop more insidiously with the onset of mood disorders in mid-adolescence following an abnormal early childhood characterized by significant difficulties with social and/or academic functioning (Figures 16.1 and 16.2).

Other (co-morbid) psychiatric disorders in these children tend to include anxiety and sleep disorders that, in the children of lithium responders, antecede the mood disorder, while in the children of lithium non-responders they

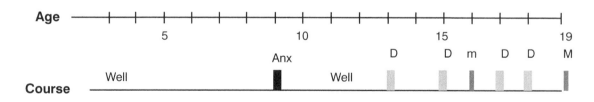

Figure 16.1   Offspring of lithium responder: course of illness. Anx, anxiety episode; D, depressive episode; m, hypomanic episode; M, manic episode

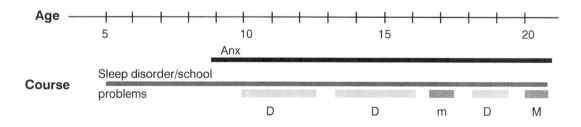

Figure 16.2   Offspring of lithium non-responder: course of illness. Anx, anxiety episode; D, depressive episode; m, hypomanic episode; M, manic episode

Table 16.1 Offspring with bipolar spectrum disorders treated with mood stabilizers (minimum of 1-year post-stabilization)

Offspring no.	Clinical course	Mood disorder onset (years)	Index episode	Major lifetime episodes	Parent treatment response	Offspring treatment response	Alda scores*
01	Episodic	19	D	4	LiR	Li	7
02	Episodic	18	D	3	LiR	Li	10
03	Episodic	16	D	3	LiR	Li	8
04	Episodic	16	D	5	LiR	Li	10
05	Episodic	15	D	7	LiR	Li	7
06	Episodic	13	D	5	LiR	Li	8
07	Episodic	25	D	2	LiR	LTL	9
08	Episodic	11	D	6	LiR	Li	9
09	Episodic	16	D	4	LiR	Li	8
10	Episodic	16	D	3	LiR	Li	10
11	Chronic	15	D	Chronic	LiNR	LiNR	2
						QTP	?
12	Chronic	13	D	Chronic	LiNR	QTP	7
13	Chronic	18	D	Chronic	LiNR	QTP	8
14	Chronic	18	D	Chronic	LiNR	LiNR	0
						QTP	9
15	Chronic	18	D	Chronic	LiNR	DVP	8

D, depressive episode; LiR, lithium responsive; LiNR, lithium non-responsive; Li, lithium; LTL, lamotrigine; QTP, quetiapine, DV; divalproex sodium.

*Alda score responder is ≥ 7/10 – this scale considers the completeness of response out of 10, with points taken off for confounding factors including decreased compliance and adjunctive use of medications

continue alongside the mood disorder. The nature of the early psychopathology overlaps in terms of anxiety and sleep problems, but among the offspring of lithium non-responders includes neurodevelopmental problems such as learning disabilities, problems with attention and cluster A traits.

More recently, we have been studying the response to a systematic open trial of mood stabilizers in offspring affected with a bipolar spectrum disorder[6]. Blind retrospective ratings of openly treated offspring suggest that the majority of early-onset bipolar patients can be stabilized and on monotherapy (Table 16.1). Furthermore, there is the suggestion of a differential response with identifiable pre-dictive variables. For example, those offspring who responded to long-term lithium (minimum of 1 year) after acute stabilization came from lithium-responsive parents and experienced an episodic remitting clinical course. Those who responded to an atypical antipsychotic came from lithium non-responsive parents (mostly stabilized on antipsychotics) and experienced a non-remitting course with significant residual symptoms prior to treatment. These residual symptoms have been characterized on Minnesota Multiphasic Personality Inventory (MMPI) profiles taken at clinical optimum, showing elevations in scales of measuring social introversion, odd and rigid beliefs and anxiety[30].

Of major significance in our experience of treating young people in the early stages of a mood disorder has been their own conceptualization of the underlying problem and the preference not to use prescribed medication to stabilize the symptoms. In a recent survey of our population of offspring of affected parents, the clear majority indicated that they did not consider their own mood disorder to be related to that of their parent[31]. Furthermore, these affected offspring ranked lifestyle changes, social rhythm, exercise, massage therapy and psychotherapy as acceptable treatment modalities, but not prescribed medication. This reluctance to take medication is borne out by the fact that the majority of responders in the case series discontinued the trial of mood stabilizer, despite showing an excellent remission and reporting no adverse effects of the medication. All of these offspring agreed to restart the medication upon relapse, but this discontinuity was associated with an additional median 2 years (2–7-year range) in starting an adequate trial of maintenance treatment.

An additional challenge has been the diagnostic approach to patients in the early stages of illness. In the above-mentioned case series, the median time from the onset of the mood disorder until the start of the rated prophylactic treatment trial was 6 years. However, those with a latency of 5 years or more had all been assessed by a health professional (family doctor, pediatrician, psychiatrist) within the first 2 years of the mood disorder. In seven out of eight cases, the diagnosis was one of reactive depression or adjustment and seemingly failed to consider the family history and risk of bipolar disorder.

Summary

There is a significant gap in our knowledge about the prophylactic efficacy of lithium in early-onset bipolar disorder and about when to intervene with long-term treatment. Given the clear evidence of prophylactic efficacy and anti-suicidal properties of long-term lithium treatment in bipolar adults, this lack of data is worrisome and requires urgent attention. While data from some studies including young children with complex psychopathology suggest that long-term lithium monotherapy may not be successful and combination therapy may be required, these conclusions are premature. Evidence of heterogeneity within the early-onset bipolar domain and associated differential treatment response warrants systematic study. Additional aspects of treatment that need due attention are factors contributing to non-compliance in this population.

LITHIUM IN THE AFFECTED OFFSPRING OF LITHIUM-RESPONSIVE PARENTS

There have been a limited number of case reports of the benefit of lithium among offspring of lithium-responsive parents which were based on the hypothesis that an important inherited factor was involved in the disorder, and that the early stages of illness may present in childhood. Dyson and Barcai[32] reported on two children from lithium-responsive manic-depressive parents each manifesting a broad range of sub-threshold symptoms including: hyperactivity, shortened attention span, low frustration tolerance, explosive anger, guilt and depression, and not meeting their potential academically. A trial of stimulant followed by a trial of lithium was instituted. In both cases there was initial improvement to the stimulant that was then lost. On lithium both achieved sustained improvement that was lost on discontinuation.

In a small double-blind cross-over trial of lithium among a heterogeneous sample of psychiatrically affected children of lithium-responsive parents, McKnew and colleagues[33] reported that the hypothesis of inherited response to lithium regardless of psychopathology was partially supported, especially for children diagnosed with an affective disturbance.

In our own studies of the children of well-characterized bipolar parents controlling for assortative mating, we have reported that anxiety, sleep and cognitive disturbances in childhood appear to be antecedents to evolving mood disorders in these offspring[29]. Therefore, it is possible that the complex psychopathology manifesting early in the course of illness may reflect one underlying disease process requiring a specific and unitary treatment approach.

Preliminary evidence in our high-risk studies to support this hypothesis comes from a consecutive small case series of offspring who were treated initially for presenting psychopathology other than bipolar disorder (sleep, attention, anxiety, depressive disorders) on the recommendation of a psychiatrist for adolescents based on blindly reviewed case descriptions and standard of practice guidelines (Table 16.2). Based on symptom rating scale scores and clinical global impression scale scores, essentially all offspring in the initial few weeks of prospective treatment appeared to benefit or at least not feel worse on the medication (antidepressant, methylphenidate, tryptophan, benzodiazepine). However, after a minimum of 8 weeks of treatment, all subjects either discontinued the medication or were clinically deemed no longer to benefit. Of these, eight offspring have subsequently gone on to stabilize on long-term prophylactic treatment of bipolar spectrum disorder. In those affected offspring who responded to a minimum 1-year adequate trial of lithium monotherapy, all had lithium-responsive parents.

Summary

There is anecdotal and case series evidence to suggest that psychiatrically affected offspring of lithium-responsive parents may themselves benefit from lithium. This is supported by both family studies of adult relatives[34] and small case series of offspring. Predicting lithium response in the early course of psychiatric illness would be of great value in reducing morbidity and mortality. It appears that the family history of treatment response is a major clue, along with other predictors that require systematic study in the early-onset population such as clinical course and family history of psychopathology.

OTHER INDICATIONS FOR LITHIUM IN CHILDREN AND ADOLESCENTS

There are a number of small case series reporting the effectiveness of lithium in diagnostically heterogeneous samples of children[35,36]. In an early case series described by Annell[37] the children who were deemed to benefit from lithium were described as having periodic psychopathology often with depressive spectrum problems and a positive family history of manic-depressive disorder. In a detailed review of these early studies (mostly case reports) Campbell and colleagues[19] concluded that lithium was justified for certain patient categories when more conventional treatments had failed. These conditions included bipolar disorder, conduct disorder (especially with severe aggression, and in mentally retarded patients with severe aggression and explosive affect; see Chapter 19) and in children with behavioral symptoms whose parents responded to lithium.

Later studies have gone on to prove that lithium is an effective anti-aggressive agent in a number of pediatric patient populations. More

Table 16.2 Consecutive series of psychiatrically affected offspring openly treated according to diagnosis and standard of practice guidelines

Offspring no.	Parent	Diagnosis	Medication	Response	Subsequent diagnosis	Stabilized
01	LiNR	Sleep/Anx	SSRI	No	Chronic D/Anx	QTP
02	LiNR	Anx	SSRI	No	Chronic D/Anx	QTP
03	LiNR	Anx/sleep	Tryp	No	Anx/sleep	No trial
04	LiNR	Anx/D	SSRI	Partial	Anx/D	No trial
05	LiNR	ADD/Anx	Stim SSRI	No Partial	Chronic Anx/D	No trial
06	LiNR	Anx Rec D	SSRI	Partial	Rec D/Anx	No trial
07	LiNR	Anx/D	SSRI	No	BP nos	QTP (failed Li)
08	LiNR	Anx/D	SSRI	No	BP nos	QTP? (failed Li)
09	LiR	Rec D	RIMA	No	BP II	Li
10	LiR	Rec D	SSRI	No – Switch	BP I	Li
11	LiR	ADD D	Stim SSRI	No Partial (rcyc)	BP nos	No trial
12	LiR	Anx/D	SNRI	Partial (rcyc)	BP nos	Refused trial
13	LiR	Sleep Adj	Zop	No	Rec d	Refused trial
14	LiR	D	SSRI	No – Switch	BP I	Li
15	LiR	D	SNRI	No – Switch	BP II	Li

Anx, anxiety disorder; ADD, attention deficit disorder; D, major depression; d, minor depression; adj, adjustment disorder; SSRI, selective serotonin reuptake inhibitor; stim, stimulant; RIMA, reversible inhibitor of monoamine oxidase; SNRI, selective serotonin norepinephrine reuptake inhibitor; Tryp, tryptophan; Zop, zopiclone; QTP, quetiapine; Li, lithium; rcyc, rapid cycling; Switch, switching into hypomania/mania; Rec D, recurrent major depressive disorder; Rec d, recurrent minor depressive disorder

recent case reports have observed the effectiveness of lithium in treating aggression, self-injury and manic-like symptoms in autistic children[38]. Several double-blind placebo-controlled short-term trials of lithium for treating aggression in pediatric patients diagnosed with conduct disorder demonstrated benefit[19,39,40]. In one recent review it was concluded that lithium was the most well-documented medication for treating conduct disorder in youth[41].

Summary

In clearly defined circumstances, as in the long-term treatment of classical bipolar disorder, lithium has been reported to have a number of benefits, some seemingly specific and some seemingly non-specific, as in the calming anti-aggressive properties and antipsychotic effects[42]. The latter effects have been conceptually linked to the serotonin enhancing actions of lithium in the limbic forebrain.

CONCLUDING REMARKS

It is clear, even from the early observations, that for specific subgroups of pediatric patients lithium is an important and possibly life-saving medication. The challenge remains to define more clearly the pediatric patient populations in which lithium is efficacious and within these populations to identify reliable factors predicting lithium response. The latter point is essential, given the broadness of the current diagnostic criteria for mood disorders. Further, the importance of reliable and valid predictive factors for lithium response is underscored by the recent observations from earlier investigators and our own studies that presenting phenomenology has little to do with the evolving underlying disorder, at least as far as bipolar disorder is concerned.

Adult studies have demonstrated that lithium response clusters in bipolar families, and can be predicted in individual patients on the basis of clinical course, co-morbidity and family history. Provocative preliminary research suggests that, within the early-onset bipolar domain, a subset respond to long-term lithium monotherapy and show reliable predictive features including an episodic course of illness and a positive family history of lithium response.

The hypothesis of differential response to long-term mood stabilizers including lithium among early-onset bipolar patients is important and requires systematic study. Further the specific effects of lithium on suicidal behavior and mortality require investigation in the early-onset population. While large-scale randomized trials are ultimately important to proving a hypothesis, we need to understand more about the predictive factors of treatment response in this population and address the issues of heterogeneity. In other words, more thoughtful study designs in homogeneous populations seem a necessary interim step. Otherwise, we are at risk for repeating the non-informative and expensive experience demonstrated by failed antidepressant trials in depressed adolescents and more recent negative trials of some putative mood stabilizers in adults.

REFERENCES

1. Youngerman J, Canino IA. Lithium carbonate use in children and adolescents. Arch Gen Psychiatry 1978; 35: 216–24
2. Campbell M, Schulman D, Rapoport JL. The current status of lithium therapy in child and adolescent psychiatry. A report of the Committee on Biological Aspects of Child Psychiatry of the American Academy of Child Psychiatry, December 1977. J Am Acad Child Psychiatry 1978; 17: 717–20
3. Schou M. Lithium prophylaxis: myths and realities. Am J Psychiatry 1989; 146: 573–6
4. Grof P, Alda M, Grof E, et al. The challenge of predicting response to stabilizing lithium treatment: the importance of patient selection. Br J Psychiatry 1993; 163 (Suppl 21): 16–19
5. Grof P. Selecting effective long-term treatment for bipolar patients: monotherapy and combination therapy. J Clin Psychiatry 2002; 63: 2723
6. Duffy A, Deshauer D, Alda M, Grof P. Long-term treatment of early-onset bipolar disorder with mood stabilizers: observations from a case series of affected offspring of well characterized bipolar parents. Bipolar Disord 2005; in press
7. Alessi NE, Naylor MW, Ghaziuddin M, Zubieta JK. Update on lithium carbonate therapy in children and adolescents. J Am Acad Child Adolesc Psychiatry 1994; 33: 291–304

8. Kafantaris V. Treatment of bipolar disorder in children and adolescents. J Am Acad Child Adolesc Psychiatry 1995; 34: 732–41

9. Rajeev J, Srinath S, Girimaji S, et al. A systematic chart review of the naturalistic course and treatment of early-onset bipolar disorder in a child and adolescent psychiatry center. Compr Psychiatry 2004; 45: 148–54

10. Strober M, Morrell W, Burroughs J, et al. A family study of bipolar I disorder in adolescence: early onset of symptoms linked to increased familial loading and lithium resistance. J Affect Disord 1988; 15: 255–68

11. Strober M, DeAntonio M, Schmidt-Lackner S, et al. Early childhood attention deficit hyperactivity disorder predicts poorer response to acute lithium therapy in adolescent mania. J Affect Disord 1998; 51: 145–51

12. Kafantaris V, Coletti DJ, Dicker R, et al. Are childhood psychiatric histories of bipolar adolescents associated with family history, psychosis, and response to lithium treatment? J Affect Disord 1998; 51: 153–64

13. Kowatch RA, Suppes T, Carmody TJ, et al. Effect size of lithium, divalproex sodium, and carbamazepine in children and adolescents with bipolar disorder. J Am Acad Child Adolesc Psychiatry 2000; 39: 713–20

14. Geller B, Cooper TB, Sun K, et al. Double-blind and placebo-controlled study of lithium for adolescent bipolar disorders with secondary substance dependence. J Am Acad Child Adolesc Psychiatry 1998; 37: 3171–9

15. Kafantaris V, Coletti DJ, Dicker R, et al. Adjunctive antipsychotic treatment of adolescents with bipolar psychosis. J Am Acad Child Adolesc Psychiatry 2001; 40: 1448–56

16. Kafantaris V, Coletti DJ, Dicker R, et al. Lithium treatment of acute mania in adolescents: a placebo-controlled discontinuation study. J Am Acad Child Adolesc Psychiatry 2004; 43: 984–883

17. Licht RW, Vestergaard P, Kessing LV, et al. Psychopharmacological treatment with lithium and antiepliptic drugs: suggested guidelines from the Danish Psychiatric Association and the Child and Adolescent Psychiatric Association in Denmark. Acta Psychiatr Scand 2003; 108: 1–22

18. Kowatch R, Sethuraman G, Hume JH, et al. Combination pharmacotherapy in children and adolescents with bipolar disorder. Biol Psychiatry 2003; 53: 978–84

19. Campbell M, Perry R, Green WH. Use of lithium in children and adolescents. Psychosomatics 1984; 25: 95–106

20. Delong GR, Aldershof AL. Long-term experience with lithium treatment in childhood: correlation with clinical diagnosis. J Am Acad Child Adolesc Psychiatry 1987; 26: 389–94

21. Strober M, Morrell W, Lampert C, Burroughs J. Relapse following discontinuation of lithium maintenance therapy in adolescents with bipolar I illness: a naturalistic study. Am J Psychiatry 1990; 147: 457–61

22. Jairam R, Srinath S, Girimaji SC, Seshadri SP. A prospective 4–5 year follow-up of juvenile onset bipolar disorder. Bipolar Disord 2004; 6: 386-394

23. Biederman J, Mick E, Prince J, et al. Systematic chart review of the pharmacologic treatment of comorbid attention deficit hyperactivity disorder in youth with bipolar disorder. J Child Adolesc Psychopharmaco 1999; 9: 247–56

24. Reichart CG, Nolen WA. Earlier onset of bipolar disorder in children by antidepressants or stimulants? An hypothesis. J Affect Disord 2004; 78: 81–4

25. Geller B, Luby J. Child and adolescent bipolar disorder: a review of the past 10 years. J Am Acad Child Adolesc Psychiatry 1997; 36: 1168–76

26. Geller B, Sun K, Zimerman B, et al. Complex and rapid-cycling in bipolar children and adolescents: a preliminary study. J Affect Disord 1995; 34: 259–68

27. Alda M. The phenotypic spectra of bipolar disorder. Eur Neuropsychopharmacol 2004; 14: S94–S99

28. Duffy A, Alda M, Kutcher S, et al. Psychiatric symptoms and syndromes among adolescent children of parents with lithium-responsive or lithium-nonresponsive bipolar disorder. Am J Psychiatry 1998; 155: 431–3

29. Duffy A, Alda M, Kutcher S, et al. A prospective study of the offspring of bipolar parents responsive and non-responsive to lithium treatment. J Clin Psychiatry 2002; 63: 1171–8

30. Demidenko N, Grof P, Alda M, et al. MMPI as a measure of subthreshold residual psycho-pathology among the offspring of lithium responsive and non-responsive bipolar parents. Bipolar Disord 2004; 6: 1–6

31. Strategies for longterm management of bipolar disorder. In Improving Quality of Life in Bipolar Disorder (Highlights of a Symposium Presented at the Annual Meeting of the Canadian Psychiatric Association, October 2004, Halifax, Nova Scotia

32. Dyson WL, Barcai A. Treatment of children of lithium-responding parents. Curr Ther Res 1970; 12: 286–90

33. McKnew DH, Cytryn L, Buchsbaum MS, et al. Lithium in children of lithium-responding parents. Psychiatry Res 1981; 4: 171–80

34. Grof P, Duffy A, Cavazzoni P, et al. Is response to prophylactic lithium a familial trait? J Clin Psychiatry 2002; 63: 942–7

35. Annell AL. Lithium in the treatment of children and adolescents. Acta Psychiatr Scand 1969; 207: 19–30

36. Frommer EA. Depressive Illness in Childhood. 1979: 117–36

37. Annell AL. Manic–depressive illness in children and effect of treatment with lithium carbonate. Acta Paedopsychiatr 1969; 36: 292–301

38. McDougle CJ, Stigler KA, Posey DJ. Treatment of aggression in children and adolescents with autism and conduct disorder. J Clin Psychiatry 2003; 64 (Suppl 4): 16–25

39. Campbell M, Adams PB, Small AM, et al. Lithium in hospitalized aggressive children with conduct disorder: a double-blind and placebo-controlled study. J Am Acad Child Adolesc Psychiatry 1995; 34: 445–53

40. Malone R, Delaney M, Luebbert J, et al. A -double-blind placebo-controlled study of lithium in hospitalized aggressive children and adolescents with conduct disorder. Arch Gen Psychiatry 2000; 57: 649–54

41. Geradin P, Cohen D, Mazet P, Flament MF. Drug treatment of conduct disorder in young people. Eur Neuropsychopharmacol 2002; 12: 361–70

42. Grof P, Grof E. Varieties of lithium benefit. Prog Neuropsychopharmacol Biol Psychiatry 1990; 14: 689–96

17 Lithium in the elderly

Laszlo Gyulai, Robert C Young, Johanna Sasse

Contents   Introduction • Pharmacology • Treatment of bipolar disorder in the elderly • Treatment of unipolar depression in the elderly • Clinical recommendations

INTRODUCTION

When lithium was discovered by Cade in 1949 as a treatment of mania ('excited psychosis'), three elderly subjects among the ten manic patients treated with lithium responded well to lithium citrate[1], although all three developed side-effects. In two, dose adjustment reduced the side-effects and lithium remained effective. In the third patient the side-effects mandated discontinuation of the treatment. Today, these cases still illustrate the key issues of administering lithium in the elderly: its efficacy in this age group, the need for dose adjustments and sensitivity to side-effects. Treatment of bipolar disorder in the elderly is not based on strong scientific evidence but rather on open-label prospective or retrospective studies[2]. Interestingly, although lithium has been the treatment of choice for bipolar disorder, its efficacy as an augmenting agent in the treatment of unipolar depression has been studied more rigorously in this age group. The discovery that lithium may have neuroprotective potential[3–5] has reinvigorated interest in the biology of lithium and its use in geriatric patients.

PHARMACOLOGY

Pharmacokinetics

Since the pharmacokinetics of lithium in the elderly are different from those in younger adults, more careful dosing and monitoring of serum level is required. Lithium dosage is generally 20–40% lower in the elderly than in younger patients[6,7]. Greil et al.[8] found that the ratio of weight-related lithium dose to plasma level may decline with age. The decrease in dose/plasma level starts at approximately age 50, with a mild decline thereafter. The lower lithium dose/plasma level reflects the lower volume of distribution in the elderly, which is due to lower total body water and decreased renal clearance[7]. Lithium clearance decreases with age by up to 60%[9]. The decline in renal function and lithium clearance in the elderly is exacerbated by hypertension and compensated heart failure and thus leaves these patients at increased risk for lithium toxicity[10]. The conservative clinical approach, based on the findings of Greil et al.[8], is to titrate lithium dosage carefully and monitor lithium levels more frequently in patients aged >50 years.

Drug–drug interactions

There have been case reports of toxicity from the combination of lithium and selective serotonin reuptake inhibitors (SSRI)[11]. Tricyclic antidepressants may increase lithium-induced tremor[12]. The combination of lithium and antipsychotic drugs can lead to serious neurotoxicity, e.g. delirium, cerebellar dysfunction and extrapyramidal symptoms. Neurotoxic side-effects such as tremor and impaired alertness develop both in the elderly and in younger patients when lithium is combined with either conventional (phenothiazines, haloperidol) or atypical antipsychotics (clozapine)[12].

Besides other psychotropic agents, drug–drug interactions can occur between lithium and medications used to treat co-morbid medical conditions[6]. There is an increased risk of lithium toxicity within a month of initiating treatment with a loop diuretic or an angiotensin-converting enzyme (ACE) inhibitor. ACE inhibitors reduce lithium clearance in hypertensive patients by 26% and increase steady-state lithium levels by 35%[13]. Thiazide diuretics, non-steroidal anti-inflammatory agents and sodium restriction can increase lithium concentration[6].

Adverse effects

Many papers have been published about lithium's side-effects and toxicity in patients of various ages, but very few are available which deal specifically with the elderly. The most frequently reported side-effects in the elderly include excessive thirst, hand tremor, excessive urination and dry mouth[14]. Lithium may cause tremor in 40% of hospitalized elderly at a serum level around or above 1 mEq/l[15]. In a recent

study by Sajatovic and colleagues[16] the most common adverse events (>10%) with lithium were dyspraxia, tremor, xerostomia, headache, infection and fatigue. Greil *et al.*[8] also noted that with comparable plasma lithium levels a higher number of older (≥ 65 years) patients (35%) developed minor adverse reactions than did their younger cohort (19%).

Lithium may be associated with cardiac conduction defect and rhythm disturbances, even on therapeutic levels of serum lithium (0.7–1.1 mEq/l)[17,18]. It has been suggested that older patients are at higher risk of developing these side-effects on therapeutic levels of lithium. Lithium-associated sick sinus syndrome may be encountered at therapeutic levels in older patients with compromised sinus node function.

Lithium antagonism of thyroid function (see Chapter 22) and the diminished reserve that accompanies aging may make the elderly vulnerable to hypothyroidism. A high proportion of geriatric lithium-treated patients receive thyroxine replacement or have elevated thyroid stimulating hormone (TSH) levels[19]. Osteoporosis is a special concern among the elderly. Since lithium can cause hyperparathyroidism and consequent bone loss[20], vigilant monitoring of parathyroid function may be needed in older patients being treated with lithium.

Toxicity

The most frequent symptoms of lithium toxicity in the elderly are ataxia, lethargy, delirium, tremor and vomiting[15]. Nevertheless, lithium did not seem to produce delirium more often than valproate in a Canadian population-based elderly cohort study[21]. Toxicity in the elderly may develop on lower serum lithium levels, especially in the presence of neurological co-morbidities[22]. However, neurotoxicity on 'therapeutic' lithium levels can develop both in the elderly and in the younger age groups[23]. In the medically ill elderly, 76% have side-effects, developing tremor, hyperactive neuromusculature, gastrointestinal problems, sedation and fatigue at a serum lithium concentration of 0.63 mmol/l and lithium dose of 484 ± 164 mg/day[24]. In particular, sodium depletion and renal diseases are identified as causative and aggravating factors leading to lithium poisoning.

TREATMENT OF BIPOLAR DISORDER IN THE ELDERLY

Research regarding lithium use in the elderly progressed at a snail's pace. No controlled trials were available for assessing the efficacy of lithium in the acute or continuation/maintenance treatment of late-life bipolar disorder (Table 17.1). The general dearth of studies can be partially explained by the fact that advanced

Table 17.1 Overview of clinical studies addressing the efficacy of lithium in bipolar disorder

	Design	n	Age (years)	Diagnosis	Duration of treatment (days)	Efficacy/ effectiveness
Himmelhoch et al.[32]	Retrospective, naturalistic	81	63.3 ± 6.9 (55–88)	BP I: 74 BP II: 7	21–56	56 (69%) responders
Chen et al.[30]	Retrospective	30	69.4 ± 8.2	BP (manic/mixed)	16.1 ± 9.9	20 (67%) improved overall
Van der Velde[53]	Retrospective	12	67 (60–74)	BP (manic)	14 (acute phase), 3 years (continuation)	4 (33%) improved in acute phase, 2 (17%) no recurrence in first year, 1 (8%) had no recurrence in second or third year
Murray et al.[6]	Prospective	37	60–78	BP 25, UP 12	14	Trend to severe/ prolonged mania in elders
Stone[54]	Retrospective	43	na	BP (manic)	22.4	Lithium did not alter the number of readmissions
Hewick et al.[5]	Retrospective	23	50–59	BP (82%) UP (9%) Other (9%)	na	Age contributed 14% to the interpatient variation
Abou-Saleh and Coppen[44]	Prospective, double-blind	22	> 59	BP MDD	12 months	Efficacy of lithium was not dependent on plasma lithium level
Schneider and Wilcox[41]	Prospective, naturalistic	4	65–81	BP I/II, rapid cycling	Acute treatment, maintenance treatment for years	All patients remitted; discontinuation of lithium led to relapse in two cases

na, not available; BP, bipolar disorder; UP, unipolar disorder; MDD, major depressive disorder age further complicates examination of the efficacy of lithium in mania, depression and maintenance treatment of bipolar disorder. These 'complexities' include medical co-morbidities, differences in the pharmaco-kinetics of lithium in the elderly compared to younger age groups, possible differences in relationship of dose/blood level and side-effects and challenges in recruitment of a sufficient number of study subjects. Guidelines for the treatment of mania are based almost exclusively on evidence gathered from mixed-age populations, and therefore not directly applicable to the treatment of mania in the elderly[25].

Treatment of mania

The need to treat acute mania in the elderly is illustrated by the fact that hospital admissions for late-onset mania after age 60 can be as high as 9.3% of all affective disorders and 4.7% of all psychiatric admissions[26]. The strength of evidence for lithium's efficacy for mania in the elderly is rather weak because the estimates are based on open-label or retrospective studies (Table 17.1). Overall, these studies indicate that lithium is efficacious in the treatment of geriatric mania. An additional limitation in delineating the efficacy of lithium in geriatric mania is that in some studies polypharmacy was used for treatment and the efficacy of lithium was not analyzed separately[27]. Elderly patients were included in some trials, but the low number of subjects did not allow sub-sample analysis. In others, the lower age limit was < 60 years, so that the patient sample included middle-aged persons as well as elderly patients. For example, Platman[28] found that lithium appeared more efficacious than chlorpromazine in the treatment of various dimensions of mania (belligerence, grandiosity, sleep, denial and overall severity) in a sample of patients of 56 ± 12.5 years of age. These studies have heuristic significance only.

There have been no systematic studies to define how the dose of lithium or serum/plasma lithium level affect the antimanic efficacy of lithium in elderly manic patients[7]. Preliminary findings from naturalistic treatments of manic elderly patients indicated that bipolar manic patients aged > 60 years with bipolar I disorder generally responded better to lithium concentrations of > 0.8 mEq/l than to lower concentrations[29]. This was also noted in a retrospective report on the manic bipolar elderly[30]. Lithium may be effective as an adjunct to other psychotropic agents in treating mania in the elderly. In a case report, Goldberg et al.[31] observed that the combination of divalproex (1250 mg/day with serum valproate level of 60–88 mg/l) and low-dose lithium (600–900 mg/day with serum lithium level of 0.4–0.6 mEq/l) may be a beneficial combination with good efficacy and low side-effect burden in two elderly (71 and 76 years old) female patients. In mixed-age adults, lithium may not be as effective for mixed episodes (depressive and manic symptoms) as for mania. In the elderly, the efficacy of acute lithium treatment for mixed episodes has not been tested in prospective controlled trials. Lithium (0.3–1.3 mmol/l serum level) appeared to be effective in controlling mixed and manic episodes in elderly subjects studied in a retrospective chart review[30], although numerically lithium seemed less effective in patients with mixed episodes than in those with manic episodes (statistical comparison was not performed).

Clinical characteristics can affect the acute antimanic effect of lithium. Elderly manic patients with co-morbid neurological illness or secondary mania may have worse acute therapeutic outcomes with lithium treatment than those without[32]. Himmelhoch et al.[32] noted that extrapyramidal impairment predicted a poorer acute antimanic effect with lithium treatment. Co-morbid dementia may worsen antimanic outcomes with lithium treatment. Executive dysfunction, which is often associated with frontostriatal pathology, was associated with attenuated acute response to pharmacotherapy in elderly manic patients[33].

Other co-morbid conditions may also have a negative influence on treatment outcomes in mania. Substance abuse is reportedly associated with poor antimanic response to lithium in the elderly. Black *et al.*[34] noted that co-morbid medical illness was also associated with poor lithium response in a patient group with a mean age of 50.8 years.

There is converging evidence that lithium is effective in the treatment of geriatric mania. It is unclear whether the effective plasma/serum level of lithium is the same as or lower than that in the younger mixed-age adults. However, some elderly patients respond to treatment with a low serum lithium level. Therefore, the starting dose of lithium could be less in the elderly than in younger mixed-age patients with bipolar disorder. It may be approximately 50% of the starting dose in mixed-age younger adults. Manic patients with neurological and other medical co-morbid conditions show a poorer response to lithium.

Treatment of acute bipolar depression

Studies on treatment research on bipolar depression in the elderly are even scarcer than those on mania. Fieve and colleagues found a mild acute antidepressant effect of lithium but only two out of 17 lithium-treated patients were ≥ 60 years old[35]. Noyes *et al.*[36] ascribed improvement of a bipolar depressive episode to lithium in a 58-year-old woman. Worrall *et al.* treated 5 bipolar and 7 unipolar depressed patients with lithium who were 59.9 ± 2.9 years old. Lithium was beneficial in lessening the intensity of depression[37]. Symptomatic bipolar disorder in the elderly, including bipolar depression and manic syndromes, may manifest a dementia-like syndrome. Cowdry and Goodwin[38] found that in a 63-year-old man a dementia syndrome masking depression was resolved using lithium at 0.6 mEq/l blood level. The clinician must vigorously pursue the diagnosis and treatment of a mood disorder despite cognitive impairment. Collateral information, general physical, neurological examination and laboratory tests contribute to an evaluation of the cognitively impaired elderly.

The extreme scarcity of studies on the efficacy of lithium in geriatric bipolar depression makes it difficult to provide clear clinical guidelines. Lithium can potentially play a useful role in the treatment of acute geriatric bipolar depression. The most important aspect of clinical management of geriatric bipolar depression is recognizing it and distinguishing it from dementia or other medical conditions masking depression.

Maintenance treatment

In a study of Murray *et al.*[6], elderly patients with bipolar disorder being maintained on lithium had the same depressive morbidity as their younger cohort with comparable plasma lithium levels. Increasing age in this study was associated with increased manic morbidity. Patients with late-onset mania may benefit from continuation/maintenance lithium treatment, since lithium reduced the frequency of affective episodes in patients with late-onset mania[39]. Recently, in two large-scale maintenance studies with mixed-age patients, the efficacy of lamotrigine was compared to that of lithium[40]. These studies included a sizeable elderly sub-set. Sajatovic *et al.*[16] conducted a secondary analysis of these studies on the elderly sub-sample. Ninety-eight patients were 55 years old or older at the time of study entry. They were randomized to 18 months of double-blind monotherapy with lamotrigine (LTG) (100–400 mg/day), lithium (Li) (serum level of 0.8–1.1 mEq/l) or placebo (PBO) after an open-label stabilization phase by lamotrigine. Efficacy outcomes (time from randomization until intervention for an emerging manic/hypomanic/mixed or depressive episode) were examined (lamotrigine $n = 33$, lithium $n = 34$, placebo $n = 31$). Lithium, but not lamotrigine, delayed time to intervention for mania compared with placebo (LTG vs. PBO, $p = 0.233$; Li vs. PBO, $p = 0.034$; LTG vs. Li, $p = 0.350$). Lithium did not delay the time to intervention for a depressive episode (Li vs. PBO, $p = 0.779$; LTG vs. PBO, $p = 0.011$; LTG vs. Li, $p = 0.011$). The fact that lithium was not effective in preventing the depressive episodes in this study may not contradict earlier studies on the efficacy of lithium in lowering depressive morbidity, because this was an enriched study design in which the randomized patient groups were lamotrigine responders in the open phase.

Clinical factors may modify the outcome of maintenance treatment for bipolar disorder in the elderly. For example, in the mixed-age population, rapid cycling bipolar illness does not particularly improve with lithium treatment. In the elderly, pertinent, systematically derived evidence on this point is lacking. In a case series, Schneider and Wilcox[41] used a combination of lithium and divalproex to treat elderly patients diagnosed with rapid cycling bipolar disorder. Two of their patients relapsed after lithium was discontinued and improved when lithium was reinstated. The authors concluded that both medications are needed to stabilize the rapid-cycling course. It is of note that all of their patients had predominantly (hypo)manic episodes, which diverges from the typical course of bipolar disorder. Therefore, this report may apply only to a subgroup of elderly patients with rapid-cycling bipolar disorder.

Cognitive and neurological impairment can also adversely affect maintenance treatment outcome in the elderly. Elderly bipolar patients with neurological co-morbidity have a higher risk of psychiatric re-hospitalization and institutionalization. Research on pharmacological approaches to prevent suicide in the bipolar elderly is sorely lacking[42]. Long-term lithium treatment reduced mortality, including suicide, in patients with manic-depressive and schizoaffective disorder. The prophylactic treatment with lithium started at 42 years and lasted 86 months. Clearly, some of these patients were 'elderly', especially by the later part of the observation period. Therefore, this study can have limited, perhaps mostly heuristic, relevance to the elderly and stimulates further research. In a recent study in Denmark[43] those patients who purchased lithium >5 times had reduced rates of suicide compared to those who purchased lithium only once. This effect of lithium was not age dependent in the sample aged between 18 and >81 (median age 55 years).

There is evidence that lithium is effective in the prevention of manic episodes in the elderly. The efficacy of lithium in preventing depressive episodes in elderly patients with bipolar disorder is weak at this point. There is no direct evidence that lithium reduces the risk of suicide in elderly bipolar patients, but by extrapolation from results in mixed-aged patients it is a possibility requiring further studies. Cognitive impairment predicts a poor prognosis.

In summary, lithium is frequently used for the treatment of older people suffering from bipolar disorder, especially for mania and maintenance, in spite of the paucity of research about its efficacy and safety. Clearly, clinical practice has acknowledged the usefulness of lithium in the treatment of bipolar disorder, and scientific investigation must now catch up with the naturalistic practice of the clinical physician.

TREATMENT OF UNIPOLAR DEPRESSION IN THE ELDERLY

The efficacy of lithium as a single or adjunctive agent in the treatment and prophylaxis of major depressive disorder (MDD) in the elderly has perhaps been given more attention in more controlled trials than has the treatment of bipolar depression. This may reflect the higher prevalence of MDD among the elderly and perhaps less complex trial designs for studying MDD than those for studying bipolar depression.

In a mostly unipolar depressed sample (42 unipolar and five bipolar patients ≥60 years old and 75 patients <60 years old), age had no effect on affective morbidity over 4–5 years of lithium treatment[44]. In 22 elderly patients (18 unipolar and four bipolar) a plasma lithium level between 0.45 and ≥0.8 mEq/l had no effect on outcome over a 12-month period[44]. Older patients maintained on lithium are not more predisposed to increased affective morbidity; on the contrary, there is a decrease in rates of hospitalization and use of additional antidepressants[6].

Augmentation of antidepressants

Lithium augmentation of antidepressants has been a useful strategy for treatment of antidepressant-resistant depression both in the elderly and in mixed-age patients. Kushnir[45] described five cases in which addition of low-dose lithium to antidepressants led to enduring improvement in medically ill patients with major depressive episodes. The serum lithium levels, achieved with 150–300 mg daily, ranged between 0.15 and 0.30 mEq/l. In two cases, adding low-dose lithium allowed a reduction of the dose of antidepressants and thus effected a subsequent decrease in antidepressant-induced side-effects. Zimmer et al.[46] found lithium augmentation to be effective in nortriptyline-resistant unipolar elderly patients, but this effect is smaller than in younger patients[47]. The antidepressant effect of lithium is dose dependent[48].

Further proof of the efficacy of lithium augmentation is the fact that upon lithium discontinuation a significant portion of patients relapse. Those patients who had been treated with lithium for a longer time before discontinuation had a higher risk of relapse. These studies indicate that long-term lithium augmentation is beneficial for patients with major depression[49]. Low-dose lithium augmentation of antidepressants in elderly patients who were in remission on various antidepressants appeared to prevent relapse[50].

CLINICAL RECOMMENDATIONS

Lithium adjustment

The target dose of lithium in the elderly is lower than in mixed adult patients because of the lower dose/serum level ratio. It is recommended that the starting dose of lithium be 150–300 mg/day. The dosage increase depends on the patient's actual dose/serum level ratio. After initiation of lithium treatment, in 5–7 days (preferably 7 days) the serum lithium level must be measured again. The clinician may calculate the dose/serum level ratio as a guide to identify patients with an extremely low dose/serum level ratio. This is important, because these patients can be acutely sensitive to changes in lithium dosage. Lithium dose can be increased then for most patients by 150–300 mg every 5–7 days. In 5–7 days after each dose increment, serum lithium level needs to be measured and preferably the dose/serum level ratio recorded. Monitoring this ratio may also help during the maintenance phase to identify a change in risk for toxicity. During the maintenance phase, serum lithium levels should be measured every 6 months.

Drug safety

Before initiation of the treatment, physical examination is performed in every patient. Particular attention needs to be paid to cardiac status, thyroid glands, kidney areas, neurological status, hydration and dermatological conditions (especially psoriasis). Pre-treatment laboratory work-up must include serum levels of creatinine, TSH, free thyroxine and tri-iodothyronin, sodium and potassium, and urine analysis. Hematological examination is useful. An initial electrocardiogram (ECG) is strongly recommended. For patients with an abnormal creatinine count, a 24-hour creatinine clearance test should be performed. During the maintenance phase, serum lithium level, sodium, potassium and creatinine should be measured every 6 months. TSH must be measured at least every 12 months. Naturally, in elderly patients who suffer medical illnesses the frequency of these measurements should be increased as is appropriate. In patients with high blood pressure, for example, sodium, potassium and serum creatinine should be measured every 3 months and an ECG taken every 6 months or as clinically indicated. It is recommended that a full neurological examination be performed every 6 months or as clinically indicated.

Education

Education of elderly patients about treatment with lithium is especially important because they are at a higher risk of developing lithium side-effects and are more likely to have received or to be receiving treatment with multiple medications for non-psychiatric conditions[51]. In the Berlin Lithium Clinic patients with affective disorders who had been followed for 12.1 ± 13.9 years showed an age-dependent

decline in their knowledge about the importance of lithium treatment and its side-effects. Therapeutic drug monitoring of lithium treatment in the elderly may induce increased compliance and safety. In a British catchment area in 1998 a computer-based monitoring of lithium use was implemented in elders. It provided reminders to the clinicians to check lithium levels and helped identify high lithium levels and increase safety[52].

REFERENCES

1. Cade JFJ. Lithium salts in the treatment of psychotic excitement. Med J Aust 1949; 3: 349–52

2. Young RC, Gyulai L, Mulsant BH, et al. Pharmacotherapy of bipolar disorder in old age: review and recommendations. Am J Geriatr Psychiatry 2004; 12: 342–57

3. Moore GJ, Bebchuk JM, Hasanat K, et al. Lithium increases N-acetyl-aspartate in the human brain: in vivo evidence in support of bcl-2's neurotrophic effects? Biol Psychiatry 2000; 48: 1–8

4. Manji HK, Moore GJ, Chen G. Lithium at 50: Have the neuroprotective effects of this unique cation been overlooked? Biol Psychiatry 1999; 46: 929–40

5. Hewick DS, Newbug P, Hopwood S, et al. Age as a factor affecting lithium therapy. Br J Clin Pharmacol 1977; 4: 201–5

6 Murray N, Hopwood S, Balfour JK. The influence of age on lithium efficacy and side-effects in out-patients. Psychol Med 1983; 13: 53–60

7. Sproule B. Lithium in bipolar disorder: can drug concentrations predict therapeutic effect? Clinical Pharmacokinetics 2002; 4: 639–60

8. Greil W, Stoltzenburg MC, Mairhofer ML, Haag M. Lithium dosage in the elderly. A study with matched age groups. J Affect Disord 1985; 9: 1–4

9. Lehmann K, Merten K. Elimination of lithium in dependence on age in healthy subjects and

patients with renal insufficiency. Int J Clin Pharmacol Ther Toxicol 1974; 10: 292–8

10. Fliser D, Franek E, Joest M, et al. Renal function in the elderly: impact of hypertension and cardiac function. Kidney Int 1997; 51: 1196–204

11. Austin LS, Arana GW, Melvin JA. Toxicity resulting from lithium augmentation of antidepressant treatment in elderly patients. J Clin Psychiatr 1990; 51: 344–5

12. Katona CL. Psychotropics and drug interactions in the elderly patient. Int J Geriatr Psychiatry 2001; 16 (Suppl 1): 86–90

13. Finley PR, O'Brien JG, Coleman RW. Lithium and angiotensin-converting enzyme inhibitors: evaluation of a potential interaction. J Clin Psychopharmacol 1996; 16: 68–71

14. Chacko RC, Marsh BJ, Marmion J, et al. Lithium side effects in elderly bipolar outpatients. Hillside J Clin Psychiatry 1987; 9: 79–88

15. Smith RE, Helms PM. Adverse effects of lithium therapy in the acutely ill elderly patient. J Clin Psychiatry 1982; 43: 94–9

16. Sajatovic M, Gyulai L, Calabrese JR, et al. Maintenance treatment outcomes in older patients with bipolar I disorder. Am J Geriatr Psychiatry 2005; 13: 305–11

17. Roose SP, Bone S, Haidorfer C, et al. Lithium treatment in older patients. Am J Psychiatry 1979; 136: 843–4

18. Roose SP, Nurnberger JI, Dunner DL, et al. Cardiac sinus node dysfunction during lithium treatment. Am J Psychiatry 1979; 136: 804–6

19. Shulman KI, Sykora K, Gill SS, et al. New thyroxine treatment in older adults beginning lithium therapy: implications for clinical practice. Am J Geriatr Psychiatry 2005; 13: 299–304

20. Tannirandorn P, Epstein S. Drug-induced bone loss. Osteoporosis Int 2000; 11: 637–59

21. Shulman KI, Sykora K, Gill S, et al. Incidence of delirium in older adults newly prescribed lithium or valproate: a population-based cohort study. J Clin Psychiatry 2005; 66: 424–7

22. Himmelhoch JM, Neil JF, May SJ, et al. Age, dementia, dyskinesias, and lithium response. Am J Psychiatry 1980; 137: 941–5

23. Strayhorn JM Jr, Nash JL. Severe neurotoxicity despite 'therapeutic' serum lithium levels. Dis Nerv Syst 1977; 38: 107–11

24. Stoudemire A, Hill CD, Lewison BJ, et al. Lithium intolerance in a medical-psychiatric population. Gen Hosp Psychiatry 1998; 20: 85–90

25. Charney DS, Reynolds CF 3rd, Lewis L, et al., Depression and Bipolar Support Alliance. Depression and Bipolar Support Alliance consensus statement on the unmet needs in diagnostic and treatment of mood disorders in late life. Arch Gen Psychiatry 2003; 60: 664–72

26. Yassa R, Nair V, Nastase C, et al. Prevalence of bipolar disorder in a psychogeriatric population. J Affect Disord 1988; 14: 197–201

27. Wylie ME, Mulsant BH, Pollock BG, et al. Age at onset in geriatric bipolar disorder. Am J Geriatr Psychiatry 1999; 7: 77–83

28. Platman SR. A comparison of lithium carbonate and chlorpromazine in mania. Am J Psychiatry 1970; 127: 351–3

29. Young RC, Kalayam B, Tsuboyama G, et al. Mania: Response to lithium across the age spectrum. Soc Neurosci 1992; 18: 669

30. Chen ST, Altshuler LL, Melnyk KA, et al. Efficacy of lithium vs. valproate in the treatment of mania in the elderly: a retrospective study. J Clin Psychiatry 1999; 60: 181–5

31. Goldberg JF, Sachs MH, Kocsis JH. Low-dose lithium augmentation of divalproex in geriatric mania. J Clin Psychiatry 2000; 61: 304

32. Himmelhoch J, Neil JR, May SJ, et al. Age, dementia, dyskinesias, and lithium response. Am J Psychiatry 1980; 137: 941–5

33. Young RC, Gyulai L, Mulsant BH, et al. Pharmacotherapy of bipolar disorder in old age: review and recommendations. Am J Geriatr Psychiatry 2004; 12: 342–57

34. Black DW, Winokur G, Bell S, et al. Complicated mania. Arch Gen Psychiatry 1988; 45: 232–6

35. Fieve RR, Platman SR, Plutchik RR. The use of lithium in affective disorders. I. Acute endogenous depression. Am J Psychiatr 1968; 125: 487–91

36. Noyes R Jr, Dempsey GM, Blum A, Cavanaugh GL. Lithium treatment of depression. Compr Psychiatry 1974; 15: 187–93

37. Worrall EP, Moody JP, Peet M, et al. Controlled studies of the acute antidepressant effects of lithium. Br J Psychiatry 1979; 135: 255–62

38. Cowdry RW, Goodwin FK. Dementia of bipolar illness: diagnosis and response to lithium. Am J Psychiatry 1981; 138: 1118–19

39. Shulman K, Post F. Bipolar affective disorder in old age. Br J Psychiatry 1980; 136: 26–32

40. Calabrese JR, Bowden CL, Sachs G, et al., Lamictal 605 Study Group. A placebo-controlled 18-month trial of lamotrigine and lithium maintenance treatment in recently depressed patients with bipolar I disorder. J Clin Psychiatry 2003; 64: 1013–24

41. Schneider AL, Wilcox CS. Divalproate augmentation in lithium-resistant rapid cycling mania in four geriatric patients. J Affect Disord 1998; 47: 201–5

42. Shulman K. Suicide and parasuicide in old age: a review. Age Ageing 1978; 7: 201–9

43. Kessing LV, Sondergard L, Kvist K, Andersen PK. Suicide risk in patients treated with lithium. Arch Gen Psychiatry 2005; 62: 860–6

44. Abou-Saleh MT, Coppen A. Prognosis of depression in old age: the case for lithium therapy. Br J Psychiatry 1983; 143: 527–8

45. Kushnir T. Lithium-antidepressant combinations in the treatment of depressed, physically ill geriatric patients. Am J Psychiatry 1986; 143: 378–9

46. Zimmer B, Rosen J, Thornton JE, et al. Adjunctive lithium carbonate in nortriptyline-resistant elderly depressed patients. J Clin Psychopharmacol 1991; 11: 254–6

47. Flint AJ, Rifat SL. A prospective study of lithium augmentation in antidepressant-resistant geriatric depression. J Clin Psychopharmacol 1994; 14: 353–6

48. Stein G, Bernadt M. Lithium augmentation therapy in tricyclic-resistant depression. A controlled trial using lithium in low and normal doses. Br J Psychiatry 1993; 162: 634–40

49. Fahy S, Lawlor BA. Discontinuation of lithium augmentation in an elderly cohort. Int J Geriatr Psychiatr 2001; 16: 1004–9

50. Wilkinson D, Holmes C, Woolford J, et al. Prophylactic therapy with lithium in elderly patients with unipolar major depression. Int J Geriatr Psychiatry 2002; 17: 619–22

51. Dharmendra MS, Eagles JM. Factors associated with patients knowledge of attitudes towards treatment with lithium. J Affect Disord 2003; 75: 29–33

52. Head L, Dening T. Lithium in the over-65s: who is taking it and who is monitoring it? A survey of older adults on lithium in the Cambridge Mental Health Services catchment area. Int J Geriatr Psychiatry 1999; 13: 164–71

53. van der Velde CD. Effectiveness of lithium carbonate in the treatment of manic–depressive illness. Am J Psychiatry 1970; 123: 345–351

54. Stone K. Mania in the elderly. Br J Psychiatry 1989; 155: 220–4

18 Women and lithium treatment

Bettina Schmitz, Christof Schaefer, Andrea Pfennig

Contents   Introduction • Oral and other contraception • Lithium and pregnancy • Lithium toxicity in the neonate • Breast feeding • Teratogenic effects • Mood-stabilizing treatment alternatives to lithium • Additional sex-related aspects regarding treatment response and adverse effects

INTRODUCTION

This chapter discusses lithium treatment with a special focus on women's issues, including contraception, planning of pregnancy, monitoring during pregnancy, teratogenic risks and breast-feeding recommendations. Additional sex-related aspects are discussed concerning response and adverse effects related to lithium treatment.

The mean onset of bipolar disorder is during puberty. Affected women are therefore at risk for relapses throughout their reproductive years. Even if there are concerns with respect to family planning, there are no reasons why women with bipolar disorder with or without medical treatment should not have children. Unfortunately, 50% of pregnancies in women with bipolar disorder are not planned, with the associated increased risks for both the mother's and the baby's health. Women with childbearing potential who take lithium for stabilizing mood should be well informed about treatment-related risks during pregnancy and in the puerperal period. This information must be provided at the beginning of lithium treatment,

irrespective of whether the woman has immediate plans to become pregnant or not. Women should also understand their individual risk for relapses during or after pregnancy if mood-stabilizing medication has to be stopped, in order to achieve agreement on the optimal treatment strategy before pregnancy, and in order to avoid irrational and dangerous actions in the case of an unplanned pregnancy. Studies have shown that the main reason why women who become pregnant on antidepressants abruptly stop their medication is the fear of teratogenic risks. Even when these women receive reassuring counseling that it would be appropriate to continue treatment, only 61% of women choose to do so[1]. It was also shown that women who take a psychiatric drug are much more likely to discontinue their drug as compared to women on non-psychiatric medications, suggesting an additional influence of illness-associated stigma. The most important factor which influenced this decision was the initial information[2]. Unfortunately, many women with bipolar disorder are advised by their doctors to avoid pregnancy (45%). After a specialized consultation 63% of women decided to pursue pregnancy[3]. These studies highlight the importance of appropriate early counseling. Unfortunately, many psychiatrists do not only advise against pregnancy or recommend abortion, they also often automatically discontinue ongoing psychotropic medication in pregnancy without considering the impending psychiatric risks.

ORAL AND OTHER CONTRACEPTION

There are no interactions between lithium and oral contraceptive hormones[4]. Therefore, the use of lithium by itself does not limit the choice of contraceptive methods. However, pregnancies in women taking lithium should be carefully planned and, therefore, reliable contraceptive methods are recommended. A disadvantage of oral contraceptives is that their effect totally depends on compliance. In women who are likely to be non-compliant, other contraceptive methods should be discussed, such as the intrauterine device, which is generally well tolerated and may be used even in very young women, who have not given birth ('nullipara'). Another compliance-independent alternative is the 3-monthly injection of contraceptive hormones. Many women who take lithium also take other drugs, often other mood stabilizers, some of which may interact with oral contraceptives. Carbamazepine, for example, belongs to a group of drugs that lower the safety of the pill because of hepatic enzyme induction. Lamotrigine can lower hormone levels (levonorgestrel) because of competition with glucuronidation and should, therefore, only be used following a discussion with the gynecologist in charge of the patient. When combining lamotrigine and oral contraceptives there is a risk of significantly decreased serum concentrations of lamotrigine, in the order of 50%[5], which may lead to loss of efficacy of lamotrigine or to toxic symptoms when an oral contraceptive is started or stopped.

LITHIUM AND PREGNANCY

All women with childbearing potential who take lithium should be well informed about the specific risks of lithium treatment during pregnancy. These issues should be discussed early in treatment. Given the importance of this subject it is recommended to mention the topic of contraception and family planning at each consultation.

The indication for the continuation of lithium in a woman who plans a pregnancy should be individually considered, and risks of treatment versus risks of psychiatric relapse need to be weighed against each other. Whether pregnancy protects against episodes of bipolar disorder is a matter of controversy. Grof *et al.*[6] retrospectively analyzed women from a registry of lithium-responsive bipolar disorder. Only pregnancies that took place prior to lithium treatment were included. The authors found a frequency of psychiatric episodes during the 9 months before pregnancy of 0.43 compared to a frequency of 0.14 during pregnancy and 0.68 during the 9 months after pregnancy. Interestingly, all recurrences observed during pregnancy took place during the last 5 weeks. Other studies could not confirm this result. It was suggested that overall pregnancy is 'risk neutral'[7], and that, in women with milder illness, pregnancy may not be destabilizing and might even be beneficial, while patients with severe bipolar disorder with recurrent illness on maintenance treatment have a high recurrence risk. A study comparing recurrence risks after discontinuation of lithium treatment in pregnant and non-pregnant women showed similar recurrence rates in both groups (52% versus 58%), and higher recurrence rates depending on number of episodes in the past and speed of discontinuation[8]. The relapse risk was also increased after birth (3-fold). In any case, pregnancy is not protective for all women with bipolar disorder and the decision regarding discontinuing treatment needs to be based on the individual course of the illness. If lithium is discontinued, the dosage should be tapered down slowly, and women need to be carefully monitored for early signs of relapse.

The most vulnerable period with respect to teratogenic effects is the first 10 weeks after the last menstrual period. In some women it might be possible to withdraw lithium slowly prior to pregnancy and restart treatment after the first 3 months of pregnancy. It should, however, be considered that not all women who want to become pregnant conceive immediately. Therefore, the duration of a lithium pause is impossible to predict with the related risks for psychiatric relapses. Discontinuation of lithium treatment should always be slow.

If continuation of lithium treatment is indicated, this should be done using a dosage as low as possible. The minimal effective dosage can be estimated by using the lowest dose that historically has kept the patient stable. High serum concentration peaks can be avoided by distributing the daily dosage into three or four single doses. Women must be informed about the symptoms of lithium toxicity which may be induced or exacerbated by hyperemesis gravidarum. Also, lithium intoxication may present with emesis which may be misinterpreted as pregnancy related. It is recommended that lithium-treated women be seen at regular intervals during pregnancy, and lithium levels should be monitored at monthly intervals and whenever clinical signs suggest intoxication. Decreasing lithium levels may require increasing dosages. During the last month of pregnancy serum levels should be checked on a weekly basis. Approximately 1 week before birth the dosage should be reduced by 25 or 50% or even stopped, and returned to the pre-pregnancy regimen after delivery.

Women who become pregnant under lithium should also be closely monitored by gynecologists. There is no special indication for a Cesarean section. However, delivery should be planned in a multidisciplinary hospital including psychiatry and pediatrics (Table 18.1).

Table 18.1 Recommendations for lithium treatment during pregnancy

(1)	Check indication for lithium and consider therapeutic alternatives
(2)	Use minimum effective dose, distributed into 3–4 single doses
(3)	Caution: lithium toxicity induced by hyperemesis gravidarum
(4)	Caution: lithium intoxication may mimic hyperemesis gravidarum
(5)	Avoid sodium restriction and the administration of diuretics
(6)	Check lithium levels: 1–8th months, monthly; 9th months, weekly; prior to delivery, every 2 days
(7)	Adjust dose according to serum levels (based on individual recurrence risk)
(8)	Avoid lithium levels above 1.2 mmol/l
(9)	Avoid dehydration around delivery (consider intravenous fluids in prolonged labor)
(10)	Lithium level may increase after delivery (consider lowering dosage around delivery)
(11)	High-level ultrasound examination (screen for fetal heart defects)
(12)	Newborn: check for hypothyroidism, diabetes insipidus, floppy infant syndrome

LITHIUM TOXICITY IN THE NEONATE

In a recent review of published cases with neonatal toxicity related to maternal lithium treatment, the most common problems were: hypotonia, respiratory distress syndrome, cyanosis, lethargy, feeding difficulties, depressed neonatal reflexes, apnea, bradycardia and jaundice[9]. Lithium babies have a higher risk of being born premature. In an international registry 36% of lithium-exposed babies were born premature and 37% of the premature infants were large for age[10]. The reason for fetal macrosomia has been considered to be the insulin-like effects of lithium on carbohydrate metabolism. Another complication of lithium exposure is nephrogenic diabetes insipidus, which may require brief treatment with antidiuretic hormone[11].

There is an increased risk for functional abnormalities of the heart and the pulmonary vascular system leading to persistent fetal circulation, atrial flutter, tricuspid regurgitation or congestive heart failure. Because of the increased risk for cardiac and ventilatory problems following birth, lithium-related deliveries should be considered high-risk births and managed accordingly. A standby neonatology team is necessary, because babies may need immediate respiratory assistance. In order to avoid neonatal toxicity, maternal lithium dosage should be lowered or paused in the days before delivery.

Transient effects on the thyroid gland include goiter and hypothyroidism which may require thyroid hormone replacement. Because of immature renal elimination, newborns should be monitored for signs of lithium toxicity for approximately 10 days after birth.

Neonatal toxic signs were fully reversible in all reported babies. Also, neurodevelopmental delay was always transient and normalized within the first year of life.

BREAST FEEDING

Older reports mentioned lithium concentrations in the breast milk of treated mothers of up to 80% of the mother's serum level. According to a more recent study, however, in half of the mothers the infants' dose via breast milk was less than 10% compared to the maternal weight-adjusted dose[12]. As the maternal serum concentrations were checked in only three of 11 mothers, non-compliance could explain the low lithium concentration in the breast milk of some mothers.

However, there were no significant differences in the calculated infants' doses between the three mothers with known serum level, one mother taking a sustained-release formulation and those seven with questionable compliance. None of the 11 infants showed toxic symptoms. After decline of the high postpartum lithium levels, breast-fed babies have blood levels that are usually not higher than one-third of the mother's blood level, but with a wide interpatient variability. One case report described a 2-month-old infant with tremor and dyskinesia. The lithium blood level was 200% as compared to the mother's blood level. The American Academy of Pediatrics classifies lithium among 'drugs that have been associated with significant effects on some nursing infants and should be given to nursing mothers with caution'[13]. Most experts agree that breast feeding is acceptable, and suggest that the benefits of breast feeding outweigh the disadvantages, if close monitoring of the baby is guaranteed, including measurements of lithium levels in the case of any symptomatology that is suspicious for lithium adverse effects. Mothers should be well informed about the increased risk for lithium intoxication in the case of infections and dehydration.

TERATOGENIC EFFECTS

Animal data on teratogenic effects of lithium are controversial. In mammals there have been both positive and negative results (reviewed in reference 14). In Wistar rats the incidence of birth defects appeared to be dependent on the total daily dosage and the frequency of doses[15]. Lithium crosses the human placenta freely. Because of the immaturity of renal elimination the lithium clearance may be reduced in the fetus. Thus, the fetus may have toxic serum concentrations while the mother's drug levels stay within the therapeutic range.

In 1974 two babies were reported who were diagnosed with a rare congenital heart defect, known as the Ebstein anomaly, following intrauterine lithium exposure[16]. The Ebstein abnormality affects the right heart and is characterized by downward displacement of the tricuspid valve into the right ventricle and variable degrees of right ventricular hypoplasia. The association between lithium exposure and cardiac malformations was confirmed by Weinstein et al.[17,18], who described a frequency of 11% malformations in the offspring of 225 women who were reported to a lithium registry. Eighteen of the babies were diagnosed to have malformations of the heart and the great vessels, including six cases of the Ebstein anomaly. This Danish–American–Canadian registry was established in order to monitor the prenatal effects of lithium. It was initiated by Schou in Denmark in 1969, later extended to an international registry, and closed in 1979. The problem of this registry was the retrospective collection of pregnancies which favored a selection of complicated outcomes.

Later studies were unable to identify significant risks for specific malformations following lithium treatment. In a cohort study by Källén and Tandberg[19], 12% of babies born to 59 mothers treated with lithium had malformations (three were exposed to lithium monotherapy, one to polytherapy including lithium). However, there was no case of Ebstein anomaly.

In a prospective Canadian study by Jacobsen et al.[20] the incidence of major malformations in children exposed to lithium in the first trimester was 2.8%, which was not different from the incidence in the control group (2.4%). Only one case of Ebstein malformation was detected among the offspring from 148 lithium-treated women.

Three independent case–control studies looked at prenatal drug exposure in babies born with Ebstein anomalies[21–23]. Summarizing these data, in a total of 133 babies with Ebstein anomalies there was no case with prenatal lithium exposure.

In a recent review the teratogenic risk of lithium with respect to the Ebstein anomaly was described to be overrated. Reviewing all available data, the risk for lithium-exposed babies with respect to the Ebstein anomaly was calculated to be in the order of 1/1000. Compared to the prevalence in the general population, which is 1 in 20 000 births, this represents a 20-fold increased risk, which is still relatively small[24].

Schou[25] followed up 60 prenatally exposed school children and found no decrease in intellectual or psychomotor development as compared to their unexposed siblings. In another study the attainment of developmental milestones was similar for 22 lithium-exposed children compared to a non-exposed control group[20].

General recommendations with respect to the reduction of teratogenic risks include the avoidance of polypharmacy and folate supplementation (3 months before conception and continuing until the end of the first trimester). High-level ultrasound examination should be offered with special focus on cardiac malformations, including fetal echocardiography.

MOOD-STABILIZING TREATMENT ALTERNATIVES TO LITHIUM

Because of the potential teratogenicity and toxicity of lithium salts, therapeutic alternatives should be considered when a pregnancy is planned. The choice of the prophylactic agent should be guided by the treatment history of the patient. Our knowledge about the teratogenic potential of mood-stabilizing drugs is still limited and does not allow us to make straight-forward recommendations.

Among mood stabilizers from the group of anticonvulsants, valproate must strictly be avoided, because of its proven teratogenicity. Apart from other major and minor malformations it increases the risk for neural tube defects by a factor of 20–30. Carbamazepine should also be avoided because of teratogenicity, although its risk is lower than that of valproic acid. Several studies suggested an increased risk for neural tube defects in the order of a factor of 20–30 (compared to the prevalence of approximately 0.05–0.1%)[24]. Experience with about 1000 pregnancies with lamotrigine mono-therapy has so far not shown an increased risk for major malformations as compared to the general population (for example, reference 26). However, it is too early to recommend lamotrigine as being superior to lithium with respect to teratogenicity. The UK pregnancy registry is one of three large prospective registries looking at the outcomes of anticon-vulsant-exposed pregnancies. The preliminary results from this registry suggest similar low major malformation rates in babies exposed to carbamazepine (2.3%) or lamotrigine (2.1%) during pregnancy[27]. The combination of lamotrigine with valproate is contraindicated, because a high prevalence of major malfor-mations in the order of 11% was observed in two studies[26,27].

If lithium therapy cannot be interrupted until the end of the first trimester, because of a high relapse risk, it should be continued at the lowest effective dosage. A change of treatment to anticonvulsants is as yet not recommended when a pregnancy is planned. Once a pregnancy has been established, it is usually too late for changes, because most patients present to their psychiatrist only after the most vulnerable teratogenic period in the first trimester. Pregnancies with exposure to anticonvulsants in the first trimester should be reported to the European Registry of Antiepileptic Drugs in Pregnancy (www.eurapinternational.org).

There are sufficient data for many tricyclic antidepressants, selective serotonin reuptake inhibitors (SSRIs), phenothiazines and haloperidol to rule out a substantial teratogenic risk. With respect to the atypical neuroleptics, some 100–200 pregnancies exposed to either clozapine or olanzapine were evaluated, but only very few with quetiapine, risperidone and ziprasidone. These limited numbers have not suggested a special risk to date. In particular with SSRIs and neuroleptics, however, toxic symptoms may occur in the neonate. Delivery should therefore be planned in a perinatology department.

There has been speculation about develop-mental toxic effects of the underlying psychiatric disease[28,29]. These hypotheses should of course not be used to worry pregnant patients, but they may be interpreted as an additional indication to continue the treatment of a woman with bipolar disorder during pregnancy.

ADDITIONAL SEX-RELATED ASPECTS REGARDING TREATMENT RESPONSE AND ADVERSE EFFECTS

The presentation of bipolar disorder differs in women and men. Amongst others, the prevalence of rapid cycling and mixed states seems to be higher in women. The effects of phases of the reproductive cycle, menopause and postmenopause are still somewhat unclear. For example, high rates of conversion to the rapid-cycling type are described in menopause[30,31], although we have to consider that the symptoms are very similar to the perimenopausal mood instability, calling for elegant research designs to clarify the issue.

Some of the differences seen in the clinical course of bipolar disease in women compared to men could reflect inadequate mood stabilization or excessive use of antidepressants, both being reported in women[32]. Supposing that women may be per se at higher risk for antidepressant-induced hypomania or mania[33], one recommendation is to minimize the use of antidepressants and adequately adopt mood-stabilizing agents in bipolar women.

Concerning treatment response, sex-associated differences are reported for antidepressants and antipsychotic agents[34–36]. Reports have suggested that mixed states may respond less well to lithium[37] and that lithium may be less sufficient in rapid cycling[38], both features being more prevalent in women than in men. Viguera et al.[39] computed an overall proportion for the data set of 17 clinical studies assessing lithium treatment in affective disorders. They did not find significant differences in response to short-term or long-term lithium treatment in unipolar depressive or bipolar disorders between women and men. Interestingly, there was even a non-significant tendency towards slight superiority in women. Baldessarini et al.[40] studied 360 bipolar I and II patients and did not find major differences in response to long-term lithium treatment between patients suffering from rapid cycling and those having other clinical presentations. They did not report sex-related differences in response to lithium.

Regarding pharmacokinetics and dynamics, subtle differences in the elimination of lithium between women and men have been reported. Women may clear lithium less efficiently than men and vary more in lithium clearance, perhaps in association with the menstrual cycle[35,41] as well as during pregnancy[42]. Kusalic and Engelsmann[43] assessed renal function in 51 bipolar patients with long-term lithium treatment. They found sex-associated differences in urinary volume, serum creatinine and creatinine clearance values.

Women are at higher risk of some adverse effects related to lithium treatment. The prevalence of lithium-associated hypothyroidism was found to be 14% in women compared to only 5.5% in men[44]. So far, no clear explanation has been found. The rate of thyroid disease in untreated women is seven to eight times that of men, which is discussed to be potentially related to higher levels of specific antithyroid antibodies in women[45]. Women may also be at higher risk for lithium-induced thyroiditis[33].

Despite conflicting data[46], there seems to be a sex-related difference in weight gain associated with lithium treatment, with women at a disadvantage[38]. Baptista et al.[47] showed in rat experiments that all doses tested significantly increased body weight in female rats. They described the data as showing a linear relationship between body weight gain and lithium dose in females. In contrast, in male rats low doses of lithium did not affect body weight and higher doses even decreased it. They also found that the effect on weight by lithium was additive to the effects of sulpiride (D2 dopamine receptor blocker) and insulin, suggesting that lithium may enhance body weight in rats by a different mechanism from that of sulpiride or insulin.

In a recent review of the literature Burt and Rasgon[13] concluded that substantially more research was needed to clarify sex-related effects on the course of bipolar disorder, on treatment response and on adverse effects.

REFERENCES

1. Einarson A, Bonari L, Koren G. Pregnancy and antidepressant counseling. Am J Psychiatry 2004; 161: 2137

2. Einarson A, Selby P, Koren G. Abrupt discontinuation of psychotropic drugs during pregnancy: fear of teratogenic risk and impact of counselling. J Psychiatry Neurosci 2001; 26: 44–8

3. Viguera AC, Cohen LS, Bouffard S, et al. Reproductive decisions by women with bipolar disorder after prepregnancy psychiatric consultation. Am J Psychiatry 2002; 159: 2102–4

4. Chamberlain S, Hahn PM, Casson P, Reid RL. Effect of menstrual cycle phase and oral contraceptive use on serum lithium levels after a loading dose of lithium in normal women. Am J Psychiatry 1990; 147: 907–9

5. Sabers A, Buchholt JM, Uldall P, Hansen EL. Lamotrigine plasma levels reduced by oral contraceptives. Epilepsy Res 2001; 47: 151–4

6. Grof P, Robbins W, Alda M, et al. Protective effect of pregnancy in women with lithium-responsive bipolar disorder. J Affect Disord 2000; 61: 31–9

7. Viguera AC, Cohen LJ, Tondo L, Baldessarini RJ. Protective effect of pregnancy on the course of lithium-responsive bipolar I disorder. J Affect Disord 2002; 72: 107–8

8. Viguera AC, Nonacs R, Cohen LS, et al. Risk of recurrence of bipolar disorder in pregnant and nonpregnant women after discontinuing lithium maintenance. Am J Psychiatry 2000; 157: 179–84

9. Kozma C. Neonatal toxicity and transient neurodevelopmental deficits following prenatal exposure to lithium: another clinical report and a review of the literature. Am J Med Genet 2005; 132: 441–4

10. Troyer WA, Pereira GR, Lannon RA, et al. Association of maternal lithium exposure and premature delivery. J Perinatol 1993; 13: 123–7

11. Pinelli JM, Symington AJ, Cunningham KA, Paes BA. Case report and review of the perinatal implications of maternal lithium use. Am J Obstet Gynecol 2002; 187: 245–9 Rev

12. Moretti ME, Koren G, Verjee Z, et al. Monitoring lithium in breast milk: an individualized approach for breast-feeding mothers. Ther Drug Monit 2003; 25: 364–6

13. Burt VK, Rasgon N. Special considerations in treating bipolar disorder in women. Bipolar Disord 2004; 6: 2–13 Rev

14. Schardein JL. Chemically Induced Birth Defects, 4th edn. New York: Marcel Dekker, 2000

15. Smithberg M, Dixit PK. Teratogenic effects of lithium in mice. Teratology 1982; 26: 239–46

16. Nora JJ, Nora AH, Toews WH. Lithium, Ebstein's anomaly, and other congenital heart defects. Lancet 1974; 2: 594–5

17. Weinstein MR, Goldfield M. Cardiovascular malformations with lithium use during pregnancy. Am J Psychiatry 1975; 132: 529–31

18. Weinstein MR. Lithium treatment of women during pregnancy and in the postdelivery period. In: Johnson FN, ed. Handbook of Lithium Therapy. Lancaster: MTP Press, 1980: 421–9

19. Källén B, Tandberg A. Lithium and pregnancy. A cohort study on manic–depressive women. Acta Psychiatr Scand 1983; 68: 134–9

20. Jacobson SJ, Jones K, Johnson K, et al. Prospective multicentre study of pregnancy outcome after lithium exposure during first trimester. Lancet 1992; 339: 530–3

21. Källén B. Comments on teratogen update: lithium. Teratology 1988; 38: 597

22. Zalzstein E, Koren G, Einarson T, Freedom RM. A case–control study on the association between first trimester exposure to lithium and Ebstein's anomaly. Am J Cardiol 1990; 65: 817–18

23. Edmonds LD, Oakley GP. Ebstein's anomaly and maternal lithium exposure during pregnancy [Abstract]. Teratology 1990; 41: 551–2

24. Shepard TH, Brent RL, Friedman JM, et al. Update on new developments in the study of human teratogens. Teratology 2002; 65: 153–61

25. Schou M. What happened later to the lithium babies? A follow-up study of children born without malformations. Acta Psychiatr Scand 1976; 54: 193–7

26. GlaxoSmithKline. Lamotrigine-Pregnancy Registry. Interim Report, January 2005

27. Morrow JI, Russell AJC, Irwin B, et al. The safety of antiepileptic drugs in pregnancy: results of the UK epilepsy and pregnancy registry. Epilepsia 2004; 45 (Suppl 3): 51

28. Hansen D, Lou HC, Olsen J. Serious life events and congenital malformations: a national study with complete follow-up. Lancet 2000; 356: 875–80

29. Zeskind PS, Stephens LE. Maternal selective serotonin reuptake inhibitor use during pregnancy and newborn neurobehavior. Pediatrics 2004; 113: 368–75

30. Blehar MC, DePaulo JR Jr, Gershon ES, et al. Women with bipolar disorder: findings from the NIMH Genetics Initiative sample. Psychopharmacol Bull 1998; 34: 239–43

31. Kukopulos A, Reginaldi D, Laddomada P, et al. Course of the manic–depressive cycle and changes caused by treatment. Pharmakopsychiatr Neuropsychopharamakol 1980; 13: 156–67

32. Tondo L, Baldessarini RJ. Rapid cycling in women and men with bipolar manic–depressive disorders. Am J Psychiatry 1998; 155: 1434–6

33. Leibenluft E. Issues in the treatment of women with bipolar illness. J Clin Psychiatry 1997; 58 (Suppl 15): 5–11

34. Yonkers KA, Kando JC, Cole JO, Blumenthal S. Gender differences in pharmacokinetics and pharmacodynamics of psychotropic medication. Am J Psychiatry 1992; 149: 587–95

35. Dawkins K. Gender differences in psychiatry: epidemiology and drug response. CNS Drugs 1995; 3: 393–407

36. Leibenluft E. Gender differences in major depressive disorder and bipolar disorder. CNS Spectrums 1999; 4: 25–33

37. Freeman MP, McElroy SL. Clinical picture and etiologic models of mixed states. Psychiatr Clin North Am 1999; 22: 535–46, vii

38. Goodwin FK, Jamison KR. Maintenance medical treatment. In Manic-Depressive Illness. New York, NY: Oxford University Press, 1990: 665–724, 746–762

39. Viguera AC, Tondo L, Baldessarini RJ. Sex differences in response to lithium treatment. Am J Psychiatry 2000; 157: 1509–11

40. Baldessarini RJ, Tondo L, Floris G, Hennen J. Effects of rapid cycling on response to lithium maintenance treatment in 360 bipolar I and II disorder patients. J Affect Disord 2000; 61: 13–22

41. Hendrik V, Altshuler LL, Burt VK. Course of psychiatric disorders across the menstrual cycle. Harvard Rev Psychiatry 1996; 4: 200–7

42. Yonkers KA, Little BB, March D. Lithium during pregnancy: drug effects and their therapeutic implications. CNS Drugs 1998; 9: 261–9

43. Kusalic M, Engelsmann F. Renal reactions to change of lithium dosage. Neuropsychobiology 1996; 34: 113–16

44. Johnston AM, Eagles JM. Lithium-associated clinical hypothyroidism. Prevalence and risk factors. Br J Psychiatry 1999; 175: 336–9

45. Bocchetta A, Bernardi F, Pedditzi M, et al. Thyroid abnormalities during lithium treatment. Acta Psychiatr Scand 1991; 83: 193–8

46. Mathew B, Rao JM, Sundari U. Lithium-induced changes in the body mass index. Acta Psychiatr Scand 1989; 80: 538–40

47. Baptista T, Murzi E, Hernandez L, et al. Mechanisms of the sex-dependent effect of lithium on body weight in rats. Pharmacol Biochem Behav 1991; 38: 533–7

19 Therapeutic and prophylactic effects of lithium on pathological aggression

Jeffrey Bierbrauer, Agneta Nilsson,
Bruno Müller-Oerlinghausen, Michael Bauer

Contents   What does pathological aggression mean? • Early case reports • Clinical trials • Possible mechanisms of the anti-aggressive effects

WHAT DOES PATHOLOGICAL AGGRESSION MEAN?

Investigations of human aggression are complicated by methodological problems and by the lack of a standardized and adequate definition of what aggression actually means. As an example, aggression has been described as a 'concept that ranges between something highly desirable to something abhorrent, which society tries to control by its legal process'[1]. Aggression seems to be best described along a continuum between 'assertiveness' (a rather useful aspect of aggression and probably an essential condition for human survival and achievement) and 'pathological aggression' (inappropriately violent and destructive behavior following any kind of provocation). Any classification of aggression has to account for the manifold situations in which aggressive behavior occurs as well as the value system that is being offended or defended.

Many researchers have chosen to regard aggression as 'any form of behavior directed towards the goal of harming or injuring another living being who is motivated to avoid such treatment'[2]. Another definition suggests that 'aggressive behavior is physical attacks on other persons, on property, or on one's self'[3], thus extending the concept to include self-injurious acts as well as damage to property. While both definitions are reasonably serviceable, a better one would be desirable.

In 1992 the Aggression Questionnaire (AQ) was published[4]. Replicated factor analyses yielded four scales: physical aggression, verbal aggression, anger and hostility. Over time, these scales proved to be internally consistent and stable. The various scales correlated differently with various personality traits and the scale scores correlated with peer nominations of the various kinds of aggression. These findings emphasize the need to assess not only overall aggression but also its individual components.

Another rating scale, the Overt Aggression Scale (OAS)[5], divides aggressive behavior into four categories: verbal aggression and physical aggression against objects, self and others. Aggression is then rated in all categories according to observable criteria.

Both questionnaires present valuable and useful resources for tracking progress in studies evaluating aggressive behavior.

EARLY CASE REPORTS

The 'father of lithium', John F Cade, seems to have been the first to suspect that lithium might have anti-aggressive effects. The following observation was included in his famous 1949 paper on the antimanic effect of lithium: 'Prefrontal leucotomy has been performed lately on restless psychopathic mental defectives in an attempt to control their restless impulses and ungovernable tempers. It is likely that lithium medication would be effective in such cases and would be much preferred to leucotomy'[6]. This interesting recommendation was not acted upon, however, until 20 years later when a number of Scandinavian case reports with sensational news were published.

Baastrup[7] had a patient with 'severe sociopathic personality disorder', dangerous to herself and to others. She had received 'all possible kinds of treatment' to no avail. When, as a last resort, she was put on lithium, she became stable in every respect and well-adjusted to society. 'I quite fail to understand this,' reported the author, 'she is certainly not a manic-depressive patient.'

Forssman and Walinder[8] described themselves as possessed by sudden 'lithomania' when they, after having seen some amazingly good results with lithium in patients with manic-depression, tried the drug for various atypical indications. Among the 18 cases reported were three with aggression as the predominant clinical feature, most notably a 43-year-old woman with symptoms of extreme 'uneasiness, aggression, hyperactivity, and loud screams.' Her behavior had 'caused fractures' and necessitated hospitalization for more than 25 years. Her response to a wide range of treatments, including psychosurgery and 'massive pharmacotherapy' had been poor. Lithium rapidly brought a striking change in her condition, however, and all aggressiveness practically ceased.

Since then several other case reports have been published on the beneficial effects of lithium on pathological human aggression[9–11].

CLINICAL TRIALS

The systematic scientific study of lithium and human aggression has involved four major areas: adult psychiatric populations, children with behavioral disturbances, patients with mental handicaps and persons with uncontrolled outbursts of rage.

Since some case reports and studies included in this review obviously might be classified as belonging to more than one category, a somewhat arbitrary labeling has sometimes been necessary. In cases of doubt, systematic presentation was preferred over absolute stringency as an inclusion criterion.

Adult psychiatric populations

Anti-aggressive effects have not been the primary matter of interest in lithium trials carried out hitherto in psychiatric populations. Many researchers have tested lithium as a last resort in intractable patients who failed to respond to previous treatment. Others have simply sought to explore the usefulness of lithium in treating a diagnostic category other than that of classic manic-depression. Consequently, the patient selection and strategy of these trials may not be ideal for the purpose of determining the cause and effect of reduced aggressive behavior. Nevertheless, the trial findings are of considerable interest. The symptom profiles involved include aggressive behavior, and the investigators have made observations concerning the effects of the lithium treatment on this particular symptom.

Van Putten and Sanders[12] administered lithium to 35 patients with 'chronic and incapacitating mental illness who had not responded to the usual pharmacological and interpersonal therapies' and who did not have a previously diagnosed manic-depressive illness. Rifkin et al.[13] conducted a 6-week, double-blind crossover trial with random allocation, comparing lithium to placebo in emotionally unstable character disorder. Both studies showed a favorable change in aggressive behavior during lithium medication. The authors of both studies concluded that the participants either had a previously undetected manic-depressive illness or a closely related condition.

Considering child abuse as aggressive behavior, it seems appropriate to mention an open trial conducted by do Prado-Lima and colleagues in 2001[14], in which lithium was administered to eight abusive mothers. In this trial, lithium significantly reduced their abusive behavior towards their children. Compiled on the basis of the global scores of the OAS, the trial results showed a statistically significant decrease in aggressiveness with lithium medication at day 30 and day 60 of treatment compared with baseline ($p = 0.027$). A closer look at all four OAS categories reveals that there was no reduction in the mothers' verbal aggression against their children or in their physical aggression against self categories, but their scores for physical aggression towards other people and towards objects showed statistically significant reductions ($p = 0.013$ and $p = 0.006$, respectively).

Using a randomized double-blind crossover design, Dorrego et al.[15] examined the efficacy of methylphenidate (MPH) and lithium for treating attention-deficit/hyperactivity disorder (ADHD) in adults. Patients received 8 weeks of MPH treatment (up to 40 mg/day) and 8 weeks of lithium treatment (up to 1200 mg/day) by random assignment. The study also examined aggression with the OAS. The findings indicated that lithium might be beneficial in the treatment of adult ADHD and that lithium (as well as MPH) significantly alleviated certain behavioral problems including aggressive outbursts.

Regarding mood disorders, an updated review by Ernst and Goldberg[16] on the anti-suicidal properties of psychotropic drugs mentions an observed reduction in suicidal behavior with lithium medication.

Children with behavioral disturbances

Studies conducted on lithium in children with aggressive behavior were also complicated by methodological difficulties[17]. Most studies conducted in children with aggressive behavior had involved extremely heterogeneous populations, and the presence of mental handicaps in some had further complicated diagnostic and other classification issues. Since 1995, at least four double-blind and placebo-controlled studies have been published on children or adolescents suffering from conduct disorders with predominantly aggressive features[18–21]. They confirm assumptions and observations made in earlier studies or case reports that medication with lithium in some cases significantly decreases aggressive behavior in children or adolescents. Some of these studies also featured aggression rating scales not previously available. A satisfactory evaluation of therapeutic effects, however, requires that rating scales be more age specific.

Interest in investigating lithium therapy in children with aggressive behavior has been growing over the past three decades. Extensive contributions in this field have been made by Campbell and colleagues, whose new rating scales have led to fundamental methodological improvements. Sixty-one children aged 5.2–12.9 years participated in the first study[22]. Inclusion criteria were a DSM-III[23] diagnosis of conduct disorder of the under-socialized and aggressive type, and a behavioral profile of severe aggressiveness, explosiveness and disruptiveness that had not responded to previous outpatient treatment. Candidates with evidence of psychosis or mental handicap were excluded from the study. The study design was double-blind and consisted of 2 weeks of baseline assessment followed by random allocation to 4 weeks on lithium, haloperidol or placebo. Lithium and haloperidol turned out to be superior to placebo in reducing target symptoms marked by hyperactivity, aggression and hostility. While there was no difference in effectiveness between haloperidol and lithium, side-effects occurred significantly more often on haloperidol than on lithium.

Studies conducted in the early 1990s failed to replicate these favorable lithium results. Carlson et al.[24] treated 11 hospitalized children (seven children received lithium in a double-blind crossover design) for 8 weeks. Although the children improved in the areas of self-control, aggression and irritability, only three out of 11 children on lithium had improved sufficiently to be discharged (8 weeks of treatment proved to be superior to 4 weeks of treatment). Moreover, improvement seen in patients on lithium was also seen in those treated with placebo, indicating that non-pharmacological factors are also involved in aggression reduction.

Campbell et al.[18] tried to replicate their earlier findings in a group of 50 children who featured severe aggressive and impulsive symptoms as part of a conduct disorder refractory to previous treatments. This placebo-controlled double-blind study consisted of 6 weeks of lithium medication followed by 2 weeks on placebo. In terms of reducing aggression, lithium was more effective than placebo, but the results were less clear than in the prior study. Campbell et al.[25] concluded that 'there is some suggestion that behavioural symptoms, particularly aggressiveness, if accompanied by a strong affective-explosive component, decrease with lithium administration.'

Rifkin et al.[19] examined the efficacy of lithium carbonate for treating conduct disorder in adolescents. Lithium or placebo was administered for 2 weeks in a double-blind fashion to 33 inpatients aged 12–17 years. Of the patients who completed the study, 8.3% of those receiving placebo (one of 12) versus 21.4% (three of 14) of those receiving lithium were considered responders. This difference was not statistically significant. As stated by the authors themselves, their results failed to support a difference between lithium and placebo, and both treatments appeared ineffective. The major limitation of this study was the relatively short duration of lithium treatment (only 2 weeks). Commenting on the differences between their results and Campbell's findings[18,22,25], which had demonstrated lithium's efficacy for hospitalized children with conduct disorder, they surmised that extending lithium treatment for a longer period might have produced a drug effect or that the response of adolescents may be different from that of children.

Malone et al.[20] investigated whether or not the aggression subtypes derived from the AQ were related to treatment response. They conducted a double-blind placebo-controlled trial of lithium as a treatment for reducing aggression in 28 aggressive conduct-disordered children (25 males, three females) with a mean age of 12.69 years (ranging between 9.8 and 17.0 years). Using the Predatory-Affective Index of the AQ to classify subjects into 'predatory' (planned) or 'affective' (explosive) subtypes of aggression and then correlating this classification to treatment response, they concluded that treatment responsiveness was associated with a more affective and less predatory subtype of aggression.

Malone and colleagues[21] conducted another important double-blind and placebo-controlled study on lithium, assessing its efficacy in the treatment of aggression in children and adolescents using a measure specific to aggression. Subjects were inpatients with conduct disorder, hospitalized because of severe and chronic aggression. A parallel-groups design was used with randomization to lithium or placebo. Only those who met the aggression criterion during the 2-week placebo-baseline period were randomized to 4 weeks of treatment. Outcome measures included Clinical Global Impressions, the Global Clinical Judgements (Consensus) Scale and the OAS. Eighty-six inpatients enrolled in the study; 40 (33 male and seven female; median age 12.5 years) entered and completed the treatment phase. Lithium turned out to be statistically and clinically superior to placebo. Sixteen of 20 subjects in the lithium group were responders on the Consensus ratings vs. six of 20 in the placebo group ($p = 0.004$). Ratings on the OAS decreased significantly for the lithium group versus the placebo group ($p = 0.04$). However, more than half of the subjects in the lithium group experienced nausea, vomiting and urinary frequency. The authors concluded that lithium is a safe and effective short-term treatment for aggression in inpatients with conduct disorder, but that its use is associated with adverse effects.

Patients with mental handicaps

The treatment of patients with mental handicaps can sometimes be an extreme challenge to the clinician. Aggressive outbursts can complicate the lives of mentally handicapped patients and their families to the extent that hospitalization is unavoidable. Self-injurious behavior such as head-banging, biting and scratching oneself is rare in most other conditions but occurs as widely as in 10–35% of institutionalized persons with mental handicaps[26]. Lithium therapy has been included comparatively often in attempts to alleviate the most severe symptoms featured by some mentally handicapped patients. The following involves only studies in which the authors have clearly diagnosed the participants as mentally handicapped on the basis of clinical evaluations and psychometric results, and in which the indication for treatment was aggressive or self-injurious behavior.

Dostal and Zvolsky[27] were the pioneers who conducted the first lithium trial on aggression. This open study of 14 adolescent, severely mentally handicapped patients featuring aggressive behavior demonstrated a beneficial effect under lithium administration. However, the majority of the patients showed signs of toxicity such as severe polydipsia and polyuria.

This study was followed by a number of prospective clinical trials also investigating the effectiveness of lithium on mentally handicapped patients featuring aggressive behavior[28–32].

Micev and Lynch's open study[28] also showed favorable results for lithium medication. Most remarkable is the fact that six out of eight patients featuring self-injurious behavior experienced complete remission of these symptoms. The other three studies cited above were conducted double-blind and placebo-controlled and showed reductions of aggressive symptoms that were significant and of clinical interest. Lithium-induced toxicity was registered in the study by Worall et al.[29] These toxic effects did not occur in the studies of Tyrer et al.[30] or Craft et al.[31]

Luchins and Dojka[33] retrospectively assessed the anti-aggressive effect of lithium ($n = 11$) and propranolol ($n = 6$), studying the charts of persons with mental retardation featuring both aggression and self-injurious behavior. Their results supported an equal reduction in both behaviors with lithium or propranolol.

Glenn et al.[10] published case reports of ten brain-injured patients with severe, unremitting, aggressive, combative, or self-destructive behavior. Five patients showed a dramatic response that resulted in a significant increase in their participation in a rehabilitation program.

Bellus and colleagues[32] concluded that the use of lithium within the context of an intensive behavioral rehabilitation program may yield positive effects in the control of aggressive behavior, even in the long term in patients following brain injury. By recording medication dosages and behavioral acuity indicators for a 2-year period in two patients, they demonstrated the efficacy of lithium in both cases (one 4 years and the other 17 years post-injury), showing that lithium in concert with other medications not only led to a decrease in the frequency of aggressive outbursts and restrictive measures but in one case also to a significant reduction of antipsychotic medication.

Interestingly, Micev and Lynch[28], Worall and colleagues[29], as well as Glenn et al.[10] reported increased aggression in some individual patients during lithium treatment, although the overall effect of lithium on all three groups respectively was a reduction of aggression. It seems safe to agree with Craft et al.[31] that 'lithium appears to be worth a 2-month trial in any [mentally handicapped] patient whose repeated aggression and self-mutilation is proving difficult to control.'

Glenn and colleagues concluded that lithium carbonate can be a useful medication in the treatment of aggressive behavior and affective instability after brain injury, but that it has significant potential for neurotoxicity in this population, particularly when used in conjunction with antipsychotic agents.

Persons with uncontrolled rage outbursts

In order to establish that lithium has an anti-aggressive effect, methodological problems have to be solved and means found to avoid at least some of the potential confusion as to what exactly is being treated. The interpretation of results is attended by the permanent uncertainty of what lithium treatment actually affects – is it aggression itself or a hitherto undetected manic-depressive illness? One interesting approach towards this goal is to study individuals in whom 'uncontrolled rage outbursts' is the main clinical trait, i.e. to focus on well-documented aggressive behavior rather than on specific psychiatric diagnoses in the study population. Ideally these participants should have few or no signs of mental disorder other than the tendency to explode with impulsive violence. These requirements are rarely met. This research strategy was adopted in a number of classic so-called 'prison studies' conducted in the 1970s on lithium and aggression[34–37].

Sheard[34] was the first to present study results, comparing lithium to placebo in a single-blind trial of 12 inmates from a maximum security prison in Connecticut. Lithium treatment resulted in significant reductions of self-rated aggressive affect while also being associated with a lower incidence of disciplinary sanctions. In a subsequent paper, Sheard[38] described the diagnostic characteristics in this study population as 'personality disorders: aggressive, sociopathic, and schizoid.'

Tupin and colleagues[35] designed a trial aimed at replicating the findings in the study by Sheard[34]. The subjects were 27 inmates of the California Medical Facility (a branch of the

California Department of Corrections) selected because of serious repeated violent behavior. Since more than one-third of the participants turned out to suffer from schizophrenia, methodologically desirable criteria for a proper 'prison trial' were obviously not met. This trial, an open study with a mean observation period of 10 months, confirmed the anti-aggressive effect of lithium. Subjective reports by the inmates taking lithium described strikingly similar experiences: an increased capacity to reflect on the consequences of actions and to control angry feelings when provoked.

Sheard[36] has also conducted the only clinical trial on lithium and aggression involving outpatients with uncontrolled rage outbursts. Twelve inmates with habitual impulsive and aggressive behavior were recruited from a larger prison population. The subjects were described as 'a rather mixed group of diagnostic categories, the main behavioral feature in common being repetitive impulsive aggressive behavior, frequently bringing them into trouble with the law.' The trial comprised 4 months of lithium treatment inside the correctional institution. After their release the patients were followed as outpatients during 1–2 months of lithium treatment. The outpatient part of the study was difficult, owing to the unreliability of the subjects. A decreased number of serious aggressive episodes was seen inside as well as outside the prison. The observation that serious incidents were reduced with lithium, but not 'all antisocial incidents' is in agreement with the study by Tupin et al.[35].

In 1976, Sheard et al.[37] went on to conduct the most famous of the prison studies: a double-blind, placebo-controlled trial with a more adequate methodology than any other study presented in this section. Sixty-six inmates from a medium-security prison participated in this 3-month trial. The primary inclusion criterion was a history of chronic impulsive-aggressive

behaviour. Again, significantly fewer major infractions occurred in the lithium than in the placebo group during the trial. In the patients who completed the full trial, the decrease in number of infractions progressed to the point where no major infractions occurred during the third month with lithium. No similar patterns were observed in the placebo group. According to Sheard et al.[37] the prison studies are 'further evidence that lithium can have an inhibitory effect on impulsive aggressive behavior.'

POSSIBLE MECHANISMS OF THE ANTI-AGGRESSIVE EFFECTS

Attempting to discern a specific anti-aggressive effect of lithium, Sheard explored various possibilities and proposed that the anti-aggressive effect of lithium could not be explained by toxicity, motor or sensory activity change, or alteration in cognition or reaction time; the lithium effect, it was concluded, is not a placebo response, nor is it due to endocrine effects[39]. In a more recent review, McElroy and colleagues pointed to the frequently combined occurrence of impulse control disorder and bipolar disorder and noted that this finding suggested a relationship between both disorders, or that at least both disorders share an underlying pathophysiological pathway[40]. The possibility of an impulse control disorder being based on an undetected manic-depressive illness can never be fully dismissed. Any assumption of an underlying bipolar disorder would, on the other hand, imply that a high percentage of those who commit violent crimes suffer from an atypical manic-depressive illness, which would only confirm the indication of lithium therapy in these cases.

Both animal and clinical studies have suggested a critical role for central 5-hydroxytryptamine (5-HT) function in the regulation of aggressive impulses (see Chapter 29). An inverse covariation has been noted between peripheral markers of central 5-HT functions and of impulsive aggressive behavior[41,42]. Recent findings of Coccaro *et al.*[43] suggest that a reduced number of 5-HT transporters on platelets correlate with a history of aggressive behavior by patients with personality disorders. The fact that lithium has serotonin-enhancing effects[44,45] matches these findings and provides an explanation for a possible working mechanism in the reduction of aggressive behavior. However, as pointed out by Coccaro[41], other mechanisms may be involved. Thus, lithium may also reduce catecholaminergic function[46,47]. Findings by Brown *et al.*[48] suggest that an increased noradrenergic and/or dopaminergic function is associated with aggression. Therefore, it is not clear whether the anti-aggressive actions of lithium stem from an increase in serotonergic function or a decrease in catecholaminergic function.

REFERENCES

1. Gunn J. Drugs in the violence clinic. In Sandler M, ed. Psychopharmacology of Aggression. New York: Raven Press, 1979: 183–96
2. Baron RA. Human Aggression. New York: Plenum Press, 1977: 7
3. Campbell M, Cohen IL, Small AM. Drugs in aggressive behaviour. J Am Acad Child Psychiatry 1982; 21: 107–17
4. Buss AH, Perry M. The aggression questionnaire. J Pers Soc Psychol 1992; 63: 452–9
5. Yudofski SC, Silver JM, Jackson W, et al. The Overt Aggression Scale for the objective rating of verbal and physical aggression. Am J Psychiatry 1986; 143: 35–9
6. Cade JF. Lithium salts in the treatment of psychotic excitement. Med J Aust 1949; 36: 349–52
7. Baastrup P. Practical clinical viewpoints regarding treatment with lithium. Acta Psychiatr Scand 1969; (Suppl) 207: 12–18
8. Forssman H, Walinder J. Lithium treatment of atypical indications. Acta Psychatr Scand 1969; (Suppl) 207: 34–40
9. Haas JF, Cope DN. Neuropharmacologic management of behavior sequelae in head injury: a case report. Arch Phys Med Rehabil 1985; 66: 472–4
10. Glenn MB, Wroblewski B, Parziale J, et al. Lithium carbonate for aggressive behavior or affective instability in ten brain-injured patients. Am J Phys Med Rehabil 1989; 68: 221–6
11. Epperson CN, McDougle CJ, Anand A, et al. Lithium augmentation of fluvoxamine in autistic disorder: a case report. J Child Adolesc Psychopharmacol 1994; 4: 201–7
12. Van Putten T, Sanders DG. Lithium in treatment failures. J Nerv Ment Dis 1975; 161: 255–64
13. Rifkin A, Quitkin F, Carillo C, et al. Lithium carbonate in emotionally unstable character disorder. Arch Gen Psychiatry 1972; 27: 519–24
14. Do Prado-Lima P, Knijnik L, Juruena M, Padilla A. Lithium reduces maternal child abuse behavior: a preliminary report. J Clin Pharm Ther 2001; 26: 279–82
15. Dorrego MF, Canevaro L, Kuzis G, et al. A randomized, double-blind, crossover study of methylphenidate and lithium in adults with attention-deficit/hyperactivity disorder: preliminary findings. J Neuropsychiatry Clin Neurosci 2002; 14: 289–95
16. Ernst CL, Goldberg JF. Antisuicide properties of psychotropic drugs: a critical review. Harvard Rev Psychiatry 2004; 12: 14–41
17. Nilsson A. The anti-aggressive actions of lithium. Rev Contemp Pharmacother 1993; 4: 269–85
18. Campbell M, Adams PB, Small AM, et al. Lithium in hospitalized children with conduct disorder: a double-blind and placebo controlled study. J Am Acad Child Adolesc Psychiatry 1995; 34: 445–53

19. Rifkin A, Karajgi B, Dicker R, et al. Lithium treatment of conduct disorders in adolescents. Am J Psychiatry 1997; 154: 554–5

20. Malone RP, Bennett DS, Luebbert JF, et al. Aggression classification and treatment response. Psychopharmacol Bull 1998; 34: 41–5

21. Malone RP, Delaney MA, Luebbert JF, et al. A double-blind placebo-controlled study of lithium in hospitalized aggressive children and adolescents with conduct disorder. Arch Gen Psychiatry 2000; 57: 649–54

22. Campbell M, Small AM, Green WH, et al. Behavioral efficacy of haloperidol and lithium carbonate. A comparison in hospitalized aggressive children with conduct disorder. Arch Gen Psychiatry 1984; 41: 650–6

23. Spitzer RL, ed. Diagnostic and Statistical Manual of Mental Disorders (DSM-III-R), 3rd revised edn. Washington DC: American Psychiatric Association, 1980

24. Carlson GA, Rapport MD, Pataki CS, et al. Lithium in hospitalized children at 4 and 8 weeks: mood, behavior and cognitive effects. J Child Psychol Psychiatry 1992; 33: 411–25

25. Campbell M, Perry R, Green WH. Use of lithium in children and adolescents. Psychosomatics 1984; 25: 95–106

26. Sing NN, Millichamp LJ. Pharmacological treatment of self-injurious behavior in mentally retarded persons. J Autism Dev Disord 1985; 15: 257–67

27. Dostal T, Zvolsky P. Antiaggressive effect of lithium salts in severe mentally retarded adolescents. Int Pharmacopsychiatry 1970; 5: 203–7

28. Micev V, Lynch DM. Effect of lithium on disturbed severely mentally retarded patients. Br J Psychiatry 1974; 125: 111

29. Worall EP, Moody JP, Naylor GJ. Lithium in non-manic-depressives: antiaggressive effect and red blood cell lithium values. Br J Psychiatry 1975; 126: 464–8

30. Tyrer SP, Walsh A, Edwards DE, et al. Factors associated with a good response to lithium in aggressive mentally handicapped subjects. Prog Neuropsychopharmacol Biol Psychiatry 1984; 8: 751–5

31. Craft M, Ismail IA, Regan A, et al. Lithium in the treatment of aggression in mentally handicapped patients. A double-blind trial. Br J Psychiatry 1987; 150: 685–9

32. Bellus SB, Stewart D, Vergo JG, et al. The use of lithium in the treatment of aggressive behaviours with two brain-injured individuals in a state psychiatric hospital. Brain Inj 1996; 10: 849–60

33. Luchins DJ, Dojka D. Lithium and propranolol in aggression and self-injurious behaviour in the mentally retarded. Psychopharmacol Bull 1989; 25: 372–5

34. Sheard MH. Effect of lithium in human aggression. Nature 1971; 230: 113–14

35. Tupin JP, Smith DB, Clanon TL, et al. The long-term use of lithium in aggressive prisoners. Compr Psychiatry 1973; 14: 311–17

36. Sheard MH. Lithium in the treatment of aggression. J Nerv Ment Dis 1975; 160: 108–18

37. Sheard MH, Marini JL, Bridges CI, Wagner E. The effect of lithium on impulsive aggressive behavior in man. Am J Psychiatry 1976; 133: 1409–13

38. Sheard MH. Clinical pharmacology of aggressive behavior. Clin Neuropharmacol 1984; 7: 173–83

39. Sheard MH. The effect of lithium and other ions on aggressive behavior. Mod Probl Psychopharmacol 1978; 13: 53–68

40. McElroy SL, Pope HG Jr, Kede PE, et al. Are impulse-control disorders related to bipolar disorder? Compr Psychiatry 1996; 37: 229–40

41. Coccaro EF. Central serotonin and impulsive aggression. Br J Psychiatry 1989; 8 (Suppl): 52–62

42. Coccaro EF, Siever LJ, Klar HM, et al. Serotonergic studies in affective and personality disorder patients; correlates with suicidal and impulsive aggressive behavior. Arch Gen Psychiatry 1989; 46: 587–99

43. Coccaro EF, Kavoussi RJ, Sheline YI, et al. Impulsive aggression in personality disorder correlates with tritiated paroxetine binding in the platelet. Arch Gen Psychiatry 1996; 53: 531–6

44. Bunney WE, Garland-Bunney BL. Mechanisms of action of lithium in affective

illness: basic and clinical implications. In Meltzer HY, ed. Psychopharmacology: Third Generation of Progress. New York: Raven Press, 1987: 553–65

45. Müller-Oerlinghausen B. Lithium long-term treatment – does it act via serotonin? Pharmacopsychiatry 1985; 18: 214–17

46. Linnoila M, Karoum F, Rosenthal N, Potter WZ. Electroconvulsive treatment and lithium carbonate. Their effects on norepinephrine metabolism in patients with primary, major depressions. Arch Gen Psychiatry 1983; 40: 677–80

47. Linnoila M, Karoum F, Potter WZ. Effects of antidepressant treatments on dopamine turnover in depressed patients. Arch Gen Psychiatry 1983; 40: 1015–17

48. Brown WA, Laughren TP, Mueller B. Endocrine effects of lithium in manic depressive patients. In Obiols J, Ballus C, Gonzales Monclus E, Pujol J, eds. Biological Psychiatry Today. Amsterdam: Elsevier, 1979: 759–63

20 The use of lithium in non-psychiatric conditions

Tom Bschor, Ute Lewitzka, Mazda Adli

Contents Introduction • Headache • Immune system • Ménière's disease • Hyperthyroidism and thyroid cancer • Epilepsy • Movement disorders • Other neurological disorders • Kleine–Levin syndrome • Miscellaneous

INTRODUCTION

Lithium, as a very small ion, exerts its action in a complex and mainly intracellular way. It passes not only the neural membrane within the central nervous system (CNS), but also the non-neural membranes of many different cell types. It is therefore not surprising that lithium not only influences mood but also has an impact on other physiological and pathophysiological functions of the organism. It has been used in a broad spectrum of diseases. The evidence for the efficacy of lithium varies considerably depending on the particular medical condition of the patient. (See Table 20.1 for an overview.)

HEADACHE

Lithium has been used for different types of headache, with cluster headache being the subtype most widely studied.

Cluster headache

Cluster headache is characterized by repeated attacks of unilateral pain in the orbital region associated with local autonomic symptoms or signs. The attacks are brief but of a very severe, almost excruciating intensity. Attacks occur in series (so-called 'cluster periods') that are separated by pain-free intervals usually lasting for months or years (so-called episodic cluster headache). A minority of patients have attacks for more than 1 year without remission or with remissions lasting less than 14 days; these patients are diagnosed as having chronic cluster headache. Cluster headache occurs in one per thousand in the general population, with a preponderance in males.

Today, in the treatment of acute attacks, sumatriptan is the drug of choice. Inhalation of 100% oxygen can also be recommended[1].

For prophylactic treatment of cluster headache, lithium is widely used. However, results available are from non-controlled clinical trials performed mainly in the late 1970s[2–9]. These open studies suggest good efficacy, even more so in the chronic than in the episodic form of the disease. Several authors state a rapid onset of the prophylactic effect within the first week. It has been suggested that even low doses of lithium

Table 20.1   The use of lithium in non-psychiatric conditions

Indication	Evidence	References
Cluster headache	Good efficacy in several nc clinical studies for prophylactic treatment, especially in chronic cluster headache	2–9
	No effect in a 1-week, db, pc, r study	10, 11
	same prophylactic efficacy as verapamil (db, r study)	
	⇨ lithium is considered a second line prophylactic agent	
Migraine	Mostly negative results from nc studies	15, 134
	positive results for cyclic migraine (nc studies)	
Hypnic headache	Positive results from several case reports	16–20
Cancer	*In vitro studies:* lithium inhibits most types of malignant cell line, but may also stimulate certain malignant cell lines	46–53
	Clinical studies: comparable rates of cancer in lithium-treated Psychiatric patients and psychiatric controls without lithium in a large observational study	54
Leukopenia induced by cancer treatment	Improvement of leukopenia demonstrated in several clinical studies	55–66
	No impact on overall survival rate; but worsening of survival rate in patients with co-morbid cardiovascular diseases possibly due to toxic lithium effects	69
Virus infection/herpes virus infection	*In vitro* studies indicate antiviral activity on DNA viruses	70–74
	Good prophylactic effect on recurrent herpes virus infections in *clinical* observations and retrospective studies	75–78, 82, 85
	Reduction of herpes symptoms in pc studies	79–81, 83, 84
Human immunodeficiency virus (HIV)	Promising results from *in vitro* and animal studies	27, 88–90, 92
	No clear positive effects on the course of HIV infection and AIDS in cr and case series; rather poor tolerance of lithium	86, 87
Bone marrow transplantation	Animal study showed positive effect when bone marrow donors were treated with lithium	94
Ménière's disease	No effect of lithium in a db study	96
Hyperthyroidism	Effective in thyrotoxicosis, but obsolete since the introduction of thionamides	99, 100
Thyroid cancer	No beneficial effect of lithium as an adjunct to radioiodine treatment in controlled studies	104, 105
Epilepsy	Reduction in seizure frequency shown in some case reports and a case series	106–110
	Increase of seizure frequency in temporal lobe epilepsy	111, 112
	⇨ lithium should be used with caution in patients with epilepsy; use as an anticonvulsant is not justified	
Spasmodic torticollis	No effect in case reports and a case series	113–116
Kleine–Levin syndrome (periodic hypersomnia)	Positive effects in case reports and a case series	118–120
Seborrheic dermatitis	Beneficial effects of topically applied lithium in several controlled, db trials	125–128
SIADH (syndrome of inappropriate antidiuretic hormone secretion)	Lithium is possibly useful but ⇨ cannot be recommended due to increased risk of severe side-effects and difficulties to establish safe and stable serum levels in this disorder	129–131
Asthma	Slightly positive effect in two r, db studies	132, 133

db, double-blind; pc, placebo controlled; r, randomized; nc, non-controlled; cr, case report; ⇨ , conclusion

(16–24 mmol/day; 600–900 mg/day lithium carbonate) or low plasma levels (0.3–0.8 mmol/l) might be sufficient.

In the only placebo-controlled, double-blind, randomized study in the field[10], 13 male patients on lithium experienced as many and as severe cluster headache attacks as did 14 male patients on placebo. Lithium was well tolerated but serum levels were rather low. Adherence to lithium intake was only moderate and the study lasted for only 1 week.

Bussone et al.[11] compared lithium with the calcium channel antagonist verapamil in a multicenter double-blind study with 30 patients suffering from chronic cluster headache. Following a crossover design, the 24 test subjects who completed the study took lithium and verapamil in monotherapy, each for an 8-week period. The authors found no difference in efficacy between the two drugs, but verapamil was associated with fewer side-effects and a somewhat more rapid onset of the therapeutic effect. The lithium dosage was not tailored according to serum levels and the lithium serum levels were rather low (determined in 18 participants; mean serum level 0.41 ± 0.1 and 0.46 ± 0.1 mmol/l, respectively). The exact mechanisms of lithium action in cluster headache are largely unknown.

In sum, today's effective acute handling of single attacks with sumatriptan injection and/or oxygen inhalation has reduced the need for prophylactic treatment. If prophylactic treatment is indicated, the calcium channel antagonist verapamil is the first option. Its prophylactic efficacy was demonstrated in at least one placebo-controlled double-blind study[12]. Alongside corticosteroids, which may induce a remission of frequent, severe attacks, lithium is nowadays considered a second-line prophylactic agent in cluster headache and can be combined with verapamil, sumatriptan, clonazepam[13] or corticosteroids if monotherapy is insufficient.

Migraine

Lithium was used in open, non-controlled studies to treat migraine. The results were discouraging, with lithium treatment resulting rather in a worsening of symptoms (summarized by Yung[14]). Cyclic migraine is characterized by daily attacks for 2 weeks or more and has an average recurrence rate of five episodes per year interspersed with symptom-free intervals. For this type of migraine, positive results for lithium treatment have been published. Medina and Diamond[15], for example, reported on relief of migraine attacks in 19 out of 22 patients in an open case series. More recent or controlled studies on that indication for lithium are not available.

Hypnic headache

Hypnic headache is a rare and short-lasting headache subtype which occurs during sleep. Lithium has shown very potent prophylactic properties in several case reports[16–20].

IMMUNE SYSTEM

Since the late 1980s, the influence of lithium on the immune system has been investigated in numerous in vitro and in vivo studies. No doubt, lithium has significant immunoregulatory effects. However, the studies focused on distinct parts of the complex immune system. While they do in fact shed light on many isolated effects of lithium in the context of the immune system, we are far from understanding the whole picture. Results from laboratory and animal studies are given in detail in Chapter 33. Some important results are summarized here.

Consistently, in vivo[21–24] and in vitro[25,26] studies have shown that lithium increases the release of tumor necrosis factor alpha (TNFα) from human monocytes. TNFα is a proinflammatory cytokine. Other proinflammatory cytokines and soluble cytokine receptors have also been found to be increased by lithium:

- Soluble TNF receptor p75 (sTNF-R p75)[22];
- Interleukin-6 (IL-6)[22,23,26] – Maes *et al.*[24], however, did not show a significant effect of lithium on IL-6 production;
- Interleukin-2 (IL-2)[27–30];
- Interferon-gamma (IFN-γ)[24];
- Interleukin-8 (IL-8)[24];
- Soluble interleukin-2 receptor (sIL-2-R)[31] – Haack *et al.*[22], however, did not find an effect of lithium on sIL-2-R.

In addition, numerous studies in humans demonstrated that lithium increases the total leukocyte count and absolute number of neutrophils[25,32–36]. However, the enlargement of the total circulating neutrophil mass alone may not be interpreted as an activation of the immune regulatory system. With regard to lymphocytes, *in vitro* studies showed an increase of IgG and IgM production in B cells[37,38].

Interleukin-1 was not affected by lithium administration in the *in vitro* study by Kleinerman and colleagues[25]. Interestingly, inhibiting immunoregulatory cytokines or proteins have been found to be increased by lithium as well: interleukin-10 (IL-10)[24] and interleukin-1 receptor antagonist (IL-1RA)[24].

In addition, lithium decreased serum C-reactive protein (CRP) levels in depressed patients in a study by Rybakowski *et al.*[39].

From the present data, it is not easy to decide which action of lithium, i.e. the negative immunoregulatory or the proinflammatory functions, prevails in patients who are treated with the drug. At the same time, lithium appears to normalize signs of immune system activation[36,39–41] and of immunosuppression[42–45] that accompany depression or stress.

As a consequence, lithium has been used to treat different conditions associated with dysfunction of the immune system with more or less success; these include cancer, leukopenia induced by cancer treatment, herpes virus infection, HIV infection and bone marrow transplantation.

Cancer

In vitro *studies*

Several *in vitro* studies were conducted to examine the effect of lithium on malignant cells but the results were inconclusive. Lithium rather increased the DNA synthesis rate of breast epithelial tissue[46,47]. In a complex experiment lithium was effective as an adjunct to a gene therapeutical approach in colorectal cancer[48]. The lithium salt of γ-linolenic acid (LiGLA) showed a selective 50% growth inhibition of pancreatic cancer cell lines (IC50) at approximately 6–16 μmol/l[49]. In a recent experiment, Erdal and others[50] found a 70% lithium-induced growth inhibition in nine out of 12 hepatocellular carcinoma cell lines. They speculated that the growth inhibition might be the result of lithium's inhibitory effect on glycogen synthase kinase 3β (GSK3β). Contradictory results were reported on the growth stimulating effect of lithium on leukemic cells[51–53].

Clinical studies

Clinical studies in this field are rare. In a study from Israel[54] the risk of developing cancer was compared between a group of 609 lithium-treated psychiatric patients and 2396 psychiatric controls without lithium therapy. The prevalence of cancer diseases did not differ between the two groups, but was lower in both groups compared to the general population (observed vs. expected rates of cancer). However, the frequency of non-epithelial (mesenchymal) cancer types was somewhat higher in the non-lithium group of psychiatric patients compared to the lithium-treated subjects (5.0 per 1000 and 3.3 per 1000 respectively; $p = 0.09$). In addition, a significant association between a lower lithium dose and a higher cancer frequency was found – an effect that was mainly due to the patients with very low lithium doses.

Leukopenia induced by cancer treatment

Leukopenia is a common side-effect in patients receiving radiotherapy and/or chemotherapy. This complication often necessitates a delay or a complete discontinuation of the cancer treatment. Against the background of lithium's well-known capacity to increase the number of leukocytes[25,32–36] (see also section above), several, mostly controlled, studies in the late 1970s and early 1980s demonstrated that lithium ameliorates leukopenic states caused by systemic chemotherapies[55–61]. Patients receiving chemotherapy in combination with lithium treatment experienced fewer days with neutropenia, fewer episodes of severe fever and fewer infection-related deaths[62]. Subjects treated with lithium also had a lower cumulative risk of infection and tolerated more intensive chemotherapy schedules than did controls[63]. However, these findings were not supported by a randomized, controlled study with 85 patients suffering from myelogenous leukemia[64]. This study did not show any advantage of adding lithium to a therapy with cytosine arabinoside and daunorubicin as induction therapy for acute myelogenous leukemia.

In a rather large study, Chang and colleagues[65] included 111 patients who were receiving radiotherapy and/or chemotherapy for cancer and suffering from leukopenia (white blood cell (WBC) count below 3000/mm³).

Sixty-nine received lithium when leukopenia was diagnosed, and 42 patients served as controls. The WBC count normalized (> 3000/mm³) after 4.9 days on average in the lithium-treated group and after 11.8 days in the control group.

Lithium's positive effects on the leukocyte count were also described in zidovudine (AZT)-induced leukopenia (AZT mainly used to treat HIV infection)[66], in neuroleptic-induced leukopenia[67] and in carbamazepine-induced leukopenia[68].

However, to date lithium has not been shown to have an impact on the overall survival rate of patients with progressive malignant diseases. Lyman and co-workers[69] reported on 100 males from three consecutive studies who suffered from small-cell lung cancer and were treated with a standardized regimen of chemotherapy and radiation therapy. Forty patients received lithium in a non-blinded design (only 20 of the patients were randomized) to ameliorate chemotherapy-associated leukopenia. Lithium dosage was adjusted to maintain serum levels between 0.4 and 1.6 mmol/l. Fifty patients (50%) had clinical evidence of cardiovascular disease or abnormalities on electrocardiogram (ECG) at the time of study entry and were equally assigned to the lithium and the non-lithium groups. Sixty patients (60%) died before data analysis (median survival time for patients with pre-treatment cardiovascular abnormalities 182 days, and 273 days for those without such abnormalities; difference not statistically significant).

With regard to lithium treatment, patients without lithium had a longer survival time (median 293 days) than patients with lithium (median 183 days; difference not statistically significant). In patients with normal cardiovascular status at study entry, there was no difference in the median survival time between groups (lithium: 330 days vs. no lithium: 275 days). However, 11 (40%) non-lithium patients with pre-existing cardiovascular abnormalities died, as opposed to 17 (77%) lithium-treated patients ($p = 0.0072$). Of those patients at risk, the survival of subjects without lithium was significantly longer (median 420 days) than that of patients with lithium (median 154 days; $p = 0.0162$). Unexpected, sudden death occurred in 13 patients (26%) with cardiovascular abnormalities and in one patient (2%) without such abnormalities ($p < 0.001$). Among those 13 patients with pre-existing cardiovascular abnormalities, sudden death occurred in two patients (7%) without lithium as compared to 11 patients with lithium (50%) ($p = 0.0006$). The authors concluded that, apart from the malignant disease, lithium (and bronchodilator) treatment were the major risk factors of both overall mortality and sudden death in patients with pre-existing cardiovascular abnormalities. The authors also further concluded that patients suffering from small-cell lung cancer with clinical or ECG evidence of cardiovascular abnormality and who had been administered theophylline derivatives should not be given adjunctive treatment with lithium[69].

In conclusion, pre-clinical and clinical studies clearly indicate that lithium inhibits the growth of several cancer cell lines and has a positive effect on leukopenia induced by cancer treatment. Although clinical studies have shown repeatedly that lithium-treated patients have a greater recovery rate from leukopenia and fewer infections, an impact on overall survival in cancer patients has not been shown. It also remains unclear whether or not lithium – due to possible toxic effects – worsens the course of illness in cancer patients with co-morbid cardiovascular diseases.

Virus infection

Lithium has been used as an antiviral agent in humans, most frequently to treat herpes virus infections. Only few data exist on lithium in human immunodeficiency virus (HIV) infections. Its positive effects are attributed to its immunomodulatory capacities on the one hand and on a direct antiviral effect on the other.

Herpes virus

Lithium has been shown to have antiviral activity[70]. Cell-culture experiments have demonstrated that replication of DNA viruses (such as herpes virus) can be suppressed by lithium in concentrations of 5–30 mmol/l[71,72]. This effect is probably due to the inhibition of viral DNA synthesis[73,74], eventually caused by a competitive inhibition of magnesium ions or a depletion of potassium, which are both involved in the viral metabolism. The replication of RNA viruses is not inhibited by lithium[71].

Lithium has also shown antiviral activity in clinical studies and case reports[75]. In addition to a direct antiviral effect, the immunomodulatory properties of the ion – as discussed above – as well as the mood-stabilizing and consecutive stress-reductive effects may play a key role. In the late 1970s and early 1980s an improvement of herpes labialis manifestations was reported in patients treated with lithium for affective disorder[76,77]. In a large retrospective chart analysis Rybakowski and Amsterdam[78] demonstrated a significant reduction of the frequency of herpes labialis recurrences in a group of patients following lithium treatment. A positive correlation between the lithium serum level and the antiviral effect was also described[78].

Prospective, placebo-controlled studies have been conducted with patients suffering from genital or labial herpes. In two clinical studies including ten and 11 patients, respectively, with mainly the genital type of herpes (caused by herpes simplex virus 2), a slight reduction in herpes symptoms in patients receiving lithium as compared to placebo treatment was shown[79–81]. A large retrospective analysis comparing 177 lithium-treated patients with 59 subjects receiving antidepressants confirmed the result of a reduction of the herpes virus infection rate under lithium treatment[82].

Positive effects have also been reported with local treatment of herpes labialis using an 8% lithium succinate ointment as compared to placebo ointment[83,84] or to the time before treatment or as compared to no treatment[85].

Human immunodeficiency virus

The use of lithium for the treatment of HIV infection or AIDS has been subject to some research. Single cases[86] and a case series[87] of lithium treatment in males with HIV infection or AIDS have been published. In the latter, which was conducted as early as 1988, ten patients with HIV infection were treated with lithium carbonate. Lithium was not well tolerated and did not show any beneficial effects on the absolute number of CD4 lymphocytes, on the CD4/CD8 ratio or on other immunological parameters.

However, *in vitro* studies showed that the addition of lithium to immune cells of patients with AIDS was associated with an increase in interleukin-2 production[27]. In mice suffering from murine deficiency syndrome (MAIDS), a retrovirus infection comparable to human HIV infection, lithium led to longer survival times and a reduction of symptoms in treated mice compared to mice without lithium treatment (e.g. a marked reduction in the development of lymphadenopathy and splenomegaly)[88–90]. As mentioned above, lithium has been used successfully to counteract leukopenia induced by AZT treatment of HIV infection[88,91].

In addition, lithium pre-treatment seems to have beneficial neuroprotective effects against HIV-gp120-mediated toxicity in mice[92], which raises the question of whether it might not also have a preventive effect against HIV-associated cognitive impairments in humans[93].

Bone marrow transplantation

Gallicchio and colleagues[94] studied lethally irradiated mice after bone marrow cell transplantation. Donor animals were treated with lithium or buffer. Animals that had received marrow cells from lithium-treated donors demonstrated greater survival, increased recovery of peripheral indices and hematopoietic progenitors compared to buffer-treated controls. However, there are no studies on lithium-treated human donors.

MÉNIÈRE'S DISEASE

An early open trail with 30 patients showed encouraging results[95], which were not confirmed in a controlled, double-blind crossover study with 21 subjects[96].

HYPERTHYROIDISM AND THYROID CANCER

Lithium is a thyrostatic drug[97,98]. This effect is mediated through different mechanisms, as shown in detail in Chapter 22. In the 1970s lithium was used for the treatment of thyrotoxicosis[99,100], but today thionamides such as carbimazole, methimazole, or propylthiouracil are the preferred medications.

Based on the assumption that lithium increases the accumulation and retention of radioiodine in thyroid cancer and its metastatic lesions[101–103], it was investigated as a possible adjuvant to radioiodine treatment. In a recent study, Bal *et al.*[104] did not find lithium to have any beneficial effect in 175 patients with hyperthyroidism treated with radioiodine and 900 mg lithium carbonate (24.4 mmol) daily for 3 weeks compared to 175 hyperthyroid patients treated with radioiodine alone. This result agrees with a study by Ang *et al.*[105], which also did not show lithium to be effective as an adjunct in increasing radioiodine (I-131) uptake in patients with well-differentiated thyroid carcinoma.

EPILEPSY

Acute administration of lithium leads to marked electroencephalogram (EEG) changes. Increased amplitude, generalized slowing, increased theta and delta and decreased alpha wave activity and in some cases paroxysmal dysrhythmia and disorganization of the background rhythm have been described[14]. Some early case reports show a reduction in the frequency of epileptic seizures under lithium therapy[106–109]. A Russian research group reported a reduction in the frequency of attacks in 30 patients suffering from epilepsy under a combined administration of oral lithium carbonate and vitamin E injections in addition to an ongoing anticonvulsant medication[110]. However, most case reports do not indicate any therapeutic benefit of lithium in controlling seizures (summarized in reference 14). In conclusion, scientific data do not justify the use of lithium for the treatment of epilepsy. Two reports even show an aggravating effect in temporal lobe epilepsy[111,112]. To sum up, lithium should be used with caution in patients suffering from epileptic seizures, because of its evoked EEG changes.

MOVEMENT DISORDERS

For the use of lithium in Huntington's chorea, in tardive dyskinesia, in Parkinson's disease (in particular L-dopa-induced hyperkinesia and the on–off phenomenon) and in Tourette's syndrome, see Chapter 32. Case reports[113–115]

and a case series of 11 patients[116] on lithium for the treatment of spasmodic torticollis have not been encouraging.

OTHER NEUROLOGICAL DISORDERS

Lithium chloride in combination with chondroitinase ABC increased the regeneration of axotomized neurons of the rubrospinal tract in a rat model of traumatic spinal cord injury[117], described in detail in Chapter 32. For treatment of organic brain syndrome secondary to brain injury or substance abuse, pre- and post-insult treatment of stroke with lithium, retinal degeneration and neuropathic pain, see Chapter 32.

KLEINE–LEVIN SYNDROME

Kleine–Levin syndrome (periodic hypersomnia) is a rare disorder that affects mainly adolescents. Periods of extreme somnolence alternate with megaphagia, psychomental changes and behavioral symptoms. The cause and pathogenesis of Kleine–Levin syndrome are unknown. In five adolescents on lithium therapy episodes of hypersomnia were shorter and monosymptomatic, with an absence of any behavioral symptoms[118]. Positive therapeutic effects from lithium treatment are described in case reports from 1977[119] and 2002[120].

MISCELLANEOUS

Recently, lithium has been used in dental medicine in lithium disilicate-based ceramic material[121,122]. In a laboratory experiment, the addition of lithium fluoride accelerated the bioactivity of calcium aluminate cement which is used for restoring defective bone and joining natural bone with artificial prostheses. The aim of the study was to speed the process of formation of the cement[123]. Using a guinea-pig model, a French research group demonstrated that lithium treatment prior to an acoustic overexposure could to some extent prevent cochlea damage[124].

In dermatology, several controlled, double-blind trials have demonstrated that topically applied lithium is beneficial in the treatment of seborrheic dermatitis[125–128].

In the long-term treatment of chronic SIADH (syndrome of inappropriate antidiuretic hormone secretion), lithium seems to be helpful[129,130], regardless of the origin of the SIADH. Its use, however, is not recommended. Owing to the disturbed water and sodium regulation and the subsequent risk of severe side-effects, it is difficult to establish a safe and stable serum level[131].

Based on the assumption that lithium, through its effects on cell signal transduction and ion-transport pathways, would be likely to protect the airways against constrictor stimuli, a randomized, double-blind study of lithium carbonate was carried out in patients suffering from asthma (completers $n = 21$). The effect observed was only slightly positive[132]. Spitz *et al.*[133] found an effect of lithium in a placebo-controlled double-blind crossover study with five patients suffering from asthma.

REFERENCES

1. Ekbom K, Hardebo JE. Cluster headache. Aetiology, diagnosis and management. Drugs 2002; 62: 61–9
2. Bussone G, Boiardi A, Merati B, et al. Chronic cluster headache: response to lithium treatment. J Neurol 1979 Sep; 221: 181–5
3. Klimek A, Szulc-Kuberska J, Kawiorski S. Lithium therapy in cluster headache. Eur Neurol 1979; 18: 267–8
4. Ekbom K. Lithium vid kroniska symptom av cluster headache. Opusc Med 1974; 19: 148–56
5. Mathew NT. Clinical subtypes of cluster headache and response to lithium therapy. Headache 1978; 18: 26–30
6. Medina JL, Fareed J, Diamond S. Blood amines and platelet changes during treatment of cluster headache with lithium and other drugs. Headache 1978; 18: 112
7. Savoldi F, Nappi G, Bono G. I sali di litio nel trattamento della cefalea a grappolo. Riv Neurol 1979; 49: 128–39
8. Manzoni GC, Terzano MG, Trabattoni G. Il trattamento della cefalea a grappolo con carbonato di litio. Acta Biomed 1979; 50: 291–5
9. Ekbom K. Lithium for cluster headache: review of the literature and preliminary results of long-term treatment. Headache 1981; 21: 132–9
10. Steiner TJ, Hering R, Couturier EGM, et al. Double-blind placebo-controlled trial of lithium in episodic cluster headache. Cephalalgia 1997; 17: 673–5
11. Bussone G, Leone M, Peccarisi C, et al. Double blind comparison of lithium and verapamil in cluster headache prophylaxis. Headache 1990; 30: 411–17
12. Leone M, D'Amico D, Frediani F, et al. Verapamil in the prophylaxis of episodic cluster headache: a double-blind study versus placebo. Neurology 2000; 54: 1382–5
13. Takebayashi M, Fujikawa T, Kagaya A, et al. Lithium and clonazepam treatment of two cases with cluster headache. Psychiatry Clin Neurosci 1999; 53: 535–7
14. Yung CY. A review of clinical trials of lithium in neurology. Pharmacol Biochem Behav 1984; 21 (Suppl 1): 57–64
15. Medina JL, Diamond S. Cyclical migraine. Arch Neurol 1981; 38: 343–4
16. Vieira-Dias M, Esperanca P. Hypnic headache: report of two cases. Headache 2001; 41: 726–7
17. Vieira Dias M, Esperanca P. Hypnic headache: a report of four cases [in Spanish]. Rev Neurol 2002; 34: 950–1
18. Patsouros N, Laloux P, Ossemann M. Hypnic headache: a case report with polysomnography. Acta Neurol Belg 2004; 104: 37–40
19. Kocasoy Orhan E, Kayrak Ertas N, Orhan KS, Ertas M. Hypnic headache syndrome: excessive

periodic limb movements in polysomnography. Agri 2004; 16: 28–30

20. Perez-Martinez DA, Berbel-Garcia A, Puente-Munoz AI, et al. Hypnic headache: a new case [in Spanish]. Rev Neurol 1999; 28: 883–4

21. Himmerich H, Koethe D, Schuld A, et al. Plasma levels of leptin and endogenous immune modulators during treatment with carbamazepine or lithium. Psychopharmacology (Berl) 2005; 179: 447–51

22. Haack M, Hinze-Selch D, Fenzel T, et al. Plasma levels of cytokines and soluble cytokine receptors in psychiatric patients upon hospital admission: effects of confounding factors and diagnosis. J Psychiatr Res 1999; 33: 407–18

23. Merendino RA, Mancuso G, Tomasello F, et al. Effects of lithium carbonate on cytokine production in patients affected by breast cancer. J Biol Regul Homeost Agents 1994; 8: 88–91

24. Maes M, Song C, Lin AH, et al. In vitro immunoregulatory effects of lithium in healthy volunteers. Psychopharmacology (Berl) 1999; 143: 401–7

25. Kleinerman ES, Knowles RD, Blick MB, Zwelling LA. Lithium chloride stimulates human monocytes to secrete tumor necrosis factor/cachectin. J Leukoc Biol 1989; 46: 484–92

26. Arena A, Capozza AB, Orlando ME, et al. In vitro effects of lithium chloride on TNF alpha and IL-6 production by monocytes from breast cancer patients. J Chemother 1997; 9: 219–26

27. Sztein MB, Simon GL, Parenti DM, et al. In vitro effects of thymosin and lithium on lymphoproliferative responses of normal donors and HIV seropositive male homosexuals with AIDS-related complex. Clin Immunol Immunopathol 1987; 44: 51–62

28. Wilson R, Fraser WD, McKillop JH, et al. The 'in vitro' effects of lithium on the immune system. Autoimmunity 1989; 4: 109–14

29. Wu YY, Yang XH. Enhancement of inter-leukin 2 production in human and gibbon T cells after in vitro treatment with lithium. Proc Soc Exp Biol Med 1991; 198: 620–4

30. Kucharz EJ, Sierakowski SJ, Goodwin JS. Lithium in vitro enhances interleukin-2 production by T cells from patients with systemic lupus erythematosus. Immuno-pharmacol Immunotoxicol 1993; 5: 515–23

31. Rapaport MH, Schmidt ME, Risinger R, Manji H. The effects of prolonged lithium exposure on the immune system of normal control subjects: serial serum soluble interleukin-2 receptor and antithyroid antibody measurements. Biol Psychiatry 1994; 35761–6

32. Rothstein G, Clarkson DR, Larsen W, et al. Effect of lithium on neutrophil mass and production. N Engl J Med 1978; 26: 178–80

33. Blicharski J, Aleksandrowicz J, Bodzon A, et al. Effect of lithium carbonate on the function and enzyme content of the neutrophils in patients with granulocytopenia. Folia Med Cracov 1980; 22: 367–73

34. Friedenberg WR, Marx JJ. The bactericidal defect of neutrophil function with lithium therapy. Adv Exp Med Biol 1980; 127: 389–99

35. Ridgway D, Wolff LJ, Neerhout RC. Enhanced lymphocyte response to PHA among leukemia patients taking oral lithium carbonate. Cancer Invest 1986; 4: 513–17

36. Sluzewska A, Wiktorowicz K, Mackiewicz SH, Rybakowski JK. The effect of short term treatment with lithium and carbamazepine on some immunological indices in depressed patients. Lithium 1994; 5: 41–6

37. Wilson R, Fraser WD, McKillop JH, et al. The 'in vitro' effects of lithium on the immune system. Autoimmunity 1989; 4: 109–14

38. Weetman AP, McGregor AM, Lazarus JH, et al. The enhancement of immunglobulin synthesis by human lymphocytes with lithium. J Immunopathol 1982; 22: 400–7

39. Rybakowski J, Sluzewska A, Sobieska M, Wiktorowicz K. The effect of lithium and carbamazepine on alpha-1 acid glycoprotein in affective patients. Poland–Israel Symposium on Biological Psychiatry, Program and Abstract Book, Krakow, 1993: 101–3

40. Sluzewska A, Sobieska M, Rybakowski JK. Changes in acute phase proteins during lithium potentiation of antidepressants in refractory depression. Neuropsychobiology 1997; 35: 123–7

41. Hornig M, Goodman DB, Kamoun M, Amsterdam JD. Positive and negative acute

phase proteins in affective subtypes. J Affect Disord 1998; 49: 9–18

42. Bubak-Satora M, Skowron-Cendrzak A, Kubera M. The effect of lithium chloride treatment on cell-mediated immunity in mice. Folia Biol 1991; 39: 21–4

43. Bubak-Satora M, Skowron-Cendrzak A, Kubera M, Holan V. Protective effect of lithium on the stress-induced depression of cell-mediated immunity in mice. Int J Immuno-pharmacol 1994; 16: 233–7

44. Kubera M, Bubak-Satora M, Holan V, et al. Modulation of cell-mediated immunity by lithium chloride. Z Naturforsch 1994; 49: 679–83

45. Song C, Leonard BE. The effects of chronic lithium chloride administration on some behavioral and immunological changes in the bilaterally olfactory bulbectomized rat. J Psychopharmacol 1994; 8: 40–7

46. Hori C, Oka T. Induction by lithium ion of multiplication of mouse mammary epithelium in culture. Proc Natl Acad Sci USA 1979; 76: 2823–7

47. Ptashnem K, Stockdalem FE, Conlon S. Initiation of DNA synthesis in mammary epithelium and mammary tumors by lithium ions. J Cell Physiol 1980; 103: 41–6

48. Bordonaro M, Lazarova DL, Carbone R, Sartorelli AC. Modulation of Wnt-specific colon cancer cell kill by butyrate and lithium. Oncol Res 2004; 14: 427–38

49. Ravichandran D, Cooper A, Johnson CD. Growth inhibitory effect of lithium gammali-nolenate on pancreatic cancer cell lines: the influence of albumin and iron. Eur J Cancer 1998; 34: 188–92

50. Erdal E, Ozturk N, Cagatay T, et al. Lithium-mediated downregulation of PKB/Akt and cyclin E with growth inhibition in hepato-cellular carcinoma cells. Int J Cancer 2005; 115: 903–10

51. Zaricznyi C, Macara IG. Lithium inhibits terminal differentiation of erythroleukemia cells. Evidence for a precommitment 'priming' effect. Exp Cell Res 1987; 168: 402–10

52. Moreb J, Hershko C. Increased leucocyte alka-line phosphatase and transcobalamine III in chronic myeloid leukemia associated with lithium therapy. Scand J Haematol 1985; 34: 238–41

53. Gauwerk C, Golde DW. Lithium enhances growth of human leukemia cells in vitro. Br J Haematol 1988; 51: 431–8

54. Cohen Y, Chetrit A, Cohen Y, et al. Cancer morbidity in psychiatric patients: influence of lithium carbonate treatment. Med Oncol 1998; 15: 32–6

55. Stein RS, Beaman C, Ali MY, et al. Lithium carbonate attenuation of chemotherapy-induced neutropenia. N Engl J Med 1977; 297: 430–1

56. Stein RS, Flexner JM, Graber SE. Lithium and granulocytopenia during induction therapy of acute myelogenous leukemia. Blood 1979; 54: 636–41

57. Catane R, Kaufman J, Mittelman A, Murphy GP. Attenuation of myelosuppression with lithium. N Engl J Med 1977; 297: 452–3

58. Greco FA, Brereton HD. Effect of lithium carbonate on the neutropenia caused by chemotherapy: a preliminary clinical trial. Oncology 1977; 34: 153–5

59. Turner AR, MacDonald RN, McPherson TA. Reduction of chemotherapy-induced neutro-penia complications with a short course of lithi-um carbonate. Clin Invest Med 1979; 2: 51–3

60. Lahousen M, Pickel H, Haas J. Lithium carbonate – a preventive agent against leuko-penia during cytostatic therapy [in German]. Wien Klin Wochenschr 1984; 96: 739–41

61. Steinherz PG, Rosen G, Ghavimi F, et al. The effect of lithium carbonate on leukopenia after chemotherapy. J Pediatr 1980; 96: 923–7

62. Lyman GH, Williams CC, Preston D. The use of lithium carbonate to reduce infection and leukopenia during systemic chemotherapy. N Engl J Med 1980; 302: 257–60

63. Lyman GH, Williams CC, Preston D, et al. Lithium carbonate in patients with small cell lung cancer receiving combination chemo-therapy. Am J Med 1981; 70: 1222–9

64. Stein RS, Vogler WR, Lefante J. Failure of lithium to limit neutropenia significantly during induction therapy of acute myelogenous

leukemia. A Southeastern Cancer Study Group study. Am J Clin Oncol 1984; 7: 365–9

65. Chang KH, Tan R, Chung CH. The use of lithium carbonate to correct leukopenia during cancer treatment. Zhonghua Yi Xue Za Zhi (Taipei) 1989; 43: 165–70

66. Gallicchio VS, Hughes NK, Tse KF. Modulation of the haematopoietic toxicity associated with zidovudine *in vivo* with lithium carbonate. J Intern Med 1993; 233: 259–68

67. Yassa R, Ananth J. Treatment of neuroleptic-induced leukopenia with lithium carbonate. Can J Psychiatry 1981; 26: 487–9

68. Kramlinger KG, Post RM. Addition of lithium carbonate to carbamazepine: hematological and thyroid effects. Am J Psychiatry 1990; 147: 615–20

69. Lyman GH, Williams CC, Dinwoodie WR, Schocken DD. Sudden death in cancer patients receiving lithium. J Clin Oncol 1984; 2: 1270–6

70. Rybakowski JK. Antiviral and immunomodulatory effect of lithium. Pharmacopsychiatry 2000; 33: 159–64

71. Randall S, Hartley CE, Buchan A, et al. Effect of lithium on viral replication. In Birch NJ, ed. Lithium and the Cell: Pharmacology and Biochemistry. London: Academic Press, 1991: 99–112

72. Ziaie Z, Kefalides NA. Lithium chloride restores host protein synthesis in herpes simplex virus-infected endothelial cells. Biochem Biophys Res Commun 1989; 160: 1073–8

73. Buchan A, Randall S, Hartley CE, et al. Effect of lithium salts on the replication of viruses and non-viral microorganisms. In Birch NJ, ed. Lithium: Inorganic Pharmacology and Psychiatric Use. Oxford: IRL Press, 1988: 83–90

74. Ziaie Z, Brinker JM, Kefalides NA. Lithium chloride suppresses the synthesis of messenger RNA for infected cell protein-4 and viral deoxyribonucleic acid polymerase in herpes simplex virus-1 infected endothelial cells. Lab Invest 1994; 70: 29–38

75. Bschor T. Complete suppression of recurrent herpes labialis with lithium carbonate. Pharmacopsychiatry 1999; 32: 158

76. Lieb J. Remission of recurrent herpes infection during therapy with lithium. N Engl J Med 1979; 301: 942

77. Gillis A. Lithium in herpes simplex. Lancet 1983; 2: 516

78. Rybakowski JK, Amsterdam JD. Lithium prophylaxis and recurrent labial herpes infections. Lithium 1991; 2: 43–7

79. Amsterdam JD, Maislin G, Potter L, Giuntoli R. Reduced rate of recurrent genital herpes infections with lithium carbonate. Psychopharmacol Bull 1990; 26: 343–7

80. Amsterdam JD, Maislin G, Potter L, et al. Suppression of recurrent genital herpes infections with lithium carbonate: a randomized, placebo-controlled trial. Lithium 1991; 2: 17–25

81. Amsterdam JD, Maislin G, Hooper MB. Suppression of herpes simplex virus infections with oral lithium carbonate – a possible antiviral activity. Pharmacotherapy 1996; 16: 1070–5

82. Amsterdam JD, Maislin G, Rybakowski J. A possible antiviral action of lithium carbonate in herpes simplex virus infections. Biol Psychiatry 1990; 27: 447–53

83. Skinner GR. Lithium ointment for genital herpes. Lancet 1983; 2: 288

84. Horrobin DF. Lithium in the control of herpesvirus infections. In Bach RO, ed. Lithium. Current Applications in Science, Medicine and Technology. New York: John Wiley & Sons, 1985: 397–406

85. Rybakowski J, Gwiezdzinski Z, Urbanowski S. Lithium succinate ointment in topical treatment of herpes simplex infections. Lithium 1991; 2: 117–18

86. Jordan WC. Use of lithium in maintaining T-cell functions in persons with documented acquired immunodeficiency syndrome. J Natl Med Assoc 1992; 84: 1044–6

87. Parenti DM, Simon GL, Scheib RG, et al. Effect of lithium carbonate in HIV-infected patients with immune dysfunction. J Acquir Immune Defic Syndr 1988; 1: 119–24

88. Gallicchio VS, Hughes NK, Tse KF. Modulation of the haematopoietic toxicity

associated with zidovudine in vivo with lithium carbonate. J Intern Med 1993; 233: 259–68

89. Gallicchio VS, Hughes NK, Tse KF, et al. Effect of lithium in immunodeficiency: improved blood cell formation in mice with decreased hematopoiesis as the result of LP-BM5 MuLV infection. Antiviral Res 1995; 26: 189–202

90. Gallicchio VS, Hughes NK, Tse KF, et al. Lithium and anti-viral drug toxicity III: further studies on the ability of lithium to exert anti-viral, anti-tumor effects and modulate the toxicity associated with anti-viral drug therapy in normal and immunodeficient retrovirus-infected mice. In Gallicchio VS, Birch NJ, eds. Lithium: Biochemical and Clinical Advances. Cheshire, CT: Weidner Publishing Group, 1996: 85–102

91. Gallicchio VS, Hughes NK, Hulette BC, Noblitt L. Effect of interleukin-1, GM-CSF, erythropoietin, and lithium on the toxicity associated with 3′-azido-3′-deoxythymidine (AZT) in vitro on hematopoietic progenitors (CFU-GM, CFU-MEG, and BFU-E) using murine retrovirus-infected hematopoietic cells. J Leukoc Biol 1991; 50: 580–6

92. Everall IP, Bell C, Mallory M. Lithium ameliorates HIV-gp120-mediated neurotoxicity. Mol Cell Neurosci 2002; 21: 493–501

93. Harvey BH, Meyer CL, Gallicchio VS, Manji HK. Lithium salts in AIDS and AIDS-related dementia. Psychopharmacol Bull 2002; 36: 5–26

94. Gallicchio VS, Messino MJ, Hulette BC, Hughes NK. Lithium and hematopoiesis: effective experimental use of lithium as an agent to improve bone marrow transplantation. J Med 1992; 23: 195–216

95. Thomsen J, Bech P, Geisler A, et al. Meniere's disease. Preliminary report of lithium treatment. Acta Otolaryngol 1974; 78: 59–64

96. Thomsen J, Bech P, Geisler A, et al. Lithium treatment of meniere's disease. Results of a double-blind cross-over trial. Acta Otolaryngol 1976; 82: 294–6

97. Bschor T, Bauer M. Thyroid gland function in lithium treatment [in German]. Nervenarzt 1998; 69: 189–95

98. Bschor T, Baethge C, Adli M, et al. Hypothalamic–pituitary–thyroid system activity during lithium augmentation in unipolar major depression. J Psychiatry Neurosci 2003; 28: 210–16

99. Gerdes H, Littmann KP, Joseph K, et al. Successful treatment of thyrotoxicosis by lithium. Acta Endocrinol 1973; 173 (Suppl): 23

100. Lazarus JH, Richards AR, Addison GM, Owen GM. Treatment of thyrotoxicosis with lithium carbonate. Lancet 1974; 2: 1160–3

101. Gershengorn MC, Izumi M, Robbins J. Use of lithium as an adjunct to radioiodine therapy of thyroid carcinoma. J Clin Endocrinol Metab 1976; 42: 105–11

102. Pons F, Carrio I, Estorch M, et al. Lithium as an adjuvant of iodine-131 uptake when treating patients with well-differentiated thyroid carcinoma. Clin Nucl Med 1987; 12: 644–7

103. Koong SS, Reynolds JC, Movius EG, et al. Lithium as a potential adjuvant to 131I therapy of metastatic, well differentiated thyroid carcinoma. J Clin Endocrinol Metab 1999; 84: 912–16

104. Bal CS, Kumar A, Pandey RM. A randomized controlled trial to evaluate the adjuvant effect of lithium on radioiodine treatment of hyperthyroidism. Thyroid 2002; 12: 399–405

105. Ang ES, Teh HS, Sundram FX, Lee KO. Effect of lithium and oral thyrotrophin-releasing hormone (TRH) on serum thyrotrophin (TSH) and radioiodine uptake in patients with well differentiated thyroid carcinoma. Singapore Med J 1995; 36: 606–8

106. Gershon S. Use of liium salts in psychiatric disorders. Dis Nerv Syst 1968; 29: 51–5

107. Erwin CW, Gerber CJ, Morrison SD, James JF. Lithium carbonate and convulsive disorders. Arch Gen Psychiatry 1973; 28: 646–8

108. Morrison SD, Erwin CW, Gianturco DT, Gerber CJ. Effect of lithium on combative behavior in humans. Dis Nerv Syst 1973; 34: 186–9

109. Shukla S, Mukherjee S, Decina P. Lithium in the treatment of bipolar disorders associated with epilepsy: an open study. J Clin Psychopharmacol 1988; 8: 201–4

110. Megrabian AA, Mkhitarian VG, Amadian MG, et al. Use of lithium carbonate and vitamin E in the complex treatment of epileptics [in Russian]. Zh Nevropatol Psikhiatr Im S S Korsakova 1986; 86: 1407–10

111. Demers R, Lukesh R, Prichard J. Convulsion during lithium therapy. Lancet 1970; 2: 315–16

112. Jus A, Villeneuve A, Gautier J, et al. Some remarks on the influence of lithium carbonate on patients with temporal epilepsy. Int J Clin Pharmacol 1973; 7: 67–74

113. Couper-Smartt J. Lithium in spasmodic torticollis. Lancet 1973; 2: 741–2

114. Foerster K, Regli F. Lithium therapy of extrapyramidal movement disorders – an attempt [in German]. Nervenarzt 1977; 48: 228–32

115. Lippmann S, Kareus J. Lithium for spasmodic torticollis. Am J Psychiatry 1983; 140: 946

116. McCaul JA, Stern GM. Lithium and haloperidol in movement disorders [Letter]. Lancet 1974; 1: 1058

117. Yick LW, So KF, Cheung PT, Wu WT. Lithium chloride reinforces the regeneration-promoting effect of chondroitinase ABC on rubrospinal neurons after spinal cord injury. J Neurotrauma 2004; 21: 932–43

118. Poppe M, Friebel D, Reuner U, et al. The Kleine–Levin syndrome – effects of treatment with lithium. Neuropediatrics 2003; 34: 113–19

119. Abe K. Lithium prophylaxis of periodic hypersomnia. Br J Psychiatry 1977; 130: 312–13

120. Muratori F, Bertini N, Masi G. Efficacy of lithium treatment in Kleine–Levin syndrome. Eur Psychiatry 2002; 17: 232–3

121. Akgungor G, Akkayan B, Gaucher H. Influence of ceramic thickness and polymerization mode of a resin luting agent on early bond strength and durability with a lithium disilicate-based ceramic system. J Prosthet Dent 2005; 94: 234–41

122. Nagai T, Kawamoto Y, Kakehashi Y, Matsumura H. Adhesive bonding of a lithium disilicate ceramic material with resin-based luting agents. J Oral Rehabil 2005; 32: 598–605

123. Oh SH, Choi SY, Lee YK, et al. Effects of lithium fluoride and maleic acid on the bioactivity of calcium aluminate cement: Formation of hydroxyapatite in simulated body fluid. J Biomed Mater Res A 2003; 67: 104–11

124. Horner KC, Higueret D, Cazals Y. Efferent-mediated protection of the cochlear base from acoustic overexposure by low doses of lithium. Eur J Neurosci 1998; 10: 1524–7

125. Efalith Multicenter Trial Group. A double-blind, placebo-controlled, multicenter trial of lithium succinate ointment in the treatment of seborrheic dermatitis. J Am Acad Dermatol 1992; 26: 452–7

126. Dreno B, Chosidow O, Revuz J, Moyse D. The Study Investigator Group. Lithium gluconate 8% vs ketoconazole 2% in the treatment of seborrhoeic dermatitis: a multicentre, randomized study. Br J Dermatol 2003; 148: 1230–6

127. Dreno B, Moyse D. Lithium gluconate in the treatment of seborrhoeic dermatitis: a multicenter, randomised, double-blind study versus placebo. Eur J Dermatol 2002; 12: 549–52

128. Sparsa A, Bonnetblanc JM. Lithium [in French]. Ann Dermatol Venereol 2004; 131: 255–61

129. Finsterer U, Beyer A, Jensen U, et al. The syndrome of inappropriate secretion of antidiuretic hormone (SIADH) – treatment with lithium. Intens Care Med 1982; 8: 223–9

130. Baker RS, Hurley RM, Feldman W. Treatment of recurrent syndrome of inappropriate secretion of antidiuretic hormone with lithium. J Pediatr 1977; 90: 480–1

131. Miyagawa CI. The pharmacologic management of the syndrome of inappropriate secretion of antidiuretic hormone. Drug Intell Clin Pharm 1986; 20: 527–31

132. Knox AJ, Higgins BG, Hall IP, Tattersfield AE. Effect of oral lithium on bronchial reactivity in asthma. Clin Sci (Lond) 1992; 82: 407–12

133. Spitz E, Saltz H, Bearman J. A double blind crossover trial of lithium carbonate in asthma. Ann Allergy 1982; 49: 165–8

134. Peatfield RC, Rose FC. Exacerbation of migraine by treatment with lithium. Headache 1981; 21: 140–2

21 Lithium and the kidneys

Mogens Schou, Dieter Kampf

Contents   Lithium and kidney function • Renal side-effects of lithium • Conclusions and recommendations

LITHIUM AND KIDNEY FUNCTION

The serum lithium concentration depends on the daily lithium intake and the renal elimination of lithium: lithium clearance. The lithium ion is filtered freely through the glomerular membrane and is reabsorbed in the proximal tubule to almost the same extent as sodium and water; only under special circumstances is some lithium reabsorbed in the distal nephron. Lithium clearance varies proportionally with and is usually 20–30% of the glomerular filtration rate. Lithium clearance is calculated as the daily dosage of lithium in millimoles divided by 1.44 and divided by the serum lithium concentration in millimoles per liter.

A constant serum lithium concentration can be maintained only when circumstances leading to a change of lithium clearance are avoided. If that is not possible, lithium intake must be adjusted to lithium clearance. Lithium clearance may change when the glomerular filtration rate changes, when there is activation of sodium-retaining or sodium-excreting mechanisms, and when there is induction of lithium reabsorption in the distal nephron (Tables 21.1 and 21.2)[1].

Change of glomerular filtration rate

Glomerular filtration rate and lithium clearance increase gradually and proportionally during pregnancy, and they reach a value about 30–50% above pre-pregnancy values immediately before the delivery[2]. At the time of delivery they fall abruptly to the levels they had before the patient became pregnant. This means that the lithium dosage must be raised gradually during pregnancy in order to maintain a constant serum concentration. After delivery the dosage must be reduced and serum lithium concentration determined frequently. Since the risk of manic and depressive recurrences is very high after delivery, lithium treatment is particularly important during the puerperium (Table 21.1).

When the number of functioning nephrons is low, the glomerular filtration rate and lithium clearance are also low, for example in old age and in chronic kidney disease. Since the change

Table 21.1 Factors that may increase renal lithium elimination

	Main cause
Pregnancy	Glomerular filtration rate ↑
Nifedipine	Glomerular perfusion ↑ +
Isradipine	Proximal tubule lithium reabsorption ↓
Theophylline	Glomerular perfusion ↑
Excessive caffeine intake	Glomerular perfusion ↑

with advancing years is slow, old age does not contraindicate lithium treatment. The patients should be given gradually lower lithium doses. During chronic kidney disease the number of functioning nephrons may be not only low but also unstable, and such illness is usually considered a contraindication. If in rare cases a high risk of recurrences makes prophylactic lithium treatment urgently needed, the serum lithium concentration should be determined at short intervals and the dosage adjusted accordingly.

Glomerular filtration and lithium clearance are reduced during lithium intoxication, rarely when it is the outcome of a suicide attempt and the exposure to lithium usually short-lasting, more frequently when it has developed gradually and the exposure has persisted for a longer time (Table 21.2).

Activation of sodium-retaining or sodium-excreting mechanisms

In everyday life the most important determinant of lithium clearance is the balance between sodium-retaining (antinatriuretic) and sodium-excreting (natriuretic) mechanisms. During activation of sodium-retaining mechanisms the proximal tubular sodium reabsorption is stimulated, leading to a decrease of lithium clearance. During activation of sodium-

excreting mechanisms the proximal tubular sodium reabsorption is inhibited, leading to an increase of lithium clearance.

Sodium-retaining mechanisms are activated during threatening or manifest dehydration or low sodium intake (Table 21.2). Polyuric patients are at particular risk because their ability to produce concentrated urine is reduced, and they continue to produce dilute urine without always being able to consume a corresponding volume of fluid. Fluid and electrolyte balances become easily disturbed during physical illness with high fever. The patients eat and drink little and lose water and salt when they sweat. Under these circumstances renal elimination of lithium is lowered and serum lithium concentration increased. Continuation of lithium treatment with unaltered dosage during physical illness with fever is one of the commonest causes of lithium poisoning. Protracted vomiting and diarrhea and unconsciousness for several hours may lead to dehydration. Unless the treatment is stopped temporarily, the lithium dosage reduced, or the dehydration corrected, the patients may become intoxicated. If a polyuric patient needs major surgery with narcosis, it may also be necessary to infuse fluid during the night before the operation when intake by mouth is prohibited[3]. Treatment should be resumed as soon as fluid and electrolyte balances are restored. The intake of

Table 21.2 Factors that may decrease renal lithium elimination

	Main cause
Old age	Glomerular filtration rate ↓
Lithium intoxication	Glomerular filtration rate ↓
Protracted vomiting/diarrhea	Proximal tubule lithium reabsorption ↑
High fever	Proximal tubule lithium reabsorption ↑
Low-salt diet	Proximal tubule lithium reabsorption ↑
Edema formation	Proximal tubule lithium reabsorption ↑
Diuretics	Proximal tubule lithium reabsorption ↑
NSAIDs	Distal tubule lithium reabsorption ↑
ACE inhibitors	Glomerular perfusion pressure ↓
Beta blockers	Glomerular perfusion pressure ↓
Verapamil	Glomerular perfusion pressure ↓

sodium falls if patients go on a rigorous slimming diet or are given a low-salt diet because they have heart failure or hypertension.

Lithium clearance is lowered under conditions associated with edema formation. It may for example fall in congestive heart failure, liver cirrhosis with ascites and nephrotic syndrome. The kidneys continue to retain sodium and water because sodium-retaining mechanisms are activated. Lithium treatment should be given with caution or not at all.

Treatment with diuretic drugs such as amiloride, thiazides and spironolactone leads to sodium loss and activation of sodium-retaining mechanisms (Table 21.2). These drugs are given to patients with edema or with lithium-induced polyuria, but the combination with lithium may induce lithium intoxication, and serum lithium concentration must be determined frequently.

Lithium clearance may also fall during treatment with drugs that lower the blood pressure such as angiotensin converting enzyme (ACE) inhibitors, beta-blocking agents, methyldopa and the calcium entry blocker verapamil. The mechanism is a reduction of renal perfusion pressure. Frequent checking of serum lithium concentration is required.

Lithium clearance increases when sodium-excreting mechanisms are activated. It is moderately increased when sodium intake is high. When sodium intake is subsequently normalized, lithium clearance falls. Serum lithium should therefore be determined frequently when patients change dietary habits. A high fluid intake is without effect on lithium clearance because the excess water is excreted very efficiently, and no marked overhydration develops.

An increase of lithium clearance and a decrease of serum lithium concentration may be seen during treatment with the calcium entry blockers nifedipine and isradipine (Table 21.1). The mechanism is afferent arteriolar vasodilatation and possibly also a direct inhibition of proximal tubular sodium reabsorption[4].

Treatment with theophylline leads to afferent arteriolar vasodilatation resulting in increased lithium clearance and decreased serum lithium concentration. A similar effect is seen during excessive caffeine intake. If the dosage of lithium is not reduced, patients in whom theophylline is discontinued and patients who abruptly stop excessive drinking of coffee or tea are at substantial risk of developing intoxication.

Induction of distal nephron lithium reabsorption

Treatment with non-steroidal anti-inflammatory drugs (NSAIDs) is the only known condition in which lithium may be reabsorbed in the distal nephron (Table 21.2). These drugs produce a severe reduction of lithium clearance, and treatment has, in several cases, led to intoxication. There is no convincing evidence that aspirin affects the serum lithium level to a clinically significant degree, and this drug may therefore be the first choice when combined administration of NSAIDs and lithium is necessary[5]. All NSAIDs should nevertheless be used with caution.

RENAL SIDE-EFFECTS OF LITHIUM

Nephrogenic diabetes insipidus

During lithium treatment the kidneys of some patients are unable to concentrate the urine to a normal extent, and the patients consequently develop polyuria and polydipsia (Table 21.3). In almost all patients the underlying mechanism is a nephrogenic diabetes insipidus, and only in a few patients may primary polydipsia or central diabetes insipidus be identified[6].

The extent of the concentrating defect can be assessed by measurement of the urine concentration after administration of a modified antidiuretic hormone (DDAVP). After lithium treatment for some years, 30–80% of patients have a concentrating defect[7–13]. Complaints of nycturia and thirst are 60% more frequent when patients are on lithium than when they are not. During lithium treatment urine volumes are 10–60% higher and concentrating abilities 10–30% lower than before the patients began lithium treatment. The changes are larger when the serum lithium concentration is maintained at a higher level than when it is maintained at a lower level[10]. Nephrogenic diabetes insipidus is caused by inhibition of vasopressin-stimulated adenylate cyclase, decreased mRNA expression of aquaporin-2, and diminished density of vasopressin receptors in the collecting tubules[14–16].

Drugs used to treat nephrogenic diabetes insipidus include amiloride, thiazides and NSAIDs. Treatment with vasopressin (DDAVP) may be tried. Use of diuretics and NSAIDs is, however, not without risk, because proximal tubular reabsorption is stimulated and lithium clearance lowered. Intoxications have been seen. If diuretics are nevertheless used, serum lithium concentration should be determined frequently.

Chronic lithium nephropathy

Clinical studies

As mentioned above, prophylactic lithium treatment was for a number of years observed to produce polyuria and increased thirst. These side-effects were regarded as inconvenient but fully reversible and not dangerous. The situation changed when pathologists discovered morphological changes in both tubuli and glomeruli of lithium-treated patients[13,17–20] (Table 21.3). A number of the centers that had been studying lithium-induced nephrogenic diabetes insipidus decided to subject this matter to systematic scrutiny[7–13]. The outcome of the studies was on the whole reassuring. In a review, Walker and Kincaid-Smith[21] concluded that, when episodes of lithium intoxication are

Table 21.3 Adverse effects of lithium on the kidneys

	Frequency	Clinical findings	Morphology	Treatment	Prognosis	Prevention
Nephrogenic diabetes insipidus	Frequent	Polyuria Nocturia Lowered concentration ability	Normal	Lower lithium concentration if possible amiloride, thiazides, NSAIDs or DDAVP	Good regarding the kidney function	Lowest effective lithium concentration possible
Chronic lithium nephropathy	Rare	Polyuria Lowered concentration ability GFR ↓	Chronic interstitial nephropathy	Lithium withdrawal Symptomatic	Progression to terminal renal failure may occur	Lowest effective lithium concentration possible Avoid lithium intoxication Avoid other nephrotoxic substances
Nephrotic syndrome	Very rare	Edema, proteinuria, hyperlipidemia	Minimal change disease or focal segmental glomerulo-sclerosis	Lithium withdrawal Corticosteroids if persistent Symptomatic	Good regarding the kidney function	Unknown

NSAIDs, non-steroidal anti-inflammatory drugs; DDAVP, desmopression; GFR, glomerular filtration rate

avoided, there is little evidence of progressive morphological changes.

During recent years large patient groups have been followed for still longer periods of lithium treatment[22–27]. These studies have shown that 15–20% of such patients experience an irreversible lowering of urinary concentrating ability[24]. In about 5–10%, glomerular function falls slowly. In the study by Presne and associates[25], 16% of patients with chronic lithium nephropathy after lithium treatment for an average of 20 years needed regular dialysis treatment. According to Markowitz and co-workers[27], advanced lithium nephropathy (serum creatinine level higher than 25 mg/l) may progress to end-stage renal disease despite discontinuation of lithium.

There are no absolutely specific clinical signs of chronic lithium nephropathy. A lowering of urinary concentrating ability may be the only warning, but very often this is caused merely by nephrogenic diabetes insipidus. Provided that other causes of kidney damage have been excluded, it is in fact only a fall in the glomerular filtration rate that reveals that a chronic lithium nephropathy has developed.

Morphologic changes

The morphologic changes correspond to a chronic interstitial nephropathy and include focally accentuated tubular changes (flattened epithelial cells, tubular dilatation, tubular atrophy), interstitial fibrosis and moderate mononuclear cell infiltration. Microcysts originating from distal tubules or collecting ducts are predominantly located in the renal cortex. Specific glomerular changes are usually absent. Only around severely damaged tubules some glomeruli may show segmental or global sclerosis[20,28].

Assessment of the literature

When the literature is assessed, one notes that the investigators did not always distinguish between renal side-effects in well-treated patients and in patients having been given lithium in rather large doses without proper monitoring. For the individual patient it may also be difficult to decide whether renal disease or administration of other medications with an effect on the kidneys may have contributed to the renal insufficiency. Without careful and critical examination, such patients may have been considered 'damaged by lithium'. It is important to have access to renal baseline information prior to lithium treatment[29].

Nephrotic syndrome

A lithium-induced nephrotic syndrome is a very rare occurrence (Table 21.3). As far as the authors have been able to ascertain, such a syndrome has been reported in only 22 patients[30–32]. In most of the patients, minimal change disease has been found; in only a few has focal segmental glomerulosclerosis been found. The prognosis of the former is good, with complete remission within a few weeks after discontinuation of lithium. The prognosis of focal segmental glomerulosclerosis is less favorable. If it persists after discontinuation of lithium, treatment with glucocorticosteroids may be considered.

CONCLUSIONS AND RECOMMENDATIONS

Effective and safe lithium treatment requires that the serum lithium concentration be maintained at the lowest level that is compatible with absence of manic and depressive recurrences. During long-term lithium treatment it is particularly important that the kidney function is followed regularly. If the function shows signs of deterioration, the patient should be given a nephrologic checkup.

Gitlin[33] suggested a medical consultation when the serum creatinine level rises above $140\,\mu mol/l$. However, nowadays nephrologists do not rely on the serum creatinine concentration. The National Kidney Foundation in the USA recommends estimation of the glomerular filtration rate*, and this can be done with use of the MDRD formula[34]:

Glomerular filtration rate (ml/min/1.73 m^2) = 186.3 × serum creatinine (mg/dl) $^{-1.154}$ × age $^{-0.203}$ (×0.742 if female)

Simpler in calculation but also less precise is the Cockcroft–Gault formula[35]:

$$Creatinine\ clearance\ (ml/min) = \frac{(140 - age) \times body\ weight\ (kg)}{72 \times serum\ creatinine\ (mg/dl)}$$

In women this value should be multiplied by 0.85.

If the glomerular filtration rate estimated by one of these equations is lower than 60 ml/min per 1.73 m^2, a nephrologist should be consulted.

A simple and elegant way of obtaining an impression of changes in kidney function is to calculate the ratio: daily lithium dosage divided by serum lithium concentration[36]. If this ratio changes, there is reason to look for an explanation. Calculating the ratio is an expedient way of ensuring not only that the

---

*The website *http://www.kidney.org/professionals/kdoqi/cap.cfm* provides calculators and downloads for both formulas.

psychiatrist watches the serum lithium concentration but also that he remembers to take the daily lithium dosage into consideration. Mistakes have arisen when, for example, the serum lithium concentration was found to be unchanged in spite of a previous change of the dosage. Then there was reason to look for an explanation.

REFERENCES

1. Thomsen K, Schou M. Avoidance of lithium intoxication: advice based on knowledge about the renal lithium clearance under various circumstances. Pharmacopsychiatry 1999; 32: 83–6

2. Schou M. Treating recurrent affective disorders during and after pregnancy: what can be taken safely? Drug Safety 1998; 18: 143–52

3. Schou M, Hippius H. Guidelines for patients receiving lithium treatment who require major surgery. Br J Anesth 1997; 59: 809–10

4. Wang W, Kwon TH, Li C, et al. Altered expression of renal aqaporins and Na(+) transporters in rats treated with L-type calcium-blocker. Am J Physiol Regul Integr Comp Physiol 2001; 280: R1632–R1641

5. Reimann IW, Diener U, Frolich JC. Indomethacin but not aspirin increases plasma lithium ion levels. Arch Gen Psychiatry 1983; 40: 283–6

6. Baylis PH, Heath DA. Water disturbances in patients treated with oral lithium carbonate. Ann Intern Med 1978; 88: 607–9

7. Bucht G, Wahlin A. Renal concentrating capacity in long-term lithium treatment and after withdrawal. Acta Med Scand 1980; 207: 309–14

8. Vestergaard P, Amdisen A. Lithium treatment and kidney function. A follow-up study of 237 patients in long-term treatment. Acta Psychiatr Scand 1981; 63: 333–45

9. Løkkegaard H, Andersen NF, Henriksen E, et al. Renal function in 153 manic–depressive patients treated with lithium for more than five years. Acta Psychiatr Scand 1985; 71: 347–55

10. Schou M, Vestergaard P. Prospective studies on a lithium cohort. 2. Renal function. Water and electrolyte metabolism. Acta Psychiatr Scand 1988; 78: 427–33

11. Christensen S, Schou M. Lithium and the kidney. Conclusions and clinical implications. In Christensen S, ed. Lithium and the Kidney. Stuttgart: Karger, 1990: 179–83

12. Kallner G, Petterson U. Renal, thyroid and parathyroid function during lithium treatment: laboratory tests in 207 people treated for 1–30 years. Acta Psychiatr Scand 1995; 91: 48–51

13. Albrecht J, Kampf D, Müller-Oerlinghausen B. Renal function and biopsy in patients on lithium-therapy. Pharmakopsykiatry 1980; 13: 228–34

14. Hensen J, Haenelt M, Gross P. Lithium induced polyuria and renal vasopressin receptor density. Nephrol Dial Transplant 1996; 11: 622–9

15. Laursen UH, Pilhakaski-Maunsbach K, Kwon TH, et al. Change of rat kidney AQP2 and Na,K-ATPase mRNA expression in lithium-induced nephrogenic diabetes insipidus. Nephron Exp Nephrol 2004; 97: e1–16

16. Walker RJ, Weggery S, Bedford JJ, et al. Lithium-induced reduction in urinary concentrating ability and urinary aquaporin 2 (APQ2) excretion in healthy volunteers. Kidney Int 2005; 67: 291–4

17. Hestbech J, Hansen HE, Amdisen A, et al. Chronic renal lesions following long-term treatment with lithium. Kidney Int 1977; 12: 203–13

18. Rafaelsen OJ, Bolwig TG, Ladefoged J, et al. C. Kidney function & morphology in long-term lithium treatment. In Cooper TB, Gershon S, Kline NS, Schou M, eds. Lithium: Controversies and Unresolved Issues. Amsterdam: Excerpta Medica, 1979: 578–83

19. Hansen HE, Hestbech J, Sørensen JL, et al. Chronic interstitial nephropathy in patients on long-term lithium treatment. Q J Med 1979; 48: 577–91

20. Walker RG, Dowling JP, Alcorn D, et al. Renal pathology associated with lithium therapy. Pathology 1983; 15: 403–11

21. Walker RG, Kincaid-Smith P. Morphological changes observed in patients on lithium therapy. In Christensen S, ed. Lithium and the Kidney. Stuttgart: Karger, 1990: 95–105

22. Bendz H, Aurell M, Lanke J. A historical cohort study of kidney damage in long-term lithium patients: continued surveillance needed. Eur Psychiatry 2001; 16: 199–206

23. Turan, T, Esel E, Tokgöz B, et al. Effects of short- and long-term lithium treatment on kidney functioning in patients with bipolar mood disorder. Prog Neuropsychopharmacol Biol Psychiatry 2002; 26: 561–5

24. Bendz H. Renal and Parathyroid Function in Psychiatric Patients on Lithium Treatment. PLD thesis, Göteborg University, Göteborg, 2002

25. Presne C, Fakhouri F, Noël L-H, et al. Lithium-induced nephropathy: rate of progression and prognostic factors. Kidney Int 2003; 64: 585–92

26. Lepkifker E, Sverdlik A, Iancu I, et al. Renal insufficiency in long-term lithium treatment. J Clin Psychiatry 2004; 65: 850–6

27. Markowitz GS, Rhadakrishnan J, Kambham N, et al. Lithium nephrotoxicity: a progressive combined glomerular and tubulointerstitial nephropathy. J Am Soc Nephrol 2000; 11: 1439–48

28. Kampf D. Lithium und Nierenfunktion. In Müller-Oerlinghausen B, Greil W, Berghöfer A, eds. Die Lithiumtherapie. 2. Auflage. Berlin: Springer-Verlag, 1986: 368–81

29. Povlsen UJ, Hetmar O, Ladefoged J, Bolwig TG. Kidney functioning during lithium treatment: a prospective study of patients treated with lithium for up to ten years. Acta Psychiatr Scand 1992; 85: 56–60

30. Bosquet S, Descombes E, Gauthier T, et al. Nephrotic syndrome during lithium therapy. Nephrol Dial Transplant 1997; 12: 2728–31

31. Gill DS. Nephrotic syndrome associated with lithium therapy. Am J Psychiatry 1997; 154: 1318

32. Sakarcan A, Thomas DB, O'Reilly KP, et al. Lithium-induced nephrotic syndrome in a young pediatric patient. Pediatr Nephrol 2002; 17: 290–2

33. Gitlin M. Lithium and the kidney. An updated review. Drug Safety 1999; 20: 231–43

34. National Kidney Foundation. K/DOQI Clinical Practice Guidelines for Chronic Kidney Disease: evaluation, classification and stratification. Am J Kidney Dis 2002; 39 (Suppl 1): S1

35. Cockroft DW, Gault MH. Prediction of creatinine clearance from serum creatinine. Nephron 1976; 16: 31–42

36. Thomsen K. Renal lithium excretion in man and its role for development of lithium intoxication. In Birch NJ, Galicchio VS, Becker R, eds. Lithium: 50 years of Psychopharmacology. Cheshire, CT: Weidner Publishing Group, 1990: 100–15

22 Effect of lithium on the thyroid and endocrine glands

John H Lazarus, George Kirov, Brian B Harris

Contents   Effect of lithium on thyroid physiology • Effect on the hypothalamic–pituitary axis • Clinical effects of lithium on the thyroid • Lithium and other endocrine glands

EFFECT OF LITHIUM ON THYROID PHYSIOLOGY

Lithium has many actions on thyroid physiology. The most important clinically relevant action is the inhibition of thyroid hormone release. This may result in the development of goiter and hypothyroidism. Independent effects on the hypothalamic–pituitary–thyroid axis and the receptor-mediated mechanism of thyroid hormone action may contribute to this picture. The effect of lithium on inhibition of cyclic AMP-mediated cellular events and its inhibitory effect on the phosphoinositol pathway help to explain the intracellular disturbances, but the full mechanisms are still not clear. The immunological influence of lithium on thyroid antibody concentrations leads to a more rapid onset of thyroid autoimmunity characterized usually by goiter and hypothyroidism but possibly also a state of hyperthyroidism in some cases.

In 1967 the occurrence of goiter in patients receiving lithium was mentioned at a conference in Denmark and these data were reported in 1968[1]. Since then the physiology and clinical effects of lithium on thyroid function in animals and humans have been extensively investigated[2–6]. This chapter discusses the effects of lithium on thyroid physiology and the clinical effects on thyroid function in psychiatric patients. The effect of lithium on other endocrine glands is also described.

Lithium is concentrated by the thyroid at levels three to four times that in plasma[7], but reduces the radioiodine uptake into rat thyroid and the thyroid of other species. The relationship of the thyroidal lithium-concentrating mechanism to the iodide-concentrating process is not clear, but lithium has also been found to be concentrated in mouse salivary glands, which also actively concentrate iodine, perhaps suggesting a common pathway. Iodide is known to be concentrated in the thyroid by the sodium–iodide symporter[8], but the relation of lithium in this system is not known. In humans, lithium administration has been reported to result in both a reduced as well as an increased thyroidal radioiodine uptake. The possible reasons for this are that lithium may compete for iodide transport resulting in low thyroid iodine uptake; it also causes iodide retention. The increase in uptake may also be due to thyroid stimulating hormone (TSH) secreted as a result of lithium-induced hypothyroidism. Although lithium can impair some aspects of intrathyroidal metabolism as determined *in vitro*, the net effect in humans is modest. The ion may increase the thyroidal sensitivity to iodine exposure in humans but the resulting block in iodine organification is mild.

An important thyroidal action of lithium is to inhibit thyroid hormone release in both euthyroid and hyperthyroid humans[9]. The mechanism of inhibition of hormone release involves an alteration in tubulin polymerization as well as inhibition of the action of TSH on cyclic AMP[3].

Under physiological conditions deiodination accounts for 80% of total thyroxine (T4) turnover, this process being mediated by three specific deiodinase enzymes[10]. Three iodothyronine deiodinases have been identified with distinct tissue distributions, catalytic specificities and regulations. Briefly, the type I deiodinase (expressed mainly in liver and kidney) converts T4 to triiodothyronine (T3), thus mediating plasma T3. The type II deiodinase (expressed in brain, pituitary and skeletal muscle) mediates local T3 production by the deiodination of T4 while the type III enzyme (expressed in brain, placenta and fetal tissues) mediates T3 degradation. The significant decrease in T4 clearance from plasma in patients receiving lithium may be due to inhibition of thyroid hormone secretion, thereby inducing a decrease in type I 5′ deiodinase activity. Lithium causes a decrease in T4 deiodination in rat liver, and inhibitory effects of lithium on T4 to T3 conversion have been demonstrated in mouse neuroblastoma cells and GH3 cells[11]. Similar data have been obtained in rats; their relevance to the clinical situation may be questioned, because of the high doses of lithium used in some experiments, although suggestive data have been obtained in humans[12]. Administration of lithium to rats for 14 days has been shown to affect the intracellular metabolism of thyroid hormones in the frontal cortex of the rat by increasing the type II deiodinase and decreasing the type III enzyme[13]. This raises the question as to whether these effects of lithium on thyroid hormone metabolism in the central nervous system (CNS) may be involved in the mood-stabilizing effects of the drug similar to data obtained for other psychotropic agents. Lithium has been shown to reduce both the deiodinase type II and type III (converting T3 to inactive 3′-3T2) in rat brain[14]. However, in further animal experiments it has been noted that 5′-DII activity and thyroid hormone concentrations in the CNS are highly sensitive to many influences that cause changes in neuronal activity (such as brain region studied and time of day)[15]. However, it is still not clear whether these changes in deiodinase activity result from a direct action of lithium on the brain or perhaps from a reduction in serum T4 levels leading in turn to a rise in 5′-DII activity. In this connection it is interesting to note that T3 levels in synaptosomes of the amygdala are raised in rats treated with lithium for 14 days[16].

EFFECT ON THE HYPOTHALAMIC–PITUITARY AXIS

Lithium is concentrated in the pituitary gland as well as the hypothalamus[17] and may interfere with cell metabolism in those tissues as a result of this. In cross-sectional studies lithium therapy in psychiatric patients has resulted in an

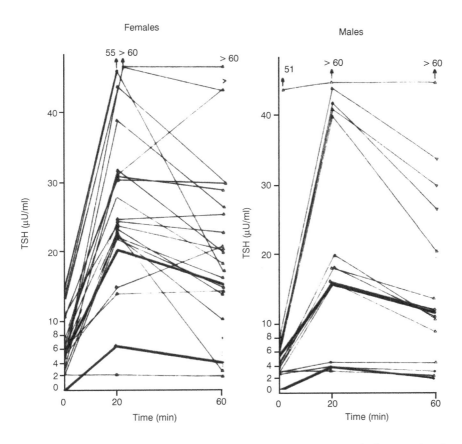

Figure 22.1 Serum thyroid stimulating hormone (TSH) response to 200 μg iv thyrotropin releasing hormone in 73 patients (34 M, 39 F) receiving lithium therapy (mean duration of therapy 37.2 months, mean serum lithium level 0.72 mmol/l). Only abnormal responses are shown (in 49.3% of patients). Limits of normal response are shown by the dark lines. (From Lazarus *et al.*, reference 18. Reproduced with permission from Cambridge University Press)

exaggerated TSH response to thyrotropin releasing hormone (TRH) in at least 50% of patients (Figure 22.1), rising to 100% in others[18]. Approximately 10% of patients so studied will have an elevated basal TSH and non-manic patients treated with lithium also have high basal and stimulated TSH levels. Basal prolactin concentrations are not raised in manic and non-manic patients on lithium but they do show exaggerated responses to TRH.

In a longitudinal study, a significant rise in basal TSH was found in 83% of 12 patients and a rise of TRH-stimulated TSH was observed in 11 patients after 12 months of therapy. The impairment of the hypothalamic axis was temporary in most cases, suggesting that the hypothalamic–pituitary–thyroid (HPT) axis adjusts to a new level of control (or 'stat') during lithium therapy[19]. In rapid-cycling bipolar disorder a latent hypofunction of the HPT system has been shown even with short-term (4 weeks) lithium challenge[20]. In 28 patients receiving lithium for 12 months, TSH levels were normal and only levels of reverse T3 (rT3) were raised[21]. The efficacy of lithium prophylaxis was significantly correlated with serum T3 suggesting an interaction with thyroid hormone metabolism in the brain. The effect of lithium on the activity and thyroid hormone binding to thyroid hormone receptors in the brain may be a partial explanation for these findings. Lithium increases thyroid hormone nuclear binding of T3 in the rat brain[22]. It regulates thyroid receptor gene expression *in vitro* in cultured cells of pituitary origin[23] and does so in an isoform- and region-specific manner within the brain[24] as well as affecting the cytoplasmic availability of T4[25].

CLINICAL EFFECTS OF LITHIUM ON THE THYROID

Goiter and hypothyroidism

The initial inhibition of the thyroid hormone secretion rate by lithium results in an increase in TSH concentration, leading to thyroid enlargement. This is not the only mechanism, as lithium alters intracellular signal transduction and the function of insulin-like growth factor. It also activates a tyrosine kinase to induce cell proliferation[26]. In normal females thyroid volume increases significantly after 28 days of lithium treatment, although no change was noted in males, suggesting a difference in susceptibility between the sexes to small increments in TSH[27]. In the rat the main histologic feature is an increase in follicular diameter and a decrease in follicle cell height[28], whereas in humans all follicles have pronounced pleomorphism of the epithelial cells and marked nuclear changes[29].

Schou *et al.*[1] reported the occurrence of 12 patients with goiter out of 330 manic-depressive patients treated with lithium for 5 months to 2 years. The calculated incidence of goiter was 4% per year per 100 patients on continuous lithium and this was compared to a 1% incidence in the general population of a separate community (Copenhagen). There is considerable variation in the estimates due to the population sample, observer experience, duration of lithium therapy and method of diagnosing goiter. An overall prevalence in 876 patients was 6.1%[30] and 5.6% in 1257 patients reported by Mannisto[31]. Some groups, however, have found no goiter while others have found incidence rates of 30–60%[6]. If imaging techniques such as scintiscanning or ultrasound are used, significant thyroid enlargement was noted when thyroid volume after 3 months of lithium treatment was compared to pre-treatment values[32]. Further cross-sectional studies employing ultrasonic measurement of thyroid volume have shown that goiter occurred in 40% of 100 patients treated for 1–5 years and in 50% of those treated for more than 10 years compared to 16% in control subjects[33]. In four recent studies the goiter rates ranged between 30 and 55% in study populations ranging from 20 to 96 patients[34–37]. The latter two studies confirmed higher goiter rates than in controls. The goiter incidence reflects the patient gender, duration of treatment and the goiter rate in the population where the patient lives. Clinically the goiter is smooth and non-tender. It may develop within weeks of starting lithium therapy or take months to years of lithium treatment before becoming evident[31].

The management of a patient receiving lithium in whom a goiter is detected is similar to that of any patient with a goiter. A diffuse enlargement suggests lithium as an etiology in a patient receiving the drug. If there is recent enlargement of a nodule or the finding of an irregularly shaped thyroid gland appropriate investigation must be performed, as the goiter may not be due to lithium therapy. In this situation fine needle aspiration cytology is an important diagnostic aid, especially in relation to thyroid malignancy. Imaging such as the use of ultrasound is useful to delineate the extent of the enlargement, but is not a reliable tool for diagnosis of cancer. Evidence of autoimmunity may, however, be observed by ultrasound. As thyroxine treatment may protect against lithium-induced goiter[37], it is reasonable to give levothyroxine to patients with significant thyroid enlargement, especially if this is associated with symptoms of neck compression. The latter clinical situation is rare in lithium-treated patients. Thyroxine should be given in a dose such that the TSH is not totally suppressed and the serum T4 and serum T3 are within normal limits. Serum T4 may occasionally be allowed to exceed the normal range, but T3 should not. Thyroxine therapy is often not effective in patients with goiter of long duration, because of fibrotic changes. When the goiter size does not reduce with T4 therapy or the compressive symptoms are predominant, surgery by an experienced thyroid surgeon should be advised.

Hypothyroidism was not a feature of the first patients to be recorded who had goiter associated with lithium therapy, but subsequent case reports then started to appear[38]. The clinical presentation of hypothyroidism in lithium-treated patients is not different from that seen in other causes of hypothyroidism. Sub-clinical hypothyroidism (elevated TSH with normal circulating thyroid hormone concentrations) may also occur, and this should be considered in a patient who is not showing a good response to lithium. Symptoms of the condition may appear within weeks of starting lithium treatment but may not occur for many months or even years, and may include unusual or atypical features such as myxedema coma[39]. The female/male ratio is about 5:1 and it appears that there is a significantly higher incidence of hypothyroidism in females even when compared to the normally expected higher incidence of this condition in the general population. Prevalence figures for lithium-induced hypothyroidism vary widely, depending on the population studied and differences in clinical and laboratory evaluation. In a review of 16 reports totaling 4681 patients up to 1986 the prevalence was 3.4% (range 0–23.3%)[3] and since then figures have ranged from 6 to 39.6% (Table 22.1)[3,34,35,40–46]. While it is clear that female gender and starting lithium at a later age are the main risk factors, potential sources of bias in

Table 22.1 Prevalence of hypothyroidism in lithium-treated patients

No. of patients	% Hypothyroid	Reference
4681	3.4	Lazarus 1986[3]
207	6	Kallner and Petterson 1995[40]
209	9.6	Kirov 1998[41]
132	39	Deodhar et al. 1999[42]
101	39.6	Kusalic and Engelsmann 1999[43]
718	10.4	Johnston and Eagles 1999[44]
49	14	Ozpoyraz et al. 2002[34]
42	7.1	Caykoylu et al. 2002[35]
82	24.4	Gracious et al. 2004[45]
159	17	Kirov et al. 2005[46]

these cross-sectional studies could skew the estimates of the incidence of this disorder in either direction. Prospective studies have found hypothyroid rates of 21.7/1000 survivor years[44], 23/1000 years[47] and 27.4/1000 years[46]. These rates are substantially greater than that observed in middle-aged women not on lithium during a 20-year follow-up[48].

The etiology of lithium-associated hypothyroidism is related to the inhibition of thyroid hormone secretion described above and may occur in those without thyroid enlargement as well as those with goiter. In early reports of lithium-associated hypothyroidism the presence of thyroid antibodies (usually microsomal, now known as thyroid peroxidase) was noted. Thyroid biopsies in some patients showed evidence of autoimmune thyroiditis[3]. Clinical studies have shown that lithium can accelerate the development of existing thyroiditis, as evidenced by an increase in circulating antibody titer. The drug does not seem to be able to stimulate the production of thyroid antibodies *de novo* in the human but there is evidence that lithium therapy is associated with a rise in antibody titer in patients who already are antibody-positive at the start of treatment[49]. Cross-sectional studies have shown a higher prevalence of thyroid antibodies in lithium-treated patients (ranging from 10 to 33%) than in control populations[3]. In 116 patients followed for 2 years, Bocchetta *et al.*[50] concluded that while elevated TSH concentrations were transitory in most patients the risk of developing hypothyroidism was higher in women with thyroid antibodies. These workers have also concluded that lithium exposure may represent an additional risk factor for hypothyroidism in women in the presence of thyroid auto-immunity[47]. Hypothyroidism has been shown to occur predominantly in females with an odds ratio of 5.89 (95% CI 1.57–22)[51].

Clearly, the presence of thyroid antibodies is an important determinant of hypothyroidism in lithium-treated patients, although the inhibitory action of the drug on thyroid hormone release may account for those cases of hypothyroidism which recover to the euthyroid state. The situation is also complicated by the fact that the prevalence of thyroid antibodies is more common in patients with bipolar disorders (e.g. rapid cyclers) before they start lithium treatment[52]. With regard to other factors which may influence the development of hypothyroidism, it has been shown that iodine and lithium can act synergistically to produce hypothyroidism[53]. Variations in iodine status, dietary goitrogens, immunogenetic make-up and their interactions in the setting of chronic lithium therapy contribute to the variable pattern of expression of hypothyroidism in different ethnic groups and areas[54].

Thus, the pathogenesis of lithium-induced hypothyroidism is either autoimmune or by direct action of lithium on hormone secretion leading to goiter and hypothyroidism. The high incidence of lithium-induced hypothyroidism has implications for the long-term monitoring of lithium therapy. For example, in 1705 new users of lithium the rate of thyroxine treatment per 100 person-years was 5.65, that is almost 6% of lithium-treated patients. This suggests that hypothyroidism develops twice as frequently as would be expected among a mixed-age population[55].

There is a strong case for measuring thyroid function and antibodies in all patients prior to lithium therapy regardless of gender or age. It is reasonable to perform annual thyroid function tests in patients receiving lithium; in older women who are thyroid antibody-positive it is suggested that thyroid testing be performed more frequently[46]. Although a recent consensus[56] recommended that patients with subclinical hypothyroidism with a TSH value less than 10 mU/l should not be treated, treatment of such a patient with thyroxine is justified[57]. When administering thyroxine to lithium patients it is important to emphasize that the lithium should not be stopped or the dose altered unless the serum level is outside the therapeutic range. Drugs that alter the bio-availability of thyroxine, such as iron, soya and some indigestion remedies, should be avoided if possible or these substances given as far apart in time from the thyroxine as feasible. In patients with autoimmune thyroiditis, lack of response to thyroxine may be due to concomitant pernicious anemia, Addison's disease or celiac disease.

Hyperthyroidism

Despite the general suppressive effect of lithium on thyroid function, a significant number of cases of hyperthyroidism have been reported. The first case was reported from New Zealand in 1974 and up to 1986 a further 40–50 cases were noted (described in reference 3). The condition occurs after many years of lithium therapy in most but not all patients[5,58]. The etiology of the hyperthyroidism included Graves' disease, toxic nodular goiter and silent thyroiditis. Granulomatous thyroiditis asso-ciated with lithium therapy has been described[59] and the thyroid histology in another case[60] showed extensive follicular destruction with no lymphocytic infiltration. A large retrospective review demonstrated that lithium-associated silent thyroiditis and lithium-associated thyrotoxicosis had a much higher incidence (1.3 and 2.7 cases per 1000 person-years, respect-ively) than that seen in the general population (0.03–0.28 and 0.8–1.2, respectively)[61]. Lithium might therefore directly damage thyroid cells with consequent release of thyroglobulin and thyroid hormones into the circulation; there-fore, thyrotoxicosis caused by silent thyroiditis might be associated with lithium use. It is clearly probable that lithium treatment could mask underlying hyperthyroidism by reduction of thyroid hormones such that when lithium is

stopped hyperthyroidism will appear. Whether lithium induces autoimmune hyperthyroidism by, for example, producing thyroid-stimulating antibodies is not known, and the reported cases have been thought to be chance events. However, an epidemiological study of 14 cases of lithium-associated thyrotoxicosis from New Zealand[56] concluded that long-term lithium therapy was associated with an increased risk of thyrotoxicosis. Nine of the 14 patients in this series had autoimmune thyrotoxicosis, although TSH-receptor antibody measurements were not available, while the others had toxic nodular goiter. There is no information on the pro-pensity of lithium to increase the titer of TSH-receptor-stimulating antibody in a manner similar to its action on anti-thyroid peroxidase antibody. It seems that the probable etiology of many of the patients developing thyrotoxicosis on lithium is a transient destructive granu-lomatous thyroiditis rather than Graves' disease. As Graves' disease is common, at least in women, the chance development of this condition in women receiving lithium is to be expected.

The management of a patient with lithium-associated thyrotoxicosis will depend on the cause of the thyroid overactivity. The radio-iodine uptake will be low in lymphocytic or granulomatous thyroiditis thus precluding the use of radioiodine therapy. Antithyroid drug therapy may be tried, but steroid treatment may also be indicated. Graves' disease should be treated by radioiodine or surgery in a patient receiving lithium, as compliance may be a problem with antithyroid drugs. A toxic nodular goiter may well require surgical resection, especially if it is causing compressive neck symptoms.

From the forgoing discussion it will be appreciated that thyroid disorders are the commonest endocrine side-effect of lithium therapy. Their age dependence is illustrated in Figure 22.2 which is derived from a study on

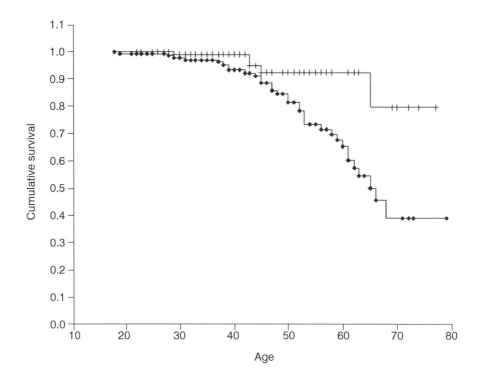

Figure 22.2   Kaplan–Meyer analysis for the development of thyroid disorders (hypo- and hyperthyroidism) in a cohort of 115 males (ı) and 159 females (♦) prospectively followed for 53.1 months (range 14–87). The vertical axis clearly indicates the increasing number of women developing thyroid disease with age. (From Kirov *et al.*, reference 46, reproduced with permission)

115 males and 159 females treated with lithium for an average of 6.3 years[46].

An intriguing report of the association of lithium therapy with exophthalmos in 10% of patients was made in 1973[62] and 25% of 73 patients in another study[18]. Both of these reports did not have accurate measurement of the eye changes, and the possible mechanisms are unclear. Nevertheless, it is interesting that, recently in a case of a bipolar patient who developed thyrotoxicosis with severe exophthalmos while on lithium, the eye signs regressed when lithium was discontinued[63].

LITHIUM AND OTHER ENDOCRINE GLANDS

Hyperparathyroidism has been described in patients on lithium therapy[40,64] and it has been shown that lithium stimulates the release of human parathyroid hormone (PTH) *in vitro*[65], thus increasing the set point release for PTH in response to calcium. There are now convincing *in vivo* human data showing that there is a clear alteration in PTH dynamics in patients on lithium such that the set point is also shifted to the right[66]. This suggests a direct effect of the cation on the parathyroid gland which may in some cases result in hyperparathyroidism. The pathology of these tumors may be single adenomas but parathyroid hyperplasia has been described more often than expected[67]. The tumorigenesis in these cases showed that the majority did not contain gross chromosomal alterations. In practice serum calcium concentrations should be measured periodically in lithium-treated patients. If hyperparathyroidism occurs, the only therapy is surgical.

Lithium is concentrated in the hypothalamic–pituitary area where it may cause structural damage at high concentrations at least in the rat[68]. The effect on the HPT axis has already been described. The effect on growth hormone is difficult to evaluate, since there are altered growth hormone secretory dynamics in depressive illness. Changes noted in humans are mild and not clinically significant. Minor changes in gonadal function and fertility have been shown in animals, but there are no convincing data in humans on these topics. Lithium may affect the Leydig cell directly rather than through the pituitary–gonadal axis[69]. Although there are changes in water handling, cortisol, aldosterone and the renin–angiotensin system during the first week of lithium administration, the main clinical consequence is diabetes insipidus (reviewed in Chapter 21). There are no significant clinical effects on adrenal function.

REFERENCES

1. Schou M, Amdisen A, Jensen S, Olsen T. Occurrence of goiter during lithium treatment. Br Med J 1968; iii: 710–13
2. Williams JA, Berens SC, Wolff J. Thyroid secretion in vitro: inhibition of TSH and dibutyryl cyclic-AMP stimulated 131-I release by Li+1. Endocrinology 1971; 88: 1385–8
3. Lazarus JH. Lithium and the thyroid gland. In Lazarus JH, ed. Endocrine and Metabolic Effects of Lithium. New York: Plenum Medical Book Company, 1986; 99–124
4. Kushner JP, Wartofsky L, Lithium–thyroid interactions. An overview. In Johnnson NF, ed. Lithium and the Endocrine System. Basel, Switzerland: Karger, 1998: 74–88
5. Chow CC, Cockram CS. Thyroid disorders induced by lithium and amiodarone: an overview. Adverse Drug React Acute Poisoning Rev 1990; 4: 207–22
6. Lazarus JH. Effect of lithium on the thyroid gland. In Weetman AP, Grossman A, eds. Pharmacotherapeutics of the Thyroid Gland. Berlin: Springer-Verlag, 1997: 207–18
7. Berens SC, Wolff J, Murphy DL. Lithium concentration by the thyroid. Endocrinology 1970; 87: 1085–7
8. Eskandari S, Loo DD, Dai G, et al. Thyroid Na+I- symporter. Mechanism, stoichiometry, and specificity. J Biol Chem 1997; 272: 27230–8
9. Spaulding SW, Burrow G, Bermudez F, Himmelhoch J. The inhibitory effect of lithium on thyroid hormone release in both euthyroid and thyrotoxic patients. J Clin Endocr Metab 1972; 35: 905–11
10. Bianco AC, Larsen PR. Intracellular pathways of iodothyronine metabolism. In Braverman LE, Utiger RD, eds. Werner and Ingbar's The Thyroid: a Fundamental and Clinical Text. Philadelphia: Lippincott Williams & Wilkins, 2005: 109–33
11. St Germain DL. Thyroid hormone metabolism. In Johnson NF, ed. Lithium and the Endocrine System. Basel, Switzerland: Karger: 1988; 123–33
12. Terao T, Oga T, Nozaki S, et al. Possible inhibitory effect of lithium on peripheral conversion of thyroxine to triiodothyronine – a prospective study. Int Clin Psychopharmacol 1995; 10: 103–5
13. Baumgartner A, Campos-Barros A, Gaio U, et al. Effects of lithium on thyroid hormone metabolism in rat frontal-cortex. Biol Psychiatry 1994; 36: 771–4
14. Baumgartner A, Pinna G, Hiedra L, et al. Effects of lithium and carbomazepine on thyroid hormone metabolism in rat brain. Neuropsychopharmacology 1997; 1: 25–41

15. Eravci M, Pinna G, Meinhold H, Baumgartner A. Effects of pharmacological and nonpharmacological treatments on thyroid hormone metabolism and concentrations in rat brain. Endocrinol 2000; 141: 1027–40

16. Pinna G, Broedel O, Eravci M, et al. Thyroid hormones in the rate amygdala as common targets for antidepressant drugs, mood stabilizers and sleep deprivation. Biol Psychiatry 2003; 54: 1049–59

17. Pfeifer WD, Davis LC, Van der Velde CD. Lithium accumulation in some endocrine tissues. Acta Biol Med Ger 1976; 35: 1519–23

18. Lazarus JH, John R, Bennie EH, et al. Lithium therapy and thyroid function a long-term study. Psychol Med 1981; 11: 85–92

19. Lomabardi G, Panza N, Biondi L, et al. Effects of lithium treatment on hypothalamic–pituitary–thyroid axis – a longitudinal study. J Endocrinol Invest 1993; 16: 259–63

20. Gyulai L, Lauer M, Bauer MS, et al. Thyroid hypofunction in patients with rapid-cycling bipolar disorder after lithium challenge. Biol Psychiatry 2003; 53: 899–905

21. Baumgartner A, Vonstuckrad M, Muller-Oerlinghausen B, et al. The hypothalamic–pituitary–thyroid axis in patients maintained on lithium prophylaxis for years – high tri-iodothyronine serum concentrations are correlated to the prophylactic efficacy. J Affect Disord 1995; 34: 211–18

22. Bolaris S, Margarity M, Valcana T. Effects of LiCl on triiodothyronin (T3) binding to nuclei from rat cerebral hemispheres. Biol Psychiatry 1995; 37: 106–11

23. Hahn CG, Pawlyk AC, Whybrow PC, Tejani-Butt SM. Differential expression of thyroid hormone receptor isoforms by thyroid hormone and lithium in rat GH3 and B103 cells. Biol Psychiatry 1999; 45: 1004–12

24. Hahn CG, Pawlyk AC, Whybrow PC, et al. Lithium administration affects gene expression of thyroid hormone receptors in rat brain. Life Sci 1999; 64: 1793–802

25. Constantiou C, Bolaris S, Valcana T, Margarity M. Acute LiCl-treatment affects the cyto-plasmic T4 availability and the expression pattern of thyroid hormone receptors in adult rat cerebral hemispheres. Neurosci Res 2004; 51: 235–41

26. Takano T, Takada K, Tada H, et al. Genistein but not staurosporine can inhibit the mitogenic signal evoked by lithium in rat-thyroid cells (FRTL-5). J Endocrinol 1994; 143: 221–6

27. Perrild H, Hegedus L, Arnung K. Sex related goitrogenic effect of lithium carbonate in healthy young subjects. Acta Endocrinol 1984; 106: 203–8

28. Heltne CE, Ollerich DA. Morphometric and electron microscopic studies of goiter induced by lithium in the rat. Am J Anat 1973; 136: 297

29. Fauerholdt L, Vendsborg P. Thyroid gland morphology after lithium treatment. Acta Pathol Microbiol Scand 1981; 89: 339–41

30. Wolff J. Lithium interactions with the thyroid gland. In Cooper TB, Gershon S, Kline NS et al., eds. Lithium Controversies and Unresolved Issues. Amsterdam: Excerpta Medica, 1978: 552–64

31. Mannisto PT. Endocrine side-effets of lithium. In Johnson FN, ed. Handbook of Lithium Therapy. Lancaster: MTP Press, 1980: 310–22

32. Lazarus JH, Bennie EH. The effect of lithium on thyroid function in man. Acta Endocrinol 1972; 70: 266–72

33. Perrild H, Hegedus L, Baastrup PC, et al. Thyroid function and ultrasonically determined thyroid size in patients receiving long-term lithium treatment. Am J Psychiatry 1990; 147: 1518–20

34. Ozpoyraz N, Tamam L, Kulan E. Thyroid abnormalities in lithium treated patients. Adv Ther 2002; 19: 176–84

35. Caykoylu A, Capoglu I, Unuyvar N, et al. Thyroid abnormalities in lithium-treated patients with bipolar affective disorder. J Int Med Res 2002; 30: 80–4

36. Schiemann U, Hengst K. Thyroid echogenicity in manic-depressive patients receiving lithium therapy. J Affect Disord 2002; 70: 85–90

37. Bauer M, Berghofer A, Blumentritt H, et al. Ultrasonographycally determined thyroid size and prevalence of goiter in lithium-treated patients with affective disorders and controls. 2006, submitted

38. Rogers M, Whybrow P. Clinical hypothyroidism occurring during lithium treatment. Two case histories and a review of thyroid function in 19 patients. Am J Psychiatry 1971; 128: 50–5

39. Waldman SA, Park D. Myxedema coma associated with lithium therapy. Am J Med 1989; 87: 355–6

40. Kallner G, Petterson U. Renal, thyroid and parathyroid function during lithium treatment: laboratory tests in 207 people treated for 1–30 years. Acta Psychiatr Scand 1995; 91: 48–51

41. Kirov G. Thyroid disorders in lithium-treated patients. J Affect Disord 1998; 50: 33–40

42. Deodhar SD, Singh B, Pathak CM, et al. Thyroid functions in lithium-treated psychiatric patients: a cross-sectional study. Biol Trace Elem Res 1999; 67: 151–63

43. Kusalic M, Engelsmann F. Effect of lithium maintenance therapy on thyroid and parathyroid function. J Psychiatry Neurosci 1999; 24: 227–33

44. Johnston AM, Eagles JM. Lithium-associated clinical hypothyroidism. Prevalence and risk factors. Br J Psychiatry 1999; 175: 336–9

45. Gracious BL, Findling RL, Seman C, et al. Elevated thyrotropin in bipolar youths prescribed both lithium and divalproex sodium. J Am Acad Child Adolesc Psychiatry 2004; 43: 215–20

46. Kirov, G, Tredget J, John R, et al. A cross-sectional and a prospective study of thyroid disorders in lithium-treated patients. J Affect Disord 2005; 87: 313–17

47. Bocchetta A, Mossa P, Velluzzi F, et al. Ten-year follow-up of thyroid function in lithium patients. J Clin Psychopharmacol 2001; 21: 594–8

48. Vanderpump MPJ, Tunbridge WMG, French JM, et al. The incidence of thyroid disorders in the community: a twenty-year follow-up of the Whickham Survey. Clin Endocrinol 1995; 43: 55–68

49. Lazarus JH, Ludgate M, McGregor A, et al. Lithium therapy induces autoimmune thyroid disease. In Walfish PG, Wall JR, Volpe R, eds. Autoimmunity and the Thyroid. London: Academic Press, 1985: 319–20

50. Bocchetta A, Bernardi F, Burrai C, et al. The course of thyroid abnormalities during lithium treatment – a 2-year follow-up study. Acta Psychiatr Scand 1992; 86: 38–41

51. Ahmadi-Abhari A, Ghaeli P, Fahimi F, et al. Risk factors of thyroid abnormalities in bipolar patients receiving lithium: a case control study. BMC Psychiatry 2003; 3: 4

52. Kupka RW, Nolen WA, Post RM, et al. High rate of autoimmune thyroiditis in bipolar disorder: lack of association with lithium exposure. Biol Psychiatry 2002; 51: 305–11

53. Shopsin B, Shenkman L, Blum M, Hollander C. Iodine and lithium-induced hypothyroidism. Documentation of synergism. Am J Med 1973; 55: 695-9

54. Lee S, Chow CC, Wing YK, Shek CC. Thyroid abnormalities during chronic lithium treatment in Hong-Kong Chinese – a controlled study. J Affect Disord 1992; 26: 173–8

55. Shulman KI, Sykora K, Gill SS. New thyroxine treatment in older adults beginning lithium therapy. Am J Geriatr Psychiatry 2005; 13: 299–304

56. Surks MI, Ortiz E, Daniels GH, et al. Subclinical thyroid disease: scientific review and guidelines for diagnosis and management. JAMA 2004; 291: 228–38

57. Kleiner J, Altshuler L, Hendrick V, Hershman JM. Lithium-induced sublinical hypothyroidism: review of the literature and guidelines for treatment. J Clin Psychiatry 1990; 60: 249–55

58. Barclay ML, Brownlie BEW, Turner JG, Wells EJ. Lithium associated thyrotoxicosis: a report of 14 cases, with statistical analysis of incidence. Clin Endocrinol 1994; 40: 759–64

59. Sinnott MJ, McIntyre HD, Pond SM. Granulomatous thyroiditis and lithium therapy. Aust NZ J Med 1992; 22: 84

60. Mizukami Y, Michigishi T, Nonomura A, et al. Histological features of the thyroid gland in a patient with lithium induced thyrotoxicosis. J Clin Pathol 1995; 48: 582–4

61. Miller KK, Daniels GH. Association between lithium use and thyrotoxicosis caused by silent thyroiditis. Clin Endocrinol 2001; 55: 501–8

62. Segal RL, Rosenblatt S, Eliasoph I. Endocrine exophthalmos during lithium therapy of manic depressive disease. N Engl J Med 1973; 289: 136–8

63. Byrne AP, Delaney WJ. Regression of thyrotoxic ophthalmopathy following lithium withdrawal. Can J Psychiatry 1993; 38: 383–90

64. Christiansen C, Baastrup PC, Lindgreen P, Transbol I. Endocrine effects of lithium. II Primary hyperparathyroidism. Acta Endocrinol 1978; 88: 528–34

65. Birnbaum J, Klandorf H, Guiliano A, Van Herle A. Lithium stimulates the release of human parathyroid hormone in vitro. J Clin Endocrinol Metab 1988; 66: 1187–91

66. Haden ST, Stoll AL, McCormick S, et al. Alterations in parathyroid dynamics in lithium-treated subjects. J Clin Endocrinol Metab 1997; 82: 2844–8

67. Dwight T, Kytola S, Teh BT, et al. Genetic analysis of lithium-associated parathyroid tumors. Eur J Endocrinol 2002; 146: 619–27

68. Rosnowska M, Gajkowska B, Borowicz J. Ultrastructure of rat hypophyseal system in chronic lithium carbonate intoxication. Acta Med Pol 1981; 23: 310–18

69. Collins TJ, Chatterjee S, LeGate LS, Banerji TK. Lithium: evidence for reduction in circulating testosterone levels in mice following chronic administration. Life Sci 1988; 43: 1501–5

23 Adverse neurological and neurotoxic effects of lithium therapy

Oliver Pogarell, Malte Folkerts, Ulrich Hegerl

Contents   Introduction • Common, usually mild, adverse neurological effects

INTRODUCTION

The discovery of the episode-preventive effects of long-term lithium treatment in affective disorders led to its widespread use, particularly since monitoring can easily be performed by measuring lithium blood concentrations.

Longstanding experience with the chronic administration of lithium, alone or in combination with other psychotropic drugs, now allows better estimation of the specific risks of this treatment to be obtained. Neurological symptoms during lithium treatment comprise fine tremor, slurred speech, blurred vision, dizziness, nystagmus and ataxia, but also stupor and coma. Mild neurological signs and symptoms are among the most frequent side-effects of lithium medication, even under therapeutic blood serum concentrations and especially if the dose is increased too rapidly.

This chapter summarizes important adverse effects of lithium on the nervous system comprising commonly occurring symptoms such as lithium-induced fine action tremor, as well as less frequent neurotoxic effects such as clouding of consciousness, dizziness, confusion, stupor and coma (sometimes with convulsions), often but not necessarily associated with excessive (toxic) lithium serum levels (Table 23.1).

COMMON, USUALLY MILD, ADVERSE NEUROLOGICAL EFFECTS

Tremor

A fine tremor of the upper limbs is one of the most frequent adverse effects occurring even at therapeutic lithium serum levels, both upon initiation and during the course of chronic lithium administration. Lithium-induced tremor presents as a postural and/or action tremor of high frequency, which occurs when the limbs are actively maintained in a posture against

Table 23.1 Adverse neurological effects of lithium

Common adverse effects

Unspecific symptoms
    weakness, sedation, concentration deficits,
    distractibility
Lithium-induced tremor
    usually harmless, but disturbing – may cause
    problems with compliance
EEG alterations
    frequent, in most cases clinically irrelevant

Neurotoxic adverse effects – central nervous system

Cognitive dysfunction
Extrapyramidal and cerebellar signs and symptoms
Oculomotor symptoms
Pseudotumor cerebri

Neurotoxic adverse effects – peripheral

Muscle weakness
Reduction in nerve conduction velocities

gravity (postural tremor) or during any type of active movements (action tremor). This tremor seems to be an exaggeration of physiologic tremors with a similar frequency range between 8 and 13 Hz. Usually these tremors can clearly be separated from a parkinsonian tremor or tremors induced by neuroleptic drugs, with a markedly lower frequency of 4–6 Hz and presenting as resting tremors, suppressed or reduced during action.

The reported incidence rates of lithium-induced tremor in the literature show a wide range between 4% for patients under chronic lithium administration and 65% in lithium-treated healthy subjects[1,2]. Koufen and Consbruch found a 20% prevalence of lithium-induced tremor in 124 patients who had received lithium for more than 8 years, both at the beginning of lithium medication and during follow-up[3]. Vestergaard *et al.* reported tremors in 16% of patients under lithium; however, tremor had already been described in about 10%

of the patients before initiation of lithium therapy[4]. Although the reported data are not conclusive and show a rather wide range of tremor incidence, there is no doubt that tremor is a frequent adverse event under lithium treatment. The intra-individual occurrence of lithium-induced tremor depends on the dosage of lithium and correlates with the respective serum levels[5–7]. The elderly seem to be most susceptible, even at serum lithium levels in the lower therapeutic range[2,8]. Regarding the course of tremor during long-term treatment, the published data are partially conflicting. Lyskowski *et al.*[9] and also Volk and Müller-Oerlinghausen[10] did not find a reduction in tremor occurrence and severity in long-term catamnestic studies, whereas other authors[4,11] reported a clear decrease in the prevalence of tremor during the course of a chronic administration of lithium at stable serum levels.

Patients with pre-existing tremors before initiation of lithium medication and patients with a positive family history of essential tremor seem to be prone to develop tremor under lithium[12,13]. Other factors increasing the risk of lithium-induced tremor are excessive caffeine consumption, distress and anxiety[14].

The intensity of lithium-induced tremor occasionally increases under concomitant use of other psychotropic agents, especially antidepressants and antipsychotics. Perenyi *et al.* found a significant difference regarding the occurrence of lithium-induced tremor between patients under lithium monotherapy (25%) and patients co-medicated with antidepressants (48%)[15]. They speculated that these differences could either be due to the tremor-inducing effects of the antidepressants themselves or via an assumed increase in intracellular lithium levels caused by tricyclic agents.

The combination of lithium and anti-psychotics seems to enhance the lithium-induced tremor as well. In a study of 130 lithium-treated patients Ghadirian *et al.*

reported a prevalence of tremor in 21% of the patients under lithium monotherapy versus 42% of patients who additionally received neuroleptics[16].

Lithium-induced tremor is usually mild and harmless, and often disappears after dose reduction or after a switch to a controlled-release lithium preparation. However, if a reduction of the lithium dosage is not possible and if the tremor is considered as clinically relevant, i.e. interfering with the patients' daily activities, co-administration of low-dose beta-blockers might be considered. Floru was one of the first who reported on a successful application of low-dose propranolol for the treatment of lithium-induced tremor[17]. Kirk *et al.* again documented the positive effects of 30–80 mg propranolol in lithium-treated patients who had experienced tremor-related social distress and job-related impairments[18]. The efficacy of propranolol was validated in a placebo-controlled study presented by Kellett *et al.*[19]. Similar positive effects on lithium tremor were reported for pindolol, which turned out to be more effective than practolol[20].

Patients with lithium-induced tremor and a history of obstructive pulmonary disorder (bronchospasms) were successfully treated with the β_1-receptor selective agent metoprolol[21], and Zubenko *et al.* reported favorable anti-tremor effects of metoprolol in daily doses of up to 400 mg[22]. Furthermore, successful treatment approaches have been reported for potassium salts and primidone[23,24].

In summary, the application of low-dose propranolol seems to be the most successful and best validated treatment strategy for lithium-induced tremor, unless there are general contraindications for a medication with beta-blockers. In individual cases even a single dose application 'on demand' instead of a chronic medication might be helpful.

According to our own experience lithium-induced tremor is a mild but often sustained side-effect and therefore might affect the patients' job-related and social activities. The decision in favor of a drug treatment of this adverse effect should be made in close cooperation with the patients themselves. Given a successful overall effect of the lithium therapy, it should be taken into account that lithium-induced tremor often is tolerated by many patients without any further interventions.

Abnormalities of EEG activity

The occurrence of various, unspecific electro-encephalogram (EEG) abnormalities is a frequent finding even at therapeutic serum lithium levels. The degree of these changes is at least in part dependent on serum lithium levels and has to be interpreted in relation to the baseline EEG recordings.

A reduction of EEG background activity by 1 to 3/s has frequently been described in patients under therapeutic serum lithium levels[6,25–29]. An increase in bilateral slow activity especially in frontal derivations has been reported as well, often in combination with an intermittent occurrence of slow waves in left anterior brain regions[25,26,30–36]. Usually there are no underlying structural correlates and therefore these focal abnormalities are interpreted as the local expression of a global brain dysfunction[37]. Helmchen and Kanowski[38], as well as Czernik[39] reported an increase in the occurrence of epileptiform activity such as sharp waves and spike-wave complexes, and some patients showed a tendency towards synchronization by presenting an increase in alpha wave amplitudes[30–32,40,41]. Occasionally a slowing of background activity, dysrhythmia and irregular slow activity under lithium therapy, for example as a result of lithium overdosage, can be a first sign of an upcoming lithium intoxication.

Regarding the effects on somatosensory evoked cortical potentials, Hegerl described an increase in amplitudes of early somatosensory and auditory evoked potentials[42], which is in line with the increased synchronization reported by other authors. Furthermore, an influence of lithium on the intensity dependence of somatosensory evoked potentials has been reported, and this might be associated with the serotonergic effects of lithium[42].

Infrequent, neurotoxic effects of lithium

The occurrence of neurotoxic symptoms at therapeutic serum lithium levels, at the beginning or during the course of treatment, has been reported in case reports. Neurotoxic effects of lithium comprise extrapyramidal symptoms, cognitive dysfunction, nystagmus and pseudotumor cerebri. Furthermore, peripheral neurotoxicity (i.e. lithium neuropathy) has been reported. Lithium neurotoxicity at therapeutic serum levels has been associated with several risk factors (Table 23.2).

- Pre-existing cerebral abnormalities[43,44].
- Aging[45–49]. Vredeveld and Morre report on two elderly women (above age 75) with therapeutic serum lithium levels, who developed a reversible neurotoxic syndrome with an increase in muscle tone, diffuse tremor, cerebellar signs such as ataxia, instability of posture and gait, dysarthria, aphasia and apraxia[50]. The symptoms rapidly and almost completely disappeared after discontinuation of lithium medication.
- Concomitant use of lithium and tricyclic agents (antidepressants or neuroleptics). Especially effects such as akathisia, dyskinesia and memory disturbances have been reported to be frequently associated with additional neuroleptic treatment[51–54]. Addonizio et al. discussed the possible underlying pathomechanisms of neurotoxic extrapyramidal symptoms under a combination of both lithium and neuroleptics. They hypothesized that either neuroleptic treatment could lead to an increase in intracellular lithium concentrations or, via inhibition of striatal dopamine synthesis, lithium might cause an amplification of dopamine antagonistic neuroleptic effects[55]. However, the exact mechanisms of the development of extrapyramidal motor dysfunction under lithium with or without additional neuroleptics remains unclear.

Regarding experimental neuropathological and/or animal studies, there is only limited evidence for neurotoxic effects of lithium under therapeutic serum levels. Peiffer investigated a case of a female patient who died at the age of 61 under long-term lithium treatment[56]. The author reported on cerebellar damage in combination with some minor alterations within the substantia nigra and the neostriatum. The assumption of direct lithium-induced alterations of brain structures was supported by similar observations in animal experiments; however, the lithium doses in these studies were far beyond the therapeutic range of lithium in humans[57–59]. According to neuropathological data by Francis and Traill, the highest lithium concentrations in brain tissue were found in brainstem (pons) and white matter[60]. Therefore, Sansone and Ziegler concluded that neurotoxic activity of lithium might well occur even within therapeutic serum lithium levels[61]. Animal experiments by Scelsi et al. and Janka et al. did not show any morphological changes under lithium[58,62]. Also, a study by Licht et al. in 25

Table 23.2 Risk factors for lithium neurotoxicity

Pre-existing cerebral disorders and structural damage
Aging
Co-medication with psychotropic drugs
    tricyclic antidepressants
    tricyclic neuroleptics

rats under a 30-week administration of lithium, alone or in combination with haloperidol, did not demonstrate neurocortical lesions[63]. Nevertheless, neurotoxic symptoms at therapeutic doses of lithium have repeatedly been discussed in the literature and will be presented in detail below.

Extrapyramidal symptoms

Extrapyramidal symptoms (EPS) other than tremor, such as hypokinesia, akathisia, dystonia, rigidity (with or without the cogwheel phenomenon) are occasional findings under lithium. Lithium-induced EPS often do not respond to anti-parkinsonian agents and were first reported by Shopsin and Gershon, who described an increase in muscle tone with rigidity in 15 out of 27 lithium-treated outpatients[64]. None of these patients received additional neuroleptic medication. The occurrence of EPS was associated with long-term lithium medication of at least 1–2 years, whereas patients with short-term lithium treatment (less than 8 months) did not present with extrapyramidal symptoms. Another interesting result was that intravenous application of anticholinergic agents improved the symptoms (rigidity) in only two out of nine patients. Branchey et al. investigated 36 lithium-treated outpatients (not having received neuroleptics for ≥6 months) with a duration of lithium medication between 6 months and 7 years and found a lower prevalence of EPS[65]. Only six patients with a treatment duration of more than 2 years suffered from significant rigidity. Kane et al. found EPS in only two out of 38 patients (5%), whereas Asnis et al. investigated 79 patients and six (7.6%) showed a marked rigidity and 22 (28%) a mild increase in muscle tonus[45,66].

A lithium-induced akathisia has been reported by Channabassavanna and Goswami and Price and Zimmer[67,68]. According to these reports akathisia seems to be dose-dependent and responds well to anti-parkinsonian agents.

The prevalence of tardive dyskinesias under lithium is controversial. On the one hand, there are some reports of successful use of lithium in dyskinetic extrapyramidal disorders such as neuroleptic-induced tardive dyskinesias or Huntington's chorea[69]. On the other hand, lithium has been shown to increase tardive dyskinesias and to facilitate their development[70,71]. In a study of 130 lithium outpatients by Ghardirian et al., 12 patients (9.2%) showed mild tardive dyskinesias especially of the orofacial regions. Further extrapyramidal symptoms comprised akathisia (4.6%), hypokinesia (7.7%) as well as dystonic syndromes (3.8%)[16]. The incidence of EPS was clearly higher in patients who received a co-treatment of lithium with neuroleptics.

Cognitive dysfunction

The issue of lithium-induced cognitive dysfunctions such as memory loss and concentration deficits is discussed controversially in the literature. An excellent review has been given by Pachet and Wisniewski[72]. In summary, there are consistent reports on mild effects of lithium (at therapeutic serum levels) on cognition. In these cases most of the patients complained of 'mental slowness' and there might be a subtle negative effect on psychomotor speed. In addition, mild effects on verbal memory have occasionally been present, but there were no consistent effects on visuospatial constructional abilities, attention and concentration. Furthermore, the lithium, induced cognitive alterations did not seem to have negative cumulative effects (see Chapter 37).

Oculomotor symptoms, nystagmus

Coppetto et al. reported the case of a 67-year-old patient who developed a downbeat nystagmus under therapeutic serum lithium levels[73]. After lithium dose reduction the nystagmus remitted completely. Gracia *et al.* reported the case of a 58-year-old male patient treated with lithium for more than 4 years with a serum concentration range between 0.96 and 1.4 mmol/l[74]. The patient developed a downbeat nystagmus without any additional symptoms and the nystagmus repeatedly decreased on reduction of the lithium dose. Further case reports of downbeat nystagmus under therapeutic serum lithium levels have been published[75–78].

The pathomechanisms of lithium-induced vertical nystagmus syndromes are unclear. Hereditary or acquired brain abnormalities such as cerebellar atrophy, brainstem lesions, Arnold–Chiari malformations as well as low serum levels of magnesium or intoxications with antiepileptic (and other) drugs were reported to facilitate vertical nystagmus[79]. Therefore, lithium-induced nystagmus has been related with spinovestibular and/or cerebellar-vestibular alterations. Clinically the nystagmus is usually reversible under dose reduction or discontinuation of lithium medication; however, remission has been reported to last between months and several years.

Pseudotumor cerebri

The association between lithium medication and the development of a pseudotumor cerebri, characterized by chronic headache, bilateral papilledema, increase in intracranial pressure without any further neurological signs and symptoms, has been reported by Lobo *et al.*[80]. They presented the case of a 29-year-old female patient who developed these symptoms including papilledema after 9 months on lithium at therapeutic serum levels. The symptoms were reversible, but the fundoscopic alterations did not remit until 1.5 years after discontinuation of lithium. Other cases of an association of pseudotumor cerebri and lithium

have been reported by Saul *et al.*, Levine and Puchalski, Dommisse, and Ames *et al.*[81–84], but controlled investigations regarding these associations are lacking. Pseudotumor cerebri can be caused by various conditions such as hypo- or hyperthyroidism, vitamin A intoxication, chronic medication with cortisole, application of carbamazepine and various other drugs, but a clear association between lithium and pseudotumor cerebri has not been established. Nevertheless, in patients with unclear long-term headaches, this diagnosis has to be taken into account and fundoscopy should be performed.

Peripheral neuromuscular effects

There are several reports on neuromuscular effects of chronic lithium medication. Helmchen *et al.* reported the development of a paroxysmal muscle weakness in a 30-year-old woman after a 7-week lithium medication at normal lithium serum levels, whereas potassium serum levels were lowered[85]. Neil *et al.* reported a 25-year-old female patient who developed myasthenia gravis on lithium medication for severe bipolar disorder[86].

Podnar *et al.* compared bipolar patients under lithium with a mean serum lithium level of 0.69 ± 0.15 mmol/l with lithium-free bipolar patients and healthy subjects[87]. They reported that the lithium-treated patients had markedly lower amplitudes of muscle action potentials as compared to healthy subjects. However, since the difference between bipolar patients with and without lithium was small, the authors concluded that patients with bipolar disorder show subclinical neuromuscular abnormalities that might be further impaired by lithium. The authors did not find any significant differences of nerve conduction velocities between bipolar patients and healthy controls.

A subtle decrease of motor nerve conduction velocity in both bipolar patients under long-term lithium treatment and healthy subjects after 1 week of lithium medication was described by Girke et al.[88]. This finding was replicated by Chang et al. who investigated 28 bipolar patients with serum lithium concentrations between 0.32 and 0.98 mmol/l[89]. Presslich et al. compared patients with long- and short-term lithium medication and again found a significant reduction in nerve conduction velocity in both groups[90].

However, a clear and clinically relevant impairment of the peripheral nervous system by lithium remains to be validated. It has nevertheless been recommended that special attention should be given to patients with muscular disorders or peripheral neuropathies in case lithium treatment is indicated[61].

Lithium intoxication

Neurological adverse effects as well as neurotoxic effects can occur within therapeutic serum lithium levels as presented above. During intoxication, symptoms will markedly increase and finally lead to a loss of consciousness, occasionally in combination with the occurrence of convulsions[41,42,91,92] (see Chapter 41).

Table 23.3 presents the wide range of clinical manifestations and highlights the large variability of the clinical presentation of lithium intoxication.

However, most lithium-intoxicated patients show both 'psychomotor/cognitive' and neurological symptoms. Initial 'psychomotor/cognitive symptoms' are a general slowing and reduction of alertness. The patients often present with fatigue and weakness with or without increase in irritability. Further initial symptoms are short-term memory dysfunctions and mild amnesia. All quantitative states of a reduction in consciousness and in individual cases the occurrence of (optical) hallucinations have been reported[91–95]. In more than 80% of intoxicated patients neurological alterations with a wide range of symptoms, especially cerebellar signs such as tremor, nystagmus, dysarthria, vertigo, ataxia, or extrapyramidal dysfunctions such as parkinsonian or choreoathetotic motor symptoms, could be found. In addition, pathological reflexes and other symptoms of pyramidal pathway dysfunction, but

Table 23.3 Clinical presentation of symptoms of lithium intoxication

Central nervous system	Peripheral neuromuscular system
Clouding of consciousness (any severity)	Myopathy: fasciculations; fibrillations; myoclonia
Cerebellar symptoms: tremor dysarthria ataxia nystagmus	Polyneuropathy
Extrapyramidal motor symptoms	
Parkinsonian or choreatic movements	
EEG abnormalities (unspecific and epileptiform patterns), cerebral convulsions, seizures	

also neuropsychological symptoms such as aphasia or apraxia have been reported incidentally. Another common symptom are EEG abnormalities, which often outlast the period of lithium intoxication; occasionally the patients develop epileptic seizures[76,77,93–95].

Neuromuscular symptoms including electromyographic changes often occur at early stages of lithium intoxication. First muscular fasciculations can be observed, later and at higher serum lithium levels fibrillations and myoclonia are additional symptoms. In individual cases sensomotor polyneuropathy has been described[61,94,96].

In recent years much attention has been paid to the phenomenon of persisting neurological deficits following lithium intoxication. Short-term memory disturbances, cerebellar dysfunctions (especially ataxia) and extrapyramidal symptoms have been reported as the most frequent lithium-induced persistent deficits[97–101]. Accordingly, the neuropathological findings in patients who died of lithium intoxication were alterations within the cerebellum (including vermis, Purkinje cells or dentate nucleus), mesencephalon and brainstem[56,100,102,103]. In view of potentially permanent CNS disturbances, attention should be paid to the detection and adequate treatment of early symptoms of lithium intoxication[91] (see Chapter 41).

REFERENCES

1. Schou M, Baastrup PC, Grof P, et al. Pharmacological and clinical problems of lithium prophylaxis. Br J Psychiatry 1970; 116: 615–19

2. Bech P, Thomsen J, Prytz S, et al. The profile and severity of lithium-induced side effects in mentally healthy subjects. Neuropsychobiology 1979; 5: 160–6

3. Koufen H, Consbruch U. Long-term catamnesis on the topic of uses and side effects of lithium prevention of phasic psychoses. Fortschr Neurol Psychiatr 1989; 57: 374–82

4. Vestergaard P, Poulstrup I, Schou M. Prospective studies on a lithium cohort. 3. Tremor, weight gain, diarrhea, psychological complaints. Acta Psychiatr Scand 1988; 78: 434–41

5. Schou M. Current status of prevention of endogenous affective diseases using lithium. Nervenarzt 1974; 45: 397–418

6. Müller-Oerlinghausen B, Bauer H, Girke W, et al. Impairment of vigilance and performance under lithium-treatment. Studies in patients and normal volunteers. Pharmakopsychiatr Neuropsychopharmakol 1977; 10: 67–78

7. Abou-Saleh MT, Coppen A. The efficacy of low-dose lithium: clinical, psychological and biological correlates. J Psychiatr Res 1989; 23: 157–62

8. Salzman C. A primer on geriatric psychopharmacology. Am J Psychiatry 1982; 139: 67–74

9. Lyskowski J, Nasrallah HA, Dunner FJ, Bucher K. A longitudinal survey of side effects in a lithium clinic. J Clin Psychiatry 1982; 43: 284–6

10. Volk J, Müller-Oerlinghausen B. Time course of AMP-documented side-effects in patients under long-term lithium treatment. Pharmacopsychiatry 1986; 19: 286–7

11. Jefferson JW. Lithium and affective disorder in the elderly. Compr Psychiatry 1983; 24: 166–78

12. Van Putten T. Lithium-induced disabling tremor. Psychosomatics 1978; 19: 27–31

13. Gelenberg AJ, Jefferson JW. Lithium tremor. J Clin Psychiatry 1995; 56: 283–7

14. Jefferson JW. Lithium tremor and caffeine intake: two cases of drinking less and shaking more. J Clin Psychiatry 1988; 49: 72–3

15. Perenyi A, Rihmer Z, Banki CM. Parkinsonian symptoms with lithium, lithium-neuroleptic, and lithium-antidepressant treatment. J Affect Disord 1983; 5: 171–7

16. Ghadirian AM, Annable L, Belanger MC, Chouinard G. A cross-sectional study of parkinsonism and tardive dyskinesia in lithium-treated affective disordered patients. J Clin Psychiatry 1996; 57: 22–8

17. Floru L. Clinical treatment of lithium induced tremors with a beta receptor antagonist (propranolol). Int Pharmacopsychiatry 1971; 6: 197–222

18. Kirk L, Baastrup PC, Schou M. Propranolol treatment of lithium tremor [Letter]. Nervenarzt 1973; 44: 657–8

19. Kellett JM, Metcalfe M, Bailey J, Coppen AJ. Beta blockade in lithium tremor. J Neurol Neurosurg Psychiatry 1975; 38: 719–21

20. Floru L, Tegeler J. Effect of beta receptor blockaders (pindolol and practolol) on lithium induced tremor. Clinical study and theoretical considerations. Arzneimittelforschung 1974; 24: 1122–5

21. Gaby NS, Lefkowitz DS, Israel JR. Treatment of lithium tremor with metoprolol. Am J Psychiatry 1983; 140: 593–5

22. Zubenko GS, Cohen BM, Lipinski JF Jr. Comparison of metoprolol and propranolol in the treatment of lithium tremor. Psychiatry Res 1984; 11: 163–4

23. Cummings MA, Cummings KL, Haviland MG. Use of potassium to treat lithium's side effects. Am J Psychiatry 1988; 145: 895

24. Goumentouk AD, Hurwitz TA, Zis AP. Primidone in drug-induced tremor. J Clin Psychopharmacol 1989; 9: 451

25. Mayfield D, Brown RG. The clinical laboratory and electroencephalographic effects of lithium. J Psychiatr Res 1966; 4: 207–19

26. Platman SR, Fieve RR. The effect of lithium carbonate on the electroencephalogram of patients with affective disorders. Br J Psychiatry 1969; 115: 1185–8

27. Small JG, Small IF, Perez HC. EEG, evoked potential, and contingent negative variations with lithium in manic depressive disease. Biol Psychiatry 1971; 3: 47–58

28. Zakowska-Dabrowska T, Rybakowski J. Lithium-induced EEG changes: relation to lithium levels in serum and red blood cells. Acta Psychiatr Scand 1973; 49: 457–65

29. Heninger GR. Lithium carbonate and brain function. I. Cerebral-evoked potentials, EEG, and symptom changes during lithium carbonate treatment. Arch Gen Psychiatry 1978; 35: 228–33

30. Andreani G, Caselli G, Martelli G. Clinical and electroencephalographic findings during treatment of mental disorders with lithium salts. G Psichiatr Neuropatol 1958; 86: 273–328

31. Johnson G. Lithium and the EEG: an analysis of behavioral, biochemical and electrographic changes. Electroencephalogr Clin Neurophysiol 1969; 27: 656–7

32. Johnson G, Maccario M, Gershon S, Korein J. The effects of lithium on electroencephalogram, behavior and serum electrolytes. J Nerv Ment Dis 1970; 151: 273–89

33. Ulrich G, Frick K, Stieglitz RD, Müller-Oerlinghausen B. Interindividual variability of lithium-induced EEG changes in healthy volunteers. Psychiatry Res 1987; 20: 117–27

34. Ulrich G, Herrmann WM, Hegerl U, Müller-Oerlinghausen B. Effect of lithium on the dynamics of electroencephalographic vigilance in healthy subjects. J Affect Disord 1990; 20: 19–25

35. Thau K, Rappelsberger P, Lovrek A, et al. Effect of lithium on the EEG of healthy males and females. A probability mapping study. Neuropsychobiology 1989; 20: 158–63

36. Schulz C, Mavrogiorgou P, Schroter A, et al. Lithium-induced EEG changes in patients with affective disorders. Neuropsychobiology 2000; 42 (Suppl 1): 33–7

37. Ulrich G. Electroencephalographic response prediction of antipsychotic drug treatment in acutely ill patients and of long-term prophylactic treatment with lithium salts. Pharmacopsychiatry 1994; 27 (Suppl 1): 24–6

38. Helmchen H, Kanowski S. EEG-changes during lithium therapy. Nervenarzt 1971; 42: 144–8

39. Czernik A. EEG changes induced by long-term lithium therapy. Psychiatr Clin (Basel) 1978; 11: 189–97

40. Passouant D, Maurel H. L'electroencéphalographic en cours du traitement par le carbonate de lithium. Montpell Med 1953; 43: 38

41. Heninger GR. Lithium effects on cerebral cortical function in manic depressive patients. Electroencephalogr Clin Neurophysiol 1969; 27: 670

42. Hegerl U. Einfluß von Lithium auf die evozierten kortikalen Potentiale. In Müller-Oerlinghausen B, Greil W, eds. Die Lithiumtherapie: Nutzen, Risiken, Alternativen. Berlin: Springer, 1986: 97–105

43. Kelwala S, Pomara N, Stanley M, et al. Lithium-induced accentuation of extrapyramidal symptoms in individuals with Alzheimer's disease. J Clin Psychiatry 1984; 45: 342–4

44. Coffey CE, Ross DR, Massey EW, Olanow CW. Dyskinesias associated with lithium therapy in parkinsonism. Clin Neuropharmacol 1984; 7: 223–9

45. Asnis GM, Asnis D, Dunner DL, Fieve RR. Cogwheel rigidity during chronic lithium therapy. Am J Psychiatry 1979; 136: 1225–6

46. Himmelhoch JM, Neil JF, May SJ, et al. Age, dementia, dyskinesias, and lithium response. Am J Psychiatry 1980; 137: 941–5

47. Miller F, Menninger J, Whitcup SM. Lithium-neuroleptic neurotoxicity in the elderly bipolar patient. J Clin Psychopharmacol 1986; 6: 176–8

48. Austin LS, Arana GW, Melvin JA. Toxicity resulting from lithium augmentation of antidepressant treatment in elderly patients. J Clin Psychiatry 1990; 51: 344–5

49. Flint AJ, Rifat SL. A prospective study of lithium augmentation in antidepressant-resistant geriatric depression. J Clin Psychopharmacol 1994; 14: 353–6

50. Vredeveld CJ, Morre HH. Lithium neurotoxicity in advanced age. 2 case reports with a literature review. Nervenarzt 1983; 54: 377–80

51. Cohen WJ, Cohen NH. Lithium carbonate, haloperidol, and irreversible brain damage. JAMA 1974; 230: 1283–7

52. Spring GK. Neurotoxicity with combined use of lithium and thioridazine. J Clin Psychiatry 1979; 40: 135–8

53. Prakash R, Kelwala S, Ban TA. Neurotoxicity in patients with schizophrenia during lithium therapy. Compr Psychiatry 1982; 23: 271–3

54. Addonizio G. Rapid induction of extrapyramidal side effects with combined use of lithium and neuroleptics. J Clin Psychopharmacol 1985; 5: 296–8

55. Addonizio G, Roth SD, Stokes PE, Stoll PM. Increased extrapyramidal symptoms with addition of lithium to neuroleptics. J Nerv Ment Dis 1988; 176: 682–5

56. Peiffer J. Clinical and neuropathological aspects of long-term damage to the central nervous system after lithium medication. Arch Psychiatr Nervenkr 1981; 231: 41–60

57. Roizin L, Akai K, Lawler HC, Liu J. Lithium neurotoxicologic effects. 1. Acute phase (preliminary observations). Dis Nerv Syst 1970; 31 (Suppl): 38–44

58. Janka Z, Szentistvanyi I, Kiraly E, et al. Preferential vulnerability of dendrites to lithium ion in rat brain and in nerve cell culture. Acta Neuropathol Suppl (Berl) 1981; 7: 44–7

59. Dixit PK, Smithberg M. Toxic effect of lithium in mouse brain. Proc Soc Exp Biol Med 1988; 187: 2–6

60. Francis RI, Traill MA. Lithium distribution in the brains of two manic patients. Lancet 1970; 2: 523–4

61. Sansone ME, Ziegler DK. Lithium toxicity: a review of neurologic complications. Clin Neuropharmacol 1985; 8: 242–8

62. Scelsi R, Arrigoni E, Moglia A, et al. Effects of lithium administration on central and peripheral nervous system in rats. Biochemical and morphological findings. Pharmacopsychiatria 1981; 14: 213–16

63. Licht RW, Larsen JO, Smith D, Braendgaard H. Effect of chronic lithium treatment with or without haloperidol on number and sizes of neurons in rat neocortex. Psychopharmacology (Berl) 1994; 115: 371–4

64. Shopsin B, Gershon S. Cogwheel rigidity related to lithium maintenance. Am J Psychiatry 1975; 132: 536–8

65. Branchey MH, Charles J, Simpson GM. Extrapyramidal side effects in lithium maintenance therapy. Am J Psychiatry 1976; 133: 444–5

66. Kane J, Rifkin A, Quitkin F, Klein DF. Extrapyramidal side effects with lithium treatment. Am J Psychiatry 1978; 135: 851–3

67. Channabasavanna SM, Goswami U. Akathisia during lithium prophylaxis. Br J Psychiatry 1984; 144: 555–6

68. Price WA, Zimmer B. Lithium-induced akathisia. J Clin Psychiatry 1987; 48: 81

69. Foerster K, Regli F. Lithium therapy of extrapyramidal movement disorders – an attempt (author's transl). Nervenarzt 1977; 48: 228–32

70. Crews EL, Carpenter AE. Lithium-induced aggravation of tardive dyskinesia. Am J Psychiatry 1977; 134: 933

71. Beitman BD. Tardive dyskinesia reinduced by lithium carbonate. Am J Psychiatry 1978; 135: 1229–30

72. Pachet AK, Wisniewski AM. The effects of lithium on cognition: an updated review. Psychopharmacology (Berl) 2003; 170: 225–34

73. Coppeto JR, Monteiro ML, Lessell S, et al. Downbeat nystagmus. Long-term therapy with moderate-dose lithium carbonate. Arch Neurol 1983; 40: 754–5

74. Gracia F, Koch J, Aziz N. Downbeat nystagmus as a side effect of lithium carbonate: case report. J Clin Psychiatry 1985; 46: 292–3

75. Williams DP, Troost BT, Rogers J. Lithium-induced downbeat nystagmus. Arch Neurol 1988; 45: 1022–3

76. Engelhardt A, Neundorfer B. Downbeat nystagmus in lithium medication. Nervenarzt 1988; 59: 624–7

77. Corbett JJ, Jacobson DM, Thompson HS, et al. Downbeating nystagmus and other ocular motor defects caused by lithium toxicity. Neurology 1989; 39: 481–7

78. Rosenberg ML. Permanent lithium-induced downbeating nystagmus. Arch Neurol 1989; 46: 839

79. Halmagyi GM, Rudge P, Gresty MA, Sanders MD. Downbeating nystagmus. A review of 62 cases. Arch Neurol 1983; 40: 777–84

80. Lobo A, Pilek E, Stokes PE. Papilledema following therapeutic dosages of lithium carbonate. J Nerv Ment Dis 1978; 166: 526–9

81. Saul RF, Hamburger HA, Selhorst JB. Pseudotumor cerebri secondary to lithium carbonate. JAMA 1985; 253: 2869–70

82. Levine SH, Puchalski C. Pseudotumor cerebri associated with lithium therapy in two patients. J Clin Psychiatry 1990; 51: 251–3

83. Dommisse J. Pseudotumor cerebri associated with lithium therapy in two patients. J Clin Psychiatry 1991; 52: 239

84. Ames D, Wirshing WC, Cokely HT, Lo LL. The natural course of pseudotumor cerebri in lithium-treated patients. J Clin Psychopharmacol 1994; 14: 286–7

85. Helmchen H, Hoffmann I, Kanowski S. Paroxysmale Muskelschwäche bei Lithiumtherapie. Pharmacopsychiatry 1969; 4: 269–73

86. Neil JF, Himmelhoch JM, Licata SM. Emergence of myasthenia gravis during treatment with lithium carbonate. Arch Gen Psychiatry 1976; 33: 1090–2

87. Podnar S, Vodusek DB, Zvan V. Lithium and peripheral nervous system function in manic-depressive patients. Acta Neurol Scand 1993; 88: 417–21

88. Girke W, Krebs FA, Müller-Oerlinghausen B. Effects of lithium on electromyographic recordings in man. Studies in manic–depressive patients and normal volunteers. Int Pharmacopsychiatry 1975; 10: 24–36

89. Chang YC, Lin HN, Deng HC. Subclinical lithium neurotoxicity: correlation of neural conduction abnormalities and serum lithium level in manic–depressive patients with lithium treatment. Acta Neurol Scand 1990; 82: 82–6

90. Presslich O, Mairhofer ML, Opgenoorth E, Schuster P. Maximal motor nerve conduction rate with lithium. Bibl Psychiatr 1981: 121–8

91. Kaschka WP. Die Lithiumintoxikation. In Muller-Oerlinghausen B, Greil W, Berghöfer A, eds. Die Lithiumtherapie. Nutzen, Risiken, Alternativen. Berlin: Springer, 1997: 424–34

92. Mavrogiorgou P, Hegerl U. Neurologische, neuromuskuläre und neurotoxische Effekte der Lithiumbehandlung. In Müller-Oerlinghausen B, Greil W, Berghöfer A, eds. Die Lithiumtherapie. Nutzen, Risiken, Alternativen. Berlin: Springer, 1997: 329–41

93. Goddard J, Bloom SR, Frackowiak RS, et al. Lithium intoxication. Br Med J 1991; 302: 1267–9

94. Kaschka WP. Klinik der Lithiumbehandlung. In Riederer P, Laux G, Pöldinger W, eds. Neuro-Psychopharmaka. Ein Therapie-Handbuch Vienna: Springer, 1993; 3: 493–523

95. Okusa MD, Crystal LJ. Clinical manifestations and management of acute lithium intoxication. Am J Med 1994; 97: 383–9

96. Vanhooren G, Dehaene I, Van Zandycke M, et al. Polyneuropathy in lithium intoxication. Muscle Nerve 1990; 13: 204–8

97. Apte SN, Langston JW. Permanent neurological deficits due to lithium toxicity. Ann Neurol 1983; 13: 453–5

98. Schou M. Long-lasting neurological sequelae after lithium intoxication. Acta Psychiatr Scand 1984; 70: 594–602

99. Ferbert A, Czernik A. [Persistent cerebellar syndrome following lithium poisoning]. Nervenarzt 1987; 58: 764–70

100. Nagaraja D, Taly AB, Sahu RN, et al. Permanent neurological sequelae due to lithium toxicity. Clin Neurol Neurosurg 1987; 89: 31–4

101. Manto M, Godaux E, Seillier M, et al. Cerebellar syndrome secondary to lithium poisoning: a cinematic and electromyographic study of 2 cases. Rev Neurol (Paris) 1994; 150: 467–70

102. Naramoto A, Koizumi N, Itoh N, Shigematsu H. An autopsy case of cerebellar degeneration following lithium intoxication with neuroleptic malignant syndrome. Acta Pathol Jpn 1993; 43: 55–8

103. Schneider JA, Mirra SS. Neuropathologic correlates of persistent neurologic deficit in lithium intoxication. Ann Neurol 1994; 36: 928–31

24 Gastrointestinal, metabolic and body-weight changes during treatment with lithium

Janusz K Rybakowski, Aleksandra Suwalska

Contents   Introduction • Gastrointestinal effects of lithium • Effect of lithium on carbohydrate metabolism • Weight changes during treatment with lithium

INTRODUCTION

The effect of lithium on the gastrointestinal system and carbohydrate metabolism was primarily covered in the first major textbook on lithium research and therapy, which appeared in 1976[1]. The issue of weight gain was included in the chapter on lithium and carbohydrate metabolism written by Mellerup and Rafaelsen[2]. It has been thought that gastrointestinal side-effects are common during a short period after the initiation of lithium therapy but rather rare during long-term lithium treatment. The origin of lithium-induced weight gain has been mainly attributed to the effect of lithium on carbohydrate metabolism; the problem has been recognized in a number of lithium-treated patients, especially females. The following 30 years documented the importance and management of these two side-effects in the process of lithium therapy and have also given some new clues regarding the effects of lithium on carbohydrate metabolism in bipolar illness.

GASTROINTESTINAL EFFECTS OF LITHIUM

Prevalence and intensity of gastrointestinal disturbances on lithium

Gastrointestinal symptoms are common side-effects of lithium. They include anorexia, nausea, vomiting, diarrhea, abdominal pains and a metallic taste. Some of them were described as early as in the original work of Cade[3] and may be regarded to be as a result of gastrointestinal irritation by lithium salt. Surprisingly, however, constipation occurring allegedly in up to 20% of long-term lithium-treated patients was also reported[4].

Diarrhea is the most frequent gastrointestinal effect of lithium. Complaints of diarrhea (loose stools, defecation urge) were received from up to 6% of patients during the first 6 months of lithium treatment, and from up to 20% of patients on long-term lithium therapy[5,6]. In a well-documented sample of 254 patients from the Berlin Lithium Clinic it was demonstrated that the frequency of diarrhea did not significantly change during 10 years of lithium therapy[7]. The frequency of diarrhea was reported to rise steeply at serum lithium concentrations over 0.8 mmol/l[6,8]. However, Persson[9] found no association between abdominal pain and loose bowels and lithium doses, or plasma lithium levels. It should be added that the patients' statements on diarrhea are sometimes quite vague and unreliable, with symptoms arising and disappearing without any predictable course.

It may also be mentioned that lithium, in spite of its laxative effect, can also act as a potential antidiarrheal agent under specific pathological conditions[10]. The mechanism of the constipating or rather the anti-diarrhea effect of lithium may be due to the inhibition of cyclic adenosine monophosphate (cAMP) synthesis. There are case reports on patients with severe chronic secretory diarrhea refractory to other drugs who responded to oral lithium carbonate[11].

Gastrointestinal side-effects of lithium are usually minor and often transient. Gastrointestinal discomfort may diminish under prolonged lithium treatment. In the study of Schou et al.,[12] ten (33%) of 30 patients experienced gastrointestinal irritation during the first 2 weeks of lithium treatment as compared to none of 100 patients taking lithium for up to 2 years. In older medical-psychiatric patients gastrointestinal side-effects were reported to be more frequent and severe. Stoudemire et al.[13] reported that three-quarters of depressed unipolar patients were unable to tolerate lithium added to antidepressant treatment, owing to side-effects (mainly gastrointestinal disturbances and tremor). Sajatovic et al.[14] retrospectively evaluated response to lamotrigine, lithium and placebo in 98 older bipolar I patients who participated in maintenance studies: in the lithium group ($n = 34$) diarrhea,

nausea and xerostomia were among the most common adverse events occurring in more than 10% of patients.

Management of gastrointestinal side-effects of lithium

Gastrointestinal side-effects are related to the time course of gastrointestinal absorption, and various lithium preparations may show differences in this respect. It was shown that nausea and vomiting were more frequent with standard preparations, coinciding with serum lithium peaks, and disappeared when serum concentration decreased. The side-effects may be minimized by taking fewer tablets or capsules at a time and by taking them with meals to slow the absorption[15].

Data concerning the usefulness of slow-release lithium tablets are, however, inconsistent. It appears plausible that diarrhea or loose stools should occur more frequently with the more slowly absorbed preparations, owing to the presence of unabsorbed lithium ion in distal portions of the intestine. In a study by Edstrom and Persson[16], slow-release lithium sulfate tablets more often produced laxative side-effects than medium–slow-release and rapidly dissolving preparations. However, in another study evaluating the side-effects of sustained-release lithium carbonate taken once daily compared to placebo, nausea constituted one of the principal symptoms and diarrhea was reported infrequently in both groups[17]. In the same study constipation was reported significantly more often in the lithium group. The difference in frequency of diarrhea in patients taking sustained-release lithium versus those taking a conventional preparation was not found in the study by Vestergaard et al.[5]. It should, however, be noted that there exist 'sustained-release' preparations which, according to experimental pharmaceutical investigations do not deserve this label[18].

Moreover, the intensity of gastrointestinal side-effects may be decreased by lithium administration after meals[19]. Jeppsson and Sjogren[20] administered 24 mmol of lithium sulfate in a single dose of slow-release tablets to 30 healthy volunteers, both fasting and after a standardized meal. Postprandial administration of lithium induced practically no side-effects, while lithium on an empty stomach resulted in diarrhea in about 20% of the subjects. Lithium was completely absorbed when given after food, but when given on an empty stomach the absorption was lower in some subjects due to rapid gastrointestinal passage and frequent diarrhea. In addition, the definition of diarrhea and gastric discomfort may vary from study to study.

Other possible causes of gastrointestinal disturbances such as concomitant medications (both psychotropic and somatic) and somatic causes (food, alcohol and viral infections, other somatic diseases) should be taken into account. If one wants to distinguish lithium-related causes from other causes, lithium should be temporarily discontinued or the dose lowered.

While most gastrointestinal symptoms caused by lithium are mild and occur at normal serum levels, more severe or persistent symptoms (vomiting, diarrhea) may be associated with impending lithium intoxication. Failure to discontinue lithium in the face of prodromal symptoms may be followed by severe neurotoxicity[15].

EFFECT OF LITHIUM ON CARBOHYDRATE METABOLISM

Insulin-like effect of lithium?

Lithium may exert insulin-like effects, increasing glucose utilization and glycogen synthesis. The lithium ion influences enzymes involved in glycolysis, gluconeogenesis and glucose uptake by the cells[21]. Both insulin and lithium inactivate glycogen synthase kinase 3 (GSK3) and thus activate glycogen synthase. Lithium is thought to have an insulin-like effect on glucose transport and metabolism in skeletal muscle and adipocytes[22]. Tabata et al.[23] found that lithium had only a minimal effect on basal glucose transport activity in rat epitrochlearis muscles but markedly increased the sensitivity of glucose transport to insulin, so that the increase in glucose transport activity induced by 300 pmol/l insulin was approximately 2.5-fold greater in the presence of lithium than in its absence. These data suggest that lithium might be useful in the treatment of insulin resistance in patients with non-insulin-dependent diabetes mellitus. It should be mentioned that an anti-diabetic effect of lithium was postulated as early as 1924[24].

Glucose tolerance in lithium-treated patients

Bipolar illness may by itself be associated with abnormal glucose metabolism. In 1943, before lithium had been introduced into psychiatric therapy, Gildea et al.[25] reported impaired glucose tolerance test results after oral, but not intravenous, administration of dextrose in 30 manic-depressive subjects. Van der Velde and Gordon[26] reported abnormal glucose tolerance in nine of 17 manic-depressive patients over the age of 40 who had never been treated with lithium, and concluded that diabetes mellitus might be a consequence of longstanding affective disorder. In the study by Cassidy et al.[27], the prevalence of diabetes mellitus among hospitalized patients with bipolar disorder was higher than in the general population. Also, bipolar patients with diabetes mellitus had a more severe course of their psychiatric illness. Possible reasons for this co-morbidity could include a genetic association between the disorders, a causal relationship in which hypercortisolemia induces diabetes or diabetic vascular lesions contribute to mania, an overlapping functional disturbance affecting similar regions of the brain, or the effect of psychotropic medications.

Lithium does not significantly affect blood glucose concentration in bipolar patients. In most studies, normal blood glucose concentrations in lithium-treated subjects were reported[28,29], both in association with hyperinsulinemia[30] and with unchanged plasma insulin levels[31]. In the study of Mellerup et al.[32], plasma glucose levels were assessed during a 24-hour period in 62 lithium-treated patients, 59 healthy control persons and 80 psychiatric controls. Euthymic patients on lithium showed higher maximal glucose and higher mean plasma glucose levels, whereas in depressed lithium-treated patients lower mean plasma glucose levels were found than in the euthymic lithium-treated patients. Vestergaard and Schou[33] assessed fasting plasma glucose concentration in bipolar patients before and during lithium treatment for up to 6 years. Total duration of lithium exposure was 495.5 years. Mean glucose levels remained unchanged from the beginning and weight gain did not influence glucose concentration. Only in one patient was diabetes mellitus diagnosed.

The results of studies investigating lithium effects on glucose tolerance are inconsistent. This may be partly due to the methodological problems connected particularly with the interpretation of the results as a predictor for the risk of manifest diabetes. In a study by Vendsborg and Prytz[29], lithium treatment for 6 months had no influence on glucose tolerance. Vendsborg[34] studied intravenous glucose tolerance in bipolar patients given once daily lithium and found that glucose tolerance was increased for some hours after each lithium administration. In the first week of treatment, glucose disposal rate was increased up to 12 hours after lithium ingestion. In long-term lithium-treated patients glucose tolerance was increased 2 hours after administration but not after 12 hours. Shah et al.[35] performed a 5-hour oral glucose tolerance test (GTT) in nine euthymic bipolar patients on lithium and seven untreated euthymic bipolar patients. During the GTT the mean nadir of serum glucose in the lithium-treated patients was significantly lower than in untreated subjects. Seven of nine lithium-treated patients, but none of the control patients, experienced hypoglycemic symptoms coinciding with low serum glucose concentration. Their findings suggest that chronic lithium treatment is associated with a symptomatic and biochemical hypoglycemia during the GTT, which is characterized by a rise in serum cortisol level but by a lack of the appropriate rise in plasma glucagon concentration.

Müller-Oerlinghausen et al.[36] performed the oral glucose tolerance test twice in a group of patients receiving long-term lithium treatment. The frequency of impaired glucose tolerance in the patients was three times higher than expected on the basis of the studies in normal populations. The results suggested mild disturbances of carbohydrate metabolism (mild diabetes) in some patients that could be attributed partially to the affective state and/or to lithium-induced weight gain. In another study by the same authors, in 24.5–30.6% of long-term lithium-treated patients a pathological oral GTT was observed and positively correlated with age and overweight[37]. The authors suggested that the oral GTT should be carried out periodically in long-term lithium-treated patients over the age of 40 years, in order to detect abnormalities in their carbohydrate metabolism.

There have been a few reports on diabetes mellitus associated with lithium treatment, including exacerbation and de novo onset of diabetes[15]. Most patients were obese, middle-aged women. In one case, withdrawal of lithium led to a normalization of glucose tolerance which deteriorated again within 5–6 weeks after lithium was reinstituted. A

41-year-old man with no personal or family history of diabetes developed diabetic keto-acidosis 4 months after starting lithium for the treatment of major depression[38]. A moderately obese patient who developed massive polyuria (24-hour urine volume 15 l) was diagnosed as having diabetes mellitus. Insulin treatment led to a rapid reduction in blood glucose level and urine volume. At 2-month follow-up, the 24-hour urine volume had fallen to 2.5 l on a regimen of lithium, perphenazine, alprazolam and insulin[39].

Other studies have also shown that lithium may acutely impair insulin release. However, high glucose and glucagon levels stimulate a compensatory increase in insulin secretion, resulting in a normalization of glucose meta-bolism. These compensatory mechanisms may be inadequate in individuals predisposed to develop type 2 diabetes, because of obesity, age, concurrent administration of other medications, affective state, or genetic factors. In such cases, glucose intolerance and manifest diabetes may develop.

Lithium administration to patients with diabetes mellitus

There are few case reports on the use of lithium in bipolar patients with pre-existing diabetes mellitus. Waziri and Nelson[40] observed hyperglycemic effects of lithium in a patient with type 1 diabetes mellitus and mania on stable insulin dosage. Serum lithium levels were correlated with fasting blood glucose levels, and lowering of the lithium level led to a lowering of the fasting glucose concentrations. On the other hand, Lippmann et al.[41] reported that lithium administration to a diabetic hemo-dialysis patient with end-stage renal disease was safe. According to Russell and Johnson[21], metabolic complications of diabetes, such as hyperosmolality and salt depletion can increase lithium absorption and the risk of toxicity even at generally acceptable serum lithium levels.

There are also case reports describing anti-diabetic effects of lithium. In a female bipolar patient with type 2 diabetes, lithium carbonate administration was associated with lowered blood glucose levels without change of other variables possibly influencing blood glucose level[42].

In two studies the effect of short-term lithium carbonate treatment on glucose meta-bolism in diabetic patients was examined. Jones et al.[43] assessed the metabolic response to a standard 50-g carbohydrate breakfast in six patients with type 2 diabetes before and after 1 week of lithium carbonate administration. The plasma glucose response was significantly lower after lithium between 60 and 180 minutes and plasma insulin level did not change. Hu et al.[44] investigated the influence of a short-term lithium carbonate treatment on fasting blood glucose (FBG) and 1-hour postprandial blood glucose (PBG) in a group of 38 diabetic patients. Group I was treated with diet only, group II with oral hypoglycemic agents and group III with insulin. The FBG and PBG levels of all three groups decreased significantly after lithium treatment, except for the FBG level in group I. These data suggest that, combined with other therapy, lithium can improve glucose metabolism in patients with diabetes and has an assisting hypoglycemic effect on anti-diabetic treatment.

WEIGHT CHANGES DURING TREATMENT WITH LITHIUM

Frequency of weight gain in lithium-treated patients

In lithium-treated patients, an important cause of relapse is non-compliance. Probably, the most often encountered reason for stopping treatment is the patient's refusal to continue, typically following several years of affective stability[45]. A second cause may be intolerance of adverse effects. Weight gain is a significant undesirable side-effect of long-term lithium administration which might interfere with treatment compliance[46,47].

In the majority of studies it was found that lithium prophylaxis led to weight gain in a high proportion of patients treated, with up to a quarter becoming clinically obese[48]. The findings seem to indicate that weight gain is a direct effect of lithium treatment. In one study, weight gain of at least 5% occurred in one-third to two-thirds of patients treated with lithium[49]. In another, among 49 lithium-treated out-patients 69% were overweight[37]. Schou et al.[12] reported that 11 of 100 patients taking lithium for 1– 2 years gained over 5 kg of body weight. Peselow et al.[50] compared bipolar patients on lithium and on placebo over a 12-month period and found that 11 of 21 patients on lithium gained more than 5 kg, whereas only one of 12 placebo-treated patients did so. Thirteen of 21 lithium-treated patients showed a gain of 5% total body weight compared to only two of 12 placebo-treated patients. In a study by Vestergaard et al.[5] in a group of 237 patients on long-term lithium treatment, one-fifth of the patients complained of weight gain exceeding 10 kg. McCreadie and Morrison[4] found that 43% of 40 patients on lithium monotherapy reported weight gain. In another study, lithium maintenance therapy stimulated weight gains of over 10 kg in 20% of patients[46]. Chengappa et al.[51] performed a chart-review study and found that 70 patients receiving lithium gained a mean 6.3 kg (>8% of their baseline body weight) and experienced an increase in body mass index (BMI) of 2.1. Fifty-four patients (77.1%) gained weight, 14 (20%) lost weight and weight in two patients (2.9%) did not change.

However, in some studies only moderate weight gain on lithium has been reported.

Moral Iglesias et al.[52] found that, among 80 patients during 1-year lithium maintenance treatment, only 28 patients gained weight, mostly less than 10% of initial weight, which did not cause discontinuation of treatment. In a prospective study by Vestergaard et al.[6], the average weight gain in bipolar patients on lithium treatment for up to 7 years was 4 kg. Data from a 1-year monotherapy study of relapse prevention comparing lithium, divalproex and placebo demonstrated a 14% increase of weight gain over placebo in divalproex-treated patients, but only 6% in the lithium group[53]. Comparison of lithium with olanzapine in 1-year monotherapy, following 6–12 weeks co-treatment with mean weight gain of 2.7 kg, showed significantly greater weight gain with olanzapine (+ 1.8 kg) than with lithium (−1.4 kg)[54]. However, in an 18-month study comparing lithium, lamotrigine and placebo, the mean weight changes were + 4.2 kg, + 1.2 kg and −2.2 kg, respectively[55]. Finally, the results of the study by Mathew et al.[56] in 117 bipolar patients who had been on lithium for a mean duration of 4.7 years indicated that, although there was a non-significant increase in BMI for the whole population, lithium and gender were not significant predictors of any increase in BMI. In 27% of patients, the BMI actually slightly decreased during lithium therapy[4–6,12,50–58] (Table 24.1).

Risk factors and mechanisms of lithium-induced weight gain

There may be several factors predisposing to lithium-induced weight gain. In the study of Vestergaard et al.[6], weight gain occurred primarily in the first 1–2 years of treatment, and then the weight remained constant. The effect was positively correlated with the patient's body weight before treatment[6,57]. In a study of Vendsborg et al.[58] in a group of 70 bipolar

Table 24.1 Frequency of weight gain in lithium-treated patients

Authors	Subjects (n)	Duration (years)	Weight gain
Schou et al., 1970[12]	100	1–2	11% > 5 kg
Grof et al., 1973[57]	42	> 1	Responders – mean 4.5 kg Non-responders – no gain
Vendsborg et al., 1976[58]	70	2–10	64% – weight gain mean 7.5 kg
Peselow et al., 1980[50]	21 – lithium 12 – placebo	1	> 5 kg: 11/21 lithium, 1/12 placebo
Vestergaard et al., 1980[5]	237	Several	> 10 kg: 20% of patients
McCreadie and Morrison, 1985[4]	40	Several	43% – weight gain mostly less than 10% of initial weight
Vestergaard et al., 1988[6]	548 patient-years	Up to 7	Mean weight gain 4 kg, mostly in the first 1–2 years
Moral Iglesias et al., 1989[52]	80	1	35% – weight gain
Mathew et al., 1989[56]	117	Mean 4.7	Non-significant increase in body mass index
Bowden et al., 2000[53]	Lithium, valproate, placebo	1	Weight gain over placebo 6% of lithium 14% of valproate
Chengappa et al., 2002[51]	70	Hospital chart review	77% – weight gain, mean 6.3 kg 20% – weight loss
Calabrese et al., 2003[55]	Lithium, lamotrigine, placebo	1.5	Mean weight change: lithium + 4.2 kg, lamotrigine – 2.2 kg, placebo + 1.2 kg
Tohen et al., 2005[54]	Lithium, olanzapine	1	Weight gain during 6–12-week co-therapy, 2.7 kg 1-year monotherapy olanzapine: + 1.8 kg, lithium: – 1.4 kg

patients treated with lithium for 2–10 years, 45 patients who increased in weight on lithium were overweight at baseline and reached a weight about 20% higher than their ideal weight. No connection between a history of infant obesity and weight gain was found. Weight gain was positively correlated with the concurrent administration of tricyclic antidepressant drugs[6], but this was not found in another study[5]. In a study by Meyer[59], in patients under 60 years of age treated with both risperidone and olanzapine, concurrent use of lithium or valproate led to more pronounced weight gain, but this difference was statistically significant only for the olanzapine cohort. While in some reports no association was found between weight gain and the sex of lithium-treated patients[5,58], in a study by Henry[60], weight gain during the first year of treatment was more frequent in women than men (47% vs. 18%). Cabral et al.[61] also found a statistically greater weight increase in women treated chronically with lithium than in men, and these results were not explained by abnormalities in thyroid function.

Grof et al.[57] found a positive correlation between lithium response and weight gain. Excellent responders (without relapses during the 2-year period) had weight increased by over 6% of their pre-lithium weight; non-responders did not change weight; weight gain of partial responders was intermediate.

Weight gain on lithium appears to be dose-related[8]. In a study by Abou-Saleh and Coppen[62], affective patients on lithium treatment were randomly allocated to two groups over a period of 1 year, either continuing their lithium regimen or decreasing their lithium dosage by up to 50%. There was an association between lower dosage/serum level of lithium and lower side-effects, including weight gain. Similarly, Gelenberg et al.[8] found that weight gain was more frequent in the group with high lithium levels (0.8–1.0 mmol/l) than in the group with low lithium levels (0.4–0.6 mmol/l).

The mechanism of weight gain obviously is complex and multifactorial. The effects of lithium on the endocrine system, neuro-transmitters, metabolism, electrolyte regulation and eating behavior might underlie the influence of this ion on body weight[63]. It may be mediated by increased intake of high-caloric fluids due to lithium-induced thirst, by increased carbohydrate and/or lipid storage, or by lithium-induced hypothyroidism, but it is as yet unclear which if any of these factors is clinically most relevant[49].

Increased calorie intake, particularly in the form of high caloric drinks, has been implicated in the mechanism of weight gain on lithium[50]. However, some studies did not find a connection between weight gain and increased thirst or edema[52], and no unambiguous evidence that fluid retention plays a major role in weight gain was found[64]. In the careful study by Greil[65], using daily protocols of eating and drinking over a period of 14 days, a distinctly higher caloric intake (from solid food, not fluids) and the typical eating pattern of obese subjects were observed in ten patients who gained weight during lithium therapy as compared to ten lithium-treated patients without weight gain. On the other hand, Vendsborg et al.[58] found increased appetite in only one-third of the patients and this increase had only a weak influence on the degree of weight gain. Nearly all the patients felt an increased thirst, and a correlation between liquid intake and weight gain was found. In the study by Vestergaard et al.[5], weight gain was associated with increased thirst and fluid output and with significantly increased blood pressure. According to Garland et al.[46], mechanisms of lithium-induced weight gain include insulin-like actions on carbohydrate and fat metabolism, polydipsia and sodium retention. In a study by Atmaca et al.[66] in inpatients with bipolar I disorder, the changes in fasting serum leptin levels were observed after 8 weeks of lithium treatment, suggesting that leptins may be associated with lithium-induced weight gain. However, Himmerich et al.[67] found an increase in the BMI and in tumor necrosis factor-alpha (TNF-α) and its soluble receptor levels, but not in leptin levels over 4 weeks of treatment with lithium or carbamazepine (Table 24.2).

Management of lithium-induced weight gain

According to Sachs and Guille[68], even after patients stop taking lithium, body weight gained during treatment may be difficult to lose. The best strategy is certainly to prevent weight gain when feasible, possibly through continuous dietary counseling, to avoid unnecessary drug combination and to intervene as soon as weight gain becomes evident. Remedial steps such as adjusting the lithium dose and giving appropriate dietary advice

Table 24.2 Potential risk factors of lithium-induced weight gain

Risk factor	Reference
Female sex	Cabral et al., 1983[61]; Vestergaard et al., 1988[6]; Henry, 2002[60]
Overweight before treatment	Grof et al., 1973[57]; Vendsborg et al., 1976[58]; Vestergaard et al., 1988[6]
Higher lithium dose/serum level	Vendsborg et al., 1976[58]; Gelenberg et al., 1989[8]; Abou-Saleh and Coppen, 1989[62]
Concomitant use of tricyclic antidepressants or atypical neuroleptics (olanzapine)	Vestergaard et al., 1988[6]; Meyer, 2002[59]; Tohen et al., 2005[54]
Increased calorie intake	Peselow et al., 1980[50]; Greil, 1981[65]; Elmslie et al., 2001[70]
Increased sweet fluid intake	Vendsborg et al., 1976[58]; Keck et al, 2003[69]
Good response to lithium	Grof et al., 1973[57]

should be taken at the first sign of weight gain. It is recommended that all patients be repeatedly warned of the risks involved in satisfying their increased thirst on lithium by fluids rich in calories[69]. In this respect, the typical eating and drinking behavior of the various populations in different countries should be considered critically. The study by Elmslie et al.[70] confirmed that drug-induced changes in food preference can lead to an excessive energy intake largely as a result of a high intake of sucrose. Dietary advice regarding the use of energy-rich beverages along with encouragement to increase levels of physical activity may help prevent weight gain in bipolar patients. Dieticians can play an important role as part of a multidisciplinary team in the treatment of patients. Such a role includes nutrition assessment and monitoring, nutrition interventions, patient and staff education and some forms of psychotherapy[71].

According to Baptista et al.[63], therapeutic options in lithium-induced weight gain include, in the long term, dietary control and physical activity and, in the short term, choosing among several drugs that have been tested either in patients or in animal models of obesity. If weight gain still cannot be controlled and treatment compliance is at risk, another mood stabilizer might be substituted for lithium treatment.

In selected cases, adjunctive treatment with the anticonvulsant topiramate may be beneficial in reducing lithium-induced weight gain. Data show that patients treated with topiramate in combination with lithium lost on average several kilograms over weeks[72,73]. Topiramate could be considered in the treatment of lithium-treated bipolar patients showing good response, who are overweight, or whose concerns about weight gain compromise their compliance with long-term prophylactic medication. However, such a combination should be given with caution (i.e. not exceeding the dose of topiramate of 200 mg/day) because topiramate itself may be associated with a range of side-effects and controversies exist about possible untoward pharmacokinetic interactions between the two drugs[74,75].

REFERENCES

1. Johnson FN, ed. Lithium Research and Therapy. London: Academic Press, 1976

2. Mellerup ET, Rafaelsen OJ. Lithium and carbohydrate metabolism. In Johnson FN, ed. Lithium Research and Therapy. London: Academic Press, 1976: 381–9

3. Cade JFK. Lithium salts in the treatment of psychotic excitement. Med J Aust 1949; 36: 349–52

4. McCreadie RG, Morrison DP. The impact of lithium in South-west Scotland. I. Demographic and clinical findings. Br J Psychiatry 1985; 146: 70–4

5. Vestergaard P, Amdisen A, Schou M. Clinically significant side effects of lithium treatment. A survey of 237 patients in long-term treatment. Acta Psychiatr Scand 1980; 62: 193–200

6. Vestergaard P, Poulstrup I, Schou M. Prospective studies on a lithium cohort. 3. Tremor, weight gain, diarrhea, psychological complaints. Acta Psychiatr Scand 1988; 78: 434–41

7. Volk J, Müller-Oerlinghausen B. Time course of AMP-documented side effects in patients under long-term lithium treatment. Pharmacopsychiatry 1986; 19: 286–7

8. Gelenberg AJ, Kane JM, Keller MB, et al. Comparison of standard and low serum levels of lithium for maintenance treatment of bipolar disorder. N Engl J Med 1989; 321: 1489–93

9. Persson G. Lithium side effects in relation to dose and to levels and gradients of lithium in plasma. Acta Psychiatr Scand 1977; 55: 208–13

10. Fedorak RN, Field M. Antidiarrheal therapy. Prospects for new agents. Dig Dis Sci 1987; 32: 195–205

11. Owyang C. Treatment of chronic secretory diarrhea of unknown origin by lithium carbonate. Gastroenterology 1984; 87: 714–18

12. Schou M, Baastrup PC, Grof P, et al. Pharmacological and clinical problems of lithium prophylaxis. Br J Psychiatry 1970; 116: 615–19

13. Stoudemire A, Hill CD, Lewison BJ, et al. Lithium intolerance in a medical-psychiatric population. Gen Hosp Psychiatry 1998; 20: 85–90

14. Sajatovic M, Gyulai L, Calabrese JR, et al. Maintenance treatment outcomes in older patients with bipolar I disorder. Am J Geriatr Psychiatry 2005; 13: 305–11

15. Jefferson JW, Greist JH, Ackerman DL, et al. Lithium Encyclopedia for Clinical Practice, 2nd edn. Washington, DC: American Psychiatric Press, 1987

16. Edstrom A, Persson G. Comparison of side effects with coated lithium carbonate tablets and lithium sulphate preparations giving medium-slow and slow-release. Acta Psychiatr Scand 1977; 55: 153–8

17. Marini JL, Sheard MH. Sustained-release lithium carbonate in double-blind study: serum lithium levels, side effects, and placebo response. J Clin Pharmacol 1976; 16: 276–83

18. Heim W, Oelschläger H, Kreuter J, et al. Liberation of lithium from sustained release preparations. Pharmacopsychiatry 1994; 27: 27–31

19. Toothaker RD, Welling PG. The effect of food on drug bioavailability. Annu Rev Pharmacol Toxicol 1980; 20: 173–99

20. Jeppsson J, Sjogren J. The influence of food on side effects and absorption of lithium. Acta Psychiatr Scand 1975; 51: 285–8

21. Russell JD, Johnson GF. Affective disorders, diabetes mellitus and lithium. Aust NZ J Psychiatry 1981; 15: 349–53

22. MacAulay K, Hajduch E, Blair AS, et al. Use of lithium and SB-415286 to explore the role of glycogen synthase kinase-3 in the regulation of glucose transport and glycogen synthase. Eur J Biochem 2003; 270: 3829–38

23. Tabata I, Schluter J, Gulve EA, et al. Lithium increases susceptibility of muscle glucose transport to stimulation by various agents. Diabetes 1994; 43: 903–7

24. Weiss H. Über eine neue Behandlungsmethode des Diabetes mellitus und verwandter Stoffwechselstörrungen. Wien Klin Wochenschr 1924; 37: 1142

25. Gildea EF, McLean VL, Man EB. Oral and intravenous dextrose tolerance curves of

patients with manic-depressive psychosis. Arch Neurol Psychiatry 1943; 49: 852–9

26. Van der Velde CD, Gordon MW. Manic-depressive illness, diabetes mellitus, and lithium carbonate. Arch Gen Psychiatry 1969; 21: 478–85

27. Cassidy F, Ahearn E, Carroll BJ. Elevated frequency of diabetes mellitus in hospitalized manic–depressive patients. Am J Psychiatry 1999; 156: 1417–20

28. Klumpers UM, Boom K, Janssen FM, et al. Cardiovascular risk factors in outpatients with bipolar disorder. Pharmacopsychiatry 2004; 37: 211–16

29. Vendsborg PB, Prytz S. Glucose tolerance and serum lipids in man after long-term lithium administration. Acta Psychiatr Scand 1976; 53: 64–9

30. Storlien LH, Higson FM, Gleeson RM, et al. Effects of chronic lithium, amitriptyline and mianserin on glucoregulation, corticosterone and energy balance in the rat. Pharmacol Biochem Behav 1985; 22: 119–25

31. Jonderko G, Sobczyk P, Gabryel A, et al. Endocrinological aspects of long-term lithium therapy. Z Gesamte Inn Med 1981; 36: 79–82

32. Mellerup ET, Dam H, Wildschiodtz G, et al. Diurnal variation of blood glucose during lithium treatment. J Affect Disord 1983; 5: 341–7

33. Vestergaard P, Schou M. Does long-term lithium treatment induce diabetes mellitus? Neuropsychobiology 1987; 17: 130–2

34. Vendsborg PB. Lithium treatment and glucose tolerance in manic–melancholic patients. Acta Psychiatr Scand 1979; 59: 306–16

35. Shah JH, Deleon-Jones FA, Schickler R, et al. Symptomatic reactive hypoglycemia during glucose tolerance test in lithium-treated patients. Metabolism 1986; 35: 634–9

36. Müller-Oerlinghausen B, Passoth PM, Poser W, et al. Impaired glucose tolerance in long-term lithium-treated patients. Int Pharmacopsychiatry 1979; 14: 350–62

37. Müller-Oerlinghausen B, Passoth PM, Poser W, et al. [Effect of long-term treatment with neuroleptics or lithium salts on carbohydrate metabolism]. Arzneimittelforschung 1978; 28: 1522–4

38. Kondziela JR, Kaufmann MW, Klein MJ. Diabetic ketoacidosis associated with lithium: case report. J Clin Psychiatry 1985; 46: 492–3

39. Bendz H. A case of solute diuresis erroneously diagnosed as lithium-induced polyuria. Acta Psychiatr Scand 1985; 71: 92–3

40. Waziri R, Nelson J. Lithium in diabetes mellitus: a paradoxical response. J Clin Psychiatry 1978; 39: 623–5

41. Lippman SB, Manshadi MS, Gultekin A. Lithium in a patient with renal failure on hemodialysis. J Clin Psychiatry 1984; 45: 444

42. Saran AS. Antidiabetic effects of lithium. J Clin Psychiatry 1982; 43: 383–4

43. Jones GR, Lazarus JH, Davies CJ, et al. The effect of short term lithium carbonate in type II diabetes mellitus. Horm Metab Res 1983; 15: 422–4

44. Hu M, Wu H, Chao C. Assisting effects of lithium on hypoglycemic treatment in patients with diabetes. Biol Trace Elem Res 1997; 60: 131–7

45. Suppes T, Baldessarini RJ, Faedda GL, et al. Discontinuation of maintenance treatment in bipolar disorder: risks and implications. Harvard Rev Psychiatry 1993; 1: 131–44

46. Garland EJ, Remick RA, Zis AP. Weight gain with antidepressants and lithium. J Clin Psychopharmacol 1988; 8: 323–30

47. Silverstone T, Romans S. Long term treatment of bipolar disorder. Drugs 1996; 51: 367–82

48. Chen Y, Silverstone T. Lithium and weight gain. Int Clin Psychopharmacol 1990; 5: 217–25

49. Ackerman S, Nolan LJ. Bodyweight gain induced by psychotropic drugs: incidence, mechanisms and management. CNS Drugs 1998; 9: 135–51

50. Peselow ED, Dunner DL, Fieve RR, et al. Lithium carbonate and weight gain. J Affect Disord 1980; 2: 303–10

51. Chengappa KN, Chalasani L, Brar JS, et al. Changes in body weight and body mass index among psychiatric patients receiving lithium, valproate, or topiramate: an open-label, non-randomized chart review. Clin Ther 2002; 24: 1576–84

52. Moral Iglesias L, Gonzalez-Pinto Arrillaga A. Weight gain secondary to treatment with lithi-

um carbonate. Actas Luso Esp Neurol Psiquiatr Cienc Afines 1989; 17: 32–5

53. Bowden CL, Calabrese JR, McElroy SL, et al. A randomized, placebo-controlled 12 month trial of divalproex and lithium in treatment of outpatients with bipolar I disorder. Arch Gen Psychiatry 2000; 57: 208–13

54. Tohen M, Greil W, Calabrese JR, et al. Olanzapine versus lithium in the maintenance treatment of bipolar disorder: a 12-month, randomized, double-blind controlled clinical trial. Am J Psychiatry 2005; 162: 1281–90

55. Calabrese JR, Bowden CL, Sachs G, et al. A placebo-controlled 18-month trial of lamotrigine and lithium maintenance treatment in recently depressed patients with bipolar I disorder. J Clin Psychiatry 2003; 64: 1013–24

56. Mathew B, Rao JM, Sundari U. Lithium-induced changes in the body mass index. Acta Psychiatr Scand 1989; 80: 538–40

57. Grof P, Loughrey E, Saxena B, et al. Lithium stabilization and weight gain. In Ban TA, Boissier JR, Gessa GJ, et al., eds. Psychopharmacology, Sexual Disorders and Drug Abuse. Amsterdam: North-Holland, 1973: 323–7

58. Vendsborg PB, Bech P, Rafaelsen OJ. Lithium treatment and weight gain. Acta Psychiatr Scand 1976; 53: 139–47

59. Meyer JM. A retrospective comparison of weight, lipid, and glucose changes between risperidone- and olanzapine-treated inpatients: metabolic outcomes after 1 year. J Clin Psychiatry 2002; 63: 425–33

60. Henry C. Lithium side-effects and predictors of hypothyroidism in patients with bipolar disorder: sex differences. J Psychiatry Neurosci 2002; 27: 104–7

61. Cabral MA, Fernandes G, Piedra Buena AE, et al. Influence of the sex factor in weight gain caused by chronic use of lithium. Acta Psiquiatr Psicol Am Lat 1983; 29: 207–12

62. Abou-Saleh MT, Coppen A. The efficacy of low-dose lithium: clinical, psychological and biological correlates. J Psychiatr Res 1989; 23: 157–62

63. Baptista T, Teneud L, Contreras Q, et al. Lithium and body weight gain. Pharmacopsychiatry 1995; 28: 35–44

64. Dempsey M, Dunner DL, Fieve RR, et al. Treatement of excessive weight gain in patients taking lithium. Am J Psychiatry 1976; 133: 1082–4

65. Greil W. Pharmacokinetics and toxicology of lithium. Bibl Psychiatr 1981; 161: 69–103

66. Atmaca M, Kuloglu M, Tezcan E, et al. Weight gain and serum leptin levels in patients on lithium treatment. Neuropsychobiology 2002; 46: 67–9

67. Himmerich H, Koethe D, Schuld A, et al. Plasma levels of leptin and endogenous immune modulators during treatment with carbamazepine or lithium. Psychopharmacology (Berl) 2005; 179: 447–51

68. Sachs GS, Guille C. Weight gain associated with use of psychotropic medications. J Clin Psychiatry 1999; 60 (Suppl 21): 16–19

69. Keck PE, McElroy SL. Bipolar disorder, obesity, and pharmacotherapy-associated weight gain. J Clin Psychiatry 2003; 64: 1426–35

70. Elmslie JL, Mann JI, Silverstone JT, et al. Determinants of overweight and obesity in patients with bipolar disorder. J Clin Psychiatry 2001; 62: 486–91

71. Gray GE, Gray LK. Nutritional aspects of psychiatric disorders. J Am Diet Assoc 1989; 89: 1492–8

72. Chengappa KNR, Levine J, Rathore D, et al. Long-term effects of topiramate on bipolar mood instability, weight change and glycemic control: a case-series. Eur Psychiatry 2001; 16: 186–90

73. Kirov G, Tredget J. Add-on topiramate reduces weight in overweight patients with affective disorders: a clinical case series. BMC Psychiatry 2005; 5: 19

74. Bialer M, Doose DR, Murthy B, et al. Pharmacokinetic interactions of topiramate. Clin Pharmacokin 2004; 43: 763–80

75. Abraham G, Owen J. Topiramate can cause lithium toxicity. J Clin Psychopharmacol 2004; 24: 565–7

25 Lithium and its cardiovascular effects

Jeffrey Bierbrauer, Jochen Albrecht,
Bruno Müller-Oerlinghausen

Contents   Introduction • Lithium's cardiac effects • Critical assessment • Consequences for clinical practice

INTRODUCTION

Lithium's cardiovascular side-effects account for the following classification (the given order reflects the frequencies of lithium-induced side-effects):

(1) Non-specific alterations of the repolarization period in the electrocardiogram (ECG) without concomitant symptoms of clinical importance;

(2) Dysfunctions of impulse generation or conduction;

(3) Myocardial damage due to degeneration and/or inflammation (myocardiopathy, myocarditis, myocardial insufficiency);

(4) Blood pressure changes.

LITHIUM'S CARDIAC EFFECTS

Non-specific alterations of repolarization

Changes of ECG ST-T segments with reversible T-wave flattening that can reach iso-electricity and occasionally negativity are the only more or less predictable phenomena of lithium's visible cardiac influence. Studies considering this kind of alteration in ECG repolarization have reported frequencies between 13 and 100% in their subjects[1–3]. T wave depression with an incidental occurrence of prominent U waves, usually without a shift of the ST segment, seems to be a dose-dependent lithium effect[4], which is boosted by an additional administration of tricyclic antidepressants or antipsychotics. A study on 32 patients showed that lithium blood levels beyond 0.8 mmol/l resulted in an average T-wave reduction of about 50% compared to T waves before lithium application. Apparently such repolarization alterations are without clinical impact, disappear mostly after continuation of lithium medication and are fully reversible after drug discontinuation; they are generally not an indication of coronary heart disease or its beginning and therefore not a reason to stop the medication. Although these findings can still not be explained precisely from an electrophysiologic standpoint, they may be associated with changes of electrolytes.

Interferences with extra-/intracellular sodium potassium ratios can be expected, due to lithium's biochemical properties.

One possible explanation is derived from animal studies and *in vitro* experiments, interpreting ST alterations as a result of a modified potassium ratio along the cellular membrane. Sodium, which is essential for the development of an action potential, can be substituted by lithium and move into the cell in similar relations. However, lithium shows a tendency to accumulate inside the cell and is transported out of the cell in a much slower manner. Furthermore, an outward rush of lithium is not accompanied by a simultaneous inward rush of potassium, as is the case in an outward rush of sodium. The consequence is an intracellular accumulation of lithium with displacement of intracellular potassium and sodium in about the same ratio[5,6].

Dysfunctions of impulse generation and conduction

Arrhythmia in humans under lithium treatment has been reported in single case reports only. Such cases have shown as following.

Abnormalities in the sinoatrial node, sinoatrial blocks and first-degree atrioventricular blocks

In a handful of cases it has been reported that sinus node bradyarrhythmia developed with signs of a sinoatrial block under long-term lithium application within therapeutic blood levels. However, more than ten observed cases featured lithium blood levels of >1.5 mmol/l (increased occurrence of side-effects) or >2.0 mmol/l (toxic range).

Sinoatrial node and atrioventricular node dysfunctions (supra-His) have to be regarded as the most frequent type of arrhythmia under lithium treatment, in contrast to dysfunctions that have been reported under intoxication with tricyclic antidepressants. The latter affect the HV interval that defines the time range in which the impulse is being conducted from distal of the atrioventricular node in the His bundle up to the contracting myocardium.

One of the cases developing sinus node dysfunctions during lithium therapy featured concomitant use of the anticonvulsant carbamazepine. Interestingly, drug monitoring showed normal serum carbamazepine levels, whereas serum lithium levels were in the toxic range, i.e. >3.3 mmol/l[7].

As a rule, these lithium-induced cardiac dysfunctions are reversible; however, there have been reports of two cases without relevant co-morbidities that showed frequent episodes of sinoatrial node pausing with occurrence of escape rhythms, even after weeks of lithium discontinuation[8,9]. The basic principle for such persisting sinoatrial node dysfunction remains unclear.

Ventricular and supraventricular arrhythmia

Only one case of multiple ventricular extrasystoles has been reported, in a previously healthy 46-year-old man being treated with lithium (lithium blood levels between 0.6 and 0.9 mmol/l)[10]. A few more cases of ventricular extrasystoles, partly due to sinus bradyarrhythmia, have been mentioned, but they featured complicating co-variables, particularly lithium intoxication (lithium blood levels 3.0 mmol/l[11] and 2.3 mmol/l)[12].

Reports that cover a larger number of patients or volunteers arrive at differing and in part conflicting conclusions.

Middelhoff and Paschen[13] examined ECGs of 31 patients and ten volunteers, each taking lithium for a period of 3 weeks. Thirty patients had been examined before and 2 weeks after the beginning of lithium therapy (group A), and 18 patients received permanent lithium therapy (group B). The average lithium blood level was 0.96 ± 0.24 mmol/l. Within the healthy control group a discrete elongation of the PQ interval was seen from 0.15 s to 0.16 s. Extrasystoles occurred in two cases.

Group A patients' PQ intervals extended from 0.16s to 0.19s. Within the patient group that received permanent lithium therapy (group B), nine subjects showed a first-degree atrioventricular block. However, it has to be noted that more than half the patients received unknown co-medication, a fact that makes the validity of this study questionable.

In contrast to this, a study by Albrecht and Müller-Oerlinghausen[4], examining 12 healthy volunteers and 20 long-term lithium patients, did not show any severe dysfunctions of impulse generation or conduction.

Recently, Mamiya et al.[14] examined 39 inpatients with bipolar disorder or schizophrenia treated with lithium. Multiple regression analysis revealed that especially higher serum lithium concentrations were determinants for the prolongation of QTc (corrected QT).

Hsu et al.[15] performed a retrospective study with available records of lithium levels in 76 patients undergoing lithium treatment. Eleven patients had serum lithium levels of >1.2 mmol/l. Patients with lithium levels of >1.2 mmol/l had slower heart rates and longer PR, QT and QTc intervals. A QTc interval of >440 ms was more commonly found in patients with high lithium blood levels (55% vs. 8%, $p > 0.001$). Similarly, diffuse T-wave inversion was more commonly found in this patient group (73% vs. 17%, $p < 0.001$).

Hagman et al.[16] prospectively examined the prevalence of sinoatrial node dysfunctions within a group of 97 patients under monitored long-term lithium treatment. Besides inter-views, tests included ECGs under resting conditions and during carotid artery massage. Lithium as a cause for sinoatrial node depression was ruled out in all but two cases, while lithium as a reason for a complete atrioventricular block could be eliminated in all but one case. No subject showed clinical symptoms and all subjects featured lithium blood levels within the therapeutic range.

Based on a study of 12 patients, some of them inherently featuring heart dysfunction or arrhythmia, it was claimed that lithium could even lower the incidence of supraventricular extrasystoles or paroxysmal supraventricular tachycardiac arrhythmia[17]. In addition it was postulated that lithium under stress conditions does not affect heart function negatively. However, ventricular arrhythmia might be noticed for the first time or might worsen under lithium therapy.

Darbar et al.[18] concluded that lithium is a potent blocker of cardiac sodium channels and may identify patients with Brugada syndrome. The first patients ever to be diagnosed with Brugada syndrome showed distinct ECG changes, such as an up-sloping ST segment in right precordial leads in association with right bundle branch block and T-wave inversion. They all experienced cardiac arrest due to ventricular fibrillation. It was suggested that Brugada syndrome might account for up to 40–60% of cases of ventricular fibrillation previously classified as idiopathic. In this study, lithium induced transient ST segment elevation (type 1 Brugada pattern) in right precordial leads at therapeutic concentrations in two patients with bipolar disorder. Lithium withdrawal resulted in reversion to type 2 or 3 Brugada patterns or resolution of ST-T abnormalities.

Wolf et al. published a case report[19] of a patient receiving lithium treatment for more than 19 years due to bipolar disorder. The patient developed hypercalcemia, hypertension and episodes of severe bradyarrhythmia with lithium levels within the therapeutic range. An endocrine workup showed biochemical findings different from those of primary hyperparathyroidism that were attributed to direct actions of lithium in the kidneys. The authors suggested that hypercalcemia together with lithium administration increases the risk of cardiac arrhythmia. In 2000, they published a retrospective study of bipolar patients with lithium-associated hypercalcemia[20]. The authors identified 18 patients not treated with lithium and who had hypercalcemia related to malignancies or other medical conditions (group A) and 12 patients with lithium-associated hypercalcemia (group B). Since patients in group A were not comparable to those in group B, two control groups were generated: group C1 which included age- and sex-comparable lithium-treated bipolar normo-calcemic patients, and group C2, which included bipolar normocalcemic patients treated with anticonvulsant mood stabilizers. ECG findings were compared with those of patients in groups C1 and C2. It was found that these groups did not differ in their overall frequency of ECG abnormalities. However, there were significant differences in the frequency of conduction defects. Patients with hypercalcemia resulting from medical diseases and bipolar patients with lithium-associated hypercalcemia had significantly higher frequencies of conduction defects.

Myocardial damage; myocardial insufficiency

There is no systematic research on lithium causing irreversible organic damage. Some case reports, however, do connect lithium to cardiac decompensation. A causal connection remains doubtful. Dietrich et al.[21] published a case report of an adolescent developing signs of myocardiopathy 6 months after the beginning of combined therapy of lithium and imipramine. However, this combination argues rather for reversible myocardial damage due to medication-induced hypothyroidism than a cardiotoxic effect of lithium.

Shopsin et al.[22] reported four cases of 'sudden death' within 105 subjects of an outpatient lithium clinic. Yet further examination showed that cardiac mortality within patients' relatives was high and that it exceeded comparable mortality rates within the general population of New York.

CRITICAL ASSESSMENT

Altogether, cardiac arrhythmia is a rare condition under lithium therapy if criteria of a well-monitored application are met. Almost all reported cases had in common that changes after lithium discontinuation were reversible. In turn, resuming lithium therapy provokes these changes again, which certainly speaks for a triggering by lithium. After critical analysis, it remains as yet unclear whether lithium in some cases acts as a causing factor or as a sensitizing coefficient regarding the development of arrhythmia.

Besides this, pre-existing heart disease, other disorders with cardiac effects, and co-medication with antidepressants or anti-psychotics have to be considered as possible reasons for observed alterations.

At present the mechanisms of lithium function have not been explicitly resolved. Owing to largely differing test arrangements and the use of extremely high dosages exceeding therapeutic ranges, results of animal experiments are difficult to transfer to the situation in human beings.

Considering *in vitro* experiments with isolated strips of myocardial tissue and trying to integrate them into findings in human beings, lithium appears to cause a concentration-dependent significant increase in the duration of action potentials in impulse-conducting parts as well as in myocardial fibers, yet only at levels above therapeutic concentrations. The increase is characterized by a corresponding elongation of its functional refractory period together with a decrease of its depolarization rate[23]. Apparently this phenomenon can clinically manifest itself in a range between common and insignificant protractions of excitation, block formations, or downstream impulse generation including extrasystoles. The fact that another electrophysiologic study showed 17 patients having reduced maximum conduction rates of motor nerves during permanent lithium therapy would strengthen this hypothesis[24].

Effects on blood pressure

There is no prospective research available on lithium's effect on blood pressure. Within the therapeutic range in humans, lithium appears not to exert a significant influence on blood pressure. During the many years of its operation, distinctive vascular abnormalities have not been noted in the Berlin Lithium Clinic.

Vestergaard and Schou[25] reported in manic depressive patients that seasonal fluctuation of blood pressure which had existed prior to lithium therapy and was characterized by lower levels during spring/fall and higher levels during summer/winter ceased after lithium application.

Klumpers et al.[26], in their study on cardiovascular risk factors in outpatients with bipolar disorder, concluded that cardiovascular risk factors, including hypertension, were increased in a large proportion of their population on monotherapy with lithium. However, no significant relationships were observed between duration of lithium treatment or bipolar disorder and presence of hypertension.

Interactions with tricyclic antidepressants and antipsychotics

Even though many questions concerning cardiac effects of antidepressants and antipsychotics remain unsettled, a set of effects has been proven to refer to anticholinergic, sympathomimetic and chinidin-like working mechanisms: sinoatrial tachycardia, atrioventricular conductor dysfunctions, intraventricular conduction protraction, possibly in combination with ventricular tachyarrhythmia and probably decreased myocardial inotropy. Furthermore, unspecific repolarization changes, as observed with lithium, are not uncommon. Thus, additive effects of a combination of both substances are conceivable. Although there has been no systematic prospective research, case reports on the occurrence of, for example, sinoatrial bradyarrhythmia with simultaneous application of haloperidol[27] or paroxysmal left bundle branch block during initiation of anesthesia[28] have been published.

CONSEQUENCES FOR CLINICAL PRACTICE

If the following rules are followed, adverse cardiac events in patients without cardiac co-morbidities should, in general, be unlikely.

- To identify patients at special risk, a detailed clinical examination with particular consideration to the patient's cardiac situation as well as an ECG have to be provided before first-time adjustment.

- As a matter of routine, ECGs should be recorded twice a year.

Repolarization abnormalities such as T-wave depression or negative T waves are no reason to discontinue therapy. Horizontal drops of $\geq 0.2\,\text{mV}$ of the ST segment in combination with T-wave depression should alert the physician to look for signs of coronary heart disease or a hidden compensated cardiac insufficiency. Patients at risk:

- Patients with diagnosed, permanent or frequently occurring arrhythmia with or without medical conditions; this applies particularly to sinoatrial node dysfunctions, all kinds of conductor protractions and bradyarrhythmia as well as ventricular extrasystoles.

- Patients with an apparent cardiac insufficiency, since reduction of the glomerular filtration rate, long-term application of diuretics or sodium chloride restriction increases the risk of intoxication due to decreased lithium clearance.

- Patients with heart malformations that feature cumulative phenomena such as cardiac insufficiency and/or arrhythmia.

- Patients showing signs of hypercalcemia.

Treatment of patients at risk

Since there is no general rule for predicting the cardiotoxicity of lithium in an individual patient, it is impossible to formulate absolute contraindications. For each patient at risk it has to be determined individually whether discontinuation of lithium treatment and replacement by other psychotropic drugs (with more serious cardiovascular side-effects) represents the greater risk. For instance, breakthrough of a manic state with severe hyperactivity, restlessness and increased energy together with poor judgment towards the own disorder may become a greater hazard to patients with heart conditions than well-monitored lithium therapy. This has been illustrated by McKnelly *et al.*[29] and Levenson *et al.*[30]. In case of bradyarrhythmia with frequent cardiac syncopes the implantation of a pacemaker should be discussed if lithium therapy seems indispensable[9].

Patients at risk should receive initial lithium adjustment under inpatient settings. Arrhythmia occurring during lithium therapy that cannot be eliminated by dose adjustment should be evaluated by a cardiologist to consider antiarrhythmic measures. Co-medication of digitalis compounds has not caused any problems within patients of our lithium clinic, although theoretically, this combination does not seem completely harmless considering patients with extended impulse conduction[31].

REFERENCES

1. Demers RG, Heninger GR. Electrocardiographic changes during lithium treatment. Dis Nerv Syst 1970; 31: 674
2. Demers RG, Heninger GR. Electrocardiographic T-wave changes during lithium carbonate treatment. JAMA 1971; 218: 381
3. Foster JR. Use of lithium in elderly psychiatric patients: a review of the literature. Lithium 1992; 3: 77–93
4. Albrecht J, Müller-Oerlinghausen B. EKG-Veränderungen unter akuter und chronischer Applikation von Lithium. Pharmacopsychiatry 1977; 10: 325–33
5. Carmeliet EE. Influence of lithium ions on the transmembrane potential and cation content of cardiac cells. J Gen Physiol 1964; 47: 501
6. McKusick VA. The effect of lithium on the electrocardiogram of animals and relation of this effect to the ratio of the intracellular and extracellular concentrations of potassium. J Clin Invest 1954; 33: 598
7. Lai CL, Chen WJ, Huang CH, et al. Sinus node dysfunction in a patient with lithium intoxication. J Formos Med Assoc 2000; 99: 66–8
8. Palileo EV, Coelho A, Westveer D, et al. Persistent sinus node dysfunction secondary to lithium therapy. Am Heart J 1983; 106: 1443–4
9. Terao T, Abe H, Abe K. Irreversible sinus node dysfunction induced by resumption of lithium therapy. Acta Psychiatr Scand 1996; 93: 407–8

10. Tangedahl TN, Gau GT. Myocardial irritability associated with lithium carbonate therapy. N Engl J Med 1972; 287: 867

11. Worthley LIG. Lithium toxicity and refractory cardiac arrhythmia treated with intravenous magnesium. Anaesth Intensive Care 1974; 2: 357

12. Habibzadeh MA, Zeller NH. Cardiac arrhythmia and hypopotassemia in association with lithium carbonate overdose. South Med J 1977; 70: 628

13. Middelhoff HD, Paschen K. Lithiumwirkungen auf das EKG. Pharmakopsychiat Neuropsychopharmacol 1974; 7: 242

14. Mamiya K, Sadanaga T, Sekita A, et al. Lithium concentration correlates with QTc in patients with psychosis. J Electrocardiol 2005; 38: 148–51

15. Hsu CH, Liu PY, Chen JH et al. Electrocardiographic abnormalities as predictors for over-range lithium levels. Cardiology 2005; 103: 101–6

16. Hagman A, Arnman K, Rydén L. Syncope caused by lithium treatment. Acta Med Scand 1979; 205: 467–71

17. Tilkian AG, Schroeder JS, Kao J, Hultgren H. Effect of lithium on cardiovascular performance. Report on extended ambulatory monitoring and exercise testing before and during lithium therapy. Am J Cardiol 1976; 38: 701

18. Darbar D, Yang T, Churchwell K et al. Unmasking of Brugada syndrome by lithium. Circulation 2005; 112: 1527–31

19. Wolf ME, Moffat M, Mosnaim J, Dempsey S. Lithium therapy, hypercalcemia, and hyperparathyroidism. Am J Ther 1997; 4: 323–5

20. Wolf ME, Ranade V, Molnar J et al. Hypercalcemia, arrhythmia, and mood stabilizers. J Clin Psychopharmacol 2000; 20: 260–4

21. Dietrich A, Mortensen ME, Wheller J. Cardiac toxicity in an adolescent following chronic lithium and imipramine therapy. J Adolesc Health 1993; 14: 394–7

22. Shopsin B, Temple H, Ingwer M. Sudden death during lithium carbonate maintenance. Internationale Lithium-Konferenz, New York, 1978

23. Naumann D'Alnoncourt C, Delhaes R, Steinbeck G, Lüderitz B. Elektrophysiologische Untersuchungen über die kardiale Wirkung von Lithium. Verh Dt Ges KreislForsch 1976; 42: 217

24. Girke W, Krebs FA, Müller-Oerlinghausen B. Effects of lithium on electromyographic recordings in man. Int Pharmacopsychiatry 1975; 10: 24

25. Vestergaard P, Schou M. Lithium treatment and blood pressure. Pharmacopsychiatry 1986; 19: 73–4

26. Klumpers UM, Boom K, Janssem FM et al. Cardiovascular risk factors in outpatients with bipolar disorder. Pharmacopsychiatry 2004; 37: 211–16

27. Rix E, Gless KH. Bradyarrhythmie unter kombinierter Lithium-Neuroleptika-Therapie. Dtsch Med Wochenschr 1981; 106: 629–30

28. Azar I, Turndorf H. Paroxysmal left bundle branch block during nitrous oxide anesthesia in a patient on lithium carbonate: a case report. Anesth Analg 1977; 56: 868–70

29. McKnelly WV, Tupin JP, Dumm M. Lithium in hazardous circumstances with one case of lithium toxicity. Compr Psychiat 1970; 11: 279

30. Levenson JL, Mishra A, Bauernfein RA, Rea RF. Lithium treatment of mania in a patient with recurrent ventricular tachycardia. Psychosomatics 1986; 27: 594–6

31. Winters WD, Ralph DD. Digoxin–lithium drug interaction. Clin Toxicol 1977; 10: 487

26 Dermatologic effects of lithium: adverse reactions and potential therapeutic utility

Andrea Pfennig, Dorian Deshauer, Gisela Albrecht

Contents   Incidence of adverse skin reactions • Dermatoses • Clinical management of lithium-induced skin conditions • Potential therapeutic roles for lithium in dermatology

INCIDENCE OF ADVERSE SKIN REACTIONS

Since lithium came into widespread use before the advent of current regulatory policies, we do not have generalizable rate estimates for its adverse skin reactions. The existing literature is methodologically limited. At best, we can say that the risk of adverse skin reactions lies between 7 and 34%[1–3]. Among patients remaining on lithium monotherapy for over 10 years, the incidence of adverse skin reactions has been reported to be less than 7%[4], but this estimate may be explained in part by early cohort drop-outs. Studies reporting estimates at the higher end of the range are limited by retrospective design[2], recall bias[2] and referral bias[3]. On the whole, acne and psoriasis are the most frequently encountered cutaneous reactions.

DERMATOSES

Psoriasis vulgaris

Psoriasis is an immune-mediated condition, defined by epidermal hyperproliferation with dermal inflammatory infiltration. It affects 1–3% of the Caucasian population, and most frequently begins in young adults. Approximately one-third of psoriatic patients have moderate to severe disease, defined either by body surface involvement or by its impact on quality of life. A third also have joint involvement. Approximately 65% and 35% of identical and fraternal twins, respectively, are concordant for psoriasis[5]. Aside from lithium, a wide range of environmental agents including skin trauma, HIV infection, streptococcal infection, contact dermatitis, interferons, abrupt withdrawal of corticosteroids, alpha-blockers, angiotensin converting enzyme (ACE) inhibitors and anti-malarials are associated with psoriasis[5].

The pathogeneisis of psoriasis involves a complex interaction between CD4 cells and keratinocytes, mediated through pro-inflammatory factors. Interleukin (IL)-6, IL-8 and transforming growth factor α (TGFα) stimulate the proliferation of keratinocytes and/or the activation of T cells, B cells, macrophages and monocytes. IL-2 and interferon γ (IFNγ) are expressed by T helper cells (type 1) and are a sign of an active local immune reaction. Lithium seems to interfere with this network of mediators. Bloomfield and Young[6] showed that lithium salts *in vitro* could degranulate the neutrophil granulocytes of psoriatic patients, initiating psoriatic lesions[6]. Beyaert and co-workers[7] later could trigger a psoriatic reaction in mice through intradermal injection of tumor necrosis factor (TNF) and lithium chloride. Initial vasodilatation and neutrophil infiltration was followed by a mononuclear infiltration and localized increases in IL-6. Ockenfels and co-workers[8] showed that lithium led to enhanced secretion of TGFα, IL-2 and IFNγ in psoriatic but not in normal keratinocytes. In addition, lithium has been shown to inhibit adenylate cyclase at the cell surface, decreasing intracellular cyclic 3′5′-AMP and in turn supporting epidermal cell proliferation.

These mechanisms do not, however, automatically apply to all psoriatic patients. For example, seborrheic dermatitis, considered a form of psoriasis, can be treated with locally applied lithium (8% lithium succinate in the solution Efalith® (Scotia Pharmaceutical Products, Glasgow)[9]. It is thought that a totally different mechanism of action is responsible for its efficacy in this condition, possibly through an antimicrobial effect on *Pityrosporum ovale*. This member of the fungus group is quite common

and is found on healthy skin. For people with seborrheic dermatitis, the organism grows rapidly and can aggravate the skin condition.

Several published case series have described both *de novo* psoriasis as well as exacerbations of pre-existing cases attributable to therapeutic levels of lithium (0.7–1.2 mmol/l). There is one report of reversible psoriasis related to the ingestion of lithium-containing spring water[10]. Common elements in the reports are an early involvement of the scalp and treatment resistance, severe at times but reversible upon lithium discontinuation[11–17]. There are anecdotal reports of a dose-severity effect, but no randomized trials have established the relationship.

In summary, lithium can exacerbate existing psoriasis and cause new cases of the skin condition. While pre-existing psoriasis is not an absolute contraindication to lithium therapy, the psychological impact of a lithium-related flare-up should be included in the individual cost–benefit analysis when choosing psychiatric medications.

Acne and acneiform reactions

Ruiz-Maldonado and co-workers[18] described a 28-year-old woman who developed severe facial and shoulder acneiform dermatitis 1 month after taking lithium (plasma level 0.9 mmol/l). The condition resolved upon lithium discontinuation but recurred on re-challenge. Yoder[19] described four female patients in whom acne worsened or developed for the first time after lithium treatment. Müller-Oerlinghausen[4] reported on a female patient with severe acne requiring lithium discontinuation despite excellent control of her psychiatric disorder. Two of the five patients presented by Reiffers and Dick[13] suffered from acne. In one case the lithium plasma level was 0.7–0.85 mmol/l, while in the second, acneiform lesions developed, even at a plasma level of 0.4 mmol/l. In the case of a 21-year-old female patient, Okrasinski[20] described a relationship between dose and severity of typical comedones, papules, pustules and cysts. Complete remission was achieved after lithium discontinuation. Hong[21] observed several patients with acne under unusually high lithium plasma levels of 1.5–2.5 mmol/l. The skin condition, described as acne medicamentosa, had a rapid onset, no seborrhea and no comedones or cysts. Rüther[22] described acne papulopustulosa in a 22-year-old female patient (lithium plasma level below 0.7 mmol/l). Stamm and Lubach[23] reported on a 54-year-old woman in whom lithium treatment was followed by a reversible hidradenitis supurativa. Gupta and co-workers observed a similar case in 1995[24].

Most case reports of acne related to lithium describe patients between 20 and 30 years of age[2], and older patients are rarely described[25]. This may be due in part to a reporting bias. Explanations for lithium's tendency to cause pustulous reactions relate to its influence on circulating neutrophil granulocytes[26] and its stimulation of sebaceous secretion[25]. It remains unclear whether the case reports of lithium-induced acne are best interpreted as acne medicamentosa, acne vulgaris or folliculitis[27]. Fortunately, these skin blemishes reverse with lithium discontinuation in almost all cases.

While cosmetic problems are often tolerated as a trade-off for effective control of psychiatric symptoms, severe acne can pose a serious problem with self-image and may influence adherence to lithium[28].

Other dermatoses

A number of case series and isolated reports point to rare skin ulcers and maculopapular eruptions in conjunction with lithium treatment. In one early case series of five lithium-treated patients, Callaway et al.[36] demonstrated the reversibility of lithium-related skin ulcers in a challenge–dechallenge–rechallenge design.

They also noted the spontaneous resolution of maculopapular eruptions despite ongoing therapeutic lithium levels in one instance. While Callaway's case series described leg ulcers, Srebrnik et al.[37] suggested that vaginal ulcers could also occur on lithium. Similarly, case reports of mucosal ulcerations[38] and two cases of geographic tongue, also known as benign migratory glossitis, have been reported. The glossitis appeared in an 8-year-old girl using lithium as add-on therapy to risperidone[39] and in a 30-year-old male on lithium monotherapy[40].

Rifkin et al. reported 12 cases of reversible folliculitis similar to dermatosis pilaris, occurring on the extensor sides of the extremities and sometimes on the trunk[41]. The time interval between starting lithium and the skin reactions varies widely, but can be as little as 6 h[42]. Isolated reports include a severe pruritis related to a dermatitis–herpetiformis-like reaction managed by reducing lithium and topical sulfones[43], reversible exfoliative dermatitis associated with the addition of 100 mg thioridazine (Melleril®)[44] and lichen planus resolving with lithium withdrawal and successfully managed with a topical steroid while lithium was continued[45]. One patient on lithium monotherapy developed a histologically verified erythema multiforme with high fever and widespread characteristic skin alterations. Remission occurred following discontinuation of lithium and systemic cortisone. Four days later a lithium re-challenge led to itching and fever even with concomitant high-dose steroid treatment[46].

Other unusual reports include a single case of histologically verified verrucous lesions in a patient who had been on lithium for 10 years, resistant to topical treatment but resolving on lithium discontinuation[47], and two cases of Darier's disease exacerbated or induced by lithium[48,49].

Hair loss

Most case reports of reversible lithium-induced alopecia[29–31] involve loss of scalp hair[32], with one report of pre-existing alopecia areata evolving into alopecia universalis[33]. Incidence estimates for hair loss vary widely from exceedingly rare to as high as 12%, and are based on small and selected samples[32,33], with reversibility upon lithium discontinuation the rule. Muniz et al.[34] reported on a female patient receiving lithium prophylaxis with diffuse effluvium at a normal thyroxin level. In view of her psychiatric symptoms, the lithium treatment was continued. Two months later the hair loss spontaneously resolved. Hair analysis showed an accumulation of lithium, a finding that was replicated by Schrauzer and co-workers in 1992[35]. The physiologic mechanism for lithium-induced hair loss is unknown, but lithium-induced hypothyroidism, itself associated with hair loss, should be considered.

CLINICAL MANAGEMENT OF LITHIUM-INDUCED SKIN CONDITIONS

Apart from constitutional factors – especially in the development of acne or psoriasis vulgaris – lithium dose plays an important role in the onset of cutaneous reactions. For mild skin conditions, e.g. mild acne or a small number of psoriatic lesions, usual dermatological treatment is suggested. For widespread dermatoses the treating psychiatrist should be consulted to discuss the possibility of a lithium reduction. In patients with severe, treatment-resistant psoriasis pustulosa and patients with widespread acne, respectively, a concurrent treatment using fumaric acid esters or retinoids (acitretinoin/Neotigason® and 13-cis-retin

acid/Roaccutane®, respectively) may be reasonable. Reliable contraception is essential for women on retinoids, because of their teratogenic effects. This may become an issue for manic or hypomanic patients.

As an alternative treatment for some cases of psoriasis, there is limited evidence for inositol supplementation. Using a crossover trial, Allen et al.[50] have recently described a positive response to inositol supplementation in 15 cases of lithium-related psoriasis. There is also an isolated case report of two patients with lithium-associated psoriasis treated successfully with omega-3 fatty acids[51]. At this stage, the evidence for both inositol and omega-3 fatty acids should be considered preliminary, requiring more rigorous trials before general recommendations can be made. In severe skin reactions, the advantages and disadvantages of ongoing lithium therapy must be balanced with the overall therapeutic effect of switching to an alternate mood stabilizer.

POTENTIAL THERAPEUTIC ROLES FOR LITHIUM IN DERMATOLOGY

There is growing high-quality evidence for the therapeutic effects of topical lithium preparations for seborrheic dermatitis[52], and there are anecdotal reports suggesting that it may have therapeutic benefits for herpetic infections[53–55]. These diverse effects serve to underscore the complex relationship between lithium salts and the skin, and some potential therapeutic benefits of lithium beyond psychiatry.

Acknowledgment

We thank Dr John Foerster, Department of Dermatology, Charité – University Medicine Berlin, for critically reviewing the manuscript.

REFERENCES

1. Bone S, Roose SP, Dunner DL, Fieve RR. Incidence of side effects in patients on long-term lithium therapy. Am J Psychiatry 1980; 137: 103–4

2. Sarantidis D, Waters B. A review and controlled study of cutaneous conditions associated with lithium carbonate. Br J Dermatol 1983; 143: 42–50

3. Chan HHL, Wing YK, Su R, Van Krevel C, Lee S. A control study of the cutaneous side effects of chronic lithium therapy. J Affect Disord 2000; 57: 107–13

4. Müller-Oerlinghausen B. 10 Jahre Lithium-Katamnese. Nervenarzt 1977; 48: 483–93

5. Gottlieb A. Psoriasis: emerging therapeutic strategies. Nature Rev Drug Discovery 2005; 4: 19–34

6. Bloomfield FJ, Young MM. Enhanced release of inflammatory mediators from lithium-stimulated neutrophils in psoriasis. Br J Dermatol 1983; 109: 13

7. Beyaert R, Schulze-Osthoff K, Van Roy F, Fiers W. Synergistic induction of interleukin-6 by tumor necrosis factor and lithium chloride in mice: possible role in the triggering and exacerbation of psoriasis by lithium treatment. Eur J Immunol 1992; 22: 2181–4

8. Ockenfels HM, Nussbaum G, Schultewolter T, et al. Tyrosine phosphorylation in psoriatic T cells is modulated by drugs that induce or improve psoriasis. Dermatology 1995; 191: 217–25

9. Efalith Multicenter Trial Group. A double-blind, placebo-controlled, multicenter trial of lithium succinate ointment in the treatment of seborrheic dermatitis. J Am Acad Dermatol 1992; 26: 452–7

10. Hanada K, Sawamura D, Sone K, Hashimoto I. Can lithium in spring water provoke psoriasis? Lancet 1997; 350: 1522

11. Voorhees JJ, Marcels CL, Duell EA. Cyclic AMP, cyclic GMP, and glucocorticoids as potential metabolic regulators of epidermal proliferation and differentiation. J Invest Dermatol 1975; 65: 179–90

12. Skott A, Mobacken H, Starmark JE. Exacerbation of psoriasis during lithium treatment. Br J Dermatol 1977; 96, 445–8

13. Reiffers J, Dick P. Manifestations cutanees par le lithium. Dermatologica 1977; 155: 155–63

14. Skoven I, Thormann J. Lithium compound treatment and psoriasis. Arch Dermatol 1979; 115: 1185–7

15. Evans DL, Martin W. Lithium carbonate and psoriasis. Am J Psychiatry 1979; 136: 1325–7

16. Bakker JB, Pepplinkhuizen L. More about the relationship of lithium to psoriasis. Psychosomatics 1976; 17: 143–6

17. Lowe NJ, Ridgeway HB. Generalized pustular psoriasis precipitated by lithium carbonate. Arch Dermatol 1978; 114: 1788–9

18. Ruiz-Maldonado R, De Francisco CP, Tamayo L. Lithiumdermatitis. JAMA 1973; 224: 1534

19. Yoder FW. Acneiform eruption due to lithium carbonate. Arch Dermatol 1975; 111: 396–7

20. Okrasinski H. Lithium acne. Dermatologia 1977; 154: 251–3

21. Hong MCY. Cutaneous manifestations of lithium toxicity. Br J Dermatol 1982; 106: 107–9

22. Rüther H. Nebenwirkungen von Lithium an der Haut. Hautarzt 1983; 34 (Suppl VI): 272–3

23. Stamm T, Lubach D. Unerwuenschte Nebenwirkungen and der Haut durch Lithium-Therapie. Kasuistik und Literaturuebersicht. Psychiat Prax 1981; 8: 152–4

24. Gupta AK, Knowles SR, Gupka MA, et al. Lithium therapy associated with hidradenitis suppurativa: a case report and a review of the dermatologic side effects of lithium. J Am Acad Dermatol 1995; 32: 382–6

25. Strothmeyer FJ. Klinische Untersuchungen zur Beeinflussung der Talgexkretion der menschlichen Haut durch zentral wirksame Pharmaka. Perazin, L-Dihydroxyphenylalanin (L-Dopa) und Lithiumacetat. Medical Dissertation, Freie Universität Berlin, 1974

26. Webster GF. Pustular drug reactions. Clin Dermatol 1993; 11: 541–3

27. Kanzaki T. Acneiform eruption induced by lithium carbonate. J Dermatol 1991; 18: 481–3

28. Deandrea D, Walker N, Mehlmauer M, White K. Dermatological reactions to lithium: a

critical review of the literature. J Clin Psychopharmacol 1982; 2: 199–204

29. Dawber R, Mortimer P. Hair loss during lithium treatment. Br J Dermatol 1982; 107: 124–5

30. Baudhuin M, Griest JM, Jefferson JW, Ackerman DL. Lithium and hair loss. Br J Dermatol 1983; 109: 492

31. Ghadirian AM, Lalinec-Michaud M. Report of a patient with lithium-related alopecia and psoriasis. J Clin Psychiatry 1986; 47: 212–13

32. Yassa R. Hair loss during lithium therapy. Am J Psychiatry 1986; 143: 7

33. Orwin A. Hair loss following lithium therapy. Br J Dermatol 1983; 108: 503–4

34. Muniz CE, Salem RB, Director KL. Hair loss in a patient receiving lithium. Psychosomatics 1982; 23: 312–13

35. Schrauzer GN, Shrestha KP, Flores-Arce MF. Lithium in scalp hair of adults, students, and violent criminals. Effects of supplementation and evidence for interactions of lithium with vitamin B12 and with other trace elements. Biol Trace Elem Res 1992; 34: 161–76

36. Callaway CL, Hendrie HC, Luby CB, Luby ED. Cutaneous conditions observed in patients during treatment with lithium. Am J Psychiatry 1968; 124: 1124–5

37. Srebrnik A, Bar-Nathan EA, Lie B, et al. Vaginal ulcerations due to lithium carbonate therapy. Cutis 1991; 48: 65–6

38. Nathan KI. Development of mucosal ulcerations with lithium carbonate therapy. Am J Psychiatry 1995; 152: 956–7

39. Gracious BL, Llana M, Barton DD. Lithium and geographic tongue. J Am Acad Child Adolesc Psychiatry 1999; 38: 1069–70

40. Pataki AH. Geographic tongue developing in a patient on lithium carbonate therapy [Letter]. Int J Dermatol 1992; 31: 368–9

41. Rifkin A, Kurtin SB, Quitkin F, Klein DF. Lithium-induced folliculitis. Am J Psychiatry 1973; 130: 1018–19

42. Meinhold JM, West DP, Gurwich E, et al. Cutaneous reaction to lithium carbonate: a case report. J Clin Psychiat 1980; 41: 395–6

43. Posey RE. Lithium carbonate dermatitis [Letter]. JAMA 1972; 221: 1517

44. Kuhnley EJ, Granoff AL. Exfoliative dermatitis during lithium treatment. Am J Psychiatry 1979; 136: 1340–1

45. Schukla S, Mukherjee S. Lichen simplex chronicus during lithium treatment. Am J Psychiatry 1984; 141: 909–10

46. Balldin J, Berggren U, Heiger A. Erythema multiforme caused by lithium. J Am Dermatol 1991; 24: 1015–16

47. Frenk E. Entzündlich-verruköse, umschriebene Hyperplasien der Haut im Verlaufe einer Lithium-Langzeitbehandlung. Z Hautkr 1984; 59: 97–100

48. Milton GP, Peck GL, Fu JJ, et al. Exacerbation of Darier's disease by lithium carbonate. J Am Acad Dermatol 1990; 23: 926–8

49. Rubin MB. Lithium induced Darier's disease. J Am Acad Dermatol 1995; 32: 674–5

50. Allen SJ, Kavanagh GM, Herd RM, Savin JA. The effect of inositol supplements on the psoriasis of patients taking lithium: a randomized, placebo-controlled trial. Br J Dermatol 2004; 150: 966–9

51. Akkerhuis GW, Nolen WA. Lithium-associated psoriasis and omega-3 fatty acids. Am J Psychiatry 2003; 160: 1355

52. Dreno B, Chosidow O, Revuz J, Moyse D. Lithium gluconate 8% vs. ketoconazole 2% in the treatment of seborrhoeic dermatitis: a multi-centre, randomized study. Br J Dermatol 2003; 148: 1230–6

53. Jefferson JW. Antiviral therapies for long-term suppression of genital herpes [Letter]. JAMA 1999; 281: 1170–1

54. Bschor T. Complete suppression of recurrent herpes labialis with lithium carbonate. Pharmacopsychiatry 1999; 32: 158

55. Amsterdam JD, Maislin G, Hooper MB. Suppression of herpes simplex virus infections with oral lithium carbonate – a possible antiviral activity. Pharmacotherapy 1996; 16: 1070–5

Part C

PHARMACOLOGY AND MECHANISMS

27 Lithium: its chemistry, distribution and transport in the body

Nick J Birch

Contents   Chemistry of lithium • Properties of lithium in biological systems • Methods for the determination of lithium and its isotopes • Distribution and transport of lithium in biological systems • Methods for studying transport of lithium • Summary

CHEMISTRY OF LITHIUM

Lithium is an odd-ball: it is the smallest and lightest solid element, it has unusual clinical, pharmacologic and biochemical properties, it is not classified into any generally accepted group of drugs, it cannot be patented and it can be dug out of the ground very cheaply. Yet after more than 55 years of widespread clinical use, it is still interesting because of its apparent simplicity. Its physicochemical properties are by no means as complex as those of the organic drugs with which we are much more familiar. These properties also may be of particular value in our understanding of other fundamental processes in drug–receptor interactions specifically because of the relative simplicity of the interactions involved.

The place of lithium in the chemistry of the elements

Lithium was discovered by August Arfwedson in 1817 in the mineral ore pétalite[1]. Berzelius named it lithion (Greek: *lithos*, stone). Most lithium is used commercially in production of lightweight metal alloys, glass, lubrication greases and electrical batteries. Less than 1% is used in medicine. Lithium occurs naturally in biological tissues and hence in foodstuffs[2] and drinking water. Natural waters containing high concentrations of this and other metals are sold as 'mineral waters' with supposed medicinal properties. Lithium's possible essentiality and its toxicity have been reviewed[3].

Structural aspects and place in the periodic table

Lithium appears in the first row of the periodic table (Figure 27.1); it is typically anomalous in its properties. It is the lightest solid element, it has the smallest ionic radius amongst the alkali metals and the largest field density at its surface, and it is the least reactive. In solution, the very small diameter of the naked lithium ion in relation to the aqueous solvent results in a large

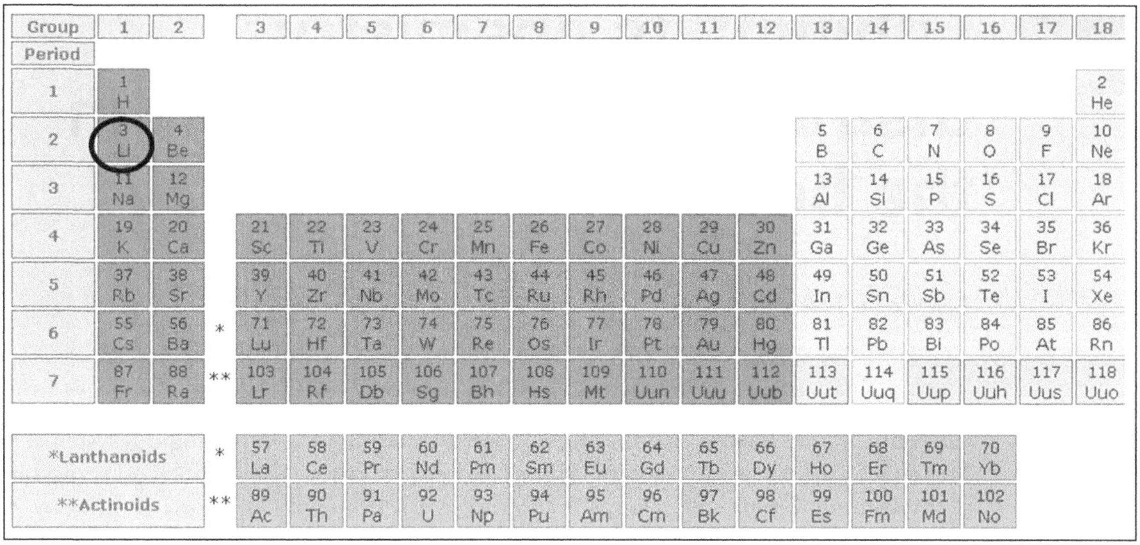

Figure 27.1 Lithium's place in the periodic table

hydration sphere the size of which is uncertain. The hydrated radius of lithium is increased out of proportion to the radius of the other alkali metal elements, resulting in poor ionic mobility, non-conformity to ideal solution behavior[4] and low lipid solubility under physiologic conditions.

The chemistry of lithium is similar to that of magnesium, being described classically by the so-called 'diagonal relationship'. Lithium may interact with magnesium- and calcium-dependent processes in physiology[5–7].

Chemistry of the element and its compounds

Lithium, like magnesium, forms covalent compounds, and organolithium compounds are formed, analogous to organomagnesium compounds. Like magnesium, lithium halides, except fluoride, are highly soluble in polar solvents and their alkyls are soluble in hydrocarbons. Both metals have water-insoluble carbonates, phosphates, oxalates and fluorides and both react directly to form a nitride and carbide. Lithium chemistry is an area of substantial commercial importance. The stable isotope ^6Li absorbs neutrons and is used in the manufacture of regulator rods for thermonuclear reactors.

PROPERTIES OF LITHIUM IN BIOLOGICAL SYSTEMS

In 1859, Garrod first described its medical use for the treatment of rheumatic conditions and gout, and particularly mentioned lithium use in 'brain gout', a depressive disorder[8]. Lithium urate is the most soluble salt of uric acid and was predicted to increase uric acid excretion to relieve gout. Lithium carbonate and citrate were in the *British Pharmacopoeia* of 1885. Lithium bromide was also considered to be the most effective of the bromide hypnotics.

It is more than 50 years since lithium became the first modern psychopharmacological agent; its clinical value in psychiatry was discovered in 1949 by John Cade, an Australian psychiatrist[9]. There was then no effective drug treatment for any major psychiatric disease and the first observation of the effect of lithium in the treatment of acute mania must have been extremely startling and exciting. Unfortunately, the serious toxic effects of lithium were first recognized quite independently at about the same time, when lithium salts were used as a salt substitute in the treatment of hypertension in the USA, and this led to a 15-year restriction by the Food and Drugs Administration (FDA) on the psychiatric use of lithium in the USA despite very strong evidence obtained in Europe of its safety and efficacy when properly regulated[10].

During the 1950s Schou and others showed that lithium could safely be used in manic-depressive disorder at lower doses than those used by Cade and, because of the paucity of other drugs, the spectrum of therapeutic activity of lithium widened for a time, to include a broad range of psychiatric disorders, including schizophrenia. It is currently used in the prophylaxis of bipolar affective disorders[11]. Additional psychiatric benefits of lithium treatment may include a reduction in actual and attempted suicide[12]. It is estimated that about between 500 000 and one million patients receive it worldwide.

METHODS FOR THE DETERMINATION OF LITHIUM AND ITS ISOTOPES

Methods for the determination of lithium in a variety of biologic situations have been extensively reviewed by Thellier and Wissocq[13]. Lithium may be determined most accurately in aqueous solutions using atomic absorption spectroscopy (AAS) or flame emission spectroscopy (FES) using the 670.8-nm spectral line or, if more sensitivity is required, flameless electrothermal atomic absorption spectroscopy (ETAAS) may be used.

There are no useful radioisotopes of lithium (isotopes ^{5}Li, ^{8}Li and ^{9}Li have half-lives of 0.8, 0.2 and 10^{-21} s). In nature, lithium occurs as a mixture of the two stable isotopes ^{7}Li (92.58%) and ^{6}Li (7.42%), which may be distinguished using isotopic shift atomic absorption spectrometry (ISAAS)[14], neutron activation analysis, nuclear reactions with neutrons or with charged particles[13], secondary ion mass spectrometry (SIMS)[15] and nuclear magnetic resonance (NMR) spectroscopy[16]. As well as imaging[17], the latter is also capable of distinguishing between lithium in the intracellular and extracellular compartments[16].

Spectroscopic methods

Lithium is most accurately determined by AAS[18], although FES is the most commonly used method in clinical laboratories. Both methods require the separation by centrifugation of blood cells from blood plasma to enable the preparation of a diluted serum or plasma sample. The advantage of AAS and FES is that, under normal conditions, they are both sensitive enough to be performed on simple aqueous dilutions of blood serum and hence do not require substantial and time-consuming sample preparation.

Flame emission spectroscopy (flame photometry)

When a sample of material in solution is sprayed into a flame, each element emits a spectrum characteristic of that element and at an intensity which is proportional to its concentration (in accordance with the Beer–Lambert Law). Therefore, it is possible to measure the concentration of any element in the sample by measuring the light emitted at each wavelength that forms part of the element's spectrum. However, in practice, many elements, particularly non-metals, are not sufficiently energized by being injected into the hot flame to emit a powerful enough signal.

Lithium is readily detected and has a strong signal, but the problem inherent in FES is that there are so many spectral lines of high intensity from sodium and potassium that there is spectral interference between the three elements. Since sodium is present at around 150 times larger concentration than lithium, the lithium spectrum is seriously disturbed. FES is inexpensive and it is possible to measure different elements simultaneously by setting up an array of detectors around the flame.

Atomic absorption spectroscopy

The converse of emission occurs when a sample of an element is irradiated by a beam of light whose frequency is one that is characteristic of that same element. Light is absorbed in proportion to the concentration of the element, again according to the Beer–Lambert Law. The major advantage of absorption spectra is, however, that they are line spectra. Emission spectra are composed of a very large number of individual emission lines which act as if they were band spectra: each spectral 'line' in emission is a broad peak and these overlap with each other to cause interference between analyses of different elements. Absorption lines are very sharp and spectral interference is highly unlikely. However, the disadvantage of the AAS analytical system is that, in order to measure the absorption resulting from a sample, it is necessary to generate the specific spectral line of that element, using a hollow cathode lamp, and have a very sensitive and spectrally stable detection system; prisms or diffraction gratings are the most common form of spectral selection. This is substantially more expensive than a simple flame photometer. The interferences in AAS are relatively minor and can be obviated by a suitable choice of diluent[18].

Atomic absorption methods for the isotopes of lithium

The two useful, non-radioactive, isotopes of lithium have absorption spectra that are doublets, the two lines being separated by 0.015 nm. By coincidence, the separation of the two isotopes is also 0.015 nm and thus 'natural lithium', which comprises 93% ^{7}Li and 7% ^{6}Li, appears to be a triplet.

The separation of the various lines is below the level of resolution of conventional absorption spectroscopy but, by having two atomic absorption hollow cathode lamps made of the two separate isotopes, it is possible to distinguish them because the atoms of each isotope absorb light most strongly from the hollow cathode lamp made of the same isotope. It is possible, therefore, to set up calibration curves for the absorbance ratio (A_6/A_7) versus the atom ratio of each isotope ($[^6Li]/[^7Li]$ atom ratio) at different concentrations[19].

Nuclear magnetic resonance spectroscopy

The NMR spectra of ^{7}Li and ^{6}Li are markedly different, but much of the work in biological systems has been carried out with ^{7}Li because the signal acquisition time for ^{6}Li spectra is long and the sensitivity is poor within the usual timescale of biological experiments. Using ^{7}Li NMR it is possible to differentiate between atoms or ions that are within the cell and those that are free in the extracellular bathing fluid[16].

The use of lithium NMR has been reviewed by Komoroski[17].

Sample collection for lithium determination

Many standard blood collection tubes contain anticoagulants that affect lithium determination. Lithium–heparin is widely used for collection of plasma samples for electrolyte and other determinations. Plasma lithium concentrations as high as 2.0 mmol/l have been reported in subjects who had not received lithium but whose blood was collected in lithium–heparin tubes[20]. It is vital that laboratories should be aware of the anticoagulant used when lithium is being determined. For this reason lithium is routinely determined in serum (i.e. clotted blood) rather than plasma. However, this is not possible for the rapid analysis using the lithium ion selective electrode, since this determination is carried out on whole blood. Such analyses are usually carried out using the calcium, sodium or ammonium salts of heparin as anticoagulant.

The problem is more likely to occur where laboratories and clinicians carry out infrequent lithium analyses. This is a potential problem in toxicologic and forensic laboratories where there may not be the routine lithium experience which is usually available in a pathology laboratory that monitors lithium patients on a regular basis.

Lithium ion selective electrodes

Lithium analysis using flame photometric methods on-site in the interview room is difficult in the presence of the patient, and thus the results of blood estimations frequently are not available to the patient and psychiatrist until a considerable time after the psychiatric interview, because of the need to send samples to a remote laboratory for estimation. The consequent delay of despatch and receipt of the report may result in poor patient compliance.

Ion selective electrode (ISE) systems are now available which allow the analysis of lithium in blood plasma in the presence of blood cells without centrifugation. The electrode measures the activity in solution of lithium ion and thus the electrical effects of the relatively large blood cells suspended in the plasma are negligible. ISEs provide individual and instant results from a small quantity of venous or capillary blood[21]. Their accuracy and reliability are comparable to those of conventional methods.

Instant lithium monitoring

The immediate feedback is a major advantage and gives the patient confidence. Unlike conventional practice where clinical review and laboratory monitoring are separate and often uncoordinated processes, ISEs enable both to be carried out simultaneously. Dosage may be changed immediately and all aspects of assessment and monitoring may be achieved in one visit[22].

The clinician no longer needs to review the medication blindly nor to rely only on results available from the last visit. A blood sample is taken and the results are discussed with the patient before the review is concluded. In addition, the patient can see the analysis as it takes place and the result as it appears on the screen of the analyzer some 30 seconds later. There can be no doubt about the ownership of the result: denials and excuses with regard to compliance are not possible, and doubtful or disputed results can be repeated immediately. Patients who have defaulted on treatment may be faced with this with confidence[22].

This instant feedback provides powerful psychological reinforcement of the advice of the physician. Since each patient visit is potentially expensive (loss of earnings or travel costs), embarrassing or traumatic, the single appointment is helpful in encouraging compliance[22]. For the psychiatrist the benefits are quickly appreciated. Time is saved because only one interview is required. Changes in medication may be more rapidly monitored and, in the initial stages of lithium treatment, the time taken to reach a stable plasma lithium concentration can be reduced by giving the new dose immediately.

DISTRIBUTION AND TRANSPORT OF LITHIUM IN BIOLOGICAL SYSTEMS

One of the problems in studying lithium action is the lack of precision in localization of the ion and the measurement of its movements between cells and tissues. This is partly because lithium is a very mobile ion, partly because of its widespread distribution in the body and partly because of the difficulties of lithium analysis. Analytical problems generally do not stem from the lack of sensitivity but from the interference of related metals and common anions present in large quantities in animal tissues.

Methods for studying distribution

The microlocalization technique with the stable isotope ^{6}Li uses a beam of neutrons in an atomic reactor. ^{6}Li nuclei absorb a neutron and immediately the nucleus undergoes fission to produce an α-particle and a ^{3}H atom, which create tracks in a suitable detector placed in contact with ^{6}Li-containing tissue. The tissue distribution in the rat[23], brain lithium distribution in the mouse[24] and rat[25], distribution in mouse embryo[26] and kinetics in mouse brain have been studied. Thellier's group, using the isotope ^{6}Li, provided visual localization of lithium in the whole body[26] and in the different

areas of the brain[27]. Recently, the lithium distribution in a single oocyte of *Xenopus* sp. was reported[15].

NMR techniques may also be used in imaging lithium in living experimental animals and in patients[17,28,29].

METHODS FOR STUDYING TRANSPORT OF LITHIUM

Cellular localization of lithium

Lithium is a very mobile, small ion and it has been difficult to define its distribution within the living cell, though attempts have been made using the stable isotopes ^{6}Li and ^{7}Li with ISAAS and NMR[16,30,31]. Direct subcellular localization using nuclear techniques has shown promising results[15]. Much of the evidence of intracellular free lithium concentration has depended on analysis of separated cells and extrapolations from lithium-transport data[32]. These techniques cannot distinguish between lithium inside cells and that attached to, or entrapped in, cellular membranes.

Studies have been performed in human and animal erythrocytes and in cells obtained from other animal sources[16,33]. Both ^{7}Li NMR and ISAAS studies were carried out on lithium-loaded erythrocytes from previously untreated subjects. The erythrocyte internal lithium concentration was under 8% of the external concentration after incubation in a range of external lithium concentrations between 2 and 40 mmol/l for up to 3 hours[34,35]. The results from NMR and ISAAS methods were in close agreement. Other workers have reported broadly comparable results[30,36–38].

It is clear from studies of erythrocytes, hepatocytes, fibroblasts and astrocytoma cells that lithium does not distribute at equilibrium according to the cellular membrane potential (in these examples between -40 and -60 mV). This may be due either to low membrane permeability or alternatively a mechanism of effective ejection of the ion from the cell interior. In all of these cell types lithium is less readily transported across the cell membrane than had been believed hitherto. These results have been broadly confirmed in SIMS and NCR experiments[39].

A number of ion channels are known to accept lithium relatively easily, and under ideal conditions these cells may show significant lithium currents. Ehrlich et al.[32] have suggested that by calculation from the Nernst equation there should be a 10-fold excess of lithium within the cell, compared with the exterior, in an excitable cell maintaining its normal potential. In practice it has never been possible to demonstrate a concentration excess higher than 4-fold. There is significant resistance to lithium influx through cell membranes.

Intracellular and extracellular lithium concentrations

Most theories of lithium action assume that the ion occurs in the fluid compartment of cells in substantial concentrations. This has not been questioned and indeed the concentration of lithium at which experiments have been carried out has ignored even the best current estimates of relevant cell lithium concentrations. Much early lithium 'pharmacology', still cited, was carried out in experiments where sodium in physiologic solution was replaced by equimolar lithium concentrations (often 150 mmol/l).

Lithium transport through cell membranes

Lithium transport across cell membranes has been studied most extensively in erythrocytes. However, these cells may not reflect accurately the uptake into other cells, since red blood cell morphology is atypical as is its metabolism. Five pathways for lithium transport in erythrocytes have been described[40].

Sodium–potassium ATPase

Lithium replaces potassium at the external surface of sodium–potassium ATPase and is transported into the cell. This is blocked by ouabain[40]. In frog skin epithelium lithium may be transported out only when sodium occupies the activator site on the inner membrane surface. The multiple intracellular sites are the same for sodium and lithium, and the stoichiometry is three lithium or three sodium ions pumped out for every two potassium ions pumped in[40].

Sodium–potassium co-transport

Lithium also enters the chloride-dependent sodium–potassium co-transport system, inhibited by furosemide[40]. Lithium and rubidium in the external medium can be simultaneously transported, and it is thought that they can replace sodium and potassium, respectively.

Leak

Leak is a downhill lithium transport system inhibited by dipyridamole (and partly by phloretin). Sodium and potassium may share this pathway[40].

Anion exchange

Anion exchange allows lithium co-transport with carbonate via an ouabain and phloretin insensitive route[40]. In solution, the divalent carbonate ion (always present in a bicarbonate solution) is capable of forming negatively charged ion pairs with sodium ($Na^+ + CO_2^{2-}$) or lithium ($Li^+ + CO_2^{2-}$) which then gain access to the anion exchange system. The single charged ion pair exchanges for a monovalent anion such as chloride. This is probably a physiologic route for sodium, but not for potassium, which is incapable of forming the ion pair with carbonate. The locus of this mechanism is probably the 'band III protein' described by Cabantchik for erythrocyte anion transport[41,42].

Sodium–lithium exchange

Lithium efflux occurs via sodium–lithium countertransport, which is ouabain insensitive, is blocked by phloretin, is independent of ATP and exhibits saturation. It is thought that lithium substitutes for sodium in a Na^+–Na^+ countertransport system whose physiologic function is unclear. A 1:1 stoichiometry occurs and the maximum affinity for both cations occurs at the internal surface, that for lithium being 20–30 times higher than for sodium[40].

Lithium transport *in vivo*

Lithium–sodium countertransport, anion exchange and the leak mechanism are thought to be the most important transport routes for lithium *in vivo*. All are potentially bidirectional, but the overall direction of flow under physiologic conditions is efflux from the cell using lithium–sodium countertransport and cell uptake with the anion exchange mechanism. A proportion of both cellular uptake and efflux of lithium can be attributed to passive diffusion.

Lithium efflux from human erythrocytes eventually becomes inhibited by approximately 50% in persons whose plasma contains lithium at prophylactically effective concentrations[43]. This involves a decrease in the apparent affinity of the countertransport mechanism for lithium associated with a 3-fold increase in the apparent

K_m, without any change in the countertransport rate V_{max}. This delayed inhibition of sodium–lithium countertransport is not due to a humoral factor or to delays in lithium entry to the cells, and is only partly due to pharmacokinetic delays. A slow process in the erythrocyte, possibly involving structural changes in the membrane or affecting membrane-bound enzymes has been suggested as the mechanism for this change[32]. These observations may explain the relatively long, but variable, period of time required for the beneficial effects of lithium to become clinically apparent, and show that lithium uptake and efflux experiments using cells from subjects who have not had recent exposure to lithium may not reflect accurately events in stabilized lithium-treated patients.

SUMMARY

The chemistry of lithium is relatively simple but it is anomalous because of the small size of the Li atom and the relatively high charge/volume ratio of the Li^+ cation. The hydrated radius, by contrast, is large because the high charge density leads to a high degree of hydration of the Li^+ ion and this leads to atypical properties in aqueous solution. Lithium chemistry is similar to that of magnesium, with which it may compete in biological systems.

Because of its lack of useful radioactive isotopes the majority of lithium studies have been carried out using spectroscopic techniques, the best of which has been atomic absorption spectroscopy. More recently, NMR spectroscopy has been applied to studies of distribution and in biochemical studies of lithium effects on enzymes and transmitter systems. Stable isotope studies using the non-radioactive isotopes ^6Li and ^7Li, though limited by their analytical complexity, may provide new insights in the future.

REFERENCES

1. Arfwedson A. Untersuchung einiger bei der Eisen-Grube von Utö vorkommenden Fosilien und von einem darin gefundenen neuen feuerfesten Alkali. Schweiggers J Chem Physik 1818; 22: 93–120

2. Anke M, Arnhold W, Muller M, Illing H. The transfer of lithium – an essential element for animals and man? – in the food chain. J Trace Microprobe Tech 1995; 13: 493

3. Shafer U. Essentiality and toxicity of lithium. J Trace Microprobe Tech 1997; 15: 341–9

4. Stern KH, Amis ES. Ionic size, a comprehensive review on radii in crystals. Chem Rev 1959; 59: 1

5. Birch NJ. Effects of lithium on plasma magnesium. Br J Psychiatry 1970; 116: 461

6. Birch NJ. Possible mechanism for biological action of lithium. Nature 1976; 264: 681

7. Fonseca CP, Montezinho LP, Nabais C, et al. Effects of Li+ transport and intracellular binding on Li+/Mg2+ competition in bovine chromaffin cells. Biochim Biophys Acta 2004; 1691: 79–90

8. Garrod AB. The Nature and Treatment of Gout and Rheumatic Gout, 1st edn. London: Walton and Maberly, 1859

9. Cade JFJ. Lithium salts in the treatment of psychotic excitement. Med J Aust 1949; 36: 349–52

10. Johnson FN. The History of Lithium Therapy, 1st edn. London: Macmillan, 1984

11. Schou M. Lithium Treatment of Manic Depressive Illness: A Practical Guide, 4th edn. Basel: Karger, 1989

12. Coppen A, Farmer R. Suicide mortality in patients on lithium maintenance therapy. J Affect Disord 1998; 50: 261–7

13. Thellier M, Wissocq J-C. Methods for the determination of the distribution of lithium at the histological and cytological levels. In Birch NJ, ed. Lithium and the Cell: Pharmacology and Biochemistry. London: Academic Press, 1991: 59–84

14. Birch NJ, Robinson D, Inie RA, Hullin RP. 6-Li: a stable isotope of lithium determined by atomic absorption spectroscopy and its use in human pharmacokinetic studies. J Pharm Pharmacol 1978; 30: 683–5

15. Thellier M, Ripoll C. NCR and SIMS study of whether lithium ions have limited intracellular access. J Trace Microprobe Tech 1995; 13: 536

16. Hughes MS. Intracellular concentrations of lithium as studied by nuclear magnetic resonance spectroscopy. In Birch NJ, ed. Lithium and the Cell. London: Academic Press, 1991: 175–84

17. Komoroski RA. Applications of (7)Li NMR in biomedicine. Magn Reson Imaging 2000; 18: 103–16

18. Birch NJ, Jenner FA. The distribution of lithium and its effects on the distribution and excretion of other ions in the rat. Br J Pharm 1973; 47: 586–94

19. Birch NJ, Hullin RP, Inie RA, Robinson D. Use of the stable isotope 6-Li in human pharmacokinetic studies. Br J Clin Pharmacol 1978; 5: 351–2

20. Lee DC, Klachko MN. Falsely elevated lithium levels in plasma obtained in lithium containing tubes. Clin Toxicol 1996; 34: 467–9

21. Greil W, Runge H, Steller B. Immediate blood lithium determination with an ion selective electrode. A new method for lithium determination for improved lithium therapy. Sofortbestimmung von Lithium im Blut mittels ionenselektiver Elektrode. Eine neue Lithiumbestimmungsmethode zur Verbesserung der Lithiumtherapie. Nervenarzt 1992; 63: 184–6

22. Srinivasan DP, Birch NJ. Lithium ion-selective electrode: field experience in a peripheral psychiatric clinic. J Trace Microprobe Tech 1995; 13: 53–7

23. Nelson SC, Herman MM, Bensch KG, et al. Localization and quantitation of lithium in rat tissue following intraperitoneal injections of lithium chloride: I. Thyroid, thymus, heart, kidney, adrenal, testis. Exp Mol Pathol 1976; 25: 38–48

24. Heurteaux C, Wissocq J-C, Stelz T, Thellier M. Microlocalisation quantitative de lithium dans le cerveau de la souris. Biol Cell 1979; 35: 251–8

25. Nelson SC, Herman MM, Bensch KG, Barchas JD. Localization and quantitation of lithium in rat tissue following intraperitoneal injections of

lithium chloride: II. Brain. J Pharmacol Exp Ther 1980; 212: 11–15

26. Wissocq J-C, Hennequin E, Heurteaux C, et al. Microlocalization of lithium in biological samples using a specific nuclear reaction: preliminary data about Li-distribution in young vertebrate embryos. In Anke M, Baumann W, Braunlich H, Bruckner C, eds. Spurenelement Symposium, Leipzig and Jena: Karl-Marx Universitat and Friedrich-Schiller Universitat, 1983; 4: 127–33

27. Hennequin E, Ouznadji H, Martini F, et al. Mapping of lithium in the brain and various organs of the mouse embryo. J Trace Microprobe Tech 1998; 16: 119–24

28. Komoroski RA, Pearce JM, Newton JE. The distribution of lithium in rat brain and muscle in vivo by 7Li NMR imaging [In Process Citation]. Magn Reson Med 1997; 38: 275–8

29. Komoroski RA, Newton JE, Sprigg JR, et al. In vivo 7Li nuclear magnetic resonance study of lithium pharmacokinetics and chemical shift imaging in psychiatric patients. Psychiatry Res 1993; 50: 67–76

30. Abraha A, Dorus E, Mota de Freitas D. Nuclear magnetic resonance study of differences between 6Li and 7Li ions in transport across human red blood cell membranes. Lithium 1991; 2: 118–21

31. Riddell FG, Bramham J. The use of lithium nuclear magnetic resonance to study biological lithium. In Birch NJ, Padgham C, Hughes MS, eds. Lithium in Medicine and Biology. Carnforth: Marius Press, 1993: 253–65

32. Ehrlich BE, Diamond JM, Fry V, Meier K. Lithium's inhibition of erythrocyte cation countertransport involves a slow process in the erythrocyte. J Membr Biol 1983; 75: 233–40

33. Thomas GMH, Hughes MS, Partridge S, et al. NMR studies of lithium transport in isolated hepatocytes. Biochem Soc Trans 1988; 16: 208

34. Partridge S, Hughes MS, Thomas GMH, Birch NJ. Lithium transport in erythrocytes. Biochem Soc Trans 1988; 16: 205–6

35. Hughes MS. Multinuclear NMR studies in lithium pharmacology. In Birch NJ, ed. Lithium: Inorganic Pharmacology and Psychiatric Use. Oxford: IRL Press, 1988: 285–8

36. Riddell FG. Studies on Li+ transport using 7-Li and 6-Li nuclear magnetic resonance. In Birch NJ, ed. Lithium and the Cell: Pharmacology and Biochemistry. London: Academic Press, 1991: 85–98

37. Mota de Freitas D, Silberberg J, Espanol MT, et al. Measurement of lithium transport in RBC from psychiatric patients receiving lithium carbonate and normal individuals by 7Li NMR spectroscopy. Biol Psychiatry 1990; 28: 415–24

38. Riddell FG, Patel A, Hughes MS. Lithium uptake rate and lithium : lithium exchange rate in human erythrocytes at a nearly pharmaco-logically normal level monitored by 7Li NMR. J Inorg Biochem 1990; 39: 187–92

39. Thellier ME, Wissocq J-C, Ripoll C. NCR and SIMS study of whether lithium ions have limited intracellular access. J Trace Microprobe Tech 1997; 15: 93–9

40. Duhm J. Pathways of lithium transport across the human erythrocyte membrane. In Thellier M, Wissocq J-C, eds. Lithium Kinetics. Carnforth: Marius Press, 1992: 27–53

41. Schofield AE, Reardon DM, Tanner MJA. Defective anion transport activity of the abnormal band-3 in hereditary ovalocytic red blood cells. Nature 1992; 355: 836–8

42. Cabantchik ZI, Knauf PA, Rothstein A. The anion transport system of the red blood cell: the role of membrane protein evaluated by the use of probes. Biochim Biophys Acta 1978; 515: 239–302

43. Phillips JD, Hughes MS, Birch NJ. Lithium–sodium countertransport and intracellular free magnesium in normal volunteers. In Lasserre B, Durlach J, eds. Magnesium – a Relevant Ion? London: John Libbey, 1991: 295–8

28 Pharmacokinetics of lithium

Martin Alda

Contents   Introduction • Absorption •Distribution • Elimination • Practical applications

INTRODUCTION

From the pharmacokinetic point of view, lithium is a simple drug. It is not metabolized, and it is not bound to proteins. Unless used in a special formulation, it is absorbed rapidly from the gastrointestinal system and eliminated almost exclusively via the kidneys in a manner mostly dependent on serum levels. For understanding the behavior of lithium in the body, it is helpful although simplifying to remember lithium as being handled similarly to sodium.

In this chapter I focus on those pharmacokinetic aspects of lithium that are clinically relevant. More basic chemical properties of lithium are addressed in Chapter 27, and practical aspects of lithium treatment including monitoring of blood levels are described in Chapter 37 of this book.

ABSORPTION

When administered orally, lithium is absorbed completely within 6–8 hours. The absorption from the gastrointestinal system is usually rapid with peak plasma levels reached between 1 and 3 hours after ingestion. Food does not interfere with lithium absorption, and thus it is often advantageous for patients to take lithium after meals in order to reduce stomach irritation that may otherwise occur.

Certain lithium preparations use a slow-release formulation to reduce the post-absorption peaks of plasma levels. Such preparations can be helpful in patients prone to gastric upset or transient side-effects (e.g. tremor) secondary to temporary increases of blood levels. On the other hand, the slower absorption may contribute to variable bioavailability of lithium, for instance in clinical states with increased gastrointestinal passage[1]. Another point to keep in mind is that 12-hour levels in patients on slow-release lithium are close to peak levels and may be more susceptible to random variation, making the laboratory monitoring more difficult (Figure 28.1). In fact, some slow-release preparations may be associated with half-lives of absorption in excess of 4 or 5 hours (which is even higher than the parameters used to generate the levels in the graph). In such cases, the 12-hour levels may correspond to still rising plasma levels and also the incomplete

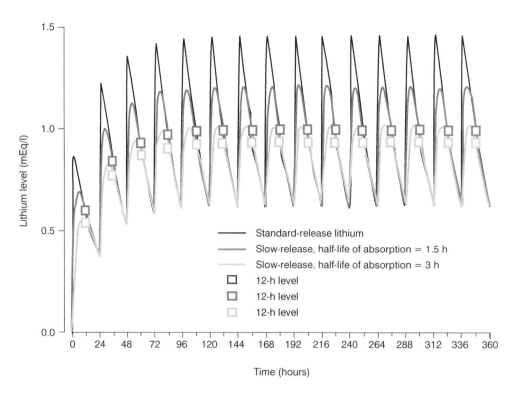

Figure 28.1 Effect of absorption rate on the course of lithium plasma levels. The illustration compares standard-release lithium with two slow-release formulations. While the expected 12-hour levels are almost identical, the preparations differ with respect to the range of levels in the course of the day

absorption from the gastrointestinal system becomes clinically relevant[1]. At the same time, it should be noted that not all sustained-release preparations on the international markets meet the accepted standards for such formulation[2]. Therefore, clinicians need to be aware of the fact that different slow-release preparations may have quite different pharmacokinetic properties.

DISTRIBUTION

Lithium is distributed quickly throughout the body/bloodstream. From the blood, lithium enters several compartments, the major one being the intracellular space. The concentration of lithium in cells is typically lower than that in the blood. The balance between blood (extra-cellular) and tissue (intracellular) concentration is maintained by several distinct transport mechanisms, described in Chapter 27. It is their relative contribution that determines the final balance. Intracellular concentrations of lithium are typically measured in erythrocytes and they correlate well with plasma levels[3], although this correlation may not be linear as the erythro-cyte/plasma lithium ratio appears to correlate with plasma levels[4,5]. The *in vivo* concentrations of lithium in the brain have been measured with

[7]Li magnetic resonance spectroscopy by several groups[6–8]. These studies indicate that the brain concentration of lithium is on average lower than the plasma concentration and that the half-life of lithium in the brain is longer than in blood[7]. This may also explain the variability of brain/plasma lithium ratios as these will obviously depend on the time of measurement. In a study examining the relationship between the brain and plasma levels, Kato *et al.* found a correlation of 0.66, higher than the correlation between erythrocyte and brain levels (0.44)[9]. However, the correlation is still relatively modest, reminding clinicians that plasma levels should be taken only as a guideline for monitoring the treatment along with clinical response and tolerability.

ELIMINATION

Most of the lithium ingested is eliminated via the kidneys. The other routes, namely sweat and stool, are usually clinically negligible. As lithium is not bound to proteins, its elimination is dependent primarily on the glomerular filtration rate and correlates reasonably well with creatinine clearance[10]. For most purposes, the elimination of lithium can be described by first-order kinetics, i.e. the rate of lithium elimination is proportional to the blood concentration of lithium. The important caveat, though, is that the elimination within the first 12–24 hours after lithium administration is faster than the rate of elimination measured in subsequent (36–48 hours) intervals. This apparent decrease in clearance is attributed to delayed redistribution between intracellular and extracellular compartments[11].

Clinically relevant is the decrease of the rate of elimination with age. On average, the half-life of elimination is 18–24 hours in otherwise physically healthy subjects, but can be well over 36 hours in the elderly. This necessitates careful monitoring of lithium treatment in older patients, especially as they are more likely to use medications that interfere with lithium elimination, and because of age-related changes in membrane transport. Thus in most cases older patients will require lower therapeutic levels. They will also achieve higher blood levels on the same dose in comparison with younger subjects.

Some authors suggested that the rate of elimination increases with the duration of treatment, which would mean that the dose of lithium should increase in the course of treatment in order to keep the levels stable[12]. However, not all studies support these observations[13].

Lithium is re-absorbed from the glomerular filtrate in the proximal tubule. For this reason, certain medications that inhibit its re-absorption in the proximal tubule, for instance carboanhydrase inhibitors or aminophyllin, may increase lithium elimination.

Conditions associated with reduced lithium clearance are among the most clinically relevant because of their potential toxicity. Various disturbances in water and electrolyte balance can lead to either faster lithium elimination or retention and toxicity. In general, lithium is retained in place of sodium in states of relative hyponatremia, or due to activation of sodium-retaining mechanisms, for instance in dehydration or edema formation[10]. Similarly, concomitant treatment with a variety of drugs including diuretics and non-steroidal anti-inflammatory agents (NSAIDs) can reduce the rate of elimination with an associated risk of side-effects and even toxicity.

Diuretics that act at the distal tubule, such as hydrochlorothiazide, spironolactone, or triamterene are more likely to increase lithium levels, while those acting at the proximal tubule may decrease them (see above). If use of a diuretic is indicated, furosemide is one that influences lithium levels minimally. Another commonly

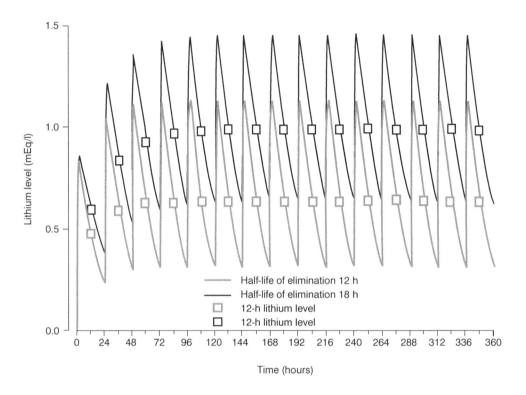

Figure 28.2 Differences in lithium levels between subjects with typical and accelerated elimination of lithium

used class of drugs, antihypertensives, including angiotensin converting enzyme (ACE) inhibitors, also have the potential of increasing lithium levels by reducing lithium clearance[14].

Examples of how altered rates of elimination affect steady-state levels are illustrated in Figures 28.2 and 28.3. Figure 28.2 shows the difference between steady-state levels in a subject with close-to-average clearance (half-life of elimination of 18 hours) and in another person with accelerated elimination (half-life of 12 hours). Figure 28.3 illustrates the effect of prolonged elimination in the course of treatment. The steady-state levels in this

example rise gradually to excessive values over a period of more than a week.

PRACTICAL APPLICATIONS

Number of daily doses

When lithium started to be used, the usual dosage schedule was twice or even three or more times daily. In recent years the practice has shifted towards once-a-day dosage, as most patients are able to tolerate such a regimen well and with better compliance. Furthermore,

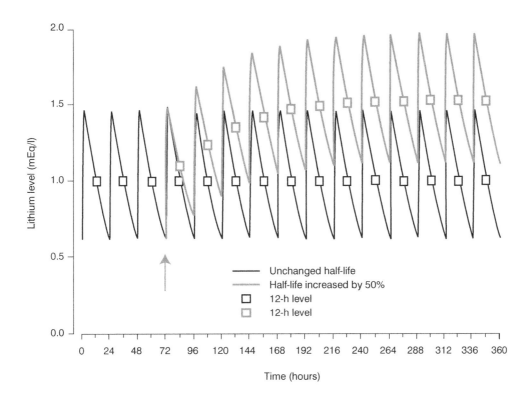

Figure 28.3 Increase in steady-state lithium levels following an increase of half-life of elimination by 50%

when given in a single daily dose, lithium treatment may be associated with less polyuria and decreased concentration capacity of the kidneys[15–17] – similar to observations of patients using lower lithium plasma levels for their maintenance treatment[18,19].

Clinicians using once-daily dosage should keep in mind that standardized 12-hour levels will be higher for the same amount of lithium given once a day in comparison with divided dosing. This point is illustrated in Figure 28.4. The recommended (therapeutic) 12-hour lithium levels are based on studies that assumed a divided dose. It is not entirely clear whether such levels might be subtherapeutic for those

taking lithium only once per day. At the same time, the ultimate measure of correct dosing in individual patients should be the therapeutic effect and tolerability.

Pharmacokinetic methods for optimizing lithium dosage

Most clinicians use gradual adjustments in dosage while checking the levels frequently enough to arrive at optimum dosage. This approach takes advantage of the almost linear relationship between the lithium dose and the blood levels. However, in specific situations it is

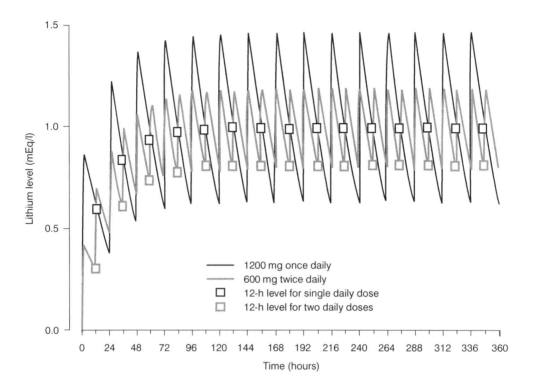

Figure 28.4 Comparison of lithium levels when lithium is given once and twice daily

helpful to predict lithium levels for a specific dosage directly and accurately. Such situations may arise when the treatment needs to be initiated (or adjusted) without a delay, or in situations where the usual assumptions about the relation between the dose and the levels do not hold – for instance in individuals with an impaired elimination of lithium due to physical illness or concurrent use of specific medications, or in patients who are non-compliant. Several methods for lithium level prediction and/or dose estimation have been developed since the early 1970s. These methods attempt to provide simple clinically applicable tools without sacrificing accuracy.

One approach is based on individualized pharmacokinetic estimations. A compromise is usually found between the accuracy of the method and the simplicity of its use. The first such method was published by Cooper *et al.*[20]. The method was based on a prior thorough pharmacokinetic analysis of lithium using multiple blood samples[21]. The detailed analysis was accurate, although not practical for clinical situations. Nevertheless, it provided essential data for development of a simplified test for estimation of lithium dosage from a single level measured 24 hours after administration of a single test dose.

Swartz and Wilcox proposed a method based on a simple first-degree kinetics model, with parameters estimated from consecutive blood levels using the least-squares method[22]. Another option is to calculate the parameters algebraically from only two levels. Alda proposed one such method and showed that it performed well in most clinical situations and was not sensitive to measurement errors[13].

A second group of methods to calculate lithium dose is based on results of typically multivariate analyses taking into account factors known to influence or rather correlate with lithium plasma levels. Such factors commonly include age, sex, body weight and/or height, concomitant medication and plasma creatinine level. These methods seem to perform quite well in typical situations – where they may not be necessary. The most popular and extensively tested method in this group has been developed by Zetin and colleagues[23]. They proposed a nomogram based on multiple linear regression that takes into account the patient's weight, concomitant medications and the lithium dose to arrive at approximate plasma levels. As the parameters of the nomogram are derived from statistical data, the method is more practical in 'average' situations – that is, when there is less need to apply such a method in the first place.

REFERENCES

1. Cihak F, Alda M. Verification of the pharmacologic properties of the preparation Contemnol Spofa [in Czech]. Cesk Psychiatr 1988; 84: 84–9

2. Heim W, Oelschlager H, Kreuter J, Müller-Oerlinghausen B. Liberation of lithium from sustained release preparations. A comparison of seven registered brands. Pharmacopsychiatry 1994; 27: 27–31

3. White K, Cohen J, Boyd J, Nelson R. Relationship between plasma, RBC, and CSF lithium concentrations in human subjects. Int Pharmacopsychiatry 1979; 14: 185–9

4. Lee CR, Hill SE, Dimitrakoudi M, et al. The relationship of plasma to erythrocyte lithium levels in patients taking lithium carbonate. Br J Psychiatry 1975; 127: 596–8

5. Schreiner HC, Dunner DL, Meltzer HL, Fieve RR. The relationship of the lithium erythrocyte: plasma ratio to plasma lithium level. Biol Psychiatry 1979; 14: 207–13

6. Kato T, Takahashi S, Inubushi T. Brain lithium concentration by ^{7}Li- and ^{1}H-magnetic resonance spectroscopy in bipolar disorder. Psychiatry Res 1992; 45: 53–63

7. Plenge P, Stensgaard A, Jensen HV, et al. 24-hour lithium concentration in human brain studied by Li-7 magnetic resonance spectroscopy. Biol Psychiatry 1994; 36: 511–16

8. Sachs GS, Renshaw PF, Lafer B, et al. Variability of brain lithium levels during maintenance treatment: a magnetic resonance spectroscopy study. Biol Psychiatry 1995; 38: 422–8

9. Kato T, Shioiri T, Inubushi T, Takahashi S. Brain lithium concentrations measured with lithium-7 magnetic resonance spectroscopy in patients with affective disorders: relationship to erythrocyte and serum concentrations. Biol Psychiatry 1993; 33: 147–52

10. Thomsen K, Schou M. Avoidance of lithium intoxication: advice based on knowledge about the renal lithium clearance under various circumstances. Pharmacopsychiatry 1999; 32: 83–6

11. Thornhill DP, Field SP. Distribution of lithium elimination rates in a selected population of psychiatric patients. Eur J Clin Pharmacol 1982; 21: 351–4

12. Goodnick PJ, Fieve RR, Meltzer HL, Dunner DL. Lithium pharmacokinetics, duration of therapy, and the adenylate cyclase system. Int Pharmacopsychiatry 1982; 17: 65–72

13. Alda M. Method for prediction of serum lithium levels. Biol Psychiatry 1988; 24: 218–24

14. Finley PR, O'Brien JG, Coleman RW. Lithium and angiotensin-converting enzyme inhibitors: evaluation of a potential interaction. J Clin Psychopharmacol 1996; 16: 68–71

15. Plenge P, Mellerup ET, Bolwig TG, et al. Lithium treatment: does the kidney prefer one daily dose instead of two? Acta Psychiatr Scand 1982; 66: 121–8

16. Hetmar O, Bolwig TG, Brun C, et al. Lithium: long-term effects on the kidney. I. Renal function in retrospect. Acta Psychiatr Scand 1986; 73: 574–81

17. Bowen RC, Grof P, Grof E. Less frequent lithium administration and lower urine volume. Am J Psychiatry 1991; 148: 189–92

18. Hullin RP, Coley VP, Birch NJ, et al. Renal function after long-term treatment with lithium. Br Med J 1979; 1: 1457–9

19. Schou M, Vestergaard P. Prospective studies on a lithium cohort. 2. Renal function. Water and electrolyte metabolism. Acta Psychiatr Scand 1988; 78: 427–33

20. Cooper TB, Bergner PE, Simpson GM. The 24-hour serum lithium level as a prognosticator of dosage requirements. Am J Psychiatry 1973; 130: 601–3

21. Bergner PE, Berniker K, Cooper TB, et al. Lithium kinetics in man: effect of variation in dosage pattern. Br J Pharmacol 1973; 49: 328–39

22. Swartz CM, Wilcox J. Characterization and prediction of lithium blood levels and clearances. Arch Gen Psychiatry 1984; 41: 1154–8

23. Zetin M, Garber D, De Antonio M, et al. Prediction of lithium dose: a mathematical alternative to the test-dose method. J Clin Psychiatry 1986; 47: 175–8

29 Interaction of lithium with neurotransmitter systems: serotonin and others

Georg Juckel, Paraskevi Mavrogiorgou

Contents   Introduction • Effects of lithium on serotonergic neurotransmission • Effects of lithium on noradrenergic neurotransmission • Effects of lithium on dopaminergic neurotransmission • Effects of lithium on cholinergic neurotransmission • Conclusions

INTRODUCTION

Lithium is an effective drug for both treatment and prophylaxis of affective disorder. The mechanism of lithium action is, however, still unknown. Over the past 50 years pre-clinical and clinical studies have focused upon the effects of both acute and chronic lithium on the regulation of neurotransmitter systems, especially the serotonergic system. In this chapter, current literature is reviewed in order to clarify the interactions of lithium with monoaminergic and cholinergic neurotransmitters.

EFFECTS OF LITHIUM ON SEROTONERGIC NEUROTRANSMISSION

It is well known that lithium in general leads to an enhancement of serotonergic neurotrans-

mission. Support for this was given by pre-clinical and clinical studies that will be presented here. Although the exact neurobiological mechanisms by which lithium induces an increase of serotonergic activity is not completely understood, it is today obvious that lithium provides its effect on serotonergic function by interacting with various parts of the brain serotonergic system, i.e. 5-hydroxytryptamine (5-HT) synthesis, 5-HT release, 5-HT receptors, etc. This is reviewed by differentiation between the acute and long-term (chronic) effects of lithium on serotonergic neurotransmission.

Pre-clinical (animal) studies

In the older pre-clinical literature, an enhanced uptake of tryptophan, the precursor of serotonin, into brain tissue and synaptosomes was found after short-term, partially high-dosage treatment with lithium[1,2]. Levels of tryptophan concentration in different brain regions were positively correlated with the duration of lithium intake[3,4].

Besides the findings of increased 5-HT synthesis induced by lithium, there is also impressive evidence from pre-clinical animal research that both acute and chronic application of lithium increases 5-HT release[4,5]. However, effects on 5-HT release by lithium differ between the different brain regions investigated. An enhanced 5-HT release was especially found in hippocampal areas, but this was significantly less pronounced in cortical areas[6,7]. Gottberg and co-workers[4], however, found no significant difference between the anterior cingulate cortex, entorhinal cortex, primary visual cortex, basal ganglia (caudate, putamen), bulbus olfactorius and hippocampus in rats concerning 5-HT release 1 hour after the application of lithium.

An explanation of the regionally different effects of lithium can be seen in regard to the different distribution of the various known 5-HT receptors. From the at least 14 5-HT receptor subtypes identified to date, the 5-HT$_{1A}$, 5-HT$_{1B}$ and 5-HT$_{2A}$ receptors seem to be specifically involved in the effects of lithium[8–11]. As long ago as 1980, Treiser and Kellar[12] reported a diminished number of 5-HT receptors in the hippocampus after lithium treatment, which they interpreted as a consequence of pre-synaptically enhanced serotonergic activity. Reduced expression of 5-HT1A receptors especially in the dorsal hippocampus of rats chronically treated with lithium was found several times in the following years[13–16]. Subhash et al.[17] observed that chronic treatment with lithium (30 days) decreased the density of 5-HT receptors in the cortex (62%), hippocampus (64%) and striatum (65%), compared to control levels.

Furthermore, short-term administration of lithium enhances the efficacy of the ascending 5-HT system in suppressing the firing rate of post-synaptic neurons in the rat dorsal hippocampus[18–20]. Subsequently, animal studies showed that, in contrast to lithium alone, lithium added to antidepressant treatments potentiated pre-synaptic 5-HTergic function in rats[21] and produced a greater disinhibition of dorsal hippocampus pyramidal neurons[22]. A subchronic lithium dosage added to chronic treatment with citalopram elevated basal levels of 5-HT in the rat ventral hippocampus, using microdialysis techniques[23]. These findings in animal studies demonstrated the efficacy of lithium as an adjunct to antidepressants in the treatment of refractory depression[24].

Further studies have shown that lithium enhanced the anti-immobility effects of the 5-HT$_{1A}$ receptor agonists gepirone and ipsapirone in mice, using the forced swimming test and tail suspension test[25–27]. In addition, studies have demonstrated that prior administration of lithium potentiated the antidepressant-like effect of the 5-HT$_{1A/B}$ receptor agonist RU 24969, together with that of the more specific 5-HT$_{1B}$ receptor agonist anpirtoline[28]. To sum up, these studies suggested that especially the 5-HT$_{1B}$ receptor may play a role in the potentiation of antidepressant effects in the forced swimming test[28]. According to the learned helplessness model of depression, chronic administration of lithium has been shown to reverse helpless behavior in rats (30 days)[29]. Another study has shown that acute administration (5 days) of lithium failed to reverse learned helplessness behavioral deficits[30].

Midbrain raphe lesions in rats are known to induce aggressive behavior including muricidal behavior[31]. A single administration of lithium slightly inhibited muricidal behavior. However, repeated treatment (5 days) significantly attenuated these behavioral abnormalities. Chronic lithium administration was also found to inhibit muricidal behavior in olfactory bulbectomized rats, also a valid animal model of depression[28]. Lithium showed a partial prophylactic effect on muricide when administered for 1 week prior to the performance of raphe lesions[31]. This inhibition of muricide by lithium was correlated with the increased 5-HT turnover rate in the brain. Previous studies showed that muricide in raphe-lesioned rats was effectively inhibited by drugs that potentiate the activity of 5-HT neurotransmission, since muricidal behavior was presumably associated with a reduction of brain 5-HT activity[32]. Taking these findings together, it seems likely that inhibition of muricide in raphe-lesioned rats by lithium is caused by activation of 5-HT neurons.

Effects of lithium on the serotonergic system in healthy subjects

In general, findings concerning the effects of lithium on serotonergic neurotransmission in healthy subjects are rather inconsistent. For example, Rudorfer and co-workers[33] found no changes related to serotonergic activity in 12 healthy male volunteers to whom lithium was administered for 1 week.

In order to investigate the influence of long-term administration of lithium on serotonergic neurotransmission, Mühlbauer and Müller-Oerlinghausen[34] used fenfluramine stimulation for the assessment of hormonal effects depending on the serotonergic tone. The cortisol plasma concentration following fenfluramine stimulation was examined in 11 healthy subjects as well as in 11 manic-depressive subjects under lithium prophylaxis and in eight untreated euthymic patients. While in the untreated patient groups no gross deviation from the expected physiological decline of morning cortisol values was found, only a subtle effect of fenfluramine stimulation in the healthy subjects was observed. However, in the lithium-treated patients, a significant inversion of the cortisol secretion was observed.

Platelet [^{3}H]5-HT uptake, [^{3}H]imipramine binding and 5-HT levels in platelets were measured in healthy volunteers during short-term (20 days) administration of lithium, followed by withdrawal[35]. In this study, the V_{max} [^{3}H]5-HT uptake was significantly decreased during lithium treatment. Following lithium withdrawal, platelet [^{3}H]5-HT uptake remained decreased and was followed by a pronounced rebound effect in some of the subjects for up to 3 months. However, binding of imipramine during the same period and platelet 5-HT levels was not affected by lithium treatment. In this line, Thies-Flechtner and co-workers[36] found no difference in the 5-HT uptake kinetics between the whole group of 37 euthymic patients (with long-term lithium treatment) and age- and sex-matched healthy controls.

On the other hand, the pharmacologic challenge test used most frequently to assess central 5-HT function is the prolactin response to intravenous L-tryptophan. Studies in healthy subjects have shown that the prolactin response to tryptophan is enhanced after both short- and long-term lithium treatment[37]. Walsh and co-workers[38] studied the effect of lithium administration (800 mg daily for 7 days) on the neuroendocrine and temperature responses to the 5-HT$_{1A}$ receptor agonist gepirone (20 mg orally) in eight healthy male volunteers. Gepirone significantly increased plasma levels of prolactin, growth hormone and cortisol, and lowered oral temperature. None of these measurements was significantly altered by lithium treatment. These results suggest that the ability of short-term administration of lithium to increase 5-HT-mediated neuroendocrine responses is unlikely to be related to changes in the sensitivity of pre- or postsynaptic 5-HT$_{1A}$ receptors. In contrast, Power *et al.* found no alteration on the prolactin response to D-fenfluramine in healthy subjects after 3 days and 3 weeks of lithium treatment[39].

Since the reported findings of the few studies in this field with healthy volunteers are inconsistent, valid conclusions on the net neurobiological effects of lithium on the serotonergic neurotransmission cannot be drawn. Further hints can, however, be obtained by studies conducted in patients with unipolar and bipolar affective disorders.

Effects of lithium on the serotonergic system in patients with affective disorders

Abnormalities of central serotonergic function are thought to be associated with the pathogenesis of affective disorders. On the other hand, there is evidence especially from animal studies, as presented, that lithium enhances serotonergic activity in terms of turnover and release. In order to obtain further information on changes of the serotonergic system by lithium in affective disorders, the release of prolactin and cortisol, which is under the influence of the serotonergic system, caused by challenges with serotonergic agonists such as fenfluramine and tryptophan was investigated in patients[2]. In the study of bipolar patients and healthy controls already presented[34], an enhanced release of cortisol stimulated by fenfluramine was found after lithium treatment. The release of cortisol was doubled in the responder group to such a treatment with lithium, as compared to the non-responders[40]. Increased release of cortisol and prolactin in patients with affective disorders under lithium medication (4–24 days) was also reported after stimulation with 5-hydroxytryptophan, tryptophan or clomipramine[41,42]. Furthermore, Price and co-workers[37] showed, in acute depressed patients, that an enhanced prolactin response to L-tryptophan was found after only 1 week of lithium intake, but not after 3 weeks.

In a recent study, Basturk and co-workers[43] studied 20 euthymic bipolar male patients on long-term lithium carbonate treatment for more than 6 months and 15 euthymic male bipolar patients on short-term lithium treatment (for shorter than 6 months) in comparison to healthy controls. Values of prolactin in serum of the long-term lithium-treated group were significantly lower than those of the control group, while there was no significant difference in prolactin values between the short-term lithium-treated group and the control group.

El Khoury and co-workers[44] measured morning plasma prolactin and cortisol values in 14 non-medicated depressed patients, 13 depressed patients treated with citalopram, 17 euthymic patients on long-term lithium treatment and 11 healthy controls. Plasma prolactin values in the lithium group were significantly lower than those of the other three groups, suggesting a net inhibitory impact of augmentative effects of lithium on serotonergic activity. Plasma cortisol values were significantly higher in non-medicated depressed patients compared to healthy controls. The authors suggested that this result might be a sign of hyperactivity of the hypothalamic–pituitary–adrenal system in depression, which seems to be a state-dependent phenomenon, and is normalized upon successful treatment with lithium.

In order to investigate whether the mood-stabilizing effects of lithium are dependent on short-term availability of serotonin, tryptophan depletion was performed in 30 patients with affective disorder (bipolar and unipolar), all psychopathologically stabilized by lithium treatment for at least 1 year[45]. In this randomized, double-blind, controlled study, plasma tryptophan was reduced by 80% in the experimental group and 16% in the control group. However, no clinically relevant mood changes were observed. Thus, it can be concluded that a transient reduction of serotonergic function presumably does not affect mood in patients with affective disorder being stabilized by long-term lithium treatment.

While the finding of reduced 5-HT uptake into blood platelets was often found in patients with affective disorders, there are inconsistent findings concerning changes of that uptake induced by lithium. Meltzer and co-workers[46] found a decrease of 5-HT uptake in platelets in 21 patients with bipolar affective disorder. This was, however, a short-term administration of lithium. A longer treatment with lithium caused enhanced 5-HT uptake in several studies. Thies-Flechtner and co-workers[36] found no changes of 5-HT uptake in 37 euthymic patients under long-term prophylactic treatment with lithium. A similar finding was reported by El Khoury and co-workers[47], who studied 29 patients with an affective disorder (bipolar and unipolar) under long-term treatment with lithium in regard to 5-HT uptake as well as densities of the serotonin transporter, $5-HT_2$ and $-\alpha2$ receptors at the platelet membrane. Only an increase of $5-HT_2$ receptors was found in these patients, while there was no significant 5-HT uptake. An enhanced density of $5-HT_{2(A)}$ receptors was also found by Pandey et al.[48] in platelets in bipolar and schizoaffective patients. The interpretation of these findings is, however, still unclear with regard to the mechanism of action of lithium.

EFFECTS OF LITHIUM ON NORADRENERGIC NEUROTRANSMISSION

Relatively less consideration has been given to the effects of lithium on measures of norepinephrine (NE), although animal studies have demonstrated that lithium also affects central noradrenergic neurotransmission[49]. However, the findings of the preclinical work do not build up a consistent picture concerning the influences of lithium on the noradrenergic system, owing to several methodological limitations[50]. Furthermore, lithium might induce different changes of noradrenergic neurotransmission due to dosage and brain region studied.

Losada and Rubio[51] investigated the acute effects of a single intravenous injection of lithium on the rat mediobasal hypothalamus and found that the concentration of NE was reduced 10 min after injection. Gottberg et al.[4,52] found that NE levels increased in several cortical areas of the rat 1 hour after the administration of lithium. In an *in vivo* electrophysiological study, Kovacs and Hernadi[53] tested the action of microiontophoretically applied lithium and NE on the firing rate of prefrontal cortical neurons in rats. They found that lithium suppressed maintained discharge activity of cortical neurons and antagonized both the inhibitory and the excitatory modulation of the firing rate by NE.

In healthy volunteers, 1 week of lithium administration did not significantly affect NE turnover[33,54]. In another study examining the effects of lithium on NE in healthy subjects, Grof et al.[55] did not find significant alterations of plasma NE or epinephrine values after 3 weeks of lithium administration. In contrast, Manji et al.[56] found significant increases in 24-hour urinary excretion of NE and normetanephrine as well as of fractional NE release, which might be comparable with increased neuronal release of NE and a lithium-induced subsensitivity of α_2-adrenergic receptor function. These changes were not statistically significant after 1 week of lithium administration in the healthy subjects investigated, suggesting that increased NE release is more characteristic of long-term rather than short-term administration of lithium.

Studies of NE turnover after lithium treatment in affective disorders have found somewhat inconsistent results. Lithium appears to decrease excretion of NE and its metabolites in manic patients while increasing NE excretion in depressed patients[57–59]. Although such data are quite inconsistent, there is considerable and consistent evidence from preclinical[60–62] and clinical studies[63–67] that lithium treatment causes a subsensitivity of α_2-adrenergic receptors. For instance, long-term lithium administration attenuates α_2-adrenergic-mediated behavioral effects and presynaptic α_2-adrenergic inhibition of NE release in animals, while enhancing potassium-evoked NE release. In humans, growth hormone responses to clonidine (post-synaptic α_2-adrenergic agonist) are blunted after lithium treatment[64,66], and there is decreased high-affinity tritiated clonidine binding to platelet α_2-adrenergic receptors after lithium treatment. Thus, increased urinary NE and normeta-nephrine excretion and increased plasma NE could be explained by a lithium-associated desensitization of presynaptic α_2-adrenergic receptors at peripheral sympathetic nerve terminals[56]. In a recent study, Ozerdem and co-workers[68] showed in ten healthy volunteers that chronic lithium administration significantly increased mean resting plasma NE levels by 53.6%. The noradrenergic responses to infusions with idazoxan (a selective α_2-adrenoceptor antagonist) were slightly enhanced after 5 days of lithium administration and significantly increased following 4 weeks of lithium intake. On the other hand, preclinical and clinical studies seem to support an action of acute lithium in reducing the β-adrenergic stimulated adenylyl cyclase response. Chronic lithium treatment seems to act by facilitating the release of NE, possibly via the effects on the presynaptic α_2-autoreceptor as well as by blocking the β-adrenergic receptor super-sensitivity after presynaptic depletion of NE[69,70].

EFFECTS OF LITHIUM ON DOPAMINERGIC NEUROTRANSMISSION

Chronic lithium treatment has been reported to prevent haloperidol-induced dopamine receptor upregulation and to induce supersensitivity to iontophoretically applied dopamine or intravenously applied apomorphine[71,72]. Interestingly, a number of studies have reported a lack of effect when lithium was administered after the induction of dopamine super-sensitivity[73–76]. D'Aquila et al.[77] studied the effect of a lithium high-dosage diet, inducing a lithium serum level in the range of therapeutic efficacy, on the development of supersensitivity to locomotor effects of the dopamine D2-like receptor agonist quinpirole. Their results showed that lithium was not able to prevent the development of such a behavioral supersensitivity.

Lithium also seems to block amphetamine-induced behavioral changes in both animals and humans[73,78–81]. Adaptive changes in the rat dopaminergic neurotransmission after repeated lithium administration were reported by Dziedzicka-Wasylewska et al.[82]. On the other hand, Kameda et al.[83] reported that lithium increased the level of the dopamine D2 receptor mRNA, and the transcription rate of the dopamine D2 receptor gene. Lithium might induce conformational changes of dopamine D2 receptors in the striatum. Fazli-Tabaei et al.[84] investigated the effect of lithium carbonate on sniffing induced by apomorphine in rats. They found that chronic lithium exposure (30–35 days), but not acute administration, decreased the behavioral response to apomorphine. Blockade of apomorphine induced sniffing by the D1 dopamine receptor antagonist SCH3390 or by the D2 dopamine receptor antagonist sulpiride was not increased in animals acutely treated with lithium. In animals that were treated chronically with lithium, blockade of the apomorphine response by sulpiride, but not by SCH3390, was potentiated. These results suggested that chronic treatment of animals with lithium is able to alter the D2 dopamine receptor-mediated behavioral response. Recently, Beaulieu and co-workers[85] have demonstrated that lithium antagonizes dopamine-dependent behaviors mediated by the AKT/glycogen synthase kinase 3 signaling cascade.

EFFECTS OF LITHIUM ON CHOLINERGIC NEUROTRANSMISSION

The cholinergic system with acetylcholine as its neurotransmitter has been subdivided into nicotinic and muscarinic receptor subtypes. Nicotinic receptors are ligand-gated ion channels, whereas muscarinic receptors belong to the family of plasma membrane-bound G-protein-coupled receptors. Currently five subtypes of muscarinic receptors have been identified. Activation of the muscarinic M1, M3 and M5 receptors stimulates a cascade of interactions including G-protein Gaq/11 and phospholipase Cβ activation, resulting in formation of the second messenger inositol triphosphate (IP3) from phospholipids, which subsequently induces release of calcium. The muscarinic M2 and M4 receptors are coupled through Ga1 and Ga0 G-proteins, and inhibit adenylate cyclase activity and reduce formation of cyclic adenosine 3′5′-monophosphate (cAMP) (for review, see reference 86). Physiologic, behavioral and neurochemical studies have all suggested that the cholinergic system is involved in affective illnesses. For example, the cholinesterase inhibitor physostigmine increased immobility in the forced swimming test, suggesting depressogenic activity[87]. Furthermore, Roundtree et al.[88] found that organophosphorous insecticides, which have cholinesterase inhibition activities, produced profound depression-like states in manic-depressive patients and healthy subjects. In contrast, cholinergic antagonists have been reported to produce euphoria and flight of ideas[89,90]. Already in 1972, Janowsky and co-workers[91] proposed the so-called cholinergic–adrenergic hypothesis of mania and depression. This hypothesis stated that hypercholinergic (or hypoadrenergic) drive produces depression, whereas hypocholinergic or hyperadrenergic drive causes mania. In line with this hypothesis, several groups have reported that cholinesterase inhibitors lessen manic symptoms in patients, whereas cholinomimetics increase depressed mood in affective disorders[86].

The effects of lithium on the cholinergic system have been extensively investigated. As found with other neurotransmitter systems, there are many reported changes of the cholinergic system produced by lithium, but it is not clear whether or not these alterations are direct effects involved in the therapeutic efficacy of lithium, or only indirect effects, i.e. an epiphenomenon[81]:

- In rat brain, lithium enhances the synaptic processing of acetylcholine[92].

- Chronic lithium treatment increases acetylcholine synthesis and uptake[93].

- Lithium enhances the expression of muscarinic M3 receptors and decreases M2 receptor levels in cultured cells[94].

- Accumulating evidence suggests that intracellular transduction pathways, rather than neurotransmitter receptors at the membranes, are targets of lithium[95].

CONCLUSIONS

A clear outcome has not been reached concerning which, if any, neurotransmitter synthesis, uptake and release processes contribute to the therapeutic action of lithium, but the reported effects on monoaminergic and cholinergic neurotransmitter systems suggest that these may make important, if as yet not completely defined, contributions. The overall consequences of these actions may be that lithium readjusts the balance between excitatory and inhibitory activities, as well as the balance between monoamines and acetylcholine, so that it is the adjusted balances by lithium, rather than actions on a single neurotransmitter, that facilitate mood recovery and stabilization[96].

REFERENCES

1. Aragon MC, Herrero E, Gimenez C. Effects of systematically administered lithium on tryptophan transport and exchange in plasma-membrane vesicles isolated from rat brain. Neurochem Res 1987; 12: 439–44
2. Müller-Oerlinghausen B. Die Wirkung von Lithium auf serotonerge Funktionen. In Müller-Oerlinghausen B, Greil W, Berghöfer A, eds. Die Lithiumtherapie, Nutzen, Risiken, Alternativen. Berlin: Springer-Verlag, 1997: 61–8
3. Berggren U. Effects of short-term lithium administration on tryptophan levels and 5-hydroxytryptamine synthesis in whole brain regions in rats. J Neural Transm 1987; 69: 115–21
4. Gottberg E, Grondin L, Reader TA. Acute effects of lithium on catecholamines, serotonin, and their major metabolites in discrete brain regions. J Neurosci Res 1989; 22: 338–45
5. Berggren U. Effects of chronic lithium treatment on brain monoamine metabolism and amphetamine-induced locomotor stimulation in rats. J Neural Transm 1985; 64: 239–50
6. Treiser SL, Cascio CS, O'Donohue TL, et al. Lithium increases serotonin release and decreases serotonin receptors in the hippocampus. Science 1981; 213: 1529–31
7. Wang HY, Friedman E. Chronic lithium: desensitization of autoreceptors mediating serotonin release. Psychopharmacology 1988; 94: 312–14
8. Moorman JM, Leslie RA. Paradoxical effects of lithium on serotonergic receptor function: an immunocytochemical, behavioural and auto radiographic study. Neuropsychopharmacology 1998; 37: 357–74
9. Massot O, Rousselle JC, Fillion MP, et al. 5-HT1B receptors: a novel target for lithium. Possible involvement in mood disorders. Neuropsychopharmacology 1999; 21: 530–41
10. Januel D, Massot O, Poirier MF, et al. Interaction of lithium with 5-HT(1B) receptors in depressed unipolar patients treated with clomipramine and lithium versus clomipramine and placebo: preliminary results. Psychiatry Res 2002; 111: 117–24
11. Hüther G, Rüther E, eds. Das serotonerge System. Bremen: UNI-MED, 2000
12. Treiser SL, Kellar KJ. Lithium: effects on serotonin receptors in rat brain. Eur J Pharmacol 1980; 64: 183–5
13. Goodwin GM, De Souza RJ, Wood AJ, et al. Lithium decreases 5-HT1A and 5-HT2 receptor and alpha-2-adrenoreceptor mediated function in mice. Psychopharmacology 1986; 90: 482–7
14. Hotta I, Yamawaki S, Segawa T. Long-term lithium treatment causes serotonin receptor down regulation via serotonergic presynapses in rat brain. Neuropsychobiology 1986; 16: 19–26
15. Friedman E, Wang HY. Effect of chronic lithium treatment on 5-hydroxytryptamine autoreceptors and release of 5-(3H) hydroxytryptamine from rat brain cortical, hippocampal, and hypothalamic slices. J Neurochem 1987; 50: 195–201
16. Mork A, Geisler A. Effects of GTP on hormone-stimulated adenylate cyclase activity in cerebral cortex, striatum, and hippocampus

from rats treated chronically with lithium. Biol Psychiatry 1989; 26: 279–88

17. Subhash MN, Vinod KY, Srinivas BN. Differential effect of lithium on 5-HT1 receptor-linked system in regions of rat brain. Neurochem Int 1999; 35: 337–43

18. Blier P, De Montigny C. Short-term lithium administration enhances serotonergic neuro-transmission: electrophysiological evidence in the rat CNS. Eur J Pharmacol 1985; 113: 69–77

19. Blier P, De Montigny C, Tardif D. Short-term lithium treatment enhances responsiveness of postsynaptic 5-HT1A receptors without altering 5-HT autoreceptor sensitivity: an electrophysiological study in the rat brain. Synapse 1987; 1: 225–32

20. McQuade R, Leitch MM, Gartside SE, et al. Effect of chronic lithium treatment on gluco-corticoid and 5-HT1A receptor messenger RNA in hippocampal and dorsal raphe nucleus regions of the rat brain. J Psychopharmacol 2004; 18: 496–501

21. Okamoto Y, Motohasi N, Hayakawa H, et al. Addition of lithium to chronic antidepressant treatment potentiates presynaptic serotonergic function without changes in serotonergic receptors in the rat cerebral cortex. Neuropsychobiology 1996; 33: 17–20

22. Haddjeri N, Szabo ST, De Montigny C, et al. Increased tonic activation of rat forebrain 5-HT(1A) receptors by lithium addition to antidepressant treatments. Neuropsycho-pharmacology 2000; 22: 346–56

23. Wegener G, Bandbey Z, Heiberg IL, et al. Increased extracellular serotonin level in rat hippocampus induced by chronic citaloprams is augmented by subchronic lithium: neuro-chemical and behavioural studies in the rat. Psychopharmacology 2003; 166: 188–94

24. Bauer M, Adli M, Baethge C, et al. Lithium augmentation therapy in refractory depression: clinical evidence and neurobiological mecha-nisms. Can J Psychiatry 2003; 48: 440–46

25. Hascoet M, Bourin M, Khimake S. Additive effect of lithium and clonidine with 5-HT1A agonists in the forced swimming test. Prog Neuropsychopharmacol Biol Psychiatry 1994; 18: 381–96

26. Bourin M, Hascoet M, Colombel MC, et al. Differential effects of clonidine, lithium and quinine in the forced swimming test in mice for antidepressants: possible roles of serotonergic systems. Eur Neuropsychopharmacol 1996; 6: 231–6

27. Redrobe JP, Bourin M. Effects of pretreatment with clonidine, lithium and quinine on the activities of antidepressants drugs in the mouse tail suspension test. Fundam Clin Pharmacol 1997; 10: 24–8

28. Redrobe JP, Bourin M. The effect of lithium administration in animal models of depression: a short review. Fundam Clin Pharmacol 1999; 13: 293–9

29. Faria MS, Teixeira NA. Reversal of learned helplesness by chronic lithium treatment at a prophylactic level. Braz J Med Biol Res 1993; 26: 1201–12

30. Teixeira NA, Pereira DG, Hermini H. Chronic but not acute lithium treatment prevents behavioural depression in rats. Braz J Med Biol Res 1995; 28: 1003–7

31. Yamamoto T, Araki H, Abe Y, et al. Effects of chronic LiCl and RbCl on muricide induced by midbrain raphe lesions in rats. Pharmacol Biochem Behav 1985; 22: 559–63

32. Yamamoto T, Ucki S. Characteristics in aggressive behavior induced by midbrain raphe lesions in rats. Physiol Behav 1977; 19: 105–10

33. Rudorfer MV, Karoum F, Ross RJ, et al. Differences in lithium effects in depressed and healthy subjects. Clin Pharmacol Ther 1985; 37: 66–71

34. Mühlbauer HD, Müller-Oerlinghausen B. Fenfluramine stimulation of serum cortisol in patients with major affective disorders and healthy controls: further evidence for a central serotonergic action of lithium in man. J Neural Transm 1985; 61: 81–94

35. Poirier MF, Galzin AM, Pimoule C, et al. Short-term lithium administration to healthy volunteers produces long-lasting pronounced changes in platelet serotonin uptake but not imipramine binding. Psychopharmacology 1988; 94: 521–6

36. Thies-Flechtner K, Weigel I, Müller-Oerlinghausen B. 5-HT uptake in platelets of

lithium-treated patients with affective disorders and of healthy controls. Pharmacopsychiatry 1994; 27 (Suppl): 4–6

37. Price LH, Charney DS, Delgado PL, et al. Lithium treatment and serotonergic function. Neuroendocrine and behavioral responses to intravenous tryptophan in affective disorder. Arch Gen Psychiatry 1989; 46: 13–19

38. Walsh AE, Ware CJ, Cowen PJ. Lithium and 5-HT1A receptor sensitivity: a neuroendocrine study in healthy volunteers. Psychopharmacology 1991; 105: 568–72

39. Power AC, Dorkins CE, Cowen PJ. Effect of lithium on the prolactin response to D-fenfluramine in healthy subjects. Biol Psychiatry 1993; 33: 801–5

40. Müller-Oerlinghausen B, Umbach C, Hegerl U, et al. Endokrinologische und psychophysiologische Befunde bei Lithium-Respondern und -Nonrespondern. In Beckmann H, Laux G, eds. Biologische Psychiatrie. Synopsis. Berlin: Springer Verlag, 1988: 281–3

41. Meltzer HY, Lowy MT, Robertson A, et al. Effect of 5-hydroxytryptophan on serum cortisol levels in major affective disorders. III: Effect of antidepressants and lithium carbonate. Arch Gen Psychiatry 1984; 41: 391–7

42. Mc Cance SL, Cohen PR, Cowen PJ. Lithium increases 5-HAT-mediated prolactin release. Psychopharmacology 1989; 99: 276–81

43. Basturk M, Karaaslan F, Esel E, et al. Effects of short and long-term lithium treatment on serum prolactin levels in patients with bipolar affective disorder. Prog Neuropsychopharmacol Biol Psychiatry 2001; 25: 315–22

44. El Khoury A, Tham A, Mathe AA, et al. Decreased plasma prolactin release in euthymic lithium-treated women with bipolar disorder. Neuropsychobiology 2003; 48: 14–18

45. Johnson L, El Khoury A, Aberg-Wistedt A, et al. Tryptophan depletion in lithium-stabilized patients with affective disorder. Int J Neuropsychopharmacol 2001; 4: 329–36

46. Meltzer HY, Arora RC, Goodnick P. Effect of lithium carbonate on serotonin uptake in blood platelets of patients with affective disorders. J Affect Disord 1983; 5: 215–21

47. El Khoury A, Johnson L, Aberg-Wistdt A, et al. Effects of long-term lithium treatment on monoaminergic function in major depression. Psychiatry Res 2001; 105: 33–44

48. Pandey GN, Pandey SC, Ren X, et al. Serotonin receptors in platelets of bipolar and schizoaffective patients: effect of lithium treatment. Psychopharmacology 2003; 170: 115–23

49. Wood AJ, Goodwin GM. A review of the biochemical and neuropharmacological actions of lithium. Psychol Med 1987; 17: 579–600

50. van Calker D, Walden J, Berger M. Effekte von Lithiumionen auf Neurotransmitter und sekundäre Botenstoffe. In Müller-Oerlinghausen B, Greil W, Berghöfer A, eds. Die Lithiumtherapie, Nutzen, Risiken, Alternativen. Berlin: Springer-Verlag Heidelberg, 1997: 35–60

51. Otero Losada ME, Rubio MC. Effects of i.c.v. lithium chloride administration on monoamine concentartion in rat mediobasal hypothalamus. Eur J Pharmacol 1992; 215: 185–9

52. Gottberg E, Montreuil B, Reader TA. Acute effects of lithium on dopaminergic responses: iontophoretic studies in the rat visual cortex. Synapse 1988; 2: 442–9

53. Kovacs P, Hernadi I. Iontophoresis of lithium antagonizes noradrenergic action on prefrontal neurons of the rat. Brain Res 2002; 947: 150–6

54. Rudorfer MV, Scheinin M, Karoum F, et al. Reduction of norepinephrine turnover by serotonergic drug in man. Biol Psychiatry 1984; 19: 179–93

55. Grof E, Brown GM, Grof P, et al. Effects of lithium administration on plasma catecholamines. Psychiatry Res 1986; 19: 87–92

56. Manji HK, Hsiao JK, Risby ED, et al. The Mechanisms of action of lithium. I: Effects on serotonergic and noradrenergic systems in normal subjects. Arch Gen Psychiatry 1991; 48: 505–12

57. Greenspan K, Schildkraut JJ, Gordon EK, et al. Catecholamine metabolsim in affective disorders. III: MHPG and other catecholamine metabolites in patients treated with lithium carbonate. J Psychiatr Res 1970; 7: 171–83

58. Beckmann H, St Laurent J, Goodwin FK. The effect of lithium on urinary MHPG in unipolar

and bipolar depressed patients. Psychopharmacology 1975; 42: 277–82

59. Bowers MB, Heninger GR. Lithium: clinical effects and cerebrospinal fluid acid monoamine metabolites. Commun Psychopharmacol 1977; 1: 135–45

60. Ebstein RP, Lerer B, Shlaufman M, et al. The effect of repeated electroconvulsive shock treatment and chronic lithium feeding on the release of norepinephrine from rat cortical vesicular preparations. Cell Mol Neurobiol 1983; 3: 191–201

61. Goodwin GM. The effects of antidepressant treatments and lithium upon 5-HT1A receptor function. Prog Neuropsychopharmacol Biol Psychiatry 1989; 13: 445–51

62. Smith DF. Lithium attenuates clonidine-induced hypoactivity: further studies in inbred mouse strains. Psychopharmacology 1988; 94: 428–30

63. Wood K, Coppen A. Prophylactic lithium treatment of patients with affective disorder is associated with decreased platelet 3H-dihydroxyergocryptine binding. J Affect Disord 1983; 5: 253–8

64. Catalano M, Bellodi L, Lucca A, et al. Lithium and alpha-2-adrenergic receptors: effects of lithium ion on clonidine-induced growth hormone release. Neuroendocrinol Lett 1984; 6: 61–5

65. Garcia-Sevilla JA, Guimon J, Garcia-Vallejo P, et al. Biochemical and functional evidence of supersensitive platelet alpha-2-adrenoreceptors in major affective disorder: effect of long-term lithium carbonate treatment. Arch Gen Psychiatry 1986; 43: 51–7

66. Brambilla F, Catalano M, Lucca A, et al. Effect of lithium treatment on the GH-clonidine test in affective disorders. Eur J Clin Pharmacol 1988; 35: 601–5

67. Pandey GN, Janicak PG, Javaid JI, et al. Increased 3H-clonidine binding in the platelets of patients with depressive and schizophrenic disorders. Psychiatry Res 1989; 28: 73–88

68. Ozerdem A, Schmidt ME, Manji HK, et al. Chronic lithium administration enhances noradrenergic responses to intravenous administration of the alpha-2-antagonist idazoxan in healthy volunteers. J Clin Psychopharmacol 2004; 24: 150–4

69. Risby ED, Hsiao JK, Manji HK, et al. The mechanisms of action of lithium. II: Effects on adenylate cyclase activity and β-adrenergic receptor binding in normal subjects. Arch Gen Psychiatry 1991; 48: 513–24

70. Lenox RH, McNamara RK, Papke RL, et al. Neurobiology of lithium: an update. J Clin Psychiatry 1998; 59: 37–47

71. Gallager DW, Pert A, Bunney WE Jr. Haloperidol-induced presynaptic dopamine supersensitivity is blocked by chronic lithium. Nature 1978; 273: 309–12

72. Verimer T, Goodale DB, Long JP, et al. Lithium effects on haloperidol-induced pre- and postsynaptic dopamine receptor supersensitivity. J Pharm Pharmacol 1980; 32: 665–6

73. Klawans HL, Weiner WJ, Nausieda PA. The effect of lithium on an animal model of tardive dyskinesia. Prog Neuropsychopharmacol 1976; 1: 53–60

74. Staunton DA, Magistretti PJ, Shoemaker WJ, et al. Effects of chronic lithium treatment on dopamine receptors in the rat corpus striatum. I: locomotor activity and behavioral supersensitivity. Brain Res 1982; 232: 391–400

75. Staunton DA, Magistretti PJ, Shoemaker WJ, et al. Effects of chronic lithium treatment on dopamine receptors in the rat corpus striatum. II: no effect on denervation or neuroleptic-induced supersensitivity. Brain Res 1982; 232: 401–12

76. Bloom FE, Baetge G, Deyo S, et al. Chemical and physiological aspects of the actions of lithium and antidepressants drugs. Neuropharmacology 1983; 22: 359–65

77. D'Aquila PS, Collu M, Deveto P, et al. Chronic lithium chloride fails to prevent imipramine-induced sensitization to the dopamine D(2)-like receptor agonist quinpirole. Eur J Pharmacol 2000; 395: 157–60

78. Pert A, Rosenblatt JE, Sivit C et al. Long-term treatment with lithium prevents the development of dopamine receptor supersensitivity. Science 1978; 201: 171–3

79. Allikmets LH, Stanley M, Gershon S. The effect of lithium on chronic haloperidol enhanced apomorphine aggression in rats. Life Sci 1979; 25: 165–70

80. Huey LY, Janowshy DS, Judd LL, et al. Effects of lithium carbonate on methylphenidate-induced mood, behavior, and cognitive processes. Psychopharmacology 1981; 73: 161–4

81. Bunney WE, Garland-Bunney BL. Mechanism of action of lithium in affective illness: basic and clinical implications. In Meltzer HY, ed. Psychopharmacology: The Third Generation of Progress. New York: Raven Press, 1987: 553–65

82. Dziedzicka-Wasylewska M, Mackowiak M, Fijat K, et al. Adaptive changes in the rat dopaminergic transmission following repeated lithium administration. J Neural Transm 1996; 103: 765–76

83. Kameda K, Miura J, Suzuki K, et al. Effects of lithium on dopamine D2 receptor expression in the rat brain striatum. J Neural Transm 2001; 108: 321–34

84. Fazli-Tabaei S, Yahyavi SH, Zarrindast MR. Effects of lithium carbonate on apomorphine-induced sniffing behaviour in rats. Pharmacol Toxicol 2002; 91: 135–9

85. Beaulieu JM, Sotnikova TD, Yao WD, et al. Lithium antagonizes dopamine-dependent behaviors mediated by an AKT/glycogen synthase kinase 3 signaling cascade. Prog Natl Acad Sci USA 2004; 101: 5099–6104

86. Bymaster FP, Felder CC. Role of the cholinergic muscarinic system in bipolar disorder and related mechanism of action of antipsychotic agents. Mol Psychiatry 2002; 7: 57–63

87. Yeomans J. Role of tegmental cholinergic neurons in dopaminergic activation, antimuscarinic psychosis and schizophrenia. Neuropsychopharmacology 1995; 12: 3–16

88. Roundtree DW, Nevin S, Wilson A. The effects of diisopropylfluorophosphonate in schizophrenia and manic depressive psychosis. J Neurol Neurosurg Psychiatry 1971; 133: 47–62

89. Safer DJ, Allen RP. The central effects of scopolamine in man. Biol Psychiatry 1971; 3: 347–55

90. Pullen GP, Best NR, Maguire J. Anticholinergic drug abuse: a common problem? Br Med J 1984; 289: 612–13

91. Janowsky DS, El-Yousef MK, Davis JM, et al. Antagonistic effects of physostigmine and methylphenidate in man. Am J Psychiatry 1972; 130: 1370–6

92. Dilsaver SC, Coffman JA. Cholinergic hypothesis of depression: a reappraisal. J Clin Psychopharmacol 1989; 9: 173–9

93. Jope RS. Effects of lithium treatment in vitro and in vivo on acetylcholine metabolism in rat brain. J Neurochem 1979; 33: 487–95

94. Gao XM, Fukamauchi F, Chuang DM. Long-term biphasic effects of lithium treatment on phospholipase C-coupled M3-muscarinic acetylcholine receptors in cultured cerebellar granule cells. Neurochem Int 1993; 22: 395–403

95. Manji HK, Chen G, Hsiao JK, et al. Regulation of signal transduction pathways by mood-stabilizing agents. Implications for the delayed onset of therapeutic efficacy. J Clin Psychiatry 1996; 57: 34–46

96. Jope RS. Anti-bipolar therapy: mechanism of action of lithium. Mol Psychiatry 1999; 4: 117–28

30 Lithium and cellular signal transduction pathways

Dietrich van Calker

INTRODUCTION

The discovery, more than half a century ago, of the antimanic action of lithium ions by John Cade and the empirical proof of its antimanic and prophylactic efficacy by Mogens Schou and collaborators (for review see reference 1) has kindled much hope that, with the advent of a specific treatment and discovery of its mechanism of action, the road would be paved to rapid progress in the elucidation of the neurobiology of bipolar illness. However, while the accumulation of data on the neurobiological actions of lithium is impressive, it has been difficult to decide which of this multitude of effects on many neurobiologic parameters are instrumental in lithium's efficacy as a mood stabilizer, and which are merely epiphenomena or responsible for side-effects. One potential solution to this problem is to identify biochemical actions that are common to several mood stabilizers, despite their different chemical structure and side-effect profile, and may therefore be most likely to be involved in their common beneficial clinical action. The presently established mood stabilizers are chemically diverse (a metal ion in the case of lithium, a simple branched-chained fatty acid in the case of valproate and a complex heterocyclic structure in the case of carbamazepine) and have thus quite different initial direct targets of action (for review see reference 2). However, recent progress in the elucidation of their downstream neurobiological actions has revealed remarkable similarities: they all have a prominent role in the regulation of neural resilience, growth and differentiation, albeit not always by virtue of similar mechanisms[2–4].

These recent findings, complemented by new insights into the molecular pathophysiology of bipolar illness[5], have provided a conceptual framework that might now allow us to assess which of the various biochemical effects of lithium are likely to be important in its mechanism of action. This recent evidence suggests that lithium, like other mood stabilizers, might act by modifying cellular signal transduction mechanisms essential for processes involved in neural resilience[5–9].

INITIAL DIRECT TARGETS OF LITHIUM

As monovalent cations Li^+ ions might be expected to act via interference with the functions of Na^+ ions in cellular physiology. However, Li^+ ions are heavily hydrated and thus acquire an ionic diameter similar to that of Mg^{2+}. Lithium's primary action therefore is the interference with the function of proteins that need for function the binding of this important co-factor at circumscribed metal ion binding sites. The enzymes inhibited by lithium ions by virtue of this mechanism comprise a quite heterogeneous group of enzymes, such as inositol monophosphatase (IMPase), phospho-glucomutase (FGM) and glycogen synthase kinase 3. Also, the acute effects of lithium on adenylyl cyclase (see below) appear to be due to competition with magnesium ions. IMPase is a member of a family of phosphomonoesterases also including inositol polyphosphate-1-phosphatase and fructose 1,6-bisphosphatase (FBPase) that are all Mg-dependent and inhibited by lithium at therapeutic concentrations. The members of this family do not show remarkable sequence similarities but are characterized by a conserved core three-dimensional structure and a conserved amino acid sequence motif, which has been used to identify the new members of this family, biphosphate-3'-nucleotidase (BNP1), and lithium-inhibited phosphomonoesterase (LPM), the function of which is unknown[10,11]. Up to now, only one member of this family, IMPase, has been strongly implicated in the potential mechanism of lithium (see below), although BNP1, also referred to as 3'-phosphoadenosine 5'-phosphate (PAP) phosphatase has now emerged as another interesting candidate[10,12,13]. With the exception of FGM and FBPase, which regulate glycogen metabolism and gluconeo-genesis, respectively, all of these lithium-sensitive enzymes, in particular adenylyl cyclase, IMPase and GSK-3, play a critical role in cellular signal transduction mechanisms. These are discussed below.

CELLULAR SIGNAL TRANSDUCTION PATHWAYS

The term 'signal transduction' denotes a process that transmits information impinging on receptors on the surface of the cell into the interior of the cell (Figure 30.1). The effects elicited there encompass both short-acting (e.g. changes in the phosphorylation of an ion channel) and long-lasting (e.g. changes of gene transcription) actions on cellular function. Particularly important components of the signal transduction system are the G-proteins, a family of guanylnucleotide-binding membrane-associated proteins, which mediate the coupling of the hormone-activated receptors to effector proteins. About 80% of all known hormones, neurotransmitters or neuromodulators act via G-proteins, which can couple to various intra-cellular effector proteins (for review see reference 14). G-proteins are heterotrimeric complexes located at the inner plasma membrane and consist of an α-subunit and the tightly associated $\beta\gamma$-subunits. The α-subunit binds guanyl nucleotides. Interaction with an activated receptor induces exchange of the

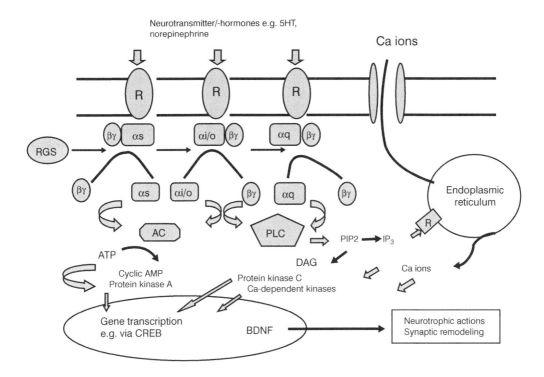

Figure 30.1 Signal transduction systems. RGS, regulators of G-protein signaling; AC, adenylyl cyclase; PLC, phospholipase DAG, diacylglycerol; CREB, cAMP-responsive element binding protein; BDNF, brain-derived neurotrophic factor; 5HT, 5-hydroxytryptamine; PIP2, phosphatidylinositolbisphosphonate; IP$_3$, inositoltriphosphate

bound guanosine diphosphate (GDP) with guanosine triphosphate (GTP) and dissociation of the heterotrimeric complex. The free α- and $\beta\gamma$-subunits subsequently activate various effectors. Activation is terminated by hydrolysis of GTP to GDP by the intrinsic GTPase activity of the α-subunit, which allows the reassociation of the heterotrimeric $\alpha\beta\gamma$-complex. This latter process of signal termination is reinforced by a separate class of proteins (regulators of G-protein signaling, RGS), which enhance the GTPase activity of the α-subunit. G-proteins comprise a family of different proteins that can be subdivided into four major classes (G_s, G_i,

G_q, G_{12}) that show some limited specificity for effector proteins. Thus, for example, G_s activates and G_i inhibits adenylyl cyclase, while G_q activates phospholipase C.

Effector proteins encompass not only enzymes such as adenylyl cyclase or various phospholipases (C, D, A$_2$), which synthesize second messenger molecules (see below) but also, for example, ion channels, the openings of which are regulated by binding to a G-protein. Second messengers are diffusible small molecules that are either water soluble, and thus easily diffuse into the cytoplasm (such as cyclic AMP, cyclic GMP or inositol polyphosphates), or lipophilic compounds that remain associated with the cell membrane, such as arachidonic acid (AA) or diacylglycerol (DAG). Second messengers often act via activation of protein kinases, which phosphorylate various target proteins, thereby modifying their functional state. Thus, for example, cyclic AMP activates protein kinase A (PKA), while DAG, together with Ca^{2+}, activates protein kinase C (PKC). Targets for these phosphorylations are ion channels, proteins of the cytoskeleton, components of the signal transduction system such as G-proteins or, in the case of long-lasting changes, transcription factors, which regulate gene transcription[15,16].

The process of G-protein-dependent signal transduction results in a several thousand-fold amplification of the original signal. Furthermore, since one type of receptor can couple with various different G-proteins, and different G-proteins can converge to modulate the function of a single effector, these signaling pathways form a complex network that accounts for the remarkable versatility of neural pathways in the integration, fine-tuning and processing of diverse signals[17,18]. Given this crucial role of signal transduction, it is not surprising that these systems are also critically involved in phenomena such as neural plasticity and memory formation[19,20], kindling[21] and behavioral sensitization[21–23], and are therefore candidates as potential targets in the mechanism of action of mood stabilizers[8]. Effects of lithium ions on signal transduction mechanisms have been a major focus of research during the past two decades[8,24–27].

EFFECTS OF LITHIUM ON THE ADENYLYL CYCLASE SYSTEM

Forn and Valdecasas[28] first described an inhibitory effect of lithium ions at near therapeutic (2 mmol/l) concentrations on the norepinephrine-stimulated accumulation of cyclic AMP. Since then, analogous effects were found in various other tissues including the brain[26,27,29]. Convincing evidence that lithium ions inhibit stimulated adenylyl cyclase also in the intact brain *in vivo* was obtained by the microdialysis technique[30]. The inhibitory action is exerted distal from the receptor and appears to be due to a competition with Mg^{2+} ions at the catalytic unit of adenylyl cyclase[26,27,29]. In contrast, the chronic inhibitory effects of lithium on the stimulation of adenylyl cyclase via β-adrenergic receptors are not influenced by Mg^{2+} ions but reversed by GTP. Thus, these chronic effects are believed to be due to actions of lithium on G-proteins (discussed below).

Early after the first description of the inhibitory effects of lithium on adenylyl cyclase, Murphy and co-workers[31] reported that the attenuating action of norepinephrine on the activity of prostaglandin E_1-stimulated adenylyl cyclase was compromised by lithium ions. This inhibitory action of norepinephrine is now known to be mediated by α_2-adrenergic receptors, which couple with the inhibitory G-protein G_i. More recent research has confirmed an inhibitory effect of lithium also on the inhibitory interaction of receptors with adenylyl cyclase[26,27,29] and revealed its mediation by an action of lithium on the G_i-protein (discussed below). This 'inhibition of inhibition' explains at least partially the increase of basal cyclic AMP in several regions of the brain that is observed after chronic lithium treatment. In addition, chronic treatment with lithium salts induces an increase in the content of protein and mRNA of two adenylyl cyclase subtypes, probably due to an increase of gene transcription (discussed below). In summary, lithium ions appear to balance signal transduction via the adenylyl cyclase system by virtue of inhibition of stimulated activity in combination with an increase in basal activity. This might preclude excessive pathologic fluctuations of signaling[32,33]. A role of cyclic AMP signal transduction abnormalities in the pathophysiology of mood disorders was indeed suggested by findings of postmortem brain studies[34].

EFFECTS OF LITHIUM ON INOSITOL PHOSPHATE SIGNALING

The great surge in interest on the effects of lithium on the processes of intracellular signaling during the last two decades was particularly stimulated by the discovery of the pivotal importance of the phosphatidylinositol (PI)-Ca^{2+} second messenger system for cellular signal transduction and the almost coincident recognition of the modulatory action of lithium ions on this system[35–37]. PI is only a minor component of the lipids in the cell membrane,

but plays an important role in the process of receptor-activated signal transduction, particularly in the central nervous system (CNS). Neurotransmitters, including norepinephrine, serotonin and acetylcholine, which are believed to be dysregulated in affective disorders, stimulate via particular receptor subtypes (e.g. $M_{1,3,5}$, α_1, 5-HT_2) and activate by G-proteins of hydrolysis of IP to two second messenger molecules, DAG and inositol-1,4,5-trisphosphate (IP_3), which activate, respectively, protein kinase C and the intracellular release of Ca^{2+} ions. The latter also enter the cytoplasm from the outside via influx through receptor-operated ion channels. IP_3 is metabolized via several phosphorylation (IP_4 and higher phosphorylated compounds) and dephosphorylation steps to myoinositol, which is used together with cytidine diphosphate (CDP)-DAG for the resynthesis of PI (Figure 30.2).

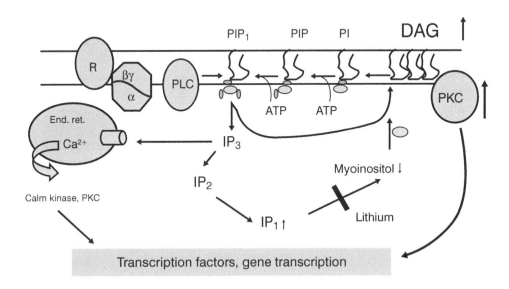

Figure 30.2 Phosphatidylinositol (PI) signal transduction – effect of lithium. DAG, diacylglycerol; PKC, protein kinase C; End. ret., endoplasmic reticulum; calm kinase, calmodulin-dependent kinase; PLC, phospholipase C

The inositol depletion hypothesis

The last step in the metabolism of IP_3, the hydrolysis of inositol monophosphate to myoinositol by IMPase, is inhibited by lithium ions in the therapeutic concentration range ($K_i = 0.8$ mmol/l). In contrast, valproate and carbamazepine, the two other established mood stabilizers, do not inhibit IMPase[38]. The now famous 'inositol depletion hypothesis'[36] postulates that the lithium-induced inhibition of IMPase leads to a depletion in the cell of myoinositol and subsequently, due to a compromised synthesis of PI, to a reduction of receptor-stimulated formation of PI-dependent second messenger molecules. This hypothesis has received considerable attention, since for the first time it appeared to offer an explanation for the most enigmatic aspect of lithium's activity, its almost specific therapeutic effects on only the pathologically altered mood of patients with affective disorders, leaving almost unaffected the psychological functioning of normal subjects. According to the hypothesis, this unique feature is due first to the uncompetitive nature of lithium's inhibition of IMPase, an unusual type of enzyme inhibition[39], which is the more pronounced the more substrate for the enzyme is available. Second, the fact that the more frequently the system is stimulated the more inositol phosphates accumulate at the expense of myoinositol could also add to the specificity of lithium's action. It was concluded from these unusual properties that a pronounced inhibition by lithium of the PI system would only occur under conditions where the respective receptors and their signal transduction system are pathologically over-activated.

From these unique features that are postulated to govern lithium's effects on PI signaling it is understandable why it has not been possible to obtain a definite proof or falsification of the inositol depletion hypothesis from experiments with experimental animals, since these 'normal' animals are not expected to show a 'pathologic overactivation' of the PI system. The extent of 'depletion' of inositol in lithium-treated rats amounts to maximally 35% and is limited to acute treatment with probably already toxic doses of lithium. Whether or not such a limited reduction in the inositol content could have functional consequences for PI signaling is open to question. It has been argued, however, that a lithium-induced depletion of inositol might be limited to selected brain areas or even cells that might be particularly vulnerable to this effect due to restricted inositol supply and/or increased activity of the PI system[25,40]. Indeed, we have shown that both the basal content of inositol and its uptake *in vivo* differ among various areas of the rat brain[41], and that a reduction in inositol levels after chronic lithium administration was limited to the hypothalamus, a brain region that might indeed be particularly activated during the stressful treatment with lithium[42,43]. Thus, further investigations specifically targeted at the effects of lithium in animal models of depression such as the 'learned helplessness' paradigm or other stress-related paradigms might provide an opportunity for detecting more meaningful lithium-induced alterations in inositol content and PI signaling.

The original inositol depletion hypothesis had assumed that inositol depletion would lead to a reduced synthesis of inositol phospholipids and thus, by virtue of substrate deprivation, to diminished production of IP_3 after receptor stimulation. However, it has now become clear that even a 90% reduction of the myoinositol content in the brain as evoked by targeted deletion of the Na^+/myoinositol co-transporter (SMIT, discussed in detail below) does not reduce the level of inositol phospholipids to an extent that could impair IP_3 signaling[44]. It is now believed that an impairment of PI signalling (if any) as a result of inositol depletion is not caused by a deficiency in inositol phospholipids, but rather by an activation of PKC due to the increased accumulation of DAG that results from diminished consumption for resynthesis of PI[45].

While earlier work with brain slices[25] and later investigations of neural cell cultures *in vitro*[46–49] had identified inhibitory effects of lithium on the agonist-stimulated release of inositol phosphates or Ca^{2+} ions, measurements of IP_3 *in vivo*[50,51] did not provide evidence for an inhibition by lithium of PI signaling. Furthermore, work by Hokin and colleagues made it clear that brain slices from species such as rats and mice were particularly vulnerable to artificial depletion of inositol during the assay procedures, and they showed that, in slices from primate brain and in neuronal cells of human origin, lithium rather increased PI signaling[52,53]. This increase was reported to be due to inhibition by lithium of glutamate uptake, which leads via stimulation of *N*-methyl-D-asparate (NMDA) receptors and subsequent Ca^{2+} influx to enhanced formation of IP_3[54].

The potential role of myoinositol in the mechanism of action of lithium has been studied also in animal behavior paradigms. Studies by Belmaker and colleagues provided evidence that effects of lithium administration on behavior (rearing) and the induction of seizures by a combination of pilocarpin and lithium could be prevented by myoinositol[55], an indication of a role of inositol depletion in these effects.

Measurements of the effects of lithium treatment on inositol levels in the human brain are partly consistent with the inositol depletion hypothesis[56,57]. Proton magnetic resonance spectroscopy (MRS) scans of bipolar patients were performed after a medication wash-out (minimum 2 weeks) at baseline and after 5 days and 4 weeks of lithium treatment. The results indicated a significant reduction of the myoinositol content in the frontal cortex already after 5 days of lithium administration, at a time when the patient's clinical state was completely unchanged[56]. Thus, while lithium indeed lowers the myoinositol content in the brain, this action alone cannot explain the therapeutic effect of lithium, but may be the initial trigger that initiates a cascade of events that ultimately account for the therapeutic effect. In contrast to these results, other investigators found in a recent study that lithium treatment rather increased myoinositol in the gray matter of the brain[58].

In summary, work of the last decade has provided evidence that, as predicted by the inositol depletion hypothesis, lithium ions indeed modify inositol content and PI signaling in neural tissue, but that the extent and even the direction of these effects apparently depend in a subtle manner on factors such as species, brain region, cell type and activation state of the cells and tissues. This provokes the question as to whether distinct neural circuits in the brain may be differentially influenced by lithium ions, and to what extent these effects might vary with the particular activation state in depressive or manic mood. Thus, a major challenge of future work is to identify the factors that stipulate the sensitivity and direction of response of a cell or neural circuit to lithium's modulating effects on cellular signaling. One of these factors is the high-affinity SMIT, which is discussed in more detail below.

Inhibition by lithium and other mood stabilizers of the high-affinity sodium/myoinositol co-transporter

The inositol content in a cell is determined by four processes[40,59] (Figure 30.3): synthesis by IMPase from myoinositol monophosphate, which is formed (1) as a final product of the hydrolysis of inositol phospholipids or (2) as an intermediate in the *de novo* synthesis of inositol from glucose-6-phosphate. The assumption that

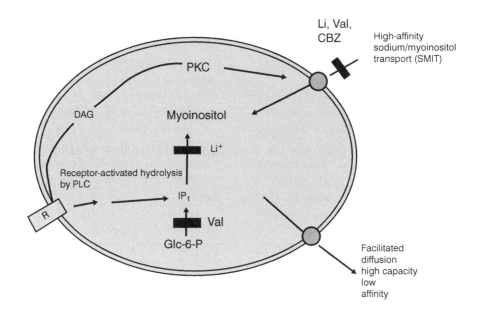

Figure 30.3 Factors determining myoinositol levels in brain cells. Li, lithium; Val, valproate; CBZ, carbamazepine; DAG, diacylglycerol; PKC, protein kinase C; Glc-6-P, glucose-6-phosphate; PLC, phospholipase C

brain cells completely rely on inositol synthesis from inositol monophosphate that is sensitive to inhibition by lithium is the central tenet of the classical inositol depletion hypothesis. However, brain cells may also acquire inositol from the extracellular space by virtue of the SMIT, a high-affinity myoinositol transport system, which has been characterized in various cell types including those of neural origin[60,61]. A fourth system involved in the regulation of cellular inositol content is a low-affinity and high-capacity facilitated diffusion system that, under normal conditions might determine the efflux of inositol. This system might, however, also mediate the entry of inositol into the cell when the extracellular inositol concentration is artificially increased to high values, for example, in experiments aimed at reversing the

inositol depletion evoked by lithium or other mood stabilizers.

The SMIT transports myoinositol against a steep concentration gradient into the cell. Among neural cells, the SMIT appears to be particularly highly expressed in astrocytes[62]. Chronic exposure of various cell types to hypertonicity leads to upregulation of the SMIT[63–65]. This effect protects the cell against hyperosmolarity, since it increases intracellular inositol concentrations and thus osmolarity without disrupting cellular functioning[66]. The expression of the SMIT and its regulation by osmolarity and corticosteroids shows remarkable differences in astrocytes cultured from distinct brain regions[61]. Both the activity of the SMIT and the expression of its mRNA in astrocytes and astrocytoma cells are down-regulated after chronic treatment with therapeutic concentrations of lithium salts, an effect which develops slowly over a time period of 8 days, in remarkable agreement with the time course of lithium's clinical effects. Furthermore, downregulation of the SMIT with a similar time course is also observed after treatment with valproate and carbamazepine, indicating that this effect might represent a common mechanism of action of all three antibipolar drugs[67,68].

The inhibition of inositol uptake by all three mood stabilizers might explain the finding that not only lithium but also valproate, after chronic application, decreased the content of myo-inositol in the brain of rats[69], although valproate does not inhibit inositol monophosphatase[38]. Valproate may deplete cells of inositol also by inhibition of myoinositol-1-phosphate synthase, which forms inositol monophosphate from glucose-6-phosphate[70] (Figure 30.3). This enzyme appears, however, to be largely restricted to the vasculature of the brain[71]. Inhibition of SMIT by all three mood stabilizers might also explain the recent finding that lithium, valproate and carbamazepine exert similar effects on growth cones of neurons from newborn rat dorsal root ganglia in culture. Growth cones are motile structures that undergo chemotaxis in response to guidance cues. All three mood stabilizers increase growth cone spreading. The effects of Li^+, valproate and carbamazepine on growth cone spreading are all reversed by the addition of myoinositol, but not by epi- and scylloinositol isomers[72].

We have recently shown that inhibition of the SMIT also occurs *in vivo* in bipolar patients chronically treated with lithium or valproate. The content of SMIT mRNA was significantly reduced in neutrophils of lithium-treated bipolar patients as compared to controls and to untreated bipolar patients. Untreated bipolar-I patients but not bipolar-II patients exhibited a significantly higher expression of SMIT mRNA than controls. Neutrophils of bipolar-I patients

treated with valproate had a significantly lower expression of SMIT mRNA than untreated bipolar-I patients, but did not differ from controls[73]. These results suggest that increased expression of the SMIT might be a risk factor for bipolar illness that is compensated for by treatment with mood stabilizers.

Effects of lithium on phosphatidylinositol signaling in humans

Since the PI system mediates the effects of hormonal agonists not only in the CNS but also in peripheral cells, potential effects of chronic lithium treatment on PI signaling as predicted by the inositol depletion hypothesis can be examined in peripheral blood cells of humans. Indeed, we have observed in neutrophils of chronically lithium-treated patients that the agonist-stimulated intracellular release of inositol phosphates and Ca^{2+} ions was compromised in comparison to untreated normal controls[74,75]. Lithium also inhibits Ca^{2+} signaling in transformed lymphocytes of bipolar patients[76]. On the other hand, neutrophils, platelets and lymphocytes of depressive or manic patients show an increased sensitivity of the PI system as compared to controls[77,78]. This may, however, not always be a trait but rather a state marker of the disorder, since this abnormality of signaling was normalized in remitted patients[79] (van Calker *et al.*, to be published). On the other hand, studies using transformed lymphocytes from bipolar patients revealed similar abnormalities, suggesting that in bipolar patients there might also be a trait-dependent component of this abnormality in Ca^{2+} signaling[76,80]. An increased sensitivity of the PI system is also suggested by the finding that PKC activation[81], PI-4,5-bisphosphate[82] and G-protein coupling[83] was increased in the platelets of bipolar patients. Also, the increased PKC activation was found to be decreased after lithium or valproate treatment[81,83]. In summary, these results provide evidence for an increased sensitivity of the PI system in peripheral cells of manic-depressive patients that is compensated or even overcompensated by treatment with lithium or valproate. A heightened state of activity of the PI signaling system is also suggested by the finding of enhanced PKC activity in post-mortem brains of bipolar subjects[84]. Recently, aberrant Ca^{2+} signaling was also shown for olfactory neurons from patients with bipolar disorder[85].

EFFECTS OF LITHIUM ON THE ARACHIDONIC ACID CASCADE IN THE BRAIN

While membrane phospholipids are best known as a substrate for the agonist-stimulated hydrolysis by phospholipase C and thus as a source for inositol phosphates and DAG as second messenger molecules (see above), they can also serve as a substrate for phospholipase A_2 (PLA_2), which is also activated by receptor–G-protein coupling. Agonist binding to certain neuroreceptors activates PLA_2 to release the second messenger arachidonic acid (AA, 20:4 n:6), from the stereospecifically numbered (sn)-2 position of membrane phospholipids[86]. Receptors that are coupled to PLA_2 via G-proteins include muscarinic $M_{1,3,5}$ receptors, dopaminergic D_2 receptors and $5\text{-}HT_{2A/2C}$ receptors[86,87]. Once released, AA has several possible metabolic fates, including conversion to eicosanoids, β-oxidation, and recycling back into phospholipids through a fatty acyl-coenzyme A (acyl-CoA) synthetase and acyl-transferase[88]. The released AA and its bioactive eicosanoid metabolites can influence many physiologic processes, including membrane excitability, gene transcription, apoptosis, sleep and behavior[89]. Initial studies of Rapoport

and collaborators showed that both chronic lithium and valproate treatment resulted in selective reductions in AA turnover rate in the brain phospholipids of the rat: 75% with lithium and 30% with valproate treatment. Lithium's effect was highly specific, since lithium did not affect PLA_2-mediated turnover of the n-3 polyunsaturated fatty acid, docosohexaenoic acid. It was further demonstrated that lithium downregulated the gene expression, protein level and activity of the AA-specific PLA_2 (cytosolic $cPLA_2$) and also reduced the level and activity of cyclo-oxygenase 2 (COX-2) and prostaglandin E_2, an AA metabolite and important messenger molecule that is formed by COX-2[90]. Valproate treatment similarly decreased the protein level of COX-2 (and also that of COX-1)[91]. Also, chronic carbamazepine treatment was recently shown to specifically downregulate $cPLA_2$ and decrease COX-2 activity and PGE_2 concentration as well as the incorporation rate and turnover of AA in the rat brain, although to a lesser extent than lithium[92,93]. Thus, there is a remarkable similarity in the actions of the three mood stabilizers on AA turnover and metabolism, which strongly argues for a potential role of these effects in their mechanism of action in bipolar disorder.

EFFECTS OF LITHIUM ON GLYCOGEN SYNTHASE-KINASE-3

Glycogen synthase-kinase-3 (GSK-3) was initially named for its role in glycogen synthesis, but is now known to be a component of diverse signaling pathways such as insulin/IGF1, neurotrophin and the Wnt signaling pathway. It is thus recognized as an important regulator of many vital cellular functions such as apoptosis, synaptic plasticity, cytoskeletal rearrangement and circadian rhythm[94–98]. GSK-3 is a constitutively active serine/threonine kinase and is found as two isoforms, GSK-3α and GSK-3β that have similar biological effects. GSK-3 is inactivated by phosphorylation on a serine residue in the N-terminal domain. Lithium inhibits GSK-3 directly by virtue of competition with Mg^{2+} ions. Li^+ also indirectly inhibits GSK-3 by virtue of increased phosphorylation on the N-terminal serine which may involve PKC[99], protein phosphatase 1 or increased protein kinase B/Akt-activity[96]. While the relevance of the inhibition by Li^+ was originally considered questionable, owing to its only marginal inhibitory effects at therapeutic concentrations, it later became evident that the Mg^{2+} concentrations utilized in the initial *in vitro* assays had been much higher than intracellular levels in brain cells. Thus, there is now convincing evidence for a relevant inhibition of GSK-3 by therapeutic lithium concentrations in the brain[98]. Also, valproate was reported to inhibit GSK-3[100], these effects are, however, controversial[98]. Carbamazepine appears not to affect GSK-3[101]. The inhibition by lithium (and perhaps valproate) of GSK-3 probably contributes to the effects of these mood stabilizers on cAMP-responsive element binding protein (CREB) DNA binding activity[102] and also to their anti-apoptotic and neuroprotective effects[95] (for review see also Chapters 31 and 32). It is, however, questionable whether inhibition of GSK-3 can be considered as a mechanism of action specific for mood stabilizers, since many other compounds and measures such as antidepressants, antipsychotics, estrogen and electroconvulsive seizures also increase inhibitory phosphorylation of GSK-3, among these several with no mood stabilizing but rather mood destabilizing activity such as imipramine or haloperidol[98]. Nevertheless, newly synthesized selective GSK-3 inhibitors such as those now developed by various industrial companies[103] for the treatment of, for example, Alzheimer's disease, are considered as potential new medications for

bipolar disorder[7]. These selective GSK-3-inhibitors were already shown to have anti-depressant-like effects on the behavior of experimental animals in acute paradigms such as the forced swimming test that predict antidepresssant efficacy[104,105].

EFFECTS OF LITHIUM ON PROTEIN KINASE ACTIVITIES AND PROTEIN PHOSPHORYLATION

As discussed above, the main effects of lithium on signal transduction are an increase in basal activity of adenylyl cyclase and a decrease of agonist-stimulated activity of this enzyme. Lithium and other mood stabilizers also exert complex modulatory actions on PI signaling, the extent and direction of which depend critically on various factors such as species, cell type and activational state. In cases of cellular depletion of inositol the subsequent decreased resynthesis of inositol phospholipids should result in a diminished consumption and thus increased accumulation of DAG and its metabolite CDP-DAG[45]. An increased cellular content of CDP-DAG is indeed now considered as a reliable indicator of inositol depletion[106]. Thus, lithium ions and, less well established, other mood stabilizing medications modulate the basal and agonist-stimulated concentrations of the second messenger molecules cyclic AMP, IP_3, Ca^{2+} and DAG and should therefore also influence the activity of the protein kinases A, C, A_2 and others that are regulated by these second messengers.

Several studies have reported that lithium can modulate protein kinase A-mediated protein phosphorylation[107–112]. Abnormalities in PKA have been found in postmortem brain studies of bipolar patients[113]. In the frontal cortex of the rat, chronic lithium treatment increases the level of DARPP-32 (32 kDa dopamine and cyclic AMP-regulated phos-phoprotein)[108]. Phosphorylation by PKA and PKG at Thr34 converts DARPP-32 into a potent inhibitor of protein phosphatase-1 (PP-1), while phosporylation at Thr75 by Cdk5 converts DARPP-32 into an inhibitor of PKA. Alterations in DARPP-32 could thus modify the phosphorylation state of several other proteins. By virtue of its ability to modulate the activity of PP-1 and PKA, DARPP-32 is critically involved in regulating electrophysio-logic, transcriptional and behavioral responses to physiologic and pharmacologic stimuli, including antidepressants, neuroleptics and drugs of abuse[114]. The specific proteins regulated by DARPP-32 phosphorylation have not been fully identified, although Na$^+$–K$^+$-ATPase represents a possible target[115]. A potential role of this enzyme in the mechanism of action of lithium has long been discussed[116,117] (for review of the older literature see reference 118).

Alterations of PKC activity by lithium were conjectured already early after the formulation of the inositol depletion hypothesis[119], since a depletion of inositol should result in a decreased consumption for PI resynthesis and thus increased accumulation of DAG, the activator of PKC. Indeed, a modulation by chronic lithium of PKC activity is now considered to play a key role in the mechanism of lithium's therapeutic effects[25,27,120–124]. PKC activity represents the action of a family of closely related subspecies, which are highly enriched in the brain. It regulates many pre- and postsyn-aptic aspects of neurotransmission including long-term alterations in gene expression and neuronal plasticity[125–127]. Persistent activation of PKC is often followed by its rapid proteolytic degradation and downregulation of enzyme activity. This explains why, in several cell systems lithium after acute or subchronic treatment induces an increase, while chronic treatment results in a decrease of PKC or PKC-

mediated processes[120]. This lithium-induced decrease in PKC activity appears to be restricted to specific isoenzymes of PKC such as α and ε, which may have a particular role in the regu-lation of neurotransmitter release[121,122,128,129]. The modulation by lithium of PKC isoenzymes in the brain is apparently not uniform but specific for particular hippocampal structures. Furthermore, the proteolytic degradation of PKC may lead to the formation of a constitu-tively active fragment ('PKM') that could be involved in the regulation of gene expression[120]. Thus, the alterations in gene expression observed after chronic lithium treatment (see below) could at least in part be mediated by effects on PKC. The modulation by lithium of PKC activity could also explain its actions on neurotransmitter systems, since PKC regulates the release of several neurotransmitters, such as serotonin and norepinephrine[130], which is also influenced by lithium[131]. Lithium's ability to potentiate in rats the seizures evoked by stimulation of muscarinic receptors might also involve modulation of PKC[25,120].

The modulation by lithium of PKC activity should result in altered phosphorylation of PKC substrates. Indeed, a major substrate of PKC in the brain, myristoylated alanine-rich C-kinase substrate (MARCKS), is downregulated by both PKC activation and chronic treatment with lithium at therapeutically relevant concentra-tions. This effect of lithium is particularly compelling, since MARCKS appears to play an important role in the restructuring of cyto-skeletal elements that are involved in the long-term alteration of processes such as signal transduction and neurotransmitter release[123,124]. Since MARCKS is involved in the regulation of PI signaling[132] its alteration by chronic lithium might also be responsible for some of the effects of lithium on signal transduction via this system. The potential importance of these effects of antibipolar drugs on PKC also becomes evident from results of the postmortem studies mentioned earlier, which suggested an increased PKC-mediated phosphorylation and elevated levels of PKC isoenzymes in the brains of patients with bipolar disorder as compared to controls[84].

The precise molecular mechanisms by which lithium modulates PKC isoenzymes are presently unclear. However, both the effects of lithium on the ε (and perhaps α) isoform of PKC[121] and the apparently PKC-mediated downregulation of MARCKS[133] by chronic lithium treatment are reversed or prevented by co-administration of myoinositol, in agreement with the principal role of inositol depletion in these effects[124]. Valproate at therapeutic concentrations has similar effects on PKC isoenzymes[134] and MARCKS protein expression[123,129,135] to those of lithium. Both drugs also inhibit at chronic application the high-affinity inositol uptake (see above) with a strikingly similar triphasic time course[67], which can be partially mimicked by PKC inhibitors (Lubrich *et al.*, unpublished). Thus, both lithium and valproate may act by way of modulation of PKC activity, which feeds back on regulation of myoinositol homeostasis and phosphoinositide signaling and also modifies proteins such as MARCKS that are involved in restructuring of the cytoskeleton and consequently the neuronal architecture.

EFFECTS OF LITHIUM ON G-PROTEINS

As discussed above, the effects of mood stabilizers on the adenylyl cyclase system and its actions on phosphoinositol signaling suggest the involvement of mechanisms beyond alterations of the catalytic subunit of adenylyl cyclase or depletion of intracellular inositol, respectively. One additional mechanism by which a mood stabilizer could modify the activity of these signal transduction systems is the alteration of activity of the heterotrimeric G-proteins, crucial molecular switches that amplify the signals impinging on the outside of a cell and relay them to the subsequent effector systems. Accordingly, early studies attracted much attention, which appeared to show a direct inhibitory influence of lithium on the coupling of various receptors to G-proteins[136,137]. However, the robustness of these findings is now questionable[26,29,138]. An influence of lithium on G-protein function can be assessed by agents that directly activate or inactivate G-proteins via specific mechanisms that bypass the receptors. Such agents are cholera toxin and pertussis toxin which, via ADP-ribosylation, activate or inhibit, respectively, the G_s-protein that stimulates and the G_i-protein that inhibits adenylyl cyclase. Using this approach it was shown by *in vivo* experiments with a micro-dialysis technique that chronic lithium treatment inhibits the function of G_i thereby increasing the basal level of cyclic AMP in the brain of rats[139,140]. Experiments with humans chronically treated with lithium also revealed an increase of basal cyclic AMP, and also of stimulated cyclic AMP accumulation, when the stimulation was performed in a way that bypassed the receptors[26,27]. Also, these effects were explained by a lithium-induced inactivation of the inhibitory G_i. On the other hand, chronic lithium treatment apparently also inhibits the function of G_s, since the inhibition by chronic lithium of the receptor-mediated activation of adenylyl cyclase is counteracted by GTP[25,29]. The acute inhibitory effect of lithium on adenylyl cyclase is, in contrast, apparently mediated by competition with Mg^{2+} ions at the catalytic subunit (see above). The biochemical mechanisms of lithium's action on the function of G_s and G_i are presently unclear. The inhibition of G_i may be due to a lithium-induced stabilization of the undissociated, inactive heterotrimeric $\alpha\beta\gamma$ state of the G_i-protein. Only this form is subject to ADP ribosylation by pertussis toxin, which was indeed increased in platelets from humans under chronic lithium therapy and in rats chronically treated with lithium[22,26,27].

Also, the gene transcription of G-proteins themselves may be modified by chronic lithium treatment. Chronic lithium application appears to downregulate the mRNAs of a number of G-protein α-subunits in the rat brain including $\alpha_{i(1,2)}$ and α_s, while varying results were reported for the respective proteins[26,27,124]. More recent studies pointed to more localized effects of chronic lithium on several different G-protein α-subunits in various regions of the rat brain[141–143].

In neutrophils of bipolar patients under chronic lithium therapy, the content of α_i mRNA is increased as compared to the content in untreated patients or controls, while lithium-treated unipolar depressive patients show no alterations of α_i mRNA[144]. In addition, the amount of α_s-mRNA[144] and α_s-protein (our unpublished results) is increased in neutrophils of bipolar but not unipolar patients. This increase is, however, also observed in untreated bipolar patients and thus independent of chronic treatment with lithium. Similarly, enhanced levels of α_s-protein were also found in postmortem brain samples[78] and in platelets of bipolar patients[145]. Since it is independent of the psychopathological state and was not found in unipolar patients, this enhanced level of α_s-mRNA may turn out to be a potential trait-marker or 'endophenotype'[146] of bipolar illness. However, although these results suggest a potential pathophysiologic role of α_s in bipolar disorder, no abnormalities in the gene for the α_s-subunit could be identified in bipolar patients[147]. Thus, the ultimate genetic alter-ations leading to an enhanced vulnerabilty for bipolar disorder may be rather found in the genes for transcription factors that regulate α_s-gene transcription. Furthermore, since only bipolar patients who show abnormal α_s

expression but not unipolar patients are sensitive to the lithium-induced upregulation of α_i mRNA (see above). This limitation of the effect of lithium to bipolar patients raises the intriguing possibility that only abnormal signal transduction may be affected by lithium and that the upregulation of α_{i2} mRNA might be related to the clinical efficacy of lithium in bipolar disorder.

EFFECTS OF LITHIUM ON GENE EXPRESSION

As already mentioned above, the activation by second messengers of protein kinases can lead to phosphorylation of nuclear transcription factors that regulate gene expression[15]. Therefore, in agreement with the effect of mood stabilizers on second messenger systems, they also affect the expression of a number of genes, probably at least in part also secondary to modulation of PKC and/or GSK3 activity[8,26,27]. The effects of chronic lithium treatment on various components of signal transduction systems such as G-proteins and adenylyl cyclase subtypes have been mentioned above. Of particular interest are the actions of mood stabilizers on so-called 'immediate early genes', members of the c-fos and c-jun families, which encode proteins that form the constituents of a family of transcription factors called AP-1 (activator protein 1). These genes are of pivotal importance for long-term changes in neuronal function[148]. Genes regulated by AP-1 include neurotrophins, neuropeptides, neurotransmitter synthesizing enzymes and other transcription factors[149]. It is now well established that lithium regulates AP-1 binding activity and func-tion[150,151]. This effect it shared by valproate[152]. There is, however, a disconcerting complexity of many apparently contradictory findings in this area of research, with reports indicating both increases and decreases as well as no changes evoked by lithium in various different *in vitro* and *in vivo* models. Jope[32] has recently attempted to integrate these data in his model of a 'bimodal mechanism of action of lithium', which suggests as the critical action of lithium a balancing of positive and negative regulators of signaling processes, thereby stabilizing signaling activities within an optimal range. The mechanisms by which lithium and valproate regulate AP-1 have not been elucidated, but a role of both PKC isoenzymes and GSK-3 (see above) can be envisaged[8]. The regulation by lithium of transcription factors is obviously not restricted to AP-1, since it also modulates two other such factors, CREB and nuclear factor (NF)-κB[153,154]. In addition, lithium alters the level of various other mRNAs in the brain and neural cell cultures (e.g. for neuropeptides, tyrosine hydroxylase, glucocorticoid type II receptor) that are important in the regulation of several aspects of neural function[27,124]. For a more comprehensive discussion of the effects of lithium on gene expression the reader is referred to Chapter 31.

EFFECTS OF LITHIUM ON CELLULAR RESILIENCE

Although the neuroprotective effects of lithium have been known for some time[155], the importance of actions of mood stabilizers on cellular resilience in the CNS was only recently fully appreciated[8,140]. The neuroprotective and anti-apoptotic effects of mood stabilizers are at least partly explained by the finding that lithium and valproate upregulate the neuroprotective and anti-apoptotic protein bcl-2[156]. Very recently it has been shown that mood stabilizers also increase BAG-1, an anti-apoptotic, glucocorticoid receptor co-chaperone protein[157]. Many of these effects may be in part mediated via inhibition of GSK-3β[95,158]. That neuroprotection could also be an important

mechanism of action of mood stabilizers *in vivo* is suggested by the findings that lithium induces neurogenesis in the adult rodent brain[159] and increases *N*-acetyl-aspartate levels (a putative marker of neuronal viability and function)[160] and total gray matter in the human brain[161]. These results are particularly important in view of the recent evidence from brain imaging and postmortem studies that mood disorders are associated with morphometric changes suggestive of cell loss and/or atrophy[8,140,162–168]. For a more comprehensive discussion of these neuroprotective effects of lithium and their potential use for the treatment of neurodegenerative diseases, the reader is referred to Chapters 31 and 32.

CONCLUSIONS

The recent progress in the unraveling of the effects of lithium and other mood stabilizers on signal transduction systems has offered a conceptual framework that might help to integrate the hitherto disconcerting and disparate actions of lithium, for example on neurotransmitters and membrane transport systems[118,169] into a comprehensive model. Thus, many of the actions of lithium on neurotransmitter release may be ultimately explained by its modulation of PKC activity, which critically depends on various factors such as acute versus chronic administration, brain region and particular isoenzyme type. On the other hand, lithium's effects on Na^+–K^+-ATPase, which may be mediated via its action on DARPP-32 (see above) illustrate how the modulating actions of lithium ions on protein phosphorylation might explain effects on mechanisms of membrane transport. Since the processes of sensitization and desensitization of receptors are determined by the function of signal transduction systems[170], it is conceivable that also the long-disputed[169] effects of lithium on receptor sensitivity are mediated by its action on second messenger systems.

However, the eventual discovery of the mechanism of action of lithium will probably depend on the identification of biochemical actions common to all or several mood stabilizers and the evaluation of the role that the respective targets play in the physiology of neural cells and the entire brain. Thus, for example, the re-evaluation of the classical inositol depletion hypothesis has revealed that depletion of inositol is a common effect of all three mood stabilizers that can be evoked by mechanisms beyond IMPase inhibition such as downregulation of the SMIT. Subsequent analysis has discovered an unexpected vital role of the SMIT in the brain. Although homozygous SMIT-1 knock-out mice show a 90% reduction of myoinositol in the brain[171], the remaining content should be sufficient to support the established functions of myoinositol as an osmolyte and a precursor of inositol phospholipids and the signaling molecules derived therefrom[44]. Nevertheless, deletion of the SMIT results in death of newborn homozygous SMIT-1 knock-out mice[171], due to central apnea as a result of dysfunction of the respiratory rhythm-generating center in the brainstem. It has therefore been postulated[44] that the reason for the unusually high content of inositol in the brain (millimoles in the brain as compared to micromoles in the liver) might be that inositol and/or SMIT serve an as yet unknown additional role in the brain essential for normal functioning of neural cells. Another unexpected common mechanism of action of these three mood stabilizers is their similar modulation of signaling through the arachidonic acid cascade. Thus, the discovery and elucidation of common actions of mood stabilizers might offer unforeseen and exciting new insights into the neurobiology of mood disorders and the functioning of neural circuits in general.

REFERENCES

1. Schou M. Lithium treatment at 52. J Affect Disord 2001; 67: 21–32
2. Gould TD, Quiroz JA, Singh J, et al. Emerging experimental therapeutics for bipolar disorder: insights from the molecular and cellular actions of current mood stabilizers. Mol Psychiatry 2004; 9: 734–55
3. van Calker D, Biber K, Walden J, et al. Carbamazepine and adenosine receptors. In Manji HK, Bowden C, Belmaker RH, eds. Bipolar Medications – Mechanism of Action. Washington, DC: American Psychiatric Press, 2000: 331–46
4. van Calker D, Biber K. The role of glial adenosine receptors in neural resilience and the neurobiology of mood disorders. Neurochemical Res 2005; 30: 1205–17
5. Quiroz JA, Singh J, Gould TD, et al. Emerging experimental therapeutics for bipolar disorder: clues from the molecular pathophysiology. Mol Psychiatry 2004; 9: 756–76
6. Coyle JT, Duman RS. Finding the intracellular signaling pathways affected by mood disorder treatments. Neuron 2003; 38: 157–60
7. Gould TD, Zarate CA, Manji HK. Glycogen synthase kinase-3: a target for novel bipolar disorder treatments. J Clin Psychiatry 2004; 65: 10–21
8. Manji HK, Moore GJ, Chen G. Bipolar disorder: leads from the molecular and cellular mechanisms of action of mood stabilizers. Br J Psychiatry 2001; 41 (Suppl): s107–19
9. Manji HK, Quiroz JA, Sporn J, et al. Enhancing neuronal plasticity and cellular resilience to develop novel, improved therapeutics for difficult-to-treat depression. Biol Psychiatry 2003; 53: 707–42
10. Spiegelberg BD, Dela Cruz J, Law TH, York JD. Alteration of lithium pharmacology through manipulation of phosphoadenosine phosphate metabolism. J Biol Chem 2005; 280: 5400–5
11. York JD, Ponder JW, Majerus PW. Definition of a metal-dependent/Li(+)-inhibited phosphomonoesterase protein family based upon a conserved three-dimensional core structure. Proc Natl Acad Sci USA 1995; 92: 5149–53

12. Shaltiel G, Kozlovsky N, Belmaker RH, Agam G. 3′(2′)-phosphoadenosine 5′-phosphate phosphatase is reduced in postmortem frontal cortex of bipolar patients. Bipolar Disord 2002; 4: 302–6

13. Agam G, Shaltiel G. Possible role of 3′(2′)-phosphoadenosine-5′-phosphate phosphatase in the etiology and therapy of bipolar disorder. Prog Neuropsychopharmacol Biol Psychiatry 2003; 27: 723–7

14. Birnbaumer L. G-proteins in signal transduction. Ann Rev Toxicol 1990; 30: 675–705

15. Karin M. Signal transduction from the surface to the nucleus through the phosphorylation of transcription factors. Curr Opin Cell Biol 1994; 6: 415–24

16. Calkhoven CF, Ab G. Multiple steps in the regulation of transcription-factor level and activity. Biochem J 1996: 317: 329–42

17. Bhalla US, Iyengar R. Emergent properties of networks of biological signaling pathways. Science 1999; 283: 381–7

18. Weng G, Bhalla US, Iyengar R. Complexity in biological signaling systems. Science 1999; 284: 92–6

19. Matzel LD, Talk AC, Muzzio IA, Rogers RF. Ubiquitous molecular substrates for associative learning and activity-dependent neuronal facilitation. Rev Neurosci 1998; 9: 129–67

20. Kandel ER. The molecular biology of memory storage: a dialogue between genes and synapses. Science 2001; 294: 1030–8

21. Ghaemi SN, Boiman EE, Goodwin FK. Kindling and second messengers: an approach to the neurobiology of recurrence in bipolar disorder. Biol Psychiatry 1999; 45: 137–44

22. Manji HK, Lenox RH. Signaling: cellular insights into the pathophysiology of bipolar disorder. Biol Psychiatry 2000; 48: 518–30

23. Gelowitz DL, Berger SP. Signal transduction mechanisms and behavioral sensitization to stimulant drugs: an overview of cAMP and PLA2. J Addict Dis 2001; 20: 33–42

24. Manji HK. G-proteins: Implications for psychiatry. Am J Psychiatry 1992; 149: 746–60

25. Jope RS, Williams MB. Lithium and brain signal transduction systems. Biochem Pharmacol 1994; 47: 429–41

26. Manji HK, Chen G, Shimon H, et al. Guanine nucleotide-binding proteins in bipolar affective disorder. Effects of long-term lithium treatment. Arch Gen Psychiatry 1995; 52: 135–44

27. Manji HK, Potter WZ, Lenox RH. Signal transduction pathways. Molecular targets for lithiums actions. Arch Gen Psychiatry 1995; 52: 531–43

28. Forn J, Veldecasas FG. Effects of lithium on brain adenyl cyclase activity. Biochem Pharmacol 1971; 20: 2773–9

29. Mork A, Geisler A, Hollund P. Effects of lithium on second messenger systems in the brain. Pharmacol Toxicol 1992; 71: 4–17

30. Masana MI, Bitran JA, Hsiao JK, et al. Lithium effects on noradrenergic-linked adenylate cyclase activity in intact rat brain: an in vivo microdialysis study. Brain Res 1991; 538: 333–6

31. Murphy DL, Donnelly C, Moskowitz J. Inhibition by lithium of prostaglandin E_1 and norepinephrine effects on cyclic adenosine monophosphate production in human platelets. Pharm Therap 1973; 14: 810–14

32. Jope RS. A bimodal model of the mechanism of action of lithium. Mol Psychiatry 1999; 4: 21–5

33. Jope RS. Anti-bipolar therapy: mechanism of action of lithium. Mol Psychiatry 1999; 4: 117–28

34. Chang A, Li PP, Warsh JJ. cAMP signal transduction abnormalities in the pathophysiology of mood disorders: contributions from postmortem brain studies. In Agam G, Everall IP, Belmaker RH. The Postmortem Brain in Psychiatric Research. Boston: Kluwer Academic Publishers, 2001: 342–62

35. Berridge MJ, Irvine RF. Inositol phosphates and cell signaling. Nature 1989; 341: 197–205

36. Berridge MJ, Downes CP, Hanley MR. Neural and developmental actions of lithium: a unifying hypothesis. Cell 1989; 59: 411–19

37. Berridge MJ. Inositol trisphosphate and calcium signaling. Nature 1993; 361: 315–25

38. Vadnal R, Parthasarathy R. Myo-inositol monophosphatase: diverse effects of lithium, carbamazepine, and valproate. Neuropsychopharmacology 1995; 12: 277–85

39. Cornish-Bowden A. Why is uncompetitive inhibition so rare? FEBS Lett 1986; 203: 3–6

40. Gani D, Downes CP, Batty I, Bramhan J. Lithium and myo-inositol homeostasis. Biochim Biophys Acta 1993; 1177: 253–69

41. Patishi Y, Lubrich B, Berger M, et al. Differential uptake of myo-inositol into rat brain areas. Eur Neuropsychopharmacology 1996; 6: 73–5

42. Lubrich B, Patishi Y, Kofman O, et al. Lithium-induced inositol depletion in rat brain after chronic treatment is restricted to the hypothalamus. Mol Psychiatry 1997; 2: 407–12

43. Belmaker RH, Agam G, van Calker D, et al. Behavioral reversal of lithium effects by four inositol isomers correlates perfectly with biochemical effects on the PI cycle: depletion by lithium of brain inositol is specific to hypothalamus, and inositol levels may be abnormal in post-mortem brain from bipolar patients. Neuropsychopharmacology 1998; 19: 220–32

44. Berry GT, Buccafusca R, Greer JJ, Eccleston E. Phosphoinositide deficiency due to inositol depletion is not a mechanism of lithium action in brain. Mol Genet Metab 2004; 82: 87–92

45. Fisher SK, Heacock AM, Agranoff BW. Inositol lipids and signal transduction in the central nervous system: an update. J Neurochem 1992; 58: 18–38

46. Varney M, Godfrey PP, Drummond AH, Watson SP. Chronic lithium treatment inhibits basal and agonist-stimulated responses in rat cerebral cortex and GH_3 pituitary cells. Mol Pharmacol 1992; 42: 671–8

47. Varney M, Galione A, Watson SP. Lithium-induced decrease in spontaneous Ca^{2+} oscillations in single GH_3 rat pituitary cells. Br J Pharmacol 1994; 112: 390–5

48. Batty IH, Downes CP. The inhibition of phosphoinositide synthesis and muscarinic-receptor-mediated phospholipase C activity by Li^+ as secondary, selective consequences of inositol depletion in 13211N1 cells. Biochem J 1994; 297: 529–37

49. Chen Y, Hertz L. Inhibition of noradrenaline stimulated increase in $[Ca^{2+}]_i$ in cultured astrocytes by chronic treatment with a therapeutically relevant lithium concentration. Brain Res 1996; 711: 245–8

50. Whitworth P, Heal DJ, Kendall DA. The effect of acute and chronic lithium treatment on pilocarpine-stimulated phosphoinositide hydrolysis in mouse brain in vivo. Br J Pharmacol 1990; 101: 39–44

51. Gur E, Lerer B, Newman ME. Acute or chronic lithium does not affect agonist-stimulated inositoltrisphosphate formation in rat brain in vivo. Neuroreport 1996; 7: 393–6

52. Dixon JF, Lee CH, Los GV, Hokin LE. Lithium enhances accumulation of [³H]inositol radioactivity and mass of second messenger inositol-1,4,5-trisphosphate in monkey cerebral cortical slices. J Neurochem 1992; 59: 2332–5

53. Los GV, Artemenko IP, Hokin LE. Time-dependent effects of lithium on the agonist-stimulated accumulation of second messenger inositol-1,4,5-trisphosphate in SH-SY5Y human neuroblastoma cells. Biochem J 1995; 311: 225–32

54. Dixon JF, Hokin LE. Lithium acutely inhibits and chronically up-regulates and stabilizes glutamate uptake by presynaptic nerve endings in mouse cerebral cortex. Proc Natl Acad Sci USA 1998; 95: 8363–8

55. Belmaker RH, Bersudsky Y, Agam G, et al. Manipulation of inositol-linked second messenger systems as a therapeutic strategy in psychiatry. In Gessa G, Fratta W, Pani L, Serra G, eds. Depression and Mania: From Neurobiology to Treatment. New York: Raven Press, 1995: 67–84

56. Moore GJ, Bebchuk JM, Parrish JK, et al. Temporal dissociation between lithium-induced changes in frontal lobe myo-inositol and clinical response in manic-depressive illness. Am J Psychiatry 1999; 156: 1902–8

57. Davanzo P, Thomas MA, Yue K, et al. Decreased anterior cingulate myo-inositol/creatine spectroscopy resonance with lithium treatment in children with bipolar disorder. Neuropsychopharmacology 2001; 24: 359–69

58. Friedman SD, Dager SR, Parow A, et al. Lithium and valproic acid treatment effects on brain chemistry in bipolar disorder. Biol Psychiatry 2004; 56: 340–8

59. van Calker D, Belmaker RH. The high affinity inositol transport system – implications for the

59. pathophysiology and treatment of bipolar disorder. Bipolar Disord 2000; 2: 102–7

60. Wiesinger H. Myo-inositol transport in mouse astroglia-rich primary cultures. J Neurochem 1991; 56: 1698–704

61. Lubrich B, Spleiss O, Gebicke-Haerter PJ, van Calker D. Differential expression and regulation of the sodium/myo-inositol cotransporter in astrocyte cultures of various regions of the rat brain. Neuropharmacology 2000; 39: 680–90

62. Glanville NT, Byers, HV, Cook MW, et al. Differences in the metabolism of inositol and phosphoinositides by cultured cells of neuronal and glial origin. Biochim Biophys Acta 1989; 1004: 169–79

63. Paredes A, McManus M, Kwon HM, Strange K. Osmoregulation of Na+/myo-inositol cotransporter activity and mRNA levels in brain glial cells. Am J Physiol 1992; 263: C1282–88

64. Kwon, HM, Yamauchi A, Schinchi U, et al. Cloning of the cDNA for a Na+/myo-inositol cotransporter, a hypertonicity stress protein. J Biol Chem 1992; 267: 6297–301

65. Cohen, DM, Wasserman JC, Gullans SR. Immediate early gene and HSP70 expression in hyperosmotic stress in MDCK cells. Am Phys Soc 1991; C: 594–601

66. Yancey PH, Clark ME, Hand SC, et al. Living with water stress: evolution of osmolyte systems. Science 1982; 217: 1214–22

67. Lubrich B, van Calker D. Inhibition of the high affinity myo-inositol uptake: a common mechanism of action of antibipolar drugs? Neuropsychopharmacology 1999; 21: 519–29

68. Wolfson M, Bersudsky Y, Zinger E, et al. Chronic treatment of human astrocytoma cells with lithium, carbamazepine or valproic acid decreases inositol uptake at high inositol concentrations but increases it at low inositol concentrations. Brain Res 2000; 855: 158–61

69. O'Donnell T, Rotzinger S, Nakashima TT, et al. Chronic lithium and sodium valproate both decrease the concentration of myo-inositol and increase the concentration of monophosphates in rat brain. Brain Res 2000; 880: 84–91

70. Shaltiel G, Shamir A, Shapiro J, et al. Valproate decreases inositol biosynthesis. Biol Psychiatry 2004; 56: 868–74

71. Wong YH, Kalmbach SJ, Hartman BK, Sherman WR. Immunohistochemical staining and enzyme activity measurements show myo-inositol-1-phosphate synthase to be localized in the vasculature of brain. J Neurochem 1987; 48: 1434–42

72. Williams RS, Cheng L, Mudge AW, Harwood AJ. A common mechanism of action for three mood-stabilizing drugs. Nature 2002; 417: 292–5

73. Willmroth F, Drieling T, Lamla U, et al. Sodium-myo-inositol-cotransporter (SMIT-1)-mRNA is increased in neutrophils of patients with bipolar 1 disorder and downregulated under treatment with mood stabilizers. Int J Neuropsychopharmacol 2006; Jan 18: 1–9

74. Greil W, Steber R, van Calker D. The agonist-stimulated accumulation of inositol phosphates is attenuated in neutrophils from male patients under chronic lithium therapy. Biol Psychiatry 1991; 30: 443–51

75. van Calker D, Förstner U, Bohus M, et al. Increased sensitivity to agonist-stimulation of the Ca^{2+} response in neutrophils of manic-depressive patients: effect of lithium therapy. Neuropsychobiology 1993; 27: 180–3

76. Wasserman MJ, Corson TW, Sibony D, et al. Chronic lithium treatment attenuates intracellular calcium mobilization. Neuropsychopharmacology 2004; 29: 759–69

77. Bohus M, Förstner U, Kiefer C, et al. Increased sensitivity of the inositol-phospholipid system in neutrophils from patients with acute major depressive episodes. Psychiatry Res 1996; 65: 45–51

78. Warsh JJ, Li PP. Second messenger systems in mood disorders. Curr Opin Psychiatry 1996; 9: 23–9

79. Bothwell RA, Eccleston D, Marshall E. Platelet intracellular calcium in patients with recurrent affective disorders. Psychopharmacology 1994; 114: 375–81

80. Emamghoreishi M, Schlichter L, Li PP, et al. High intracellular calcium concentrations in transformed lymphoblasts from subjects with

bipolar I disorder. Am J Psychiatry 1997; 154: 976–82

81. Friedman E, Wang H-Y, Levinson D, et al. Altered platelet protein kinase C activity in bipolar affective disorder, manic episode. Biol Psychiatry 1993; 33: 520–5

82. Brown AS, Mallinger AG, Renbaum LC. Elevated platelet membrane phospha-tidylinositol-4,5-bisphosphate in bipolar mania. Am J Psychiatry 1993; 150: 1252–4

83. Hahn CG, Umapathy, Wang HY, et al. Lithium and valproic acid treatments reduce PKC activation and receptor-G protein coupling in platelets of bipolar manic patients. J Psychiatr Res 2005; 39: 355–63

84. Hahn CG, Friedman E. Abnormalities in protein kinase C signaling and the patho-physiology of bipolar disorder. Bipolar Disord 1999; 1: 81–6

85. Hahn CG, Gomez G, Restrepo D, et al. Aberrant intracellular calcium signaling in olfactory neurons from patients with bipolar disorder. Am J Psychiatry 2005; 162: 616–18

86. Axelrod J. Phospholipase A$_2$ and G proteins. Trends Neurosci 1995; 18: 64–5

87. Bayon Y, Hernandez M, Alonso A, et al. Cytosolic phospholipase A$_2$ is coupled to muscarinic receptors in the human astrocytoma cell line 1321N1: characterization of the trans-ducing mechanism. Biochem J 1997; 323: 281–7

88. Rapoport SI, Chang MC, Spector AA. Delivery and turnover of plasma-derived essential PUFAs in mammalian brain. J Lipid Res 2001; 42: 678–85

89. Fitzpatrick F, Soberman R. Regulated formation of eicosanoids. J Clin Invest 2001; 107: 1347–51

90. Rapoport SI, Bosetti F. Do lithium and anticonvulsants target the brain arachidonic acid cascade in bipolar disorder? Arch Gen Psychiatry 2002; 59: 592–6

91. Bosetti F, Weerasinghe GR, Rosenberger TA, Rapoport SI. Valproic acid down-regulates the conversion of arachidonic acid to eicosanoids via cyclooxygenase-1 and -2 in rat brain. J Neurochem 2003; 85: 690–6

92. Ghelardoni S, Tomita YA, Bell JM, et al. Chronic carbamazepine selectively down-regulates cytosolic phospholipase A2 expression and cyclooxygenase activity in rat brain. Biol Psychiatry 2004; 56: 248–54

93. Bazinet RP, Rao JS, Chang L, et al. Chronic carbamazepine decreases the incorporation rate and turnover of arachidonic acid but not docosahexaenoic acid in brain phospholipids of the unanesthetized rat: relevance to bipolar disorder. Biol Psychiatry 2006 Mar 1; 59: 401–7

94. Li X, Bijur GN, Jope RS. Glycogen synthase kinase-3beta, mood stabilizers, and neuro-protection. Bipolar Disord 2002; 4: 137–44

95. Jope RS, Bijur GN. Mood stabilizers, glycogen synthase kinase-3beta and cell survival. Mol Psychiatry 2002; 7 (Suppl 1): S35–45

96. Jope RS. Lithium and GSK-3: one inhibitor, two inhibitory actions, multiple outcomes. Trends Pharmacol Sci 2003; 24: 441–3

97. Jope RS, Johnson GV. The glamour and gloom of glycogen synthase kinase-3. Trends Biochem Sci 2004; 29: 95–102

98. Gould TD, Manji HK. Glycogen synthase kinase-3: a putative molecular target for lithium mimetic drugs. Neuropsycho-pharmacology 2005; 30: 1223–37

99. Kirshenboim N, Plotkin B, Shlomo SB, et al. Lithium-mediated phosphorylation of glycogen synthase kinase-3b involves PI3 kinase-dependent activation of protein kinase C-alpha. J Mol Neurosci 2004; 24: 237–45

100. Chen G, Huang LD, Jiang YM, Manji HK. The mood-stabilizing agent valproate inhibits the activity of glycogen synthase kinase-3. J Neurochem 1999; 72: 1327–30

101. Harwood AJ, Agam G. Search for a common mechanism of mood stabilizers. Biochem Pharmacol 2003; 66: 179–89

102. Grimes CA, Jope RS. CREB DNA binding activity is inhibited by glycogen synthase kinase-3 beta and facilitated by lithium. J Neurochem 2001; 78: 1219–32

103. Cohen P, Goedert M. GSK3 inhibitors: devel-opment and therapeutic potential. Nat Rev Drug Discov 2004; 3: 479–87

104. Gould TD, Einat H, Bhat R, Manji HK. AR-A014418, a selective GSK-3 inhibitor, produces antidepressant-like effects in the forced swim test. Int J Neuropsychopharmacol 2004; 7: 387–90

105. Kaidanovich-Beilin O, Milman A, Weizman A, et al. Rapid antidepressive-like activity of specific glycogen synthase kinase-3 inhibitor and its effect on beta-catenin in mouse hippocampus. Biol Psychiatry 2004; 55: 781–4

106. Stubbs EB, Agranoff BW. Lithium enhances muscarinic receptor-stimulated CDP-diacylglycerol formation in inositol-depleted SK-N-SH neuroblastoma cells. J Neurochem 1993; 60: 1292–9

107. Casebolt TL, Jope RS. Effects of chronic lithium treatment on protein kinase C and cyclic AMP-dependent protein phosphorylation. Biol Psychiatry 1991; 29: 233–43

108. Guitard X, Nestler EJ. Chronic administration of lithium or other antidepressants increases levels of DARPP-32 in rat frontal cortex. J Neurochem 1992; 59: 1164–7

109. Jensen JB, Mork A. Altered protein phosphorylation in the rat brain following chronic lithium and carbamazepine treatments. Eur Neuropsychopharmacol 1997; 7: 173–9

110. Zanardi R, Racagni G, Smeraldi E, Perez E. Differential effects of lithium on platelet protein phosphorylation in bipolar patients and healthy subjects. Psychopharmacology 1997; 129: 44–7

111. Mori S, Zanardi R, Popoli M, et al. Inhibitory effects of lithium on cAMP dependent phosphorylation systems. Life Sci 1996; 59: 99–104

112. Mori S, Tardito D, Dorigo A, et al. Effects of lithium on cAMP-dependent protein kinase in rat brain. Neuropsychopharmacology 1998; 19: 233–40

113. Chang A, Li PP, Warsh JJ. Altered cAMP-dependent protein kinase subunit immunolabeling in post-mortem brain from patients with bipolar affective disorder. J Neurochem 2003; 84: 781–91

114. Svenningsson P, Nishi A, Fisone G, et al. DARPP-32: an integrator of neurotransmission. Annu Rev Pharmacol Toxicol 2004; 44: 269–96

115. Nishi A, Snyder GL, Fienberg AA, et al. Requirement for DARPP-32 in mediating effect of dopamine D2 receptor activation. Eur J Neurosci 1999; 11: 2589–92

116. El-Mallakh RS, Li R. Is the Na$^+$-K$^+$-ATPase the link between phosphoinositide metabolism and bipolar disorders? J Neuropsychiatry 1993; 5: 361–8

117. El-Mallakh RS, Wyatt RJ. The Na$^+$-K$^+$-ATPase hypothesis for bipolar illness. Biol Psychiatry 1995; 37: 235–44

118. Wood AJ, Goodwin GM. A review of the biochemical and neuropharmacological actions of lithium. Psychol Med 1987; 17: 579–600

119. Drummond AH. Lithium and inositol lipid-linked signaling mechanisms. Trends Pharmacol Sci 1987; 8: 129–33

120. Manji HK, Lenox RH. Long term action of lithium: a role for transcriptional and posttranscriptional factors regulated by protein kinase C. Synapse 1994; 16: 11–28

121. Manji HK, Bersudsky Y, Chen G, et al. Modulation of protein kinase C isoenzymes and substrates by lithium: the role of myo-inositol. Neuropsychopharmacology 1996; 15: 370–81

122. Manji HK, Chen G, Shimon H, et al. Regulation of signal transduction pathways by mood stabilizing agents: implications for the delayed onset of therapeutic efficacy. J Clin Psychiatry 1996; 57 (Suppl 13): 34–46

123. Lenox RH, McNamara RK, Watterson JM, Watson DG. Myristoylated alanine-rich C kinase substrate (MARCKS): a molecular target for the therapeutic action of mood stabilizers in the brain? J Clin Psychiatry 1996; 57 (Suppl 13): 23–31

124. Lenox RH, McNamara RK, Papke LR, Manji HK. Neurobiology of lithium: an update. J Clin Psychiatry 1998; 59 (Suppl 6): 37–47

125. Decker LV, Parker PJ. Protein kinase C – a question of specificity. Trends Biol Sci 1994; 19: 73–7

126. Shearman MS, Sekiguchi K, Nishizuka Y. Modulation of ion channel activity: a key function of the protein kinase C enzyme family. Pharmacol Rev 1989; 41: 211–37

127. Ben Ari Y, Aniksztejn L, Bregestovski P. Protein kinase C modulation of NMDA currents: an important link for LTP induction. Trends Neurosci 1992; 15: 333–9

128. Li X, Jope RS. Selective inhibition of expression of signal transduction proteins by lithium in

nerve growth factor-differentiated PC 12 cells. J Neurochem 1995; 65: 2500–8

129 Manji HK, Lenox RH. Protein kinase C signaling in the brain: molecular transduction of mood stabilization in the treatment of manic-depressive illness. Biol Psychiatry 1999; 46: 1328–51

130. Wang H-Y, Friedman E. Lithium inhibition of protein kinase C activation-induced serotonin release. Psychopharmacology 1989; 99: 213–18

131. Sharp T, Bramwell SR, Lambert P, Grahame-Smith DG. Effect of short- and long-term administration of lithium on the release of endogenous 5-HT in the hippocampus of the rat in vitro. Neuropharmacology 1991; 30: 977–84

132. Glaser M, Wanaski S, Buse CA, et al. Myristoylated alanine-rich C kinase substrate (MARCKS) produces reversible inhibition of phospholipase C by sequestering phosphatidylinositol 4,5-bisphosphate in lateral domains. J Biol Chem 1996; 271: 26187–93

133. Watson DG, Lenox RH. Chronic lithium-induced downregulation of MARCKS in immortalized hippocampal cells: potentiation by muscarinic receptor activation. J Neurochem 1996; 67: 767–7

134. Chen G, Manji HK, Hawver DB, et al. Chronic sodium valproate selectively decreases protein kinase C α and ε in vitro. J Neurochem 1994; 63: 2361–4

135. Watson DG, Watterson JM, Lenox RH. Sodium valproate down-regulates the myristoylated alanine-rich C kinase substrate (MARCKS) in immortalized hippocampal cells: a property of protein kinase C-mediated mood stabilizers. J Pharmacol Exp Ther 1998; 285: 307–16

136. Avissar S, Schreiber G, Danon A, Belmaker RH. Lithium inhibits adrenergic and cholinergic increases in GTP binding in rat cortex. Nature 1988; 331: 440–2

137. Drummond AH. Lithium affects G-protein receptor coupling. Nature 1988; 331: 388

138. Ellis J, Lenox RH. Receptor coupling to G-proteins: interaction not affected by lithium. Lithium 1991; 2: 141–7

139. Masana MI, Bitran JA, Hsiao JK, Potter WZ. In vivo evidence that lithium inactivates G_i

modulation of adenylate cyclase in brain. J Neurochem 1992; 59: 200–5

140. Manji HK, Moore GJ, Rajkowska G, Chen G. Neuroplasticity and cellular resilience in mood disorders. Mol Psychiatry 2000; 5: 578–93

141. McGowan S, Eastwood SL, Mead A, et al. Hippocampal and cortical G protein Gsα, Goα, Gi2α mRNA expression after electroconvulsive shock or lithium treatment. Eur J Pharmacol 1996; 306: 249–55

142. Dwivedi Y, Pandey GN. Effects of subchronic administration of antidepressants and anxiolytics on levels of the α subunits of G proteins in the rat brain. J Neural Transm 1997; 104: 747–60

143. Jakobsen SN, Wiborg O. Selective effects of long-term lithium and carbamazepine administration on G-protein subunit expression in rat brain. Brain Res 1998; 780: 46–55

144. Spleiss O, van Calker D, Schärer L, et al. Abnormal G-protein α_{i2}- and α_{o}-subunit mRNA expression in bipolar affective disorder. Mol Psychiatry 1998; 3: 512–20

145. Mitchell PB, Manji HK, Chen G, et al. High levels of $G_s\alpha$ in platelets of euthymic patients with bipolar affective disorder. Am J Psychiatry 1997; 154: 218–23

146. Lenox RH, Gould TD, Manji HK. Endophenotypes in bipolar disorder. Am J Med Genet 2002; 114: 391–406

147. Ram A, Guedj F, Cravchik A, et al. No abnormality in the gene for the G protein stimulatory α subunit in patients with bipolar disorder. Arch Gen Psychiatry 1997; 54: 44–8

148. Silva AJ, Giese KP. Plastic genes are in! Curr Opin Neurobiol 1994; 4: 413–20

149. Hughes P, Dragunow M. Induction of immediate–early genes and the control of neurotransmitter-regulated gene expression within the nervous system. Pharmacol Rev 1995, 47: 133–78

150. Yuan PX, Chen G, Huang LD, Manji HK. Lithium stimulates gene expression through the AP-1 transcription factor pathway. Brain Res Mol Brain Res 1998; 58: 225–30

151. Yuan P, Chen G, Manji HK. Lithium activates the c-Jun NH2-terminal kinases in vitro and in the CNS in vivo. J Neurochem 1999; 73: 2299–309

152. Chen G, Yuan PX, Jiang YM, et al. Valproate robustly enhances AP-1 mediated gene expression Brain Res Mol Brain Res 1999; 64: 52–8

153. Ozaki N, Chuang DM. Lithium increases transcription factor binding to AP-1 and cyclic AMP-responsive element in cultured neurons and rat brain. J Neurochem 1997; 69: 2336–44

154. Jope RS, Song L. AP-1 and NF-κB stimulated by carbachol in human neuroblastoma SH-SY5Y cells are differentially sensitive to inhibition by lithium. Mol Brain Res 1997; 50: 171–80

155. Nonaka S, Hough CJ, Chuang DM. Chronic lithium treatment robustly protects neurons in the central nervous system against excito-toxicity by inhibiting N-methyl-D-asparate receptor-mediated calcium influx. proc Natl Acad Sci USA. 1998; 95: 2642–7

156. Chen G, Zeng WZ, Yuan PX, et al. The mood-stabilizing agents lithium and valproate robustly increase the levels of the neuro-protective protein bcl-2 in the CNS. J Neurochem 1999; 72: 879–82

157. Zhou R, Gray NA, Yuan P, Li X, et al. The anti-apoptotic, glucocorticoid receptor cochaperone protein BAG-1 is a long-term target for the actions of mood stabilizers. J Neurosci 2005; 25: 4493–502

158. King TD, Bijur GN, Jope RS. Caspase-3 activation induced by inhibition of mitochondrial complex I is facilitated by glycogen synthase kinase-3beta and attenuated by lithium. Brain Res 2001; 919: 106–14

159. Chen G, Rajkowska G, Du F, et al. Enhancement of hippocampal neurogenesis by lithium. J Neurochem 2000; 75: 1729–34

160. Moore GJ, Bebchuk JM, Hasanat K, et al. Lithium increases N-acetyl-aspartate in the human brain: in vivo evidence in support of bcl-2's neurotrophic effects? Biol Psychiatry 2000; 48: 1–8

161. Moore GJ, Bebchuk JM, Wilds IB, et al. Lithium-induced increase in human brain grey matter. Lancet 2000; 356: 1241–2

162. Drevets WC, Price JL, Simpson JR Jr, et al. Subgenual prefrontal cortex abnormalities in mood disorders. Nature 1997; 386: 824–7

163. Ongur D, Drevets WC, Price JL. Glial reduction in the subgenual prefrontal cortex in mood disorders. Proc Natl Acad Sci USA 1998; 95: 13290–5

164. Rajkowska G, Miguel-Hidalgo JJ, Wei J, et al. Morphometric evidence for neuronal and glial prefrontal cell pathology in major depression. Biol Psychiatry 1999; 45: 1085–98

165. Rajkowska G. Postmortem studies in mood disorders indicate altered numbers of neurons and glial cells. Biol Psychiatry 2000; 48: 766–77

166. Rajkowska G, Halaris A, Selemon LD. Reductions in neuronal and glial density characterize the dorsolateral prefrontal cortex in bipolar disorder. Biol Psychiatry 2001; 49: 741–52

167. Drevets WC. Neuroimaging and neuro-pathological studies of depression: implications for the cognitive-emotional features of mood disorders. Curr Opin Neurobiol 2001; 11: 240–9

168. Rajkowska G. Histopathology of the prefrontal cortex in major depression: what does it tell us about dysfunctional monoaminergic circuits? Prog Brain Res 2000; 126: 397–412

169. Bunney WE, Garland-Bunney B. Mechanisms of action of lithium in affective illness: Basic and clinical implications. In Meltzer HY ed. Psychopharmacology: the third generation of progress. New York: Raven Press, 1987: 553–65

170. Hadcock JR, Malbon CC. Agonist regulation of gene expression of adrenergic receptors and G-proteins. J Neurochem 1993; 60: 1–9

171. Berry GT, Wu S, Buccafusca R, et al. Loss of murine Na+/myo-inositol cotransporter leads to brain myo-inositol depletion and central apnea. J Biol Chem 2003; 278: 18297–302

31 Effects of lithium on gene expression

Jun-Feng Wang, L Trevor Young

Contents Introduction • Transcription factors and gene expression • Lithium, gene transcription factors and gene expression • Consequences of regulation of neuroprotective genes by lithium • Conclusion and discussion

INTRODUCTION

Lithium is the gold standard treatment for bipolar disorder. Early studies on the mechanism of action of lithium focused on neurotransmitters and determined that the drug exerts effects on synthesis, turnover and release of monoaminergic neurotransmitters and their receptors in the central nervous system[1–5]. However, these effects occur only at supratherapeutic concentrations of lithium or after its acute administration. Because lithium must be administered chronically to influence the course of bipolar disorder and to prevent relapse of manic and depressive episodes, the drug's acute biochemical effects are not able to lead to a conclusive understanding of its mechanism of action. Since intracellular signaling pathways play a pivotal role in the central nervous system, recent research into lithium's mechanism of action has shifted from individual neurotransmitters and their receptors to focus on post-receptor events and mechanisms. Indeed, an increasing body of evidence has been accumulated demonstrating that chronic treatment with lithium at therapeutically relevant concentrations affects G-proteins and their effectors, including cyclic AMP and phosphoinositide signaling pathways. Chronic lithium treatment has been reported in a variety of neuronal tissues and cells to increase the basal level of cyclic AMP, to decrease agonist-induced increases in guanosine triphosphate (GTP) binding and cyclic AMP level, to induce the translocation of cyclic AMP dependent protein kinase from the cytosol to the nucleus, to increase expression of specific adenylyl cyclase isoforms and phosphorylation of DARPP-32, a substrate for cyclic AMP-dependent protein kinase[6–15].

Chronic treatment with lithium has also been shown to affect calcium and phosphoinositide signaling pathways. For example, lithium at therapeutically relevant concentrations inhibits glutamate-induced calcium influx in rat cerebellar granule cells and cerebral cortical cells[16,17]. Lithium is also a non-competitive inhibitor of intracellular inositol monophosphatase (IMPase), a key enzyme in inositol recycling[18–20]. Studies from several research groups found, that in rat brain, lithium reduced agonist-induced phosphoinositide hydrolysis secondary to inositol depletion, by inhibition of IMPase and reduction in phospho-inositide-generated second messengers[21–23]. Protein kinase C (PKC) is a major signal mediator linked to phosphoinositide-generated second messengers which influences many cell functions by protein phosphorylation. Chronic lithium treatment increased PKC translocation from cytosol to membrane and selectively decreased membrane levels of the PKC α isozyme in rat hippocampus[24–27]. Chronic lithium treatment also reduced protein levels and phosphorylation of myristoylated alanine-rich C kinase substrate (MARCKS), the prominent PKC substrate, in rat hippo-campus[26,28]. More recently chronic lithium treatment has been found to regulate other intracellular signaling pathways including mitogen-activated protein (MAP) kinase, serine/threonine kinase Akt-1, glycogen synthase kinase (GSK) and others[29–35].

Intracellular signaling actions depend on activation of protein kinases that further phosphorylate many cellular proteins including gene transcription factors. Regulation of transcription factors leads to gene expression and results in the synthesis of new proteins, which induce permanent effects that last for days or weeks. Chronic administration of lithium in the treatment and prophylaxis for bipolar disorder indicates that repeated stimulation with this drug prolongs activation of intracellular signaling pathways, resulting in alteration at the genomic level. Indeed, a growing body of evidence has shown that chronic lithium treatment regulates gene transcription factors and gene expression in neuronal cells.

TRANSCRIPTION FACTORS AND GENE EXPRESSION

Gene expression is the process whereby information coded by genes is translated into proteins[36]. This process occurs in two major steps: first is gene transcription, by which DNA is transcribed into mRNA, initiated by RNA polymerase II in the nucleus; second is RNA translation, by which the mRNA molecule is translated into corresponding amino acids to form a protein. RNA polymerase II initiates gene transcription by binding to the TATA box of the promoter region located at 25–35 bp upstream of the transcription start site. There are multiple regulatory elements called *cis*-acting DNA elements upstream of the core promoter region[37]. Transcription factors (*trans*-acting proteins) are nuclear proteins that bind to these *cis*-acting DNA elements, and interact with RNA polymerase II in order to regulate the rate of DNA transcription in the nucleus. Transcription factors are activated or inhibited by various intracellular signaling pathways through expression regulation, post-translational modification and ligand activation. Transcription factor activating protein 1 (AP-1 complex) and cyclic AMP responsive element binding protein (CREB) along with their DNA binding activities have been extensively studied in psychiatric research[38–44]. The biochemical processes regulated by complex networks of various signal trans-duction pathways such as cAMP/PKA signaling, IP$_3$/PKC, Ca^{2+}/CaM kinase, MAP kinases and GSK-3 ultimately result in gene expression mediated via activation or inhibition of the AP-1 and CREB gene transcription factors.

The AP-1 complex is a mixture of homo- and heterodimers that are composed of the Jun family of proteins (c-Jun, JunB and JunD) combined with the Fos-related proteins (Fos, FosB, Fra1 and Fra2). The AP-1 complex binds to a palindromic regulatory motif known as the AP-1 site that shows the consensus sequence (TGACTCA) to regulate gene expression. Because the specific PKC activator phorbol 12-myristate 13-acetate (TPA) markedly induces expression of genes containing the AP-1 site, the AP-1 site is also called the TPA response element (TRE)[45–47]. In the central nervous system, a wide variety of extracellular stimuli such as mitogens, hormones, extracellular matrix and genotoxic agents, can induce expression of Fos and Jun family proteins[48–51]. Although basal levels of these proteins are very low, they are induced rapidly and transiently by various stimuli, translocated to the nucleus to form the AP-1 complex and then bind the TRE/AP-1 motif to regulate gene transcription. Because each Fos and Jun family protein is regulated differently to form AP-1 complexes with subtly different functions, different AP-1 complex dimers may result in different outcomes of AP-1 activation. In addition, Jun proteins can also be phophorylated by c-Jun N-terminal kinase (JNK) and GSK-3 to positively and negatively regulate target gene transcription[52,53]. Recent research indicates that increases of Jun and Fos protein expression and JNK activity are involved in the process of neuronal cell apoptosis[54,55].

Cyclic AMP responsive element binding protein contains (1) the C-terminal basic domain responsible for DNA binding; (2) the leucine zipper domain responsible for dimerization with CREB or other members of the CREB family such as activating transcription factor (ATF) and CRE modulator (CREM); and (3) the kinase inducible domain containing the serine-133 amino acid residue that can be phosphorylated by various kinases including cAMP-dependent protein kinase A, Ca^{2+}/calmodulin-dependent protein kinases II and IV (CaMK II and IV), the extracellular regulated kinases (ERK1/2) and p38 MAP kinase[56]. In addition, the serine-129 amino acid residue of CREB protein can be phosphorylated by GSK-3[57,58]. Phosphorylated CREB interacts with CREB binding protein (CBP), binds consensus CRE sequence (TGACGTCA) and regulates expression of target genes. CREB plays a critical role in many neuronal processes such as long-term memory, synaptic plasticity and cell survival[59].

LITHIUM, GENE TRANSCRIPTION FACTORS AND GENE EXPRESSION

Effect of lithium on AP-1 and CREB gene transcription factors

Studies from numerous laboratories have indicated that lithium at therapeutically relevant concentrations regulates AP-1 and its DNA binding activity. Consistent results from a number of studies in different cell lines and rat brain regions suggest that acute lithium treatment not only increases basal expression of c-Fos and c-Jun and AP-1 DNA binding activity, but also potentiates c-Fos expression and AP-1 binding DNA activity[60–63]. However, chronic lithium treatment has shown more complex regulation in basal and stimulated AP-1 DNA binding activity. It has been reported that chronic lithium treatment increases c-Fos and c-Jun expression, and AP-1 DNA binding activity not only in human SH-SY5Y cells, rat C6 glioma cells and cultured rat cerebellar granule cells *in vitro*, but also in rat frontal cortex, hippocampus, amygdala and cerebellum *in vivo*[30,38,44,62]. Recently, lithium has been recognized as an inhibitor of glycogen synthase kinase (GSK-3)[34]. GSK-3 has been shown to phosphorylate c-Jun on Ser-239, Ser-243 and Ser-249, and further to inhibit AP-1 DNA binding activity[64,65]. Chronic lithium treatment also may increase basal AP-1 DNA binding activity by inhibiting GSK-3. To determine whether lithium regulates AP-1 responsive gene expression, Yuan et al.[44] analyzed activity of an SV40 promoter that contains AP-1 sites after lithium treatment. When SH-SY5Y or C6 cells were transfected with a reporter gene vector driven by an SV40 promoter that contains AP-1 sites, they found that lithium treatment increased the expression of a luciferase report gene. The effect of lithium on this report gene expression was also suppressed by mutations in the AP-1 sites, indicating that AP-1 transcription factor may mediate lithium-induced gene expression. Although chronic lithium treatment increased basal AP-1 binding activity, chronic treatment with the drug has also been shown to decrease glutamate-stimulated AP-1 binding activity and c-Jun expression in rat cerebellar granule cells[38]. JNK kinase usually acts synergistically with p38 to increase AP-1 DNA binding activity by phosphorylating c-Jun. Chronic lithium treatment has been shown to inhibit glutamate-induced JNK activation, c-Jun phosphorylation, p38 kinase activation and AP-1 DNA binding activation, indicating that lithium may decrease glutamate-stimulated AP-1 binding activity by regulating the MAP kinase pathway[30].

Chronic, but not acute treatment with lithium inhibited phosphorylation of CREB and CRE DNA binding activity induced by the adenylyl cyclase activator forskolin in human neuroblastoma SH-SY5Y cells[40]. Chronic lithium treatment has also been shown to suppress chronic restraint stress-induced decrease in dendritic length and glial glutamate transporter 1 mRNA expression, and increase in CREB phosphorylation in the rat hippocampus, implying that lithium may protect the hippocampus from potentially deleterious effects of chronic stress on glutamatergic activation[66]. It is interesting that chronic lithium treatment has also been found to increase basal CRE binding activity in rat

cerebellar granule cells *in vitro* and in rat frontal cortex, hippocampus, amygdala and cerebellum *in vivo*[38]. Increase in basal CRE DNA binding activity and decrease in stimulated CRE DNA binding activity by lithium are consistent with the effects of lithium in increasing the basal cyclic AMP level and blunting the agonist-increased cyclic AMP level. These results also suggest that lithium may regulate CRE DNA binding activity via the cyclic AMP signaling pathway. The biphasic effects of lithium on CRE DNA binding activity require further investigation.

Activity-dependent signaling pathway-induced gene transcription is mediated by transcription factors such as AP-1 complexes and CREB. This process is crucial for many types of longlasting neural plasticity and cellular responsiveness, and plays an important role in neuronal survival and differentiation. Regulation of transcription factors may contribute to the therapeutic efficacy of long-term treatment with lithium.

Lithium, gene expression and neuroprotection

Initial studies have shown that chronic lithium treatment regulates the expression of a number of genes including those for enzymes, receptors, G proteins and other signal transduction molecules in cultured cells and animal models. Chronic lithium treatment has been reported to reduce G-protein α-subunit mRNA levels and increase expression of adenylyl cyclase types I and II in rat cerebral cortex[14]. Lithium has also been shown to decrease MARCKS expression, a PKC substrate in the immortalized hippocampal cell line HN33[67]. This finding is consistent with downregulation of PKC by lithium. Chronic treatment with lithium for 6 weeks has been reported to decrease brain mRNA, protein and activity levels of arachidonic acid (AA)-selective cytosolic phospholipase A_2 (cPLA$_2$) and AP-2 DNA binding activity in the rat frontal cortex[68,69]. Because the AP-2 binding site has been recognized on the promoter region of the cPLA$_2$, this result suggests that chronic lithium treatment may decrease the expression of cPLA$_2$ by reducing AP-2 transcriptional activity. Chronic lithium treatment in rat C6 glioma cells for 1 week also increased gene transcription for the enzyme 2′, 3′-cyclic nucleotide 3′-phosphodiesterase type II that is a myelin-associated enzyme and is important in myelinogenesis and possibly neuronal growth and repair, indicating that lithium treatment may also be involved in this process[70]. In addition, a number of genes that include the AP-1 binding site in their promoter region were reported to be increased by lithium. Tyrosine hydroxylase that is known to be regulated by AP-1 transcription factors is increased in the rat frontal cortex, hippocampus and striatum by chronic lithium treatment[71]. Other AP-1-regulated genes including those for nitric oxide synthases (eNOS), prodynorphin and PEBP2β are also increased by lithium treatment in the rat hippocampus, basal ganglia and cerebral cortex regions[72–74]. Nonetheless, considering these numerous findings of lithium's effect on gene expression together still provides an incomplete picture of the underlying mechanism of action of this drug in bipolar disorder. Therefore, the isolation of other lithium-regulated genes is very important, particularly if these genes can be shown to be involved in the development of bipolar disorder.

Using differential display polymerase chain reaction (PCR) and DNA microarray technologies and their following studies, researchers have found that a number of lithium-regulated genes are neuroprotective. Chen et al.[74], using differential display PCR, found that chronic treatment with lithium and valproate increased mRNA levels of polyomavirus enhancer-binding protein (PEBP) 2β in the rat frontal cortex. PEBP 2β is the transcription factor that transcriptionally regulates anti-apoptotic factor Bcl-2. They also found that lithium and valproate increased the DNA binding activity of PEBP. Using immunohistochemistry, they found that chronic treatment with these two drugs increased the protein level of Bcl-2 in layers 2 and 3 of the rat frontal cortex. Nuclear protein p53 is a transcription factor that inhibits the expression of Bcl-2, but promotes the expression of the proapoptotic gene Bax. Chen and Chuang[75] found, in cultured rat cerebellar granule cells, that chronic lithium treatment not only increased mRNA and protein levels of cytoprotective Bcl-2, but also decreased mRNA and protein levels of p53 and Bax, indicating that changes in the mRNA and protein levels of Bax and Bcl-2 may result from the inhibition of p53 expression.

Wang et al.[76] also used differential display PCR to identify a number of valproate-regulated genes including the molecular chaperone GRP78 in primary cultured rat cerebral cortical cells. Later, this group found that chronic treatment with lithium at therapeutically relevant concentrations also increased mRNA and protein levels of GRP78, and the closely related molecular chaperones GRP94 and calreticulin[77,78]. In contrast to a classic GRP78 inducer thapsigargin, an inhibitor of the ER Ca^{2+}-ATPase, chronic treatment with lithium or valproate for 1 week modestly increased GRP78 expression in neuronal cells, had no effect on basal intracellular free Ca^{2+} concentration and did not induce cell death. These results indicate that lithium and valproate may increase expression of GRP78, GRP94 and calreticulin in primary cultured rat cerebral cortical cells without causing cell damage. Chronic lithium treatment has also been shown to increase GRP78 expression and inhibit thapsigargin-induced cytotoxicity in PC-12 cells, indicating that the induction of GRP78 probably contributes to lithium-induced protection against ER stress[79]. Recently Wang *et al.*[80] used microarray technology to analyze gene expression profiles after chronic valproate treatment in primary cultured rat cerebral cortical cells. They found that valproate increased the expression of glutathione *S*-transferase (GST) μ subtype, an important factor against oxidative stress. The level of GST μ protein, and GST activity, were also increased by chronic valproate treatment. In addition, chronic treatment with lithium also increased mRNA level, protein level and enzyme activity of GST μ. Zhou *et al.*[81] recently performed a series of cDNA microarray studies in order to identify changes in gene expression after chronic treatment with lithium and valproate in the rat hippocampus. They found that both drugs at therapeutically relevant concentrations increased the expression of BAG-1, and decreased dexamethasone-induced glucocorticoid receptor nuclear translocation and glucocorticoid receptor mediated transcriptional activity. Upregulation of bcl-2, BAG-1, GRP78 and GST, and downregulation of p53 and Bax suggest that chronic lithium treatment produces neuroprotective effects. The names and functions of neuroprotective genes and their regulation by lithium are summarized in Table 31.1.

CONSEQUENCES OF REGULATION OF NEUROPROTECTIVE GENES BY LITHIUM

Chronic treatment with lithium is required to generate its therapeutic effects, and this treatment has been found to regulate expression of a number of genes. Because increasing evidence indicates that chronic lithium treatment is neuroprotective both *in vitro* and *in vivo*, the most interesting targets among these genes are those that exhibit neuroprotection. Chronic lithium treatment has been found to protect cultured rat cerebellar, cerebral cortical and hippocampal neurons against glutamate-induced excitotoxicity[16,82–84]. Glutamate-induced toxicity is a consequence of induced supraphysiologically prolonged activation of glutamate receptor subtypes, resulting in an increase of cytosolic Ca^{2+} and mitochondrial depolarization, which then induces

Table 31.1 The neuroprotective genes regulated by lithium ion (Li^+)

Name	Effect of Li^+	Gene functions
Bax	Decrease	Induce cytochrome c release and activate caspase
Bcl-2	Increase	Block Bax-induced destructive effects
PEBP2β	Increase	Transcription factor for Bcl-2; increase Bcl-2 expression
p53	Decrease	Transcription factor for Bcl-2 and Bax; decrease Bcl-2 expression; increase Bax expression
GRP78, GRP94, Calreticulin	Increase	Molecular chaperone, bind calcium and fold damaged proteins
GST μ	Increase	Conjugation of GSH with oxidized products; inhibit JNK

PEBP, polyomavirus enhancer-binding protein; GRP, glucose-regulated protein; GSH, glutathione; GST; glutathione *S*-transferase; JNK, c-Jun *N*-terminal kinase mitochondrial Ca^{2+} sequestration. When accumulated Ca^{2+} is above the threshold of Ca^{2+} sequestration, excessive Ca^{2+} in mitochondria results in respiratory inhibition and generation of reactive oxygen species[85–87]. Chronic lithium treatment has recently been found to inhibit glutamate-induced oxidative damage to lipid and protein in rat cerebral cortical cells[88]. In *in vivo* study, chronic lithium treatment has been found to inhibit cerebral ischemia, quinolinic acid-induced striatal injury, excitotoxic lesions of the cholinergic system and kainic acid-induced brain damage[89–92]. Chronic lithium treatment has also been found to stimulate neurogenesis in the adult rat hippocampus, suggesting that this drug may produce a neurotrophic effect[93]. Lithium-induced neuroprotection appears to be mediated through multiple mechanisms and actions. Regulation in gene-expression of Bcl-2, p53, Bax, GRP78, GST and others implies that these gene-coded products may play a substantial role in the neuroprotection generated by lithium. The neuroprotective mechanism of lithium is currently undergoing extensive study.

The mitochondrial death pathway has been known to be regulated by Bcl-2 family proteins that consist of pro-apoptotic members and anti-apoptotic members[94,95]. Two major pro-apoptotic members of this family are Bax and Bak and two major anti-apoptotic members are Bcl-2 and Bcl-xL. Bax and Bak exert destructive effects on membrane integrity, which results in release of cytochrome c from mitochondria into the cytosol, caspase activation and DNA fragmentation. Bcl-2 and Bcl-xL are located in the outer membrane of mitochondria and maintain mitochondrial membrane integrity by blocking Bax-induced cytochrome c release and caspase activation. Transcription factor p53 increases Bax gene expression, but decreases Bcl-2 gene expression[96]. Upregulation of Bcl-2, and downregulation of p53 and Bax by lithium suggest that lithium may protect mitochondrial membrane integrity and prevent cytochrome c release in order to produce neuroprotective effects. Lithium has recently been recognized as a GSK-3 inhibitor[34]. GSK-3 plays an active role in various types of neuronal neurotoxic insult-induced apoptosis[97]. GSK-3 has been reported to phosphorylate Bax, which activates the mitochondrial death pathway by stimulating cytochrome c release from mitochondria, suggesting that lithium may also reduce Bax-promoted apoptosis by inhibiting GSK-3[98].

GRP78 functions as a molecular chaperone, binds calcium and folds damaged proteins, and has been found to produce cytoprotective effects by suppressing oxyradical accumulation and stabilizing mitochondria function[99–101]. It has been reported that blocking GRP78 increased glutamate-induced neuronal cell death, while pretreatment with 2-deoxy-D-glucose, an inducer of GRP78 expression, inhibited glutamate-induced calcium influx and cell death[102]. Glutamate has been known to cause imbalance of neuronal Ca^{2+} resulting in mitochondrial depolarization, and further induced inhibition of the mitochondrial electron transport chain and generation of reactive oxygen species. In addition, GRP78 is able to form a complex with caspase-7 and -12 and then prevent release of caspase-12 from the ER[103]. Increase of GRP78 by lithium indicates that lithium may have neuroprotective effects against oxidative stress and apoptosis. Shao *et al.*[88] recently found that chronic lithium treatment significantly inhibited lipid peroxidation and protein oxidation in rat cerebral cortical cells. Many studies have shown that lithium inhibits release of cytochrome c, activation of caspase-3 and DNA fragmentation[75,83,88]. Lithium-induced increase in GRP78 expression may collaborate with Bcl-2 to stabilize mitochondrial membrane potential and suppress oxyradical accumulation, resulting in prevention of the linkage of cytochrome c and the activation of caspase.

Supporting the effect of lithium against oxidative stress is a recent finding that GST is also a target for chronic treatment with lithium and valproate[80]. GST catalyzes the conjugation of the reduced glutathione with oxidized products generated by reactive oxygen species to form a non-toxic product[104,105]. Detoxification by GST provides protection against harmful endogenous reactive oxygen species; this enzyme is now believed to play a critical role in combating oxidative stress and cell toxicity. Increase of GST by lithium and valproate suggests that these two drugs may increase scavenging of oxidized products by increasing GST activity in order to protect oxidative stress. In addition, GST as an endogenous inhibitor of c-Jun N-terminal kinase (JNK) represses JNK-dependent oxidative stress-induced cell death[106,107]. It has been reported that chronic lithium treatment suppresses glutamate-induced JNK activation and cell death in rat cerebellar granule cells[30]. Recent findings suggest that reactive oxygen species accumulation initiates further downstream events that lead to cell death, including JNK phosphorylation, cytochrome c release, activation of caspases, and DNA fragmentation[108–110]. GST, together with Bcl-2 and GRP78, may mediate the neuroprotective effects produced by chronic lithium treatment. The neuroprotective mechanism of lithium is summarized in Figure 31.1.

The neuroprotective effect of lithum has been recognized only in the last few years. Although there are at present no available data directly indicating that neuroprotection is relevant to treatment by these drugs, the concept is supported by studies demonstrating significant reductions in regional volume and cell number in the central nervous system associated with mood disorder. It is clearly necessary to extend these studies in other mood-stabilizing drugs, to verify their neuroprotective action in animal behavioral models, and demonstrate in a longitudinal study that these treatments do indeed reduce or delay the central nervous system cell death or atrophy in mood disorder patients.

CONCLUSION AND DISCUSSION

Chronic treatment with lithium at therapeutically relevant concentrations has been found to regulate gene expression of Bax, Bcl-2, GRP78, GST and others. The pro-apoptotic factor Bax and anti-apoptotic factor Bcl-2 are members of the Bcl-2 family that regulate the mitochondrial death pathway. Decreasing Bax and increasing Bcl-2 maintain mitochondrial membrane integrity, and prevent cytochrome c release and caspase activation. GRP78 engages in molecular chaperone activity, binds Ca^{2+} and protects cells from the deleterious effects of damaged proteins. GST catalyzes conjugation of the brain major antioxidatant GSH with oxidized product, and increases the ability of reactive oxygen species scavenging. Increased BCl-2, GRP78 and GST expression and decreased Bax expression by lithium suggest that this drug may produce neuroprotective effects. Supporting this possibility are studies demonstrating cell loss and brain atrophy in patients with bipolar disorder, and a growing body of evidence that lithium does indeed exert neuroprotective effects both *in vitro* and *in vivo*. Increased BCl-2, GRP78 and GST expression and decreased Bax expression may be an important mechanism by which mood-stabilizing drugs protect vulnerable brain regions by enhancing the resistance of neuronal cells against a variety of insults.

Recent studies suggest that excitotoxicity and mitochondrial dysfunction may play important roles in the loss of brain volume and cell number in bipolar disorder patients. Mitochondria play a critical role in the regulation of cell death, and their dysfunction may mediate neuronal damage or loss in bipolar

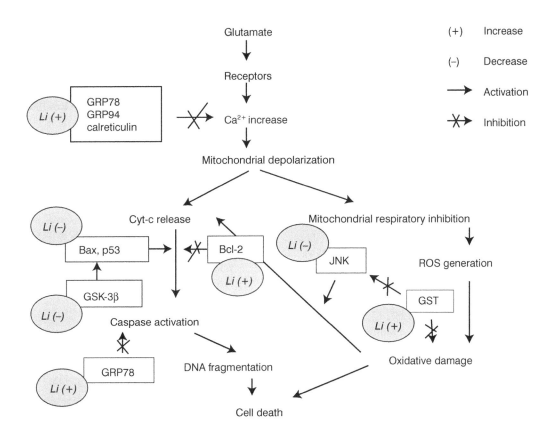

Figure 31.1 Mechanism of lithium neuroprotection. Li, lithium; GSK-3β. glycogen synthase kinase-3β; Cyt-c, cytochrome c; ROS, reactive oxygen species; GST, glutathione S-transferase; JNK, c-jun N-terminal kinase

disorder. Cell death can be initiated by excitotoxicity and reactive oxygen species, or by glucocorticoid and other insults. These toxic insults regulate multiple signaling pathways that usually converge at the mitochondria, changing mitochondrial membrane potential, increasing the release of cytochrome c and further stimulating downstream caspases. Chronic lithium treatment may produce a neuroprotective property by stabilizing mitochodrial function via multiple pathways, decreasing activities of p53, Bax and GSK-3, and increasing Bcl-2 to help protect mitochondrial membrane integrity from various insults, and prevent mitochondria dysfunction-triggered cell death. Increased GRP78 may increase ER calcium binding activity that allows cells to accommodate to stress resulting from elevated calcium, preventing calcium overtake by mitochondria which in turn stabilizes mitochondrial function and inhibits accumulation of reactive oxygen species. Increase in GST also increases the ability to scavenge oxidized products by reactive oxygen species.

REFERENCES

1. Odagaki Y, Koyama Y, Yamashita I. Lithium and serotonergic neural transmission: a review of pharmacological and biochemical aspects in animal studies. Lithium 1992; 3: 95–107

2. Price LH, Charney DS, Delgado PL, Heninger DR. Lithium and serotonin function: implications for the serotonin hypothesis of depression. Psychopharmacology 1990; 100: 3–12

3. Bunney WE Jr, Garland-Bunney BL. Mechanisms of action of lithium in affective illness: basic and clinical implications. In Meltzer HY, ed. Psychopharmacology: The Third Generation of Progress. New York: Raven Press, 1987: 553–65

4. Wood AJ, Goodwin GM. A review of the biochemical and neuropharmacological actions of lithium. Psychol Med 1987; 17: 579–600

5. Risby ED, Hsiao JK, Manji HK. The mechanisms of action of lithium. II. Effects on adenylate cyclase activity and β-adrenergic receptor binding in normal subjects. Arch Gen Psychiatry 1991; 48: 513–24

6. Forn J, Valdecasas FG. Effects of lithium on brain adenyl cyclase activity. Biochem Pharm 1971; 20: 2773–9

7. Goldberg H, Clayman P, Skorecki K. Mechanism of Li inhibition of vasopressin-sensitive adenylate cyclase in cultured renal epithelial cells. Am J Physiol 1988; 255: F995–F1002

8. Mork A, Geisler A. Effects of lithium ex vivo on the GTP-mediated inhibition of calcium-stimulated adenylate cyclase activity in rat brain. Eur J Pharmacol 1989; 168: 347–54

9. Mork A, Geisler A. Effects of GTP on hormone-stimulated adenylate cyclase activity in cerebral cortex, striatum, and hippocampus from rats treated chronically with lithium. Biol Psychiatry 1989; 26: 279–88

10. Avissar S, Schreiber G, Danon A, Belmaker RH. Lithium inhibits adrenergic and cholinergic increases in GTP binding in rat cortex. Nature 1988; 331: 440–2

11. Masana MI, Bitran JA, Hsiao JK, Potter WZ. In vivo evidence that lithium inactivates Gi modulation of adenylate cyclase in brain. J Neurochem 1992; 59: 200–5

12. Masana MI, Bitran JA, Hsiao JK, et al. Lithium effects on noradrenergic-linked adenylate cyclase activity in intact rat brain and in vivo microdialysis study. Brain Res 1991; 538: 333–6

13. Guitart X, Nestler EJ. Regulation of cyclic AMP-dependent protein phosphorylation in rat frontal cortex by chronic lithium: identification of DARPP-32 and other lithium-regulated phosphoproteins. Soc Neurosci Abstr 1992; 18: 104

14. Colin SF, Chang H-C, Mollner S, et al. Chronic lithium regulates the expression of adenylate cyclase and Gi-protein α subunit in rat cerebral cortex. Proc Natl Acad Sci USA 1991; 88: 10634–7

15. Guitart X, Nestler EJ. Chronic administration of lithium or other antidepressants increases levels of DARPP-32 in rat frontal cortex. J Neurochem 1992; 59: 1164–7

16. Nonaka S, Hough CJ, Chuang DM. Chronic lithium treatment robustly protects neurons in the central nervous system against excitotoxicity by inhibiting N-methyl-D-aspartate receptor-mediated calcium influx. Proc Natl Acad Sci USA 1998; 95: 2642–7

17. Hashimoto R, Hough C, Nakazawa T, et al. Lithium protection against glutamate excitotoxicity in rat cerebral cortical neurons: involvement of NMDA receptor inhibition possibly by decreasing NR2B tyrosine phosphorylation. J Neurochem 2002; 80: 589–97

18. Hallcher LM, Sherman WR. The effects of lithium ion and other agents on the activity of myo-inositol-1-phosphatase from bovine brain. J Biol Chem 1980; 255: 10896–901

19. Naccarato WF, Ray RE, Wells WW. Biosynthesis of myo-inositol in rat mammary gland. Isolation and properties of the enzymes. Arch Biochem Biophys 1974; 164: 194–201

20. Atack JR, Broughton HB, Pollack SJ. Inositol monophosphatase – a putative target for Li+ in the treatment of bipolar disorder. Trends Neurosci 1995; 18: 343–9

21. Berridge MJ. Inositol triphosphate, calcium, lithium and cell signalling. JAMA 1989; 262: 1834–41

22. Berridge MJ. Irvine RF. Inositol phosphates and cell signalling. Nature 1989; 341: 197–205

23. Berridge MJ, Downes CP, Hanley MR. Lithium amplifies the agonist dependent phosphatidylinositol responses in brain and salivary glands. Biochem J 1992; 206: 587–95

24. Anderson SMP, Godfrey PP, Grahame-Smith DG. The effects of phorbol esters and lithium on 5-HT release in rat hippocampal slices. Br J Pharmacol 1988; 93 (Suppl): 96P

25. Bitran JA, Gusovsky F, Manji HK, Potter W. Effects of chronic lithium treatment on signal transduction mechanisms in HL60 cells. Biol Psychiatry 1989; 25: 46A

26. Lenox RH, Watson DG. Targets for lithium action in the brain: protein kinase C substrates and muscarinic receptor regulation. Clin Neuropharmacol 1991; 15 (Suppl): 612A–13A

27. Li PP, Sibony D, Green M, Warsh JJ. Lithium modulation of the phosphoinositide signalling system in rat cortex: selective effects on phorbol ester binding. J Neurochem 1993; 61: 1722–30

28. Lenox RH, Watson DG, Patel J, Ellis J. Chronic lithium administration alters a prominent PKC substrate in rat hippocampus. Brain Res 1992; 570: 333–40

29. Einat H, Yuan P, Gould TD, et al. The role of the extracellular signal-regulated kinase signaling pathway in mood modulation. J Neurosci 2003; 23: 7311–16

30. Chen RW, Qin ZH, Ren M, et al. Regulation of c-Jun N-terminal kinase, p38 kinase and AP-1 DNA binding in cultured brain neurons: roles in glutamate excitotoxicity and lithium neuroprotection. J Neurochem 2003; 84: 566–75

31. Chalecka-Franaszek E, Chuang DM. Lithium activates the serine/threonine kinase Akt-1 and suppresses glutamate-induced inhibition of Akt-1 activity in neurons. Proc Natl Acad Sci USA 1999; 96: 8745–50

32. De Sarno P, Li X, Jope RS. Regulation of Akt and glycogen synthase kinase-3 beta phosphorylation by sodium valproate and lithium. Neuropharmacology 2002; 43: 1158–64

33. Beaulieu JM, Sotnikova TD, Yao WD, et al. Lithium antagonizes dopamine-dependent behaviors mediated by an AKT/glycogen synthase kinase 3 signaling cascade. Proc Natl Acad Sci USA 2004; 101: 5099–104

34. Stambolic V, Ruel L, Woodgett JR. Lithium inhibits glycogen synthase kinase-3 activity and mimics wingless signalling in intact cells. Curr Biol 1996; 6: 1664–8

35. Takahashi M, Yasutake K, Tomizawa K. Lithium inhibits neurite growth and tau protein kinase I/glycogen synthase kinase-3beta-dependent phosphorylation of juvenile tau in cultured hippocampal neurons. J Neurochem 1999; 73: 2073–83

36. Strachan T, Read AP. Human Molecular Genetics, 2nd edn. Oxford, UK: Bios, 1999

37. Sathya G, Li W, Klinge CM, et al. Effects of multiple estrogen responsive elements, their spacing, and location on estrogen response of reporter genes. Mol Endocrinol 1997; 11: 1994–2003

38. Ozaki N, Chuang DM. Lithium increases transcription factor binding to AP-1 and cyclic AMP-responsive element in cultured neurons and rat brain. J Neurochem 1997; 69: 2336–44

39. Jope RS, Song L. AP-1 and NF-kappaB stimulated by carbachol in human neuroblastoma SH-SY5Y cells are differentially sensitive to inhibition by lithium. Brain Res Mol Brain Res 1997; 50: 171–80

40. Wang JF, Asghari V, Rockel C, Young LT. Cyclic AMP responsive element binding protein phosphorylation and DNA binding is decreased by chronic lithium but not valproate treatment of SH-SY5Y neuroblastoma cells. Neuroscience 1999; 91: 771–6

41. Young LT, Bezchlibnyk YB, Chen B, et al. Amygdala cyclic adenosine monophosphate response element binding protein phosphorylation in patients with mood disorders: effects of diagnosis, suicide, and drug treatment. Biol Psychiatry 2004; 55: 570–7

42. Koch JM, Kell S, Hinze-Selch D, Aldenhoff JB. Changes in CREB-phosphorylation during recovery from major depression. J Psychiatr Res 2002; 36: 369–75

43. Chen AC, Shirayama Y, Shin KH, et al. Expression of the cAMP response element binding protein (CREB) in hippocampus produces an antidepressant effect. Biol Psychiatry 2001; 49: 753–62

44. Yuan PX, Chen G, Manji HK. Lithium stimulates gene expression through the AP-1 transcription factor pathway. Mol Brain Res 1998; 58: 225–30

45. Angel P, Imagawa M, Chiu R, et al. Phorbol ester-inducible genes contain a common cis element recognized by a TPA-modulated trans-acting factor. Cell 1987; 49: 729–39

46. Curran T, Vogt PK. Dangerous liaisons: Fos and Jun, oncogenic transcription factors. In McKnight SL, Yamamoto KR, eds. Transcriptional Regulation. Cold Spring Harbor: Cold Spring Harbor Laboratory Press, 1992: 797–831

47. Curran T, Morgan JI. Fos: an immediate–early transcription factor in neurons. J Neurobiol 1995; 26: 403–12

48. Kaczmarek L, Lapinska-Dzwonek J, Szymczak S. Matrix metalloproteinases in the adult brain physiology: a link between c-Fos, AP-1 and remodeling of neuronal connections? EMBO J 2002; 21: 6643–8

49. Malik RK, Roe MW, Blackshear PJ. Epidermal growth factor and other mitogens induce binding of a protein complex to the c-fos serum response element in human astrocytoma and other cells. J Biol Chem 1991; 266: 8576–82

50. Grundker C, Gunthert AR, Hellriegel M, Emons G. Gonadotropin-releasing hormone (GnRH) agonist triptorelin inhibits estradiol-induced serum response element (SRE) activation and c-fos expression in human endometrial, ovarian and breast cancer cells. Eur J Endocrinol 2004; 151: 619–28

51. Lackinger D, Eichhorn U, Kaina B. Effect of ultraviolet light, methyl methanesulfonate and ionizing radiation on the genotoxic response and apoptosis of mouse fibroblasts lacking c-Fos, p53 or both. Mutagenesis 2001; 16: 233–41

52. Dunn C, Wiltshire C, MacLaren A, Gillespie DA. Molecular mechanism and biological functions of c-Jun N-terminal kinase signalling via the c-Jun transcription factor. Cell Signal 2002; 14: 585–93

53. Liu S, Yu S, Hasegawa Y, et al. Glycogen synthase kinase 3beta is a negative regulator of growth factor-induced activation of the c-Jun N-terminal kinase. J Biol Chem 2004; 279: 51075–81

54. Lee YH, Kim S, Kim J, et al. Overexpression of phospholipase C-gamma1 suppresses UVC-induced apoptosis through inhibition of c-fos accumulation and c-Jun N-terminal kinase activation in PC12 cells. Biochim Biophys Acta 1999; 1440: 235–43

55. Filomeni G, Aquilano K, Civitareale P, et al. Activation of c-Jun-N-terminal kinase is required for apoptosis triggered by glutathione disulfide in neuroblastoma cells. Free Radic Biol Med 2005; 39: 345–54

56. Johannessen M, Delghandi MP, Moens U. What turns CREB on? Cell Signal 2004; 16: 1211–27

57. Fiol CJ, Williams JS, Chou CH, et al. A secondary phosphorylation of CREB341 at Ser129 is required for the cAMP-mediated control of gene expression. A role for glycogen synthase kinase-3 in the control of gene expression. J Biol Chem 1994; 269: 32187–93

58. Bullock BP, Habener JF. Phosphorylation of the cAMP response element binding protein CREB by cAMP-dependent protein kinase A and glycogen synthase kinase-3 alters DNA-binding affinity, conformation, and increases net charge. Biochemistry 1998; 37: 3795–809

59. Lonze BE, Ginty DD. Function and regulation of CREB family transcription factors in the nervous system. Neuron 2002; 35: 605–23

60. Divish MM, Sheftel G, Boyle A, et al. Differential effect of lithium on fos proto-oncogene expression mediated by receptor and postreceptor activators of protein kinase C and cyclic adenosine monophosphate: model for its antimanic action. J Neurosci Res 1991; 28: 40–8

61. Unlap MT, Jope RS. Lithium attenuates nerve growth factor-induced activation of AP-1 DNA binding activity in PC12 cells. Neuropsychopharmacology 1997; 17: 12–17

62. Williams MB, Jope RS. Circadian variation in rat brain AP-1 DNA binding activity after cholinergic stimulation: modulation by lithium. Psychopharmacology 1995; 122: 363–8

63. Asghari V, Wang JF, Reiach JS, Young LT. Differential effects of mood stabilizers on Fos/Jun proteins and AP-1 binding activity in human neuroblastoma SH-SY5Y cells. Mol Brain Res 1998; 58: 95–102

64. Boyle WJ, Smeal T, Defize LH, et al. Activation of protein kinase C decreases phosphorylation of c-Jun at sites that negatively regulate its DNA-binding activity. Cell 1991; 64: 573–84

65. de Groot RP, Auwerx J, Bourouis M, Sassone-Corsi P. Negative regulation of Jun/AP-1: conserved function of glycogen synthase kinase 3 and the Drosophila kinase shaggy. Mol Psychiatry 2002; 7 (Suppl 1): S35–S45

66. Wood GE, Young LT, Reagan LP, et al. Stress-induced structural remodeling in hippocampus: prevention by lithium treatment. Proc Natl Acad Sci USA 2004; 101: 3973–8

67. Wang L, Liu X, Lenox RH. Transcriptional down-regulation of MARCKS gene expression in immortalized hippocampal cells by lithium. J Neurochem 2001; 79: 816–25

68. Chang MC, Jones CR. Chronic lithium treatment decreases brain phospholipase A2 activity. Neurochem Res 1998; 23: 887–92

69. Rao JS, Rapoport SI, Bosetti F. Decrease in the AP-2 DNA-binding activity and in the protein expression of AP-2 alpha and AP-2 beta in frontal cortex of rats treated with lithium for 6 weeks. Neuropsychopharmacology 2005; 30: 2006–13

70. Wang JF, Young LT. Differential display PCR reveals increased expresssion of 2′,3′-cyclic nucleotide 3′-phosphodiesterase by lithium. FEBS Lett 1996; 386: 225–9

71. Chen G, Yuan PX, Jiang YM, et al. Lithium increases tyrosine hydroxylase levels both in vivo and in vitro. J Neurochem 1998; 70: 1768–71

72. Bagetta G, Corasaniti MT, Melino G, et al. Lithium and tacrine increase the expression of nitric oxide synthase mRNA in the hippo-campus of rat. Biochem Biophys Res Commun 1993; 197: 1132–9

73. Sivam SP, Takeuchi K, Li S, et al. Lithium increases dynorphin A(1-8) and prodynorphin mRNA levels in the basal ganglia of rats. Brain Res 1988; 427: 155–63

74. Chen G, Zeng WZ, Yuan PX, et al. The mood-stabilizing agents lithium and valproate robustly increase the levels of the neuro-protective protein bcl-2 in the CNS. J Neurochem 1999; 72: 879–82

75. Chen RW, Chuang DM. Long term lithium treatment suppresses p53 and Bax expression but increases Bcl-2 expression. A prominent role in neuroprotection against excitotoxicity. J Biol Chem 1999; 274: 6039–42

76. Wang JF, Bown C, Young LT. Differential DISPLAY PCR reveals novel targets for the mood stabilizing drug valproate including the molecular chaperone GRP78. Mol Pharmacol 1999; 55, 521–7

77. Wang JF, Young LT. Regulation of molecular chaperone GRP78 by mood stabilizing drugs. Clin Neurosci Res 2004; 4: 281–8

78. Shao L, Sun X, Xu L, et al. Mood stabilizing drug lithium increases expression of endo-plasmic reticulum stress proteins in primary cultured rat cerebral cortical cells. Life Sci 2006; 78: 1317–23

79. Hiroi T, Wei H, Hough C, et al. Protracted lithium treatment protects against the ER stress elicited by thapsigargin in rat PC12 cells: roles of intracellular calcium, GRP78 and Bcl-2. Pharmacogenomics J 2005; 5: 102–11

80. Wang JF, Shao L, Sun X, Young LT. Glutathione S-transferase is a novel target for mood stabilizing drugs in primary cultured neurons. J Neurochem 2004; 88: 1477–84

81. Zhou R, Gray NA, Yuan P, et al. The anti-apoptotic, glucocorticoid receptor cochaperone protein BAG-1 is a long-term target for the actions of mood stabilizers. J Neurosci 2005; 25: 4493–502

82. Nonaka S, Chuang DM. Neuroprotective effects of chronic lithium on focal cerebral ischemia in rats. Neuroreport 1998; 9: 2081–4

83. Nonaka S, Katsube N, Chuang DM. Lithium protects rat cerebellar granule cells against

apoptosis induced by anticonvulsants, phenytoin and carbamazepine. J Pharmacol Exp Ther 1998; 286: 39–47

84. Hashimoto R, Takei N, Shimazu K, et al. Lithium induces brain-derived neurotrophic factor and activates TrkB in rodent cortical neurons: an essential step for neuroprotection against glutamate excitotoxicity. Neuro-pharmacology 2002; 43: 1173–9

85. Coyle JT, Puttfarcken P. Oxidative stress, gluta-mate, and neurodegenerative disorders. Science 1993; 262: 689–95

86. Skaper SD, Floreani M, Ceccon M, et al. Excitotoxicity, oxidative stress, and the neuro-protective potential of melatonin. Ann NY Acad Sci 1999; 890: 107–18

87. Leist M, Nicotera P. Apoptosis, excitotoxicity, and neuropathology. Exp Cell Res 1998; 239: 183–201

88. Shao L, Young LT, Wang JF. Chronic treat-ment with mood stabilizers lithium and valproate prevents excitotoxicity by inhibiting oxidative stress in rat cerebral cortical cells. Biol Psychiatry 2005; 58: 879–84

89. Nonaka S, Chuang DM. Neuroprotective effects of chronic lithium on focal cerebral ischemia in rats. Neuroreport 1998; 9: 2081–4

90. Wei H, Qin ZH, Senatorov VV, et al. Lithium suppresses excitotoxicity-induced striatal lesions in a rat model of Huntington's disease. Neuroscience 2001; 106: 603–12

91. Pascual T, Gonzalez JL. A protective effect of lithium on rat behaviour altered by ibotenic acid lesions of the basal forebrain cholinergic system. Brain Res 1995; 695: 289–92

92. Goodenough S, Conrad S, Skutella T, Behl C. Inactivation of glycogen synthase kinase-3beta protects against kainic acid-induced neurotoxicity in vivo. Brain Res 2004; 1026: 116–25

93. Chen G, Rajkowska G, Du F, et al. Enhancement of hippocampal neurogenesis by lithium. J Neurochem 2000l; 75: 1729–34

94. Lindsten T, Zong WX, Thompson CB. Defining the role of the Bcl-2 family of proteins in the nervous system. Neuroscientist 2005; 11: 10–5

95. Breckenridge DG, Xue D. Regulation of mito-chondrial membrane permeabilization by BCL-2 family proteins and caspases. Curr Opin Cell Biol 2004; 16: 647–52

96. Miyashita T, Krajewski S, Krajewska M, et al. Tumor suppressor p53 is a regulator of bcl-2 and bax gene expression in vitro and in vivo. Oncogene 1994; 9: 1799–805

97. Jope RS, Bijur GN. Mood stabilizers, glycogen synthase kinase-3beta and cell survival. Mol Psychiatry 2002; 7 (Suppl 1): S35–S45

98. Linseman DA, Butts BD, Precht TA, et al. Glycogen synthase kinase-3beta phosphorylates Bax and promotes its mitochondrial localiza-tion during neuronal apoptosis. J Neurosci 2004; 24: 9993–10002

99. Nigam SK, Goldberg AL, Ho S, et al. A set of endoplasmic reticulum proteins possessing properties of molecular chaperones includes CA2+ binding proteins and member of the thioredoxin superfamily. J Biol Chem 1994; 269: 1744–9

100. Yu Z, Luo H, Fu W, Mattson MP. The endo-plasmic reticulum stress-responsive protein GRP78 protects neurons against excitotoxicity and apoptosis: suppression of oxidative stress and stabilization of calcium homeostasis. Exp Neurol 1999; 155: 302–14

101. Liu H, Bowes RC 3rd, van de Water B, et al. Endoplasmic reticulum chaperones GRP78 and calreticulin prevent oxidative stress, Ca2+ disturbances, and cell death in renal epithelial cells. J Biol Chem 1997; 272: 21751–9

102. Lee J, Bruce-Keller AJ, Kruman Y, et al. 2-Deoxy-D-glucose protects hippocampal neu-rons against excitotoxic and oxidative injury: evidence for the involvement of stress proteins. J Neurosci Res 1999; 57: 48–61

103. Reddy RK, Mao C, Baumeister P, et al. Endoplasmic reticulum chaperone protein GRP78 protects cells from apoptosis induced by topoisomerase inhibitors: role of ATP binding site in suppression of caspase-7 activation. J Biol Chem 2003; 278: 20915–24

104. Eaton DL, Bammler TK. Concise review of the glutathione S-transferases and their signifi-cance to toxicology. Toxicol Sci 1999; 49: 156–64

105. Hayes JD, Strange RC. Potential contribution of the glutathione S-transferase supergene family to resistance to oxidative stress. Free Radic Res 1995; 22: 193–207

106. Jang JH, Surh YJ. beta-Amyloid induces oxidative DNA damage and cell death through activation of c-Jun N terminal kinase. Ann N Y Acad Sci 2002; 973: 228–36

107. Yin Z, Ivanov VN, Habelhah H, et al. Glutathione S-transferase p elicits protection against H2O2-induced cell death via coordinated regulation of stress kinases. Cancer Res 2000; 60: 4053–7

108. Petrosillo G, Ruggiero FM, Paradies G. Role of reactive oxygen species and cardiolipin in the release of cytochrome c from mitochondria. FASEB J 2003; 17: 2202–8

109. Tan S, Wood M, Maher P. Oxidative stress induces a form of programmed cell death with characteristics of both apoptosis and necrosis in neuronal cells. J Neurochem 1998; 71: 95–105

110. Higuchi M, Honda T, Proske RJ, Yeh ET. Regulation of reactive oxygen species-induced apoptosis and necrosis by caspase 3-like proteases. Oncogene 1998; 17: 2753–60

32 Potential use of lithium in neurodegenerative disorders

De-Maw Chuang, Josef Priller

Contents   Introduction • Lithium protects against glutamate-induced neuronal apoptosis in cellular models • Neuroprotective effects of lithium in animal and cellular models of neurodegenerative diseases • Clinical trials of lithium in neurodegenerative disorders • Conclusion

INTRODUCTION

Aberrant processes of cell death have been positively linked to the pathogenesis of a number of diseases including disorders of the central nervous system (reviewed in references 1 and 2). Cell death can be broadly separated into two polar categories termed apoptosis and necrosis. In apoptosis, or programmed cell death, cells display chromatin condensation, internucleosomal DNA cleavage, cytoplasmic shrinking and plasma membrane blebbing, and are phagocytosed by neighboring cells. This contrasts with necrosis, where cells swell and rupture, eliciting an inflammatory response. Mitochondria play a pivotal role in the genesis and propagation of apoptosis via events such as mitochondrial calcium accumulation, generation of free radicals and, perhaps, activation of permeability transition pores[3]. Four mitochondrial molecules mediating downstream cell-death pathways have been identified:

cytochrome c, Smac, apoptosis-inducing factor and endonuclease G. Cytochrome c binds to Apaf-1, which, together with procaspase-9, forms apoptosomes and, in turn, causes caspase-9 and caspase-3 activation. Smac binds to inhibitors of activated caspases, resulting in further caspase activation. Apoptosis-inducing factor and endonuclease G act via caspase-independent pathways to trigger cell death[4–7]. A schematic diagram showing the apoptotic cascades is shown in Figure 32.1.

Increasingly, reports support the notion that excessive apoptosis and other types of cell death contribute to the pathophysiology of certain forms of neurodegenerative diseases. For example, in cerebral ischemia, necrotic cell death occurs in the core of the infarct, where hypoxia and energy depletion are more severe. Conversely, in the ischemic penumbra, where the insult is not as severe, apoptosis prevails and accompanying changes in gene expression and

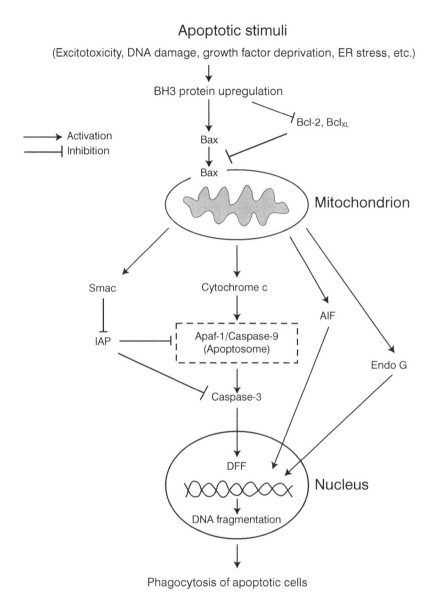

Figure 32.1 Critical molecular events involved in cell apoptosis. Following apoptotic insult, the pro-apoptotic BH3 proteins are upregulated, causing translocation of the major pro-apoptotic protein Bax to the mitochondria and this process is inhibited by Bcl-2 or Bcl$_{XL}$. The mitochondrial damage triggers the release of cytochrome c and induces caspase activation through apaf-1. In addition, Smac, apoptosis-inducing factor (AIF) and endonucleus G (Endo G) are released from injured mitochondria. Smac neutralizes the function of IAP (inhibitor of apoptosis protein) which suppresses the activities of the apaf-1/caspase-9 apoptosome and downstream caspase-3. The latter is translocated to the nucleus and, in turn, activates DFF to cause DNA fragmentation. AIF and Endo G are also translocated to the nucleus to induce apoptosis by a caspase-independent mechanism. Dead cells are phagocytosed by scavenger cells

activation of caspases 1, 3, 8, 9 and 11 have been reported[8–10]. There is a general consensus that cell death resulting from massive glutamate release plays a prominent role in brain infarction and neurological deficits. In Huntington's disease, an autosomal dominant neurodegenerative disease caused by an expansion of a polyglutamine repeat sequence in the huntingtin protein, cytochrome c release, caspase activation and apoptosis in the striatum have been documented[10]. β-Amyloid peptide, which has been strongly implicated in the pathogenesis of Alzheimer's disease, has been reported to induce apoptosis in neuronal cultures and to increase their vulnerability to death induced by conditions such as oxidative stress[9]. Moreover, hallmarks of apoptosis such as DNA fragmentation, caspase activation and induction of apoptosis-related genes have been found in neurons associated with amyloid deposits in the brain of Alzheimer's patients[11]. A growing body of data also links apoptotic cell death to other types of neurodegenerative diseases such as Parkinson's disease, amyotrophic lateral sclerosis (ALS), cerebellar degeneration, epilepsy and HIV-1-induced dementia[1,2,7,10,11].

Emerging evidence raises the possibility that apoptosis or other forms of cell death may be involved in neuropsychiatric illnesses, particularly mood disorders, and that mood stabilizing drugs may elicit their therapeutic effects in part by their neuroprotective actions. Structural imaging studies have shown a reduction in gray matter volume in several brain areas including the orbital and medial prefrontal cortices, ventral striatum and hippocampus as well as an enlargement of the third ventricles of patients with mood disorders[12–15]. Postmortem studies yield complementary results: a reduction in cortical volume and a decrease in the density of neurons/glial cells in the prefrontal, orbital and cingulated cortices, amygdala and other brain areas[15,16]. A possible relationship between these brain abnormalities and the pathological state of mood disorders is suggested by the observation that the loss of brain volume in the subgenual prefrontal cortex of patients with bipolar mood disorder is greatly suppressed in bipolar subjects chronically treated with lithium or valproate, two mainstay drugs used to treat this mood disorder[12]. An independent clinical study shows that the gray matter volume in the brain is increased by approximately 4% in bipolar patients treated with the mood stabilizer lithium[17]. The current working hypothesis concerning the evolution of mood disorder is that environmental and genetic factors (e.g. susceptibility and protective genes) interact to remodel the nervous system. Early episodes of affective disorders have been linked to psychosocial stressors[18]. In animal models, stressors have been shown to induce changes in the expression of immediate early genes and neurotrophic factors[19], and under chronic conditions, a decrease in neurogenesis[20] as well as atrophy or cell loss in the hippocampus[21]. Stress increases extracellular glutamate levels in the hippocampus, and N-methyl-D-aspartate (NMDA) receptor antagonists attenuate stress-induced hippocampal atrophy[21,22]. All together, these observations suggest that atrophy and even cell death are mediated, at least in part, by excessive glutamate neurotransmission.

LITHIUM PROTECTS AGAINST GLUTAMATE-INDUCED NEURONAL APOPTOSIS IN CELLULAR MODELS

Glutamate overflow in discrete brain areas has also been linked to a variety of neurodegenerative diseases such as stroke, Huntington's disease, ALS, spinal cord injury, brain trauma, cerebellar degeneration, and possibly

Alzheimer's disease and Parkinson's disease. The effects of lithium on glutamate-induced excitotoxicity were first studied in cultured rodent brain neurons. Exposing rat cerebellar granule neurons, cerebral cortical neurons and hippocampal neurons to glutamate induces neuronal death, largely by apoptosis, which is mediated almost exclusively by overactivation of NMDA receptors, resulting in an excessive influx of calcium through NMDA receptor channels[23,24]. Pre-treatment of these neurons with lithium causes a robust protection against glutamate-induced excitotoxicity[23,24]. The lithium-induced neuroprotective effects occur at therapeutically relevant concentrations of this drug (e.g. 1 mmol/l) and require 5–6 days' pre-treatment for complete neuroprotection. Lithium neuroprotection is closely associated with a reduction in NMDA receptor-mediated calcium entry. The NMDA receptor is made up of heteromeric assemblies of NR1 and NR2 subunits. The NR1 subunit is mandatory for receptor function, and NR2 (NR2A-D) subunits regulate NMDA receptor activity primarily by their phosphorylation states. Lithium-induced reduction of NMDA receptor-mediated intracellular calcium increase is likely to be due to a decrease in phosphorylation of NR2B at Tyr1472[24]. The phosphorylation of NR2B Tyr1472 is necessary for NMDA-receptor-mediated calcium influx[25], and this phosphorylation step is believed to be upregulated by the Src-family tyrosine kinase, whose activity is also suppressed by long-term lithium treatment[26]. The NR2B subunit has been proposed as an important target for intervening NMDA receptor-related neurodegenerative diseases[27]. Inhibition of NMDA receptor activity is a contributing factor to lithium's inhibition of glutamate-induced activation of c-Jun-N-terminal kinase (JNK) and p38 kinase; both have a key role in mediating excitotoxic neuronal death[28].

The requirement of protracted lithium pretreatment to obtain maximal neuroprotection suggests the involvement of gene expression. Indeed, a variety of neuroprotective proteins are induced by chronic or long-term lithium treatment. Among them is brain-derived neurotrophic factor (BDNF), which plays a prominent role in cortical development, synaptic plasticity and neuronal survival[29]. Chronic treatment of rats with lithium and another mood stabilizer, valproate, increases levels of BDNF in the rat frontal cortex[30,31]. In rat cortical neuronal cultures, lithium treatment also induces BDNF and, in turn, activates its receptor TrkB[32]. Pharmacologic and BDNF knock-out studies demonstrate that the lithium effect on BDNF/TrkB is necessary for neuroprotection against excitotoxicity. This trophic action is probably involved in lithium-induced activation of phosphatidylinositol 3-kinase (PI 3-kinase) and downstream Akt[33], and MEK/ERK mitogen-activated protein kinase (MAP kinase)[31,34,35]. One downstream target of both Akt and MAP kinase is cyclic AMP response element binding protein (CREB); its activation through phosphorylation increases the expression of BDNF and the key anti-apoptotic protein Bcl-2[29]. Bcl-2 can be induced *in vivo* using rats[36,37] and *in vitro* using rat primary neuronal cultures treated with lithium[38]. In cultured neurons, lithium-induced Bcl-2 expression is paralleled by down-regulation of the pro-apoptotic molecules p53 and Bax, and blocks glutamate-induced cytochrome c release and caspase activation[38].

One of the critical targets of lithium is glycogen synthase kinase-3 (GSK-3), present in α and β isoforms, which is a pro-apoptotic enzyme generally considered to be constitutively active. Lithium can directly inhibit GSK-3 possibly by competitively inhibiting Mg^{2+} binding to the active site of this kinase[39–41]. Lithium also indirectly inhibits GSK-3 through enhanced ser21 phosphorylation of GSK-3α and ser9 phosphorylation of GSK-3β. Multiple mechanisms probably contribute to lithium-induced GSK-3 phosphorylation and these include PI 3-kinase-dependent activation of Akt and protein kinase C[33,42] as well as auto-regulation resulting from inhibition of the protein phosphatase-1/inhibitor-2 complex[43]. GSK-3 activation has been linked to apoptotic cell death induced by multiple insults including glutamate excitotoxicity[44]. Thus, lithium's inhibition of GSK-3 undoubtedly constitutes part of the molecular mechanisms underlying its neuroprotective effects. Inhibition of GSK-3 leads to activation of cell-survival transcription factors such as CREB and heat-shock factor-1 (HSF-1), and inhibition of pro-apoptotic factors such as p53[44]. Figure 32.2[45,46] is a schematic illustration of the proposed multiple signaling pathways involved in the neuroprotective effects of this drug.

NEUROPROTECTIVE EFFECTS OF LITHIUM IN ANIMAL AND CELLULAR MODELS OF NEURODEGENERATIVE DISEASES

Cerebral stroke

It is becoming clear that there is a substantial increase in extracellular glutamate in the brain following cerebral ischemia, owing to energy depletion and inhibition of Na/K ATPase, and that a large portion of the brain damage is attributable to overstimulation of glutamate receptors, notably NMDA receptors. The neuroprotective effects of lithium against brain ischemic stroke have been demonstrated in a rodent model in which rats were subjected to middle cerebral artery occlusion (MCAO) by inserting a nylon suture into the left carotid artery to occlude the origin of the left middle cerebral artery. Using permanent or transient

MCAO, LiCl pre-treatment for approximately 2 weeks by daily subcutaneous injections at therapeutically relevant doses was found to decrease ischemia-induced brain infarct volume substantially[47,48]. This neuroprotection was accompanied by a suppression of caspase-3 activation and a reduction of neurologic deficits including abnormal posture and hemiplegia. Thus, lithium pre-treatment might be advantageous in controlling conditions that carry a high risk of stroke at predictable times, such as cardiac surgery, carotid endarterectomy and transient ischemic attack. A more recent report indicates that post-insult treatment of rats with therapeutic doses of lithium similarly reduces transient MCAO-induced brain infarction and DNA damage, and has a longlasting benefit in the behavioral functional outcome[49]. The treatment time window for lithium is at least 3 hours after the onset of ischemia for reducing both the infarct volume and neurologic deficit score. These observations raise the possibility of using lithium to treat patients with acute stroke.

It has been recognized that heat shock protein 70 (HSP70) plays a critical role in neuroprotection and is induced in the ischemic penumbra of the brain, where tissue damage is not as severe as in the core and can be repaired[50]. The neuroprotection elicited by post-insult lithium treatment is correlated with super-induction of HSP70 and activation of its transcription factor, HSF-1[49]. Of interest, HSP70 is also super-induced in the ischemic brain of rats subjected to MCAO and post-insult treatment with valproate[51]. It is likely that lithium protection against ischemia-induced brain injury comprises multiple mechanisms. For example, lithium was reported to inhibit ischemia-induced NMDA receptor subunit 2A tyrosine phosphorylation and its interactions with Src and Fyn mediated by PSD-95 in the rat hippocampus[52], and to attenuate hypoxia-induced serine dephosphorylation (and hence activation) of GSK-3α

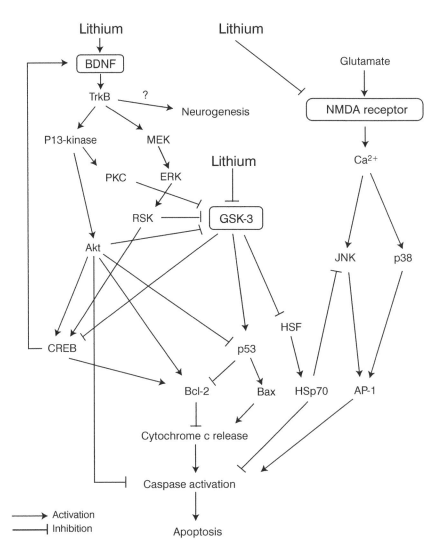

Figure 32.2 Proposed signaling pathways underlying the neuroprotective effects of lithium. Lithium-induced brain-derived neurotrophic factor (BDNF) expression and activation of its receptor TrkB is an early and essential step for the neuroprotection against glutamate excitotoxicity and probably other insults. Downstream effectors such as the phosphatidylinositol (PI)-3 kinase/Akt and MEK/ERK pathways are activated, causing phosphorylation and activation of cyclic AMP response element binding protein (CREB), a transcription factor that regulates the expression of cytoprotective Bcl-2 and BDNF. Lithium also directly and indirectly inhibits glycogen synthase kinase (GSK)-3 by multiple mechanisms, leading to changes in transcription factor activities and induction of major cytoprotective proteins such as Bcl-2, BDNF and heat shock protein (HSP)70. BDNF induction might also be involved in lithium-induced neurogenesis *in vitro* and *in vivo*. Inhibition of *N*-methyl-ᴅ-aspartate (NMDA) receptor-mediated calcium influx and suppression of c-Jun-N-terminal kinase (JNK) and p38 kinase activation, and subsequent AP-1 binding activation also contribute to lithium neuroprotection. The figure is modified from references 45 and 46

and β in the mouse brain cortex, hippocampus and striatum[53]. In organotypic cultures of rat hippocampus exposed to oxygen and glucose deprivation, lithium showed neuroprotection in the range of 0.2–1.2 mmol/l and this effect was associated with activation of HSP27[54].

Huntington's disease

Huntington's disease (HD) is a fatal neurodegenerative disorder characterized by a selective loss of medium-sized spiny neurons in the striatum, involuntary hyperkinetic movement, impaired cognition and neuropsychiatric syndromes such as depression. HD is one of a number of neurodegenerative diseases caused by an expansion of polyglutamine in the disease protein huntingtin. There are also indications that supersensitivity or hyperactivation of NMDA receptors contributes to the pathophysiology of HD. The excitotoxicity hypothesis has been supported in part by an imaging study showing elevated glutamate and glutamine in the striatum of HD patients[55], and by a clinical investigation demonstrating reduced chorea scores in HD patients treated with an NMDA antagonist, amantadine[56]. One animal model of HD is to inject quinolinic acid (QA), an NMDA receptor excitotoxin, into the striatum of rats, which causes selective degeneration of medium-sized spiny neurons and produces neuroanatomic and neurochemical manifestations of this disease. In the QA model of HD, long-term (16 days) or short-term (1 day), pre-treatment with therapeutic concentrations of LiCl reduces the QA-induced striatal lesion and the loss of medium-sized neurons that express dopamine D_1 receptors and glutamate decarboxylase[37,57]. Short-term lithium pre-treatment is sufficient to reduce the number of neurons showing DNA damage or activated caspase-3, and to upregulate Bcl-2 expression and the Bcl-2 immunostaining in striatal neurons. Interestingly, lithium pre-treatment also stimulates the proliferation of striatal cells near the site of the QA-induced injury, and some of these replicating cells have the phenotype of neurons or astroglia[57]. These data suggest that the lithium neuroprotection in the QA model involves not only anti-apoptotic action, but also the ability to stimulate proliferation of neuronal and astroglial progenitors.

The HD-causing mutation is an expansion of the CAG repeat encoding polyglutamine in exon-1 of the huntingtin gene. The effects of lithium have been examined in a cellular HD model in which, to cause cell death, neuroblastoma cells were transfected with the huntingtin exon-1 fragment with 74 glutamate repeats[58]. Pre-treatment with LiCl at relatively high concentrations reduced polyglutamine-induced nuclear fragmentation and inclusion formation. Lithium's neuroprotection involves GSK-3β inhibition, because it is mimicked by a GSK-3 inhibitor or by overexpression of a dominant-negative GSK-3β mutant. Under the conditions studied, GSK-3 activity is stimulated by the expression of expanded polyglutamine and inhibited by lithium treatment. Perhaps, the most studied transgenic mouse HD model is the R 6/2 line, which carries a 145 CAG repeat expansion in huntingtin and shows behavioral motor deficits as early as 5–6 weeks of age. Chronic lithium treatment post-, but not pre-symptomatically showed significant improvement in rotarod performance, but had no overall effect on survival time[59]. Intriguingly, the subgroup of mice that lost weight faster and died earlier benefited less from lithium treatment. The effects of lithium on other transgenic HD mouse lines have not been reported. However, it is noteworthy that in the YAC mouse model of HD expressing full-length mutant huntingtin, an increased sensitivity to NMDA receptor-mediated excitotoxicity and loss of wild-type huntingtin-induced BDNF gene transcription have been reported[60,61]. Since lithium has the potential to correct both functional deficits, its beneficial effects on other HD transgenic mouse lines may be anticipated.

Alzheimer's disease

Some evidence suggests that hyperphosphorylation of tau, a microtubule-binding protein, is an early event in the development of the neurofibrillary pathology associated with Alzheimer's disease (AD) and other neurodegenerative diseases. Two pioneering studies demonstrate that lithium reduces tau phosphorylation by inhibiting GSK-3, a major tau kinase *in vivo* and *in vitro*[62,63]. In cultured neurons, lithium-induced loss of tau phosphorylation resulted in enhanced binding of tau to microtubules and promotion of microtubule assembly. Another histopathologic hallmark of AD is the presence in the brain of amyloid plaques whose major building block is β-amyloid peptide (Aβ). Several studies have demonstrated that treating neurons with Aβ leads to hyperphosphorylation of tau protein, a decrease in Bcl-2 protein and neuronal death. All these parameters are largely suppressed by lithium treatment in cultured neurons and neurally related cell types[64,65]. Lithium also reportedly prevented Aβ-induced stress in the endoplasmic reticulum along with the resultant activation of caspase-12 and -3, NF-κB activation and GSK-3 nuclear translocation in the hippocampus of rabbits[66]. This action might be related to lithium's ability to superinduce the chaperone protein GRP 78 (glucose-regulated protein 78) in response to endoplasmic reticulum stress[67].

Aβ peptide is derived from amyloid precursor protein (APP) by sequential proteolytic processing, first by β-secretase and then by presenilin-dependent γ-secretase. A preliminary study reports that lithium inhibits Aβ secretion in COS7 cells transiently transfected with APPC100, a truncated APP fragment[68]. A subsequent detailed study shows that lithium and other GSK-3 inhibitors block the production of $A\beta_{1-40}$ and $A\beta_{1-42}$ by interfering with the reaction of γ-secretase[69]. Chronic lithium treatment also blocks Aβ accumulation in the brain of mice overproducing APP. The results in CHO cells transfected with GSK-3α or treated with GSK-3α siRNA demonstrate that Aβ production is regulated by this GSK-3 isoform. However, the results from another study, using HEK 293 cells, show that inhibition of the GSK-3β isoform can also mimic the ability of both lithium and valproate to suppress the process of Aβ formation from APP[70]. Chronic lithium treatment protects against neurodegeneration and improves spatial learning deficits in rats injected with preformed Aβ fibrils[71]. *In toto*, the research from a number of laboratories agrees sufficiently to suggest the possibility of using lithium to treat AD.

Other neurodegenerative disorders

Mitochondrial complex I inhibitors such as 1-methyl-4-phenylpyridinium (MPP) and rotenone are widely used as a tool to trigger neurochemical changes that may be associated with Parkinson's disease (PD). Caspase-3 activation induced by MPP and rotenone in human neuroblastoma cells is facilitated by GSK-3β activation and inhibited by lithium in a PI 3-kinase-dependent manner[72]. Another PD mimetic, 6-hydroxydopamine (6-OHDA) activates GSK-3β in cultured neurons and this appears to be triggered by stress on the endoplasmic reticulum[73]. Lithium and other GSK-3 inhibitors prevent 6-OHDA-induced caspase-3 activation, poly-(ADP-ribose) polymerase (PARP) cleavage, DNA fragmentation and neuronal death. In an *in vivo* study in which mice were injected with the MPP precursor, *N*-methyl-4-phenyl-1,2,3,6-tetrahydropyridine (MPTP), chronic (4-week) lithium pre-treatment at a therapeutic dose was found to prevent MPTP-induced reduction of striatal tyrosine hydroxylase and depletion of dopamine and its metabolites[74]. In addition, lithium normalizes the downregulation of Bcl-2 and upregulation of Bax elicited by MPTP in the striatum.

Lithium has also been shown to support the survival and regeneration of axons of retinal ganglion cells (RGCs) in a manner that appears to require Bcl-2 overexpression, suggesting that lithium may be used to treat degeneration of RGCs[75]. In a spinal cord injury model of rats induced by unilateral hemisection, combined lithium with chondroitinase was reported to have synergistic effects in increasing axonal regeneration of the rubrospinal tract and in improving forelimb movement[76]. Intrathecal injection of lithium can also reduce neuropathic pain responses in rats subjected to chronic constrictive injury to the sciatic nerve[77], raising its potential utility in neuropathic pain syndromes resulting from peripheral nerve injury. Murine AIDS (MAIDS) is a mouse-related syndrome that shows extensive similarities to human HIV infection and is caused by a defective murine leukemia virus. MAIDS mice treated with lithium show a marked reduction in their development of lymphadenopathy and splenomegaly[78]. A more recent study demonstrates that lithium pre-treatment protects the hippocampus of mice from HIV-gp120-induced toxicity[79]. Similarly, pre- but not post-exposure of human neuroblastoma cells to lithium reduces gp120-induced neurotoxicity and this protective effect is blocked by a PI 3-kinase inhibitor. These results are compatible with the view that prophylactic treatment with lithium may prevent or delay the onset and progression of HIV-associated cognitive impairments. Table 32.1 summarizes the reported advantageous effects of lithium in various *in vitro* and *in vivo* models of neurodegenerative diseases.

CLINICAL TRIALS OF LITHIUM IN NEURODEGENERATIVE DISORDERS

Since lithium was licensed for the treatment of bipolar disorder, numerous clinical trials have addressed its efficacy in various neurologic and psychiatric conditions. John Cade was first to make use of lithium's calming effects[80]. The extrapyramidal side-effects of the drug including tremor, rigidity and choreoathetosis later prompted its use in the treatment of movement disorders. Among others, lithium has been used in Huntington's disease, tardive dyskinesia, Gilles de la Tourette syndrome and Parkinson's disease. Moreover, lithium trials have been performed in organic brain syndromes with brain injury.

Huntington's disease

Dalén first used lithium carbonate in six HD patients and found a striking reduction in chorea with improvement of voluntary movements[81]. His findings were substantiated by another case report of four HD patients who showed marked improvement of motor function after lithium therapy[82]. Interestingly, three of these patients also benefited from the normalization of mood and temper. In several HD patients, a combined therapy of lithium and neuroleptics proved beneficial[83–87]. However, in a double-blind placebo-controlled clinical trial of lithium carbonate in nine HD patients, no change in hyperkinetic movements, mood, behavior or voluntary motor activity occurred[88]. Lithium also failed to improve the motor skills, hyperkinesias and global health condition of six HD patients in another double-blind placebo-controlled clinical trial[89]. In some instances, lithium even seemed to worsen the motor and cognitive performances, particularly when used as the sole therapeutic agent[86,90]. It should be noted that the number of patients

Table 32.1 Lithium has beneficial effects in animal and cellular models of neurodegenerative diseases

Name of disease model	Descriptions	References
Stroke and hypoxia	Suppresses ischemic-induced neurologic deficits, brain infarction, caspase-3 activation and GSK-3 dephosphorylation in rodents. Induces and activates HSPs *in vivo* and *in vitro*	47–49, 53, 54
Huntington's disease	Induces Bcl-2 and cell proliferation as well as protects against NMDA agonist-induced striatal lesion in rats. Reduces polyglutamine-induced nuclear fragmentation and inclusion formation in a cellular model. Improves rotarod performance in the R 6/2 transgenic mouse model	37, 57–59
Alzheimer's disease	Reduces tau phosphorylation by inhibiting GSK-3 *in vivo* and *in vitro*. Protects against Aβ-induced neurotoxicity *in vivo* and endoplasmic reticulum stress in the rabbit hippocampus. Blocks APP processing to form and secrete Aβ *in vitro* and *in vivo*. Decreases Aβ-induced spatial learning deficits in rats	62–66, 68–71
Parkinson's disease	Inhibits MPP, rotenone and 6-OHDA-induced caspase-3 activation and neuronal death *in vitro*. Prevents MPTP-induced striatal dopamine depletion and normalizes Bcl-2 downregulation and Bax upregulation in rats	72–74
Retinal degeneration	Supports the survival and regeneration of axons of retinal ganglion cells *in vitro*	75
Spinal cord injury	Potentiates chondroitinase-induced axonal regeneration and improves forelimb movement in a rat model	76
HIV infection	Reduces the development of lymphadenopathy and splenomegaly in murine AIDS. Decreases gp120-induced neurotoxicity *in vitro* by a PI 3-kinase-dependent mechanism	78, 79

included in these trials was small and the duration of lithium treatment too short to assess the potential neuroprotective effects of the drug. Interestingly, one study suggested that patients in early stages of disease might be more likely to benefit from lithium treatment[91]. Several clinical trials are currently underway to explore the long-term effects of lithium salts in HD. An ongoing phase II clinical trial of lithium carbonate, given alone or with the anticonvulsant divalproex, examines the efficacy of lithium in restoring BDNF concentrations in the cerebrospinal fluid of HD patients as a surrogate measure of neuroprotective activity[92].

Tardive dyskinesia

Tardive dyskinesia (TD) is clinically characterized by involuntary choreiform movements mostly of the mouth, tongue and face which disappear during sleep. TD is hypothesized to be a result of dopaminergic supersensitivity associated with the prolonged use of neuroleptics. In animal models of TD, lithium was found to prevent the supersensitivity to apomorphine[93,94], underscoring its potential prophylactic and therapeutic usefulness in TD. Numerous case report studies have suggested that lithium salts are beneficial in the treatment of drug-induced TD, particularly in combination with antidepressants[81,95–98]. However, controlled double-blind crossover studies suggested that only a subpopulation of TD patients may improve with lithium[99–101]. It is interesting to note that lithium failed to show a therapeutic effect in a trial with older patients in whom TD was of long duration[102]. A recent Cochrane review did not recommend lithium for the everyday use in TD[103].

Gilles de la Tourette syndrome

This syndrome is characterized by tics, involuntary sounds and coprolalia. The symptoms responded well to lithium carbonate in two case report trials[104,105], but not in a more recent controlled clinical trial[106].

Parkinson's disease

Most trials of lithium in PD have dealt with side-effects of L-dopa therapy, namely the 'on-off' phenomenon (alternating periods of dyskinesia and akinesia) and L-dopa-induced hyperkinesias. Despite experimental evidence to suggest that lithium may prevent striatal dopamine receptor desensitization, the few case report studies addressing the effect of lithium on L-dopa-induced hyperkinesias remain contradictory[107–109]. On the other hand, lithium did prove beneficial in the management of the 'on-off' phenomenon associated with L-dopa therapy. In a double-blind crossover study and one case report, lithium was found to reduce akinesia significantly[110,111]. However, lithium may also increase dyskinesia[110], or fail to improve the 'on-off' phenomenon[112].

Organic brain syndromes

In several independent case reports, patients with organic affective syndromes as a result of brain trauma, hemorrhage or brain tumor responded well to lithium treatment[113–116].

Alzheimer's disease

Encouraged by recent experimental findings suggesting a protective role of lithium in tau and amyloid pathology, clinical trials are underway to explore the neuroprotective potential of this drug in AD. An ongoing phase II clinical trial of lithium carbonate, given alone or with the anticonvulsant divalproex, examines the efficacy of lithium in reducing the concentrations of phosphorylated tau epitopes (Thr-181, Thr-231) in the cerebrospinal fluid of AD patients as a surrogate measure of neuroprotective activity[117]. Table 32.2 summarizes clinical trials of lithium in various forms of neurodegenerative diseases.

CONCLUSION

Lithium is an effective neuroprotective drug at therapeutically relevant doses. It protects against apoptosis induced by a variety of insults, including glutamate-induced excitotoxicity. The signaling pathways involved in lithium-induced neuroprotection comprise inactivation of NMDA receptors, inhibition of GSK-3 and activation of PI3-kinase and MAP kinase cell-survival pathways. Major neurotrophic and neuroprotective factors such as BDNF, Bcl-2 and heat shock proteins are induced by lithium. The encouraging results from pre-clinical studies in models of cerebral stroke, Huntington's disease, Alzheimer's disease and Parkinson's disease have led to a reappraisal of earlier clinical trials using lithium salts in neurodegenerative disorders. Newly designed trials

Table 32.2   Clinical trials of lithium in neurodegenerative disorders

Name of disease	Descriptions	References
Huntington's disease	Improvement of hyperkinetic movements, motor function, mood and behavior	82–87, 91
	No change or worsening of symptoms	86, 88, 90
Tardive dyskinesia	Improvement of dyskinesia	81, 95–101
	No change of symptoms	102, 103
Gilles de la Tourette syndrome	Improvement of tics, involuntary sounds and coprolalia	104, 105
	No change of symptoms	106
Parkinson's disease	Improvement of L-dopa-induced hyperkinesia and 'off' phenomenon	107, 110, 111
	No change or worsening of symptoms	109, 110, 112
Organic brain syndromes	Improvement of affective syndromes	113–116
Alzheimer's disease		117

are underway to explore the neuroprotective potential of lithium in various degenerative brain disorders.

REFERENCES

1. Chuang D-M, Hough CJ, Senatorov VV. Glyceraldehyde-3-phosphate dehydrogenase, apoptosis and neurodegenerative diseases. Annu Rev Pharmacol Toxicol 2005; 45: 296–90
2. Ekshyyan O, Aw TY. Apoptosis in acute and chronic neurological disorders. Frontiers Biosci 2004; 9: 1567–76
3. Reynolds IJ. Mitochondrial membrane potential and the permeability transition in excitotoxicity. Ann NY Acad Sci 1999; 893: 33–41
4. Horvitz HR. Genetic control of programmed cell death in the nematode Caenorhabditis elegans. Cancer Res 1999; 59 (Suppl S): 1701S–6S
5. Hengartner MO. The biochemistry of apoptosis. Nature 2000; 407: 770–6
6. Wang X. The expanding role of mitochondria in apoptosis. Genes Dev 2001; 15: 2922–33
7. Mattson MP, Kroemer G. Mitochondria in cell death: novel targets for neuroprotection and cardioprotection. Trends Mol Med 2003; 9: 196–205
8. Sharp FR, Lu AG, Tang Y, Millhorn DE. Multiple molecular penumbras after focal cerebral ischemia. J Cerebr Blood F Met 2000; 20: 1011–132
9. Love S. Apoptosis and brain ischaemia. Progr Neuropsychopharm Biol Psychiatry 2003; 27: 267–82
10. Friedlander RM. Apoptosis and caspases in neurodegenerative diseases. N Engl J Med 2003; 348: 1365–75
11. Yuan J, Yankner BA. Apoptosis in the nervous system. Nature 2000; 407: 802–29
12. Drevets WC. Neuroimaging and neuropathological studies of depression: implications for

the cognitive-emotional features of mood disorders. Curr Opin Neurobiol 2001; 11, 240–9

13. Beyer J, Krishnan RR. Volumetric brain imaging findings in mood disorders. Bipolar Disord 2002; 4: 89–104

14. Strakowski SM, Adler CM, DelBello MP. Volumetric MRI studies of mood disorders: do they distinguish unipolar and bipolar disorder? Bipolar Disorders 2002; 4: 80–8

15. Manji, HK, Quiroz JA, Sporn J, et al. Enhancing neuronal plasticity and cellular resilience to develop novel, improved therapeutics for difficult-to-treat depression. Biol Psychiatry 2003; 53: 707–42

16. Rajkowska G. Cell pathology in bipolar disorder. Bipolar Disord 2002; 4: 105–16

17. Moore GJ, Bebchuk JM, Wilds IB, et al. Lithium-induced increase in human brain grey matter. Lancet 2000; 356: 1241–2

18. Leverich GS, Perez S, Luckenbaugh DA, Post RM. Early psychosocial stressors: relationship to suicidality and course of bipolar illness. Clin Neurosci Res 2002; 2: 161–70

19. Smith MA, Makino S, Kvetansky R, Post RM. Stress and glucocorticoids affect the expression of brain-derived neurotrophic factor and neurotrophin-3 mRNAs in the hippocampus. J Neurosci 1995; 15: 1768–77

20. Gould E, Tanapat P, McEwen BS, et al. Proliferation of granule cell precursors in the dentate gyrus of adult monkeys is diminished by stress. Proc Natl Acad Sci USA 1998; 95: 3168–71

21. Sapolsky RM. Glucocorticoids and hippocampal atrophy in neuropsychiatric disorders. Arch Gen Psychiatry 2000; 57: 925–35

22. McEwen BS. Stress and hippocampal plasticity. Annu Rev Neurosci 1999; 22: 105–22

23. Nonaka S, Hough C, Chuang D-M. Chronic lithium treatment robustly protects CNS neurons against excitotoxicity by inhibiting NMDA receptor-mediated calcium influx. Proc Natl Acad Sci USA 1998; 95: 2642–7

24. Hashimoto R, Hough C, Nakazawa T, et al. Lithium protection against glutamate excitotoxicity in rat cerebral cortical neurons: involvement of NMDA receptor inhibition possibly by decreasing NR2B tyrosine phosphorylation. J Neurochem 2002; 80: 589–97

25. Takasu MA, Dalva MB, Zigmond RE, Greenberg ME. Modulation of NMDA receptor-dependent calcium influx and gene expression through EphB receptors. Science 2002; 295: 491–5

26. Hashimoto R, Fujimaki K, Jeong M-R Chuang D-M. Lithium-induced inhibition of Src tyrosine kinase in rat cerebral cortical neurons: a role in neuroprotection against N-methyl-D-aspartate receptor-mediated excitotoxicity. FEBS Lett 2003; 538: 145–8

27. Steece-collier K, Chambers LK, Jaw-Tsai SS, et al. Antiparkinsonian actions of CP-101,606, an antagonist of NR2B subunit-containing N-methyl-D-aspartate receptors. Exp Neurol 2000; 163: 239–43

28. Chen R-W, Qin Z-H, Ren M, et al. Regulation of c-Jun N-Terminal kinase, p38 kinase and AP-1 DNA binding in cultured brain neurons: roles in glutamate excitation and lithium neuroprotection. J Neurochem 2003; 84: 566–575

29. Finkbeiner S. CREB couples neurotrophin signals to survival messages. Neuron 2000; 25: 11–14

30. Fukumoto T, Morinobu S, Okamoto Y, et al. Chronic lithium treatment increases the expression of brain-derived neurotrophic factor in the rat brain. Psychopharm 2001; 158: 100–6

31. Einat H, Yuan PX, Gould TD, et al. The role of the extracellular signal-regulated kinase signaling pathway in mood modulation. J Neurosci 2003; 23: 7311–16

32. Hashimoto R, Takei N, Shimazu K, et al. Lithium induces brain-derived neurotrophic factor and activates TrkB in rodent cortical neurons: an essential step for neuroprotection against glutamate excitotoxicity. Neuropharm 2002; 43: 1173–9

33. Chalecka-Franaszek E, Chuang D-M. Lithium activates the serine/threonine kinase Akt-1 and suppresses glutamate-induced inhibition of Akt-1 activity in neurons. Proc Natl Acad Sci USA 1999; 96: 8745–50

34. Yuan PX, Huang LD, Jiang YM. The mood stabilizer valproic acid activates mitogen-

activated protein kinases and promotes neurite growth. J Biol Chem 2001; 276: 31674–83

35. Kopnisky KL, Chalecka-Franaszek E, Gonzalez-Zulueta M, Chuang D-M. Chronic lithium treatment antogonizes glutamine-induced decrease of phosphorylated CREB in neurons by reducing PP1 and increasing MEK activities. Neuroscience 2003; 116: 425–35

36. Chen G, Zeng W-Z, Yuan P-X, et al. The mood-stabilizing agents lithium and valproate robustly increase the levels of the neuro-protective protein bcl-2 in the CNS. J Neurochem 1999; 72: 879–82

37. Wei H, Qin Z-H, Senatorov V, et al. Lithium suppresses excitotoxicity-induced striatal lesions in a rat model of Huntington's disease. Neuroscience 2001; 106: 603–12

38. Chen R-W, Chuang D-M. Long term lithium treatment suppresses p53 and Bax expression but increases Bcl-2 expression: a prominent role in neuroprotection against excitotoxicity. J Biol Chem 1999; 274: 6039–42

39. Klein PS, Melton DA. A molecular mechanism for the effect of lithium on development. Proc Natl Acad Sci USA 1996; 93: 8455–9

40. Stambolic V, Ruel L, Woodgett JR. Lithium inhibits glycogen synthase kinase-3 activity and mimics wingless signalling in intact cells. Curr Biol 1996; 6: 1664–8

41. Ryves WJ, Harwood AJ. Lithium inhibits glycogen synthase kinase-3 by competition for magnesium. Biochem Biophys Res Commun 2001; 280: 720–5

42. Kirshenboim N, Plotkin E, Ben Shlomo S, et al. Lithium-mediated phosphorylation of glycogen synthase kinase-3β involves PI3 kinase-dependent activation of protein kinase C-α. J Mol Neurosci 2004; 24: 237–46

43. Zhang F, Phiel CJ, Spece L, et al. Inhibitory phosphorylation of glycogen synthase kinase-3 (GSK-3) in response to lithium: evidence for autoregulation of GSK-3. J Biol Chem 2003; 278: 33067–77

44. Grimes CA, Jope RS. The multifaceted roles of glycogen synthase kinase 3β in cellular signaling. Prog Neurobiol 2002; 65: 391–426

45. Rowe MK, Chuang D-M. Lithium neuro-protection: molecular mechanisms and clinical implications. Exp Rev Mol Med 2004; 6: 1–18

46. Chuang D-M. Neuroprotective and neuro-trophic actions of the mood stabilizer lithium: can it be used to treat neurodegenerative diseases? Crit Rev Neurobiol 2004; 16: 83–9

47. Nonaka S, Chuang D-M. Neuroprotective effects of chronic lithium on focal cerebral ischemia in rats. Neuro report 1998; 9: 2081–4

48. Xu JH, Culman J, Blume A, Brecht S, Gohlke P. Chronic treatment with a low dose of lithium protects the brain against ischemic injury by reducing apoptotic death. Stroke 2003; 34: 1287–92.

49. Ren M, Senatorov VV, Chen R-W, Chuang D-M. Post-insult treatment with lithium reduces brain damage and facilitates neurological recovery in a rat ischemia/reperfusion model. Proc Natl Acad Sci USA 2003; 100: 6210–15

50. Lipton P. Ischemic cell death in brain neurons. Physiol Rev 1999; 79: 1431–568

51. Ren M, Leng Y, Jeong MR, et al. Valproic acid reduces brain damage induced by transient focal cerebral ischemia in rats: potential roles of histone deacetylase inhibition and heat shock protein induction. J Neurochem 2004; 89: 1358–67

52. Ma J, Zhang GY. Lithium reduced N-methyl-D-aspartate receptor subunit 2A tyrosine phosphorylation and its interactions with Src and Fyn mediated by PSD-95 in rat hippo-campus following cerebral ischemia. Neurosci Lett 2003; 348, 185–9

53. Roh M-S, Eom T-Y, Zmijewska AA, et al. Hypoxia activates glycogen synthase kinase-3 in mouse brain in vivo: protection by mood stabi-lizers and imipramine. Biol Psychiatry 2005; 57: 278–86

54. Cimarosti H, Rodnight R, Tavares A, et al. An investigation of the neuroprotective effect of lithium in organotypic slice cultures of rat hippocampus exposed to oxygen and glucose deprivation. Neurosci Lett 2001; 315: 33–6

55. Taylor-Robinson SD, Weeks RA, Bryant DJ, et al. Proton magnetic resonance spectroscopy in Huntington's disease: evidence in favour of the

glutamate excitotoxic theory? Mov Disord 1996; 11: 167–73

56. Metman LV, Morris MJ, Farmer C, et al. Huntington's disease: a randomized, controlled trial using the NMDA-antagonist amantadine. Neurology 2002; 59: 694–9

57. Senatorov VV, Ren M, Kanai H, et al. Short-term lithium treatment promotes neuronal survival and proliferation in rat striatum infused with quinolinic acid, an excitotoxic model of Huntington's disease. Mol Psychiatry 2004; 9: 371–85

58. Carmichael J, Sugars KL, Bao YP, Rubinsztein DC. Glycogen synthase kinase-3beta inhibitors prevent cellular polyglutamine toxicity caused by the Huntington's disease mutation. J Biol Chem 2002; 277: 33791–8

59. Wood NI, Morton AJ. Chronic lithium chloride treatment has variable effects on motor behaviour and survival of mice transgenic for the Huntington's disease mutation. Brain Res Bull 2003; 61: 375–83

60. Zeron MM, Hansson O, Chen N, et al. Increased sensitivity to N-methyl-D-aspartate receptor-mediated excitotoxicity in a mouse model of Huntington's disease. Neuron 2002; 33: 849–60

61. Zuccato C, Ciammola A, Rigamonti D, et al. Loss of huntingtin-mediated BDNF gene transcription in Huntington's disease. Science 2001; 293: 493–8

62. Hong M, Chen DCR, Klein PS, Lee VMY. Lithium reduces tau phosphorylation by inhibition of glycogen synthase kinase-3. J Biol Chem 1997; 272: 25326–2

63. Muñoz-Montaño JR, Moreno FJ, Avila J, Díaz-Nido J. Lithium inhibits Alzheimer's disease-like tau protein phosphorylation in neurons. FEBS Lett 1997; 411: 183–8

64. Alvarez G, Muñoz-Montaño JR, Satrústegui J, et al. Lithium protects cultured neurons against β-amyloid-induced neurodegeneration. FEBS Lett 1999; 453: 260–4

65. Wei H, Leeds PR, Qian Y, et al. β-amyloid peptide-induced death of PC 12 cells and cerebellar granule cell neurons is inhibited by long-term lithium treatment. Eur J Pharmacol 2000; 392: 117–23

66. Ghribi O, Herman MM, Savory J. Lithium inhibits Aβ-induced stress in endoplasmic reticulum of rabbit hippocampus but does not prevent oxidative damage and tau phosphorylation. J Neurosci Res 2003; 71: 853–62

67. Hiroi T, Wei H, Hough C, et al. Protracted lithium treatment protects against the ER stress elicited by thapsigargin in rat PC12 cells: roles of intracellular calcium, GRP78 and Bcl-2. Pharmacogen J 2005; 5: 102–11

68. Sun X, Sato S, Murayama O, et al. Lithium inhibits amyloid secretion in COS7 cells transfected with amyloid precursor protein C100. Neurosci Lett 2002; 321: 61–4

69. Phiel CJ, Wilson CA, Lee VMY, Klein PS. GSK-3α regulates production of Alzheimer's disease amyloid-β peptides. Nature 2003; 423: 435–9

70. Su Y, Ryder J, Li B, et al. Lithium, a common drug for bipolar disorder treatment, regulates amyloid-β precursor protein processing. Biochemistry 2004; 43: 6899–908

71. De Ferrari GV, Chacón MA, Barría MI, et al. Activation of Wnt signaling rescues neurodegeneration and behavioral impairments induced by β-amyloid fibrils. Mol Psychiatry 2003; 8: 195–208

72. King TD, Bijur GN, Jope RS. Caspase-3 activation induced by inhibition of mitochondrial complex I is facilitated by glycogen synthase kinase-3β and attenuated by lithium. Brain Res 2001; 919: 106–14

73. Chen G, Bower KA, Ma CL, et al. Glycogen synthase kinase 3β (GSK3β) mediates 6-hydroxydopamine-induced neuronal death. FASEB J 2004; 18: 1162–4

74. Youdim MBH, Arraf Z. Prevention of MPTP (N-methyl-4-phenyl-1,2,3,6-tetrahydropyridine) dopaminergic neurotoxicity in mice by chronic lithium: involvements of Bcl-2 and Bax. Neuropharm 2004; 46: 1130–40

75. Huang X, Wu D-Y, Chen G, et al. Support of retinal ganglion cell survival and axon regeneration by lithium through a Bcl-2-dependent mechanism. Invest Ophthalmol Vis Sci 2003; 44: 347–54

76. Yick L-W, So K-F, Cheung P-T, Wu W-T. Lithium chloride reinforces the regeneration-

promoting effect of chondroitinase ABC on rubrospinal neurons after spinal cord injury. J Neurotrauma 2004; 21: 932–43

77. Shimizu T, Shibata M, Wakisaka S, et al. Intrathecal lithium reduces neuropathic pain responses in a rat model of peripheral neuropathy. Pain 2000; 85: 59–64

78. Gallicchio VS, Cibull ML, Hughes NK, Tse KF. Effect of lithium in murine immuno-deficiency virus-infected animals. Pathobiology 1993; 61: 216–21

79. Everall IP, Bell C, Mallory M, et al. Lithium ameliorates HIV-gp120-mediated neuro-toxicity. Mol Cell Neurosci 2002; 21: 493–501

80. Cade JFJ. Lithium salts in the treatment of psychotic excitement. Med J Aust 1949; 2: 349–52

81. Dalén P. Lithium therapy in Hungtinton's chorea and tardive dyskinesia. Lancet 1973; 1: 107–8

82. Mattsson B. Huntington's chorea and lithium therapy. Lancet 1973; 1: 718–19

83. Manyam NVB, Bravo-Fernandez E. Lithium carbonate in Huntington's chorea. Lancet 1973; 1: 1010

84. Schenk G, Leijnse-Ybema HJ. Huntington's chorea and levodopa. Lancet 1974; 1: 364

85. Andén N-E, Dalén P, Johansson B. Baclofen and lithium in Huntington's chorea. Lancet 1973; 2: 93

86. Leonard DP, Kidson MA, Shannon PJ, Brown J. Double-blind trial of lithium carbonate and haloperidol in Huntington's chorea. Lancet 1974; 2: 1208–9

87. Leonard DP, Kidson MA, Brown JGE, et al. A double blind trial of lithium carbonate and haloperidol in Huntington's chorea. Aust NZ J Psychiatry 1975; 9: 115–18

88. Aminoff MJ, Marshall J. Treatment of Huntington's chorea with lithium carbonate: a double-blind trial. Lancet 1974; 1: 107–9

89. Vestergaard P, Baastrup PC, Petersson H. Lithium treatment of Huntington's chorea. Acta Psychiatr Scand 1977; 56: 183–8

90. Carman JS, Shoulson I, Chase TN. Huntington's chorea treated with lithium carbonate. Lancet 1974; 1: 811

91. Foerster K, Regli F. Therapieversuch mit Lithium bei extrapyramidal-motorischen Störungen. Nervenarzt 1977; 48: 228–32

92. NINDS. Stimulation of tryrosine kinase and ERK signaling pathways in Huntington's disease. NCT00095355

93. Klawans HL, Weiner WJ, Nausieda PA. The effect of lithium on an animal model of tardive dyskinesia. Prog Neuropsychopharmacol 1977; 1: 53–60

94. Pert A, Rosenblatt JE, Sivit C, et al. Long-term treatment with lithium prevents the development of dopamine receptor supersensitivity. Science 1978; 201: 171–3

95. Simpson GM. Tardive dyskinesia. Br J Psychiatry 1973; 122: 618

96. Reda FA, Escobar JL, Scanlen JM. Lithium carbonate in the treatment of tardive dyskinesia. Am J Psychiatry 1975; 132: 560–2

97. Pickar D, Davis RK. Tardive dyskinesia in younger patients. Am J Psychiatry 1978; 135: 385–6

98. Rosenbaum AH, Niven RG, Hanson NP, Swanson DW. Tardive dyskinesia: relationship with a primary affective disorder. Dis Nerv Syst 1977; 38: 423–7

99. Prange AJ, Wilson IC, Morris CE, Hall CD. Preliminary experience with tryptophan and lithium in the treatment of tardive dyskinesia. Psychopharmacol Bull 1973; 9: 36–7

100. Gerlach J, Thorsen K, Munkvad I. Effect of lithium on neuroleptic-induced tardive dyskinesia compared with placebo in a double-blind crossover trial. Pharmakopsychiatr Neuropsychopharmakol 1975; 8: 51–6

101. Jus A, Villeneuve A, Gautier J, et al. Deanol, lithium and placebo in the treatment of tardive dyskinesia. Neuropsychobiology 1978; 4: 140–9

102. Simpson GM, Branchey MH, Lee JH, et al. Lithium in tardive dyskinesia. Pharmakopsychiatr Neuropsychopharmakol 1976; 9: 76–80

103. Soares-Weiser KV, Joy C. Miscellaneous treatments for neuroleptic-induced tardive dyskinesia. Cochrane Database Syst Rev 2003; 2: CD000208

104. Messiha F, Erickson HN, Goggin JE. Lithium carbonate in Gilles de la Tourette's disease. Res Commun Chem Pathol Pharmacol 1976; 15: 609–12

105. Erickson HM, Goggin JE, Messiha FS. Comparison of lithium and haloperidol therapy in Gilles de la Tourette syndrome. Adv Exp Med 1977; 90: 197–205

106. Borison RL, Ang L, Hamilton WJ, et al. Treatment approaches in Gilles de la Tourette syndrome. Brain Res Bull 1983; 11: 205–8

107. Dalén P, Steg G. Lithium and levodopa in Parkinsonism. Lancet 1973; 1: 936–7

108. Van Woert MH, Ambani LM. Lithium and L-dopa in Parkinsonism. Lancet 1973; 1: 1390–1

109. McCaul JA, Stern GM. Lithium in Parkinson's disease. Lancet 1974; 1: 1058

110. Coffey CE, Ross DR, Ferren EL, et al. Treatment of the 'on-off' phenomenon in Parkinsonism with lithium carbonate. Ann Neurol 1982; 12: 375–9

111. Ross DE. 'On-off' syndrome treated with lithium carbonate: a case report. Am J Psychiatry 1981; 138: 1626–7

112. Lieberman A. Treatment of 'on-off' phenomena with lithium. Ann Neurol 1982; 12: 402

113. Cohen CK, Wright JR, Devaul RA. Post head trauma syndrome in an adolescent treated with lithium carbonate – case report. Dis Nerv Syst 1977; 38: 630–1

114. Young LD, Taylor I, Holmstrom V. Lithium therapy of patients with affective illness associated with organic brain syndromes. Am J Psychiatry 1977; 134: 1405–7

115. Hale MS, Donaldson JO. Lithium carbonate in the treatment of organic brain syndrome. J Nerv Ment Dis 1982; 170: 362–5

116. Oyewumi LM, Lapierre YD. Efficacy of lithium in treating mood disorders occurring after brain stem injury. Am J Psychiatry 1981; 138: 110–11

117. NINDS. Glycogen synthetase kinase 3 (GSK-3) inhibition in Alzheimer's disease. NCT00088387

33 The effects of lithium on the immune system

Mohammed S Inayat, Vincent S Gallicchio

Contents   Introduction • Effect of lithium on peripheral blood cells • Effect of lithium on hematopoietic stem cells and growth factor production • Lithium potentiation of hematopoiesis via transport-related mechanisms • Lithium-induced inhibition of suppressor lymphocytes and prostaglandin production • Granulocyte function in patients receiving lithium carbonate • *In vitro* studies on granulocyte function involving lithium • Effect of lithium on B lymphocytes and immunoglobulin production • Lithium effects on T lymphocytes • Effect of lithium on natural killer and lymphocyte activator killer cells • Biochemical mechanisms for lithium effects on lymphocytes • Clinical utility of lithium as an immunomodulator

INTRODUCTION

Lithium is the lightest metal known. In nature it exists only as lithium ions or salts and is not considered to be an essential trace element for man[1,2]; however, data collected from the work of Anker using several animal species has identified several key biological and physiologic reactions that, upon elimination of lithium from the diet of these species, produced a variety of altered physiologic processes, specifically those related to reproduction, that were found to be significantly impaired. Consequently, these data provide proof that lithium must be reconsidered as a trace element.

Lithium carbonate has been widely used for psychiatric purposes[3]. Following therapeutic use of lithium, effects on the hematopoietic system have been documented, especially in the cells responsible for the body's defense systems, in particular granulocytes and lymphocytes. This chapter reviews our current understanding of the effects of lithium on blood cell development as it relates to early hematopoietic stem cells and progenitors and their subsequent differentiation into the mature cells of the blood.

Although lithium is not considered to be an important trace element for biological systems in man, this is still an issue under debate. Lithium has been postulated to play an important physiologic role in hematopoiesis[4]. Experimental data have demonstrated that lithium influences various lines of blood cell differentiation without any particular cell lineage specificity, and that effects observed either *in vivo* or *in vitro* have been observed at similar ionic concentrations. These *in vitro* observations have been documented to involve not only lithium, but also other monovalent alkali metal ions such as rubidium and cesium. Because these ions exist at either micromolar or nanomolar concentrations in human systems, they may play an important role in the mechanisms that control the formation of blood cells. The effects of lithium on blood cell formation have been previously reviewed[5–9].

The well-documented effect of lithium on blood cell formation suggested that the element may be of value in treating various hematopoietic disorders, for example following the use of anti-cancer therapy to ameliorate the bone marrow toxicity associated with the use of chemotherapeutic drugs. Although considerable research has investigated lithium in this capacity, following the discovery and purification via recombinant DNA technology of the specific hematopoietic growth factors that were shown to be increased as an indirect effect of lithium, interest in lithium in this clinical setting has gradually declined.

EFFECT OF LITHIUM ON PERIPHERAL BLOOD CELLS

Attention first focused on the ability of lithium to induce leukocytosis in manic-depressive patients receiving lithium as therapy[10]. Patients or normal subjects receiving lithium, in doses sufficient to produce a systemic lithium concentration of 0.3 mmol/l or more, usually produced a sustained elevation in the blood neutrophil concentration[11–13]. For therapeutic administration, lithium is given orally. The vast majority of human studies designed to study the hematopoietic effects of lithium have reported a dosage of 300 mg three times a day, producing a blood systemic level of 0.5–1.5 mmol/l. Serum or plasma lithium levels are checked at regular intervals and obtained 2 hours before the morning dose is administered. In experimental animal studies, either performed *in vivo* or *in vitro*, lithium chloride (LiCl) is used and is preferred over lithium carbonate (Li_2CO_3) because Li_2CO_3 is associated with inducing a higher pH.

For the majority of studies that examined eosinophils, their concentration was usually elevated[14,15], but not always. Monocytes have been reported to be increased, decreased or not affected[4,16,17]. The basophil has not been reported to be influenced following lithium administration. The ability of lithium to influence the total number of neutrophilic granulocytes has been shown by numerous studies[9]. In addition, lithium is an effective inducer of neutrophil function[18].

Blood platelet concentrations following lithium administration have been reported to be increased in some studies in humans[19] and in mice[20], but other human studies[13] did not show an effect of lithium on platelets. The functional activity of platelets as measured by bleeding time or aggregation has been reported to be unaffected by lithium administration[21].

Lithium, in non-toxic doses, does not significantly influence either blood erythrocyte or reticulocyte levels in man. Prolonged daily administration (>10 weeks) in mice when the lithium was placed directly in the drinking water did not produce a significant reduction in blood erythrocyte levels[22].

In humans receiving lithium, the neutrophil concentration has been reported not to exceed 1.5 times baseline. Neutrophilia usually develops within the first week of lithium administration, and it persists on a stable plateau. It has been difficult to determine the exact lithium dose that results in a blood lithium level producing neutrophilia[10]. A progressive increase in mean neutrophil concentrations has been observed in 56 adult patients who received either 600, 900 or 1200 mg lithium day. This regimen produced an increase in the mean neutrophil concentration as follows: 3.7×10^9 cells/kg in controls; 4.0×10^9 cells/kg in the 600-mg group; 4.8×10^9 cells in the 900-mg group; and 5.8×10^9 cells/kg in the 1200-mg group[13]. In a study performed in normal subjects there was a weak correlation between the neutrophil concentration and the blood lithium levels between 0.2 and 0.9 mmol/l, but no correlation at levels above 0.9 mmol/l[17]. There have been no reports of the presence of immature neutrophil forms or a differential shift to the left following lithium administration. Lithium has also been reported to increase the total white blood cell count and the neutrophil count in children with acute lymphoblastic leukemia receiving lithium orally[23]. This is an important finding, because of concern that lithium use in human clinical conditions associated with altered cell proliferation would be contraindicated, because of the danger that lithium would induce an undesired effect, perhaps accelerating the disease when used in these conditions. However, lithium has been shown to increase apoptosis when cultured with the K562 human leukemia cell line[24] and interacts synergistically with all-*trans*-retinoic acids thus promoting the terminal differentiation of myelomonocytic leukemia cells[25].

EFFECT OF LITHIUM ON HEMATOPOIETIC STEM CELLS AND GROWTH FACTOR PRODUCTION

The observation that lithium stimulation of leukocytosis involved a true proliferative response rather than just a shift of neutrophil populations from the marginating to the circulating pool of cells led investigators to examine the bone marrow for changes in rates of mitotic cell proliferation[26,27]. These data indicated that lithium exerts its effect on neutrophil production by influencing the progenitor and/or stem cells involved with hematopoietic cellular proliferation and differentiation. The effect of lithium on the hematopoietic stem cell and associated progenitor cells is summarized in Table 33.1[22,26,28–56] and growth factor production in Table 33.2[22,47,57–70].

LITHIUM POTENTIATION OF HEMATOPOIESIS VIA TRANSPORT-RELATED MECHANISMS

Studies focused on the role of sodium transport processes in the mechanism(s) whereby lithium influences granulopoiesis and megakaryocytopoiesis showed that, in the presence of sodium transport ionophores, but not potassium transport ionophores, lithium stimulation occurred[52]. In the presence of ouabain, a Na/K ATPase inhibitor, lithium potentiation of *in vitro* colony-forming unit– granulocyte/monocyte (CFU-GM) growth was inhibited and irreversible. Furthermore, studies conducted in the presence of the calcium ionophore A23187 blocked this effect of lithium[52]. These observations showed that, in the presence of activated calcium transport, the ability of lithium to influence granulopoiesis was restricted. In addition, studies conducted with sodium transport inhibitors were effective in blocking the effect of lithium on both granulopoietic and megakaryocytic progenitors[71]. These studies are consistent with the observation that changes in sodium influx induced by hematopoietic growth factors may be important in their target cell interactions[72].

Table 33.1 Lithium effects on hematopoietic stem and progenitor cells following either *in vivo* or *in vitro* administration

Cell	Line of differentiation	Lithium response	Reference
CFU-S	Pluripotential	Increase *in vivo*	Gallicchio and Chen, 1980[28]
CFU-S	Pluripotential	Increase *in vitro*	Gallicchio and Chen, 1981[29]
CFU-S	Pluripotential	Increase *in vitro*	Levitt and Quesenberry, 1980[30]
CFU-S	Pluripotential	Increase via diet	Gallicchio et al., 1981[29]
CFU-S	Pluripotential	Following radiation	Gallicchio et al., 1983[31] Gallicchio et al., 1984[32] Vacek et al., 1982[33] Moroz et al., 1988[34]
CFU-S	Pluripotential	Following chemotherapy	Friedenberg and Marx, 1980[35] Gallicchio et al., 1986[36] Gallicchio et al., 1987[37] Gallicchio et al., 1988[38]
CD34+/33–	Pluripotential	Increased granulocytes	Ballin et al., 1998[39]
CD34+/33–	Pluripotential	Mesenchymal stem cells	Gregory et al., 2005[40]
CFU-GM	Myeloid precursor	Bone marrow – man	Greco and Brereton, 1977[41] Joyce and Chervenick, 1980[26] Morley and Galbraith, 1978[42] Spitzer et al., 1979[43]
CFU-GM	Myeloid precursor	Bone marrow – dog	Hammond and Dale, 1980[44] Rossof and Fehir, 1979[45]
CFU-GM	Myeloid precursor	Bone marrow – mouse	Gallicchio and Chen, 1982[46] Harker et al., 1977[47] Levitt and Quesenberry, 1980[30]
CFU-GM	Myeloid precursor	Following chemotherapy	Gallicchio et al., 1985[22]
CFU-GM	Myeloid precursor	Following antiviral drug	Gallicchio et al., 1995[48]
CFU-Meg	Platelet precursor	Bone marrow – mouse	Friedenberg and Marx, 1980[35] Gamba-Vitalo et al., 1983[49]
BFU/CFU-E	Erythroid precursors	Bone marrow – human Bone marrow – mouse	Chan et al., 1980[50] Gallicchio and Chen, 1980[28] Gallicchio and Murphy, 1983[51] Levitt and Quesenberry, 1980[30]
Stroma	Marrow microenvironment	Bone marrow – normal Bone marrow – short term Bone marrow – long term Bone marrow – long term Bone marrow – human Acute radiation exposure Low-dose radiation exposure	Gallicchio et al., 1986[52] Doukas et al., 1986[53] McGrath et al., 1992[54] Quesenberry et al., 1984[55] Quang et al., 1999[56] Gallicchio et al., 1983[31] Vacek et al., 1982[33]

CFU, colony-forming unit; -S, stem cell; -GM, granulocyte/monocyte; -Meg, megakaryocyte; BFU, blood-forming unit; -E, erythrocyte

Table 33.2 Lithium effects on hematopoietic growth factor production

Growth factor	Action	Reference
GM-CSF	Responsible for increasing granulocytes and myeloid progenitor cells released from macrophages	Chatelain et al., 1983[57] Greenberg et al., 1980[58] Harker et al., 1977[47] Ramsey and Hays, 1979[59] Verma et al., 1982[60]
GM-CSF	Released from T lymphocytes	Gallicchio et al., 1984[61]
GM-CSF	Absent from serum following sub-lethal radiation	Gallicchio et al., 1985[22]
Diffusion chamber	Absence of either GM-CSF or CSF1 production	Doukas et al., 1989[62]
IL-1	Increased from activated monocytes	Kucharz et al., 1988[63]
IL-2	Increased from activated T lymphocytes Increased from normal lymphocytes – humans Increased from normal lymphocytes – primates Number of secreting cells decreased	Kucharz et al., 1988[63] Kishter et al., 1985[64] Wu and Yang, 1991[65] Boufidou et al., 2004[66]
IL-4	Inhibited by lithium	Szuster-Ciesielska et al., 2003[67]
IL-8	Inhibitor of hematopoiesis, blocked by lithium	Merendino et al., 2000[68]
IL-10	Number of secreting cells decreased	Boufidou et al., 2004[66]
IL-12	Increased in lupus patients receiving lithium	Kucharz et al., 1993[69]
IFN-γ	Number of secreting cells decreased	Boufidou et al., 2004[66] Sharma, 1982[70]

GM-CSF, granulocyte/monocyte colony-stimulating factor; IL, interleukin; IFN, interferon

LITHIUM-INDUCED INHIBITION OF SUPPRESSOR LYMPHOCYTES AND PROSTAGLANDIN PRODUCTION

Another mechanism to explain lithium effects on hematopoiesis may be attributed to the ability of lithium to inhibit the activity of suppressor T lymphocytes. These cells are thymus-derived lymphocytes that are known to limit hematopoiesis[73,74]. The therapeutic levels of lithium observed clinically are within the concentration range where lithium effectively reduces the levels of cyclic-AMP[75]. However, lithium can stimulate or enhance the responsiveness of lymphocytes to mitogens such as phytohemagglutinin[76], which can be inhibited in the presence of prostaglandin E. The effects of prostaglandins are mediated in part by increasing the activity of cyclic-AMP[77]. Therefore, lithium and prostaglandins have opposing effects, apparently on the same target cells using similar pathways. These opposing actions have been demonstrated to influence in vitro hematopoiesis[50], and, in the presence of a prostaglandin inhibitor, to stimulate lymphocytes in vitro[61]. Lithium stimulates granulopoiesis while at the same time inhibiting erythropoiesis, whereas prostaglandins are capable of the opposite effects[78]. These effects with respect to cyclic-AMP activity and lithium have been demonstrated utilizing long-term bone marrow cultures[79].

GRANULOCYTE FUNCTION IN PATIENTS RECEIVING LITHIUM CARBONATE

The importance of polymorphonuclear leukocytes (PMNs) is that they provide protection against a wide variety of microbial pathogens. A reduction in the number of neutrophils or an abnormality in their cellular function is most often associated with infection. Studies evaluating random migration, chemotaxis, phagocytosis and measurement of bactericidal ability have been evaluated from patients receiving lithium[80]. These studies observed no adverse effects among neutrophils examined either from patients receiving lithium or from cells exposed to lithium *in vitro*. Cohen and colleagues[80] concluded that such cells are capable of responding and contributing fully to the phagocytic host defense system of the body. This observation confirmed earlier studies that neutrophils harvested from lithium-treated patients were capable of ingesting yeast to the same degree as controls[81].

Lithium has been reported to decrease granulocyte adherence, although in one study this response was not due to lithium but to a plasma factor, removal of which by patient dialysis caused granulocyte adhesiveness to return[82]. Another study reported normal to increased migration of neutrophils into inflammatory sites as the result of lithium therapy[83]. These results implied that the ratio of cyclic-AMP to cyclic-GMP may affect neutrophil chemotaxis. Together with the observation that lithium is known to decrease cyclic-AMP, this suggested that lithium activity on granulocyte adhesiveness may involve alterations in cyclic-AMP concentrations.

Other studies that focused on assessing granulocyte function from neutrophils taken from patients who had been on long-term lithium treatment[21,35] demonstrated a decrease in granulocyte function tests such as nitroblue tetrazolium (NBT) reduction, chemotaxis in response to bacteria-derived factors and zymosan-induced C5a, and phagocytic and bactericidal capabilities. However, in another study assessing bactericidal capacity, five patients exposed to long-term lithium treatment were not found to have decreased activity[84]. Bipolar patients on lithium therapy have been shown repeatedly to present with higher neutrophil counts compared to individuals not receiving lithium therapy. One additional measurement that relates the action of lithium-induced neutrophilia with that of increased neutrophil function is the report showing that, in addition to elevation levels of neutrophils in patients receiving lithium, there is also the elevation in human leukocyte elastase activity, a substance responsible for the ability of leukocytes/neutrophils to adhere to vessel walls or bind to foreign antigens[85].

IN VITRO STUDIES ON GRANULOCYTE FUNCTION INVOLVING LITHIUM

Previous investigations identified lithium as capable of influencing a number of activities that involved blood mononuclear cells. These included increasing thymidine incorporation by phytohemagglutinin[18], stimulating phagocytosis of polystyrene latex particles by human monocytes, and reversing prostaglandin E- and theophylline-induced inhibition of mitogen responsiveness by mononuclear cells[86]. Similar results found using β-adrenergic agonists indicated that cyclic-AMP was involved[75]. Further investigations demonstrated both that neutrophil chemotaxis could be inhibited by agents that elevate cellular levels of cyclic-AMP, and that lithium was an effective stimulator of neutrophil chemotaxis by inhibiting cyclic-AMP-induced inhibition by all agents that are capable of elevating cyclic-AMP, except cyclic-

AMP itself. Lithium does not prevent the inhibition of chemotaxis of cells when they are directly exposed to cyclic-AMP[87]. More recent experiments have studied the effect on neutrophils of the chemotactic factor N-formyl-methionyl-leucyl phenylalanine (FMLP), which activates an amiloride-sensitive alkali metal cation-H[+] counter-transport system that exhibits a 1:1 stoichiometry. Lithium can effectively utilize this carrier system as well as sodium to promote chemotaxis, while potassium, rubidium and cesium are not effective[88]. These results indicate there is a cation-exchange mechanism operating on neutrophils, similar to mechanisms present in a wide variety of other cell types, which, when activated, can promote chemotaxis.

Studies have also examined the ability of lithium to influence the metabolic function of granulocytes. Various reports investigating a variety of homogeneous cell populations have shown that lithium can increase the adhesion of nervous system cells and interfere with the effects of colcemid in vitro, increase the intensity of platelet aggregation and prolong the duration of desegregation in vitro[89], and enhance neutrophil skin window migration in vivo[83]. Studies[26] have indicated that, within the therapeutic concentration range (0.5–1.5 mmol/l), lithium was neither toxic nor stimulating to resting neutrophils in any oxidative or membrane function measured, such as O_2 generation as an indicator of the respiratory burst of stimulated neutrophils. Glucose-1-^{14}C oxidation of resting neutrophils was not affected by the presence of lithium. However, from phagocytic activated neutrophils [14]CO_2 production was increased. Lithium is effective in elevating lysosomal enzyme release of unstimulated and phagocytic neutrophils. Also, lithium increased neutrophil cell migration as measured by in vivo skin chambers[90].

In general, within the therapeutic concentration range, lithium has no effect on O_2 generation, chemiluminescence and candida-cidal activity of optimally stimulated neutrophils. Energy and membrane-dependent activities such as aggregation and degranulation are unaffected by lithium. Lithium has been suggested in certain systems to act like calcium and can amplify calcium-mediated actions or, as was described earlier, reverse reactions dependent upon activated adenyl cyclase activity, a calcium cofactor-dependent reaction[83].

Lithium has also been speculated to serve as an effective antiviral agent in a number of different mechanisms, but one is certainly by increasing the cytotoxicity of cells chronically infected with HIV as was shown in the in vitro study reported by Mpanju and colleagues[91]. The ability of added lithium in the form of lithium γ-linoleic acid (LiGLA) was independent of the action of tumor necrosis factor (TNF)-α and was observed at concentrations as low as 5 μg/ml.

EFFECT OF LITHIUM ON B LYMPHOCYTES AND IMMUNOGLOBULIN PRODUCTION

Few studies have considered the effect of lithium on B lymphocytes. Weetman and colleagues reported a dose-dependent effect for in vitro testing of B lymphocytes using a protein A plaque-forming assay with pokeweed mitogen (PWM)[92]. Normal lymphocytes incubated with lower lithium doses of 10^{-3} to 10^{-1} mol/l showed increased production of IgG but not IgM or IgA. If, however, higher doses of lithium were used, there was less stimulation until actual suppression at 10 mmol/l. Cultures in the absence of lipopolysaccharide (LPS) showed increased IgM and IgG plaque-forming cells even at 10 mmol/l[93,94]. Spontaneous plaque-forming cells derived from controls versus patients on lithium showed an increase in all immunoglobulin types, but significance only for IgM. There was no correlation with lithium levels. The use of PWM to detect B-cell activity, however, is dependent on both T cells and macrophages, and may not be a true representation. Thus, the spontaneous plaque assay may be more reliable. The testing with a more sensitive B-cell mitogen such as LPS using human cells would be important to investigate. In murine studies lithium enhanced LPS stimulation of B cells, especially at high concentrations (10 mmol/l)[93,94]. Also, lithium could induce a partial response to LPS in previously determined LPS non-responsive cells[94]. The enhancement of LPS stimulation was believed to be linked to the cyclic nucleotide system[93]. *In vitro* lithium has been demonstrated to increase IgG and IgM production from activated B cells[95]. In a clinical study designed to determine whether lithium treatment may contribute to the development of autoimmune diseases, because of its ability to modulate the immune response, a small number of patients responded to lithium therapy by increasing B-cell activity as measured by increased IgG and IgM production and released following mitogen stimulation. However, this response was also observed following use of psychiatric medications other than lithium; therefore this antibody response was not attributed to lithium specifically[96].

LITHIUM EFFECTS ON T LYMPHOCYTES

The effect of lithium on mitogen-induced proliferation of normal lymphocytes was originally described by Shenkman *et al.*[18]. Lithium enhanced phytohemagglutinin-induced proliferation, but was effective only at concentrations greater than 1 mmol/l with the optimal level being 5–10 mmol/l. Doses greater than 10 mmol/l began to show inhibition[97]. The

concentration of mitogen to which lithium was not stimulatory seemed to be a suboptimal concentration for maximal stimulation with phytohemagglutinin alone[18]. The optimal concentration of phytohemagglutinin and the highest concentrations of lithium – when combined – produced inhibition. Similar responses to other plant lectins, e.g. concanavalin A (Con-A) and PWM have been reported[98,99]. It should be noted that lithium independently is not mitogenic[18,97].

There have been a few studies that have investigated the effect of lithium when combined with T-cell subsets. Sengar *et al.*[100] reported no change in the ratio of T cells or B cells after lithium therapy[100]. However, Wahlin and colleagues, using monoclonal antibody staining, showed consistent alteration in the mean CD4/CD8 ratio of controls or patients before lithium treatment when compared to samples taken from treated patients[101]. There was a significant reduction in CD4 cells and therefore abnormally high and low CD4/CD8 ratios. Similar findings were reported by Crockard *et al.*[102]. Dosch *et al.*[103] showed that lithium could affect suppressor cells by altering a plaque-forming assay believed to be inhibited by a suppressor cell population. These results were consistent with another study[104]. These results were similar to those described above with respect to mitogen-stimulated lymphocytes[103]. Lithium increases the CD4 helper T-cell/CD8 suppressor ratio when administered either to normal adults or in psychiatric patients receiving lithium as therapy[101]. These results conclude that in therapeutic doses lithium has immunomodulatory effects.

From clinical studies, one report by Ridgway *et al.*[23] and another by Fernandez and Fox[98] showed a significant improvement in lymphocyte response to phytohemagglutinin after therapy with lithium. Patients in these studies were being treated for either psychiatric disorders or leukemia. Other studies, which included normal human volunteers, have concluded that there is no stimulatory effect of lithium on lymphocytes when assaying these cells without the addition of lithium to the culture medium[97,100,101,105]. These results may certainly be explained by the low tolerable level of lithium in patients with respect to the high levels needed for significant proliferation.

Fernandez and MacSween reported the effects of lithium on T-cell colonies[106]. By using patients receiving lithium and comparing them to normal controls, they showed significantly fewer T-cell colonies in those receiving lithium. There were, however, no pre-lithium-colony assays performed for granulocyte colonies or lymphoid colonies and thus the results were difficult to interpret. Lithium has been reported to increase the mixed lymphocyte reaction (MLR). The concentration required for significant alternation is 5 mmol/l and therefore is a less sensitive system than mitogen proliferation[18]. Since MLR and mitogen proliferation require functional macrophages, one must consider the effect of lithium on the macrophage. Lithium may also affect the adherent cells of the bone marrow, causing these cells to secrete growth factors or other monokines/cytokines, since removal of these cells does influence lithium-stimulated granulopoiesis. Whether lithium affects the ability of the macrophage to present antigens has not been investigated. Clearly lithium cannot replace monocyte/macrophage activity in depleted population studies of lymphocyte proliferation[107].

EFFECT OF LITHIUM ON NATURAL KILLER AND LYMPHOKINE-ACTIVATED KILLER CELLS

As with other non-granulocytic cells, lithium effects cultures stimulated with phytohemagglutinin or Con-A and lithium (5 mmol/l). Sharma[70] evaluated the effect of lithium on the production of interferon from human lymphocytes. Lithium alone did not increase the production of IFNα-mediated arrest of granulopoietic differentiation. This was not T-cell mediated and appeared to be related to the dose of lithium, with nearly total reversal at the highest concentration tested (4 mmol/l). The possible mechanism of this effect might be increased cerebrospinal fluid production through the inhibition of adenyl cyclase activity decreasing the cyclic AMP levels, since interferon has the opposite effect. At this concentration lithium significantly stimulated natural killer (NK) activity. As with interferon production, lithium alone was not capable of enhancement of NK activity[70]. The synergistic effect of lithium and mitogen causing measured interferon production probably explains the increased NK activity. In a murine system, using lithium lactate rather than lithium chloride did not increase NK activity *in vitro*. However, by pre-treating mice with lithium, there was increased NK activity in the spleen. This response was believed to have been due to the increased number of NK precursors, which are derived from the bone marrow. Lithium was not able to reverse cyclophosphamide suppression of NK cell activity. Lithium was also effective in inducing NK activity by inducing the secretion of stimulators present in conditioned medium[108]. Lithium could also effectively increase NK activity following *in vivo* administration that was postulated to occur because of the capacity of lithium to increase the number of NK precursor cells[109].

The *in vitro* effect of lithium on lymphokine-activated killer cell (LAK) activity and its *in vivo* anti-tumor growth was observed[110]. LAK activity was enhanced when lithium was added during LAK cell induction, and this enhancement was observed both in human peripheral blood mononuclear cells and in mouse splenocytes used as LAK precursors. Cholera toxin, which can increase intracellular levels of cyclic AMP, decreased LAK cell activity. This negative effect was partially reversed with lithium, indicating that lithium increased LAK cell activity by decreasing cyclic AMP levels. These results suggested that lithium could be used as adjuvant therapy for treating human cancer and other related immune diseases by acting as an agent in the immunotherapy of these conditions.

BIOCHEMICAL MECHANISMS FOR LITHIUM EFFECTS ON LYMPHOCYTES

Lithium influences several key cellular systems including ion transport, adenylate cyclase and cyclic nucleotides, phosphoinositide metabolism, poly-biosynthesis and the oxygenation of arachidonic acids forming the leukotrienes. When evaluating the effect of lithium in these systems, it is imperative to keep in mind that, as with many non-granulocytic effects, these are usually seen at levels much higher than are therapeutic and thus would have considerable toxicity if attempts were made to observe these findings in patients.

The stimulatory effects of lithium can be modulated by the inhibition of Na–K ATPase, located in the cell membrane, by the inhibitor ouabain. Also, the binding of this inhibitor can be modulated by varying the concentration of lithium. These findings suggest that the transport of lithium into cells requires sodium transport. Inhibition of lithium transport with ouabain has been shown to cause a reduction in the ability of lithium to increase the granulocyte progenitors colony-forming units–granulocytes/monocytes (CFU-GM)[51]. The opposite effect is seen with erythroid precursor progenitor stem cells[52]. The binding of lithium may affect the transport of other monovalent cations and possibly divalent cations such as

calcium, which may have significant effects on cellular events. Although not as well described in lymphoid cells, it is clear that lithium does affect cation binding as demonstrated with ouabain[111,112].

Many of the effects of lithium on lymphocytes have been attributed to the well-described effect on the cyclic nucleotide system, cyclic AMP[75,103,113]. Lithium decreases the concentration of cyclic AMP. This reduction affects numerous neurohormone receptors and the effect of prostaglandin E and interferon. The result of the direct effect on prostaglandins is reduction in erythroid cells[50], whereas the effect on interferon may be the reversal of inhibition on granulocytic precursors, to increase precursor growth[60]. It is noteworthy that lithium acts synergistically with phytohemagglutinin proliferation. This occurs at an increase in cyclic AMP, not a decrease[75]. The direct stimulation of cyclic AMP production results in a dose-dependent decrease in proliferation. Since cyclic AMP is one of the major second messenger systems, it may have further implications that are currently not fully understood.

The activation of lymphocytes by mitogens is a complex phenomenon, which, very early, results in a rapid activation of the enzyme ornithine decarboxylase (ODC)[114]. ODC is the rate-limiting enzyme in polyamine synthesis. Polyamines are thought to play an important role in cell growth. Mustelin et al.[115] have shown that lithium at 1 mmol/l is capable of inhibiting the activation of ODC by the mitogen Con-A. This is done by decreasing the cellular pool of inositol needed to activate ODC by inhibiting the enzyme inositol-1-phosphatase[115]. Addition of exogenous inositol will override the inhibition. These studies correlated enzyme levels and putrescine production in the enzyme responsible for early events but did not evaluate proliferation. Despite these findings of reduction in the enzyme responsible for early events in cellular recognition, the combination of lithium and

Con-A has been shown to increase lymphocyte proliferation[99]. *In vitro* incubation with lithium for short periods of time does not have this effect. From these studies, it is evident that lithium has an effect on the principal second messenger systems, cyclic AMP and inositol phosphates, by causing downregulation.

The leukotrienes are the product of 5-lipoxygenase-catalyzed oxygenation of arachidonic acid. This class of compound is believed to participate in a variety of inflammatory diseases. Lithium in extremely high concentrations has been shown to potentiate leukotriene synthesis in human peripheral blood monocytes[116]. It is believed that these findings are due to the ability of lithium to modulate the metabolism of inositol phosphate.

CLINICAL UTILITY OF LITHIUM AS AN IMMUNOMODULATOR

There was optimism that, as the understanding of the effects of lithium increased, this would expand the clinical use of lithium. Certainly the understanding that lithium affects both second messenger systems may offer explanations for its utility in the treatment of psychiatric disorders; there was the potential that this knowledge would expand its clinical use. Although lithium does have the capability of synergistically stimulating lymphoid cells with appropriate mitogens, augmenting NK cell function and inhibiting T-suppressor cells, the intention for its use clinically to provide significant alterations was not justified. Two areas that at one time did show potential clinical promise were based upon the observations that lithium increases immunoresponsiveness and IL-2 production, especially in immunological conditions that were associated with decreased IL-2 production. Two clinical areas of interest in this regard were for patients who were HIV-infected who presented with decreased

IL-2 and patients in the transplant setting who were at risk for developing graft-versus-host-disease. Further basic research and clinical studies would be required to further develop either of these two clinical settings for potential lithium intervention. Although there is evidence that many of the actions for lithium are mediated through the action of protein kinase C (PKC), there is little evidence supporting the changes in peripheral blood elements and changes in PKC activity during lithium administration[117].

REFERENCES

1. Mertz W. The essential trace elements. Science 1981; 213: 1332–8
2. Schou M. Biology and pharmacology of the lithium ion. Pharmacol Rev 1957; 9: 17–58
3. Gershon S, Yuwiler A. Lithium ion: a specific psychopharmacological approach to the treatment of mania. J Neuropsychiatry 1960; 1: 229–41
4. Barr RD, Koekebakker M, Brown EA, Falbo MC. Putative role for lithium in human hematopoiesis. J Lab Clin Med 1987; 109: 159–63
5. Barr RD, Galbraith PR. Lithium and hematopoiesis. Can Med Assoc J 1983; 128: 123–6
6. Boggs DR, Joyce RA. The hematopoietic effects of lithium. Semin Hematol 1983; 20: 129–38
7. Gallicchio VS. Effect of lithium on blood cells and the function of granulocytes. In Birch NJ, ed. Lithium and the Cell. London: Academic Press, 1991: 185–98
8. Gallicchio VS. Effect of lithium on the formation and function of blood cells. In Gallicchio VS, ed. Lithium and the Blood. Basel: Karger AG, 1991: 1–17
9. Gallicchio VS. Lithium and the bood. Johnson FN, ed. Lithium Therapy Monographs #4. Basel: Karger AG, 1991: 1–150

10. Shopsin B, Friedmann R, Gershon S. Lithium and leukocytosis. Clin Pharmacol Ther 1971; 12: 923–8

11. Mayfield D, Brown RG. The clinical laboratory and electroencephalographic effects of lithium. J Psychiat Res 1966; 4: 207–19

12. Cruet J, Dancey JT, Waite J. Lithium effects on leukocytosis and lymphopenia. In Lithium in Medical Practice, 1st British Lithium Congress, Lancaster, UK 1978

13. Ricci P, Bandini G, Franchi P, et al. Haematological effects of lithium carbonate: a study in 56 psychiatric patients. Haematologica 1981; 66: 627–33

14. Bille PE, Jensen MK, Kaalund Jensen JP, et al. Studies on the haematologic and cytogenetic effect of lithium. Acta Med Scand 1975; 198: 281–6

15. Murphy DL, Goodwin FK, Bunney WE Jr. Leukocytosis during lithium treatment. Am J Psychiatry 1971; 127: 1559–61

16. Pointud C, Clerc CA, Manegand G. Essai de traitment du syndrome de Felty par le lithium. Semin Hosp Paris 1976; 52: 1719–23

17. Stein RS, Howard CA, Brennan M, Czorniak M. Lithium carbonate and granulocyte production: dose optimization. Cancer 1981; 48: 2697–701

18. Shenkman L, Borkowsky W, Holzman RS, Shopsin B. Enhancement of lymphocyte and macrophage function in vitro by lithium chloride. Clin Immunol Immunopathol 1978; 10: 187–92

19. Steinherz PG, Rosen G, Ghavimi F, et al. The effect of lithium carbonate on leukopenia after chemotherapy. J Pediatr 1980; 96: 923–7

20. Gallicchio VS, Gamba-Vitalo C, Watts TD, Chen MG. In vivo and in vitro modulation of megakaryocytopoiesis and stromal colony formation by lithium. J Lab Clin Med 1986; 108: 199–205

21. Friedenberg WR, Marx JJ. The bactericidal defect of neutrophil function with lithium therapy. Adv Exp Med Biol 1980; 127: 389–99

22. Gallicchio VS, Chen MG, Watts TD. Lithium-stimulated recovery of granulopoiesis after sublethal irradiation is not mediated via increased levels of colony stimulating factor

23. Ridgway D, Wolff LJ, Neerhout RC. Enhanced lymphocyte response to PHA among leukemia patients taking oral lithium carbonate. Cancer Invest 1986; 4: 513–17

24. Tang HR, He Q. Effects of lithium chloride on the proliferation and apoptosis of K562 leukemia cells. Hunan Yi Ke Da Xue Xue Bao 2003; 28: 357–60

25. Holtz KM, Rice AM, Sartorelli AC. Lithium chloride inactivates the 20S proteasome from WEHI-3B D+ leukemia cells. Biochem Biophys Res Commun 2003; 303: 1058–64

26. Joyce RA, Chervenick PA. Lithium effects on granulopoiesis in mice following cytotoxic chemotherapy. Adv Exp Med Biol 1980; 127: 145–54

27. Tisman G, Herbert V, Rosenblatt S. Evidence that lithium induces human granulocyte proliferation: elevated serum vitamin B 12 binding capacity in vivo and granulocyte colony proliferation in vitro. Br J Haematol 1973; 24: 767–71

28. Gallicchio VS, Chen MG. Modulation of murine pluripotential stem cell proliferation in vivo by lithium carbonate. Blood 1980; 56: 1150–2

29. Gallicchio VS, Chen MG. Influence of lithium on proliferation of hematopoietic stem cells. Exp Hematol 1981; 9: 804–10

30. Levitt LJ, Quesenberry PJ. The effect of lithium on murine hematopoiesis in a liquid culture system. N Engl J Med 1980; 302: 713–19

31. Gallicchio VS, Chen MG, Watts TD, Gamba-Vitalo C. Lithium stimulates the recovery of granulopoiesis following acute radiation injury. Exp Hematol 1983; 11: 553–63

32. Gallicchio VS, Chen MG, Watts TD. Ability of lithium to accelerate the recovery of granulopoiesis after subacute radiation injury. Acta Radiol Oncol 1984; 23: 361–6

33. Vacek A, Sikulova J, Bartonickova A. Radiation resistance in mice increased following chronic application of Li2CO3. Acta Radiol Oncol 1982; 21: 325–30

34. Moroz BB, Deshevoi Iu B, Tsybanev OA, Adiushkin AI. Effect of lithium carbonate on

(CSF). Int J Radiat Biol Relat Stud Phys Chem Med 1985; 47: 581–90

hematopoietic stem cells (CFUs) in acute radiation lesions. Patol Fiziol Eksp Ter 1988; 41–3

35. Friedenberg WR, Marx JJ Jr. The effect of lithium carbonate on lymphocyte, granulocyte, and platelet function Cancer 1980; 45: 91–7

36. Gallicchio VS. Lithium and hematopoietic toxicity. I. Recovery in vivo of murine hematopoietic stem cells (CFU-S and CFU-Mix) after single-dose administration of cyclophosphamide. Exp Hematol 1986; 14: 395–400

37. Gallicchio VS. Lithium and hematopoietic toxicity. II. Acceleration in vivo of murine hematopoietic progenitor cells (CFU-gm and CFU-meg) following treatment with vinblastine sulfate. Int J Cell Cloning 1987; 5: 122–33

38. Gallicchio VS. Lithium and hematopoietic toxicity. III. In vivo recovery of hematopoiesis following single-dose administration of cyclophosphamide. Acta Haematol 1988; 79: 192–7

39. Ballin A, Lehman D, Sirota P, et al. Increased number of peripheral blood CD34+ cells in lithium-treated patients. Br J Haematol 1998; 100: 219–21

40. Gregory CA, Perry AS, Reyes E, et al. Dkk-1-derived synthetic peptides and lithium chloride for the control and recovery of adult stem cells from bone marrow. J Biol Chem 2005; 280: 2309–23

41. Greco FA, Brereton HD. Effect of lithium carbonate on the neutropenia caused by chemotherapy: a preliminary clinical trial. Oncology 1977; 34: 153–5

42. Morley DC Jr, Galbraith PR. Effect of lithium on granulopoiesis in culture. Can Med Assoc J 1978; 118: 288–90

43. Spitzer G, Verma DS, Barlogie B, et al. Possible mechanisms of action of lithium on augmentation of in vitro spontaneous myeloid colony formation. Cancer Res 1979; 39: 3215–19

44. Hammond WP, Dale DC. Lithium therapy of canine cyclic hematopoiesis. Blood 1980; 55: 26–8

45. Rossof AH, Fehir KM. Lithium carbonate increases marrow granulocyte-committed colony-forming units and peripheral blood granulocytes in a canine model. Exp Hematol 1979; 7: 255–8

46. Gallicchio VS, Chen MG. Cell kinetics of lithium-induced granulopoiesis. Cell Tissue Kinet 1982; 15: 179–86

47. Harker WG, Rothstein G, Clarkson D, et al. Enhancement of colony-stimulating activity production by lithium. Blood 1977; 49: 263–7

48. Gallicchio VS, Hughes NK, Tse KF, et al. Effect of lithium in immunodeficiency: improved blood cell formation in mice with decreased hematopoiesis as the result of LP-BM5 MuLV infection. Antiviral Res 1995; 26: 189–202

49. Gamba-Vitalo C, Gallicchio VS, Watts TD, Chen MG. Lithium stimulated in vitro megakaryocytopoiesis. Exp Hematol 1983; 11: 382–8

50. Chan HS, Saunders EF, Freedman MH. Modulation of human hematopoiesis by prostaglandins and lithium. J Lab Clin Med 1980; 95: 125–32

51. Gallicchio VS, Murphy MJ Jr. Cation influences on in vitro growth of erythroid stem cells (CFU-e and BFU-e). Cell Tissue Res 1983; 233: 175–81

52. Gallicchio VS. Lithium stimulation of in vitro granulopoiesis: evidence for mediation via sodium transport pathways. Br J Haematol 1986; 62: 455–66

53. Doukas MA, Niskanen E, Quesenberry PJ. Effect of lithium on stem cell and stromal cell proliferation in vitro. Exp Hematol 1986; 14: 215–21

54. McGrath HE, Wade PM, Kister VK, Quesenberry PJ. Lithium stimulation of HPP-CFC and stromal growth factor production in murine Dexter culture. J Cell Physiol 1992; 151: 276–86

55. Quesenberry PJ, Coppola MA, Gualtieri RJ, et al. Lithium stimulation of murine hematopoiesis in liquid culture: an effect mediated by marrow stromal cells. Blood 1984; 63: 121–7

56. Quang et al. 1999

57. Chatelain C, Burstein SA, Harker LA. Lithium enhancement of megakaryocytopoiesis in

culture: mediation via accessory marrow cells. Blood 1983; 62: 172–6

58. Greenberg PL, Packard B, Steed SM. Effects of lithium chloride on human and murine marrow myeloid colony formation and colony stimulating activity. Adv Exp Med Biol 1980; 127: 137–44

59. Ramsey R, Hays EF. Factors promoting colony stimulating activity (CSA) production in macrophages and epithelial cells. Exp Hematol 1979; 7: 245–54

60. Verma DS, Johnston DA, Spitzer G, et al. The mechanism of lithium carbonate-induced augmentation of colony-stimulating activity elaboration in man. Leuk Res 1982; 6: 349–63

61. Gallicchio VS, Chen MG, Watts TD. Specificity of lithium (Li+) to enhance the production of colony stimulating factor (GM-CSF) from mitogen-stimulated lymphocytes in vitro. Cell Immunol 1984; 85: 58–66

62. Doukas MA, Shadduck RK, Waheed A, Gass C. Lithium stimulation of diffusion chamber colony growth is mediated by factors other than colony-stimulating factor. Int J Cell Cloning 1989; 7: 168–78

63. Kucharz EJ, Sierakowski S, Staite ND, Goodwin JS. Mechanism of lithium-induced augmentation of T-cell proliferation. Int J Immunopharmacol 1988; 10: 253–9

64. Kishter S, Hoffman FA, Pizzo PA. Production of and response to interleukin-2 by cultured T cells: effects of lithium chloride and other putative modulators. J Biol Response Mod 1985; 4: 185–94

65. Wu YY, Yang XH. Enhancement of interleukin 2 production in human and Gibbon T cells after in vitro treatment with lithium. Proc Soc Exp Biol Med, 1991; 198: 620–4

66. Boufidou F, Nikolaou C, Alevizos B, et al. Cytokine production in bipolar affective disorder patients under lithium treatment. J Affect Disord 2004; 82: 309–13

67. Szuster-Ciesielska A, Tustanowska-Stachura A, Slotwinska M, et al. In vitro immuno-regulatory effects of antidepressants in healthy volunteers. Pol J Pharmacol 2003; 55: 353–62

68. Merendino RA, Arena A, Gangemi S, et al. In vitro interleukin-8 production by monocytes treated with lithium chloride from breast cancer patients. Tumori 2000; 86: 149–52

69. Kucharz EJ, Sierakowski SJ, Goodwin JS. Lithium in vitro enhances interleukin-2 production by T cells from patients with systemic lupus erythematosus. Immunopharmacol Immunotoxicol 1993; 15: 515–23

70. Sharma SD. Lithium modulates mitogen induced natural killer activity and interferon production. J Immunopharmacol 1982; 4: 303–13

71. Gallicchio VS, Hughes NK, Hulette BC, Noblitt, L. Effect of interleukin-1, GM-CSF, erythropoietin, and lithium on the toxicity associated with 3'-azido-3'-deoxythymidine (AZT) in vitro on hematopoietic progenitors (CFU-GM, CFU-MEG, and BFU-E) using murine retrovirus-infected hematopoietic cells. J Leukoc Biol 1991; 50, 580–6

72. Imamura K, Kufe D. Colony-stimulating factor 1-induced Na+ influx into human monocytes involves activation of a pertussis toxin-sensitive GTP-binding protein. J Biol Chem 1988; 263: 14093–8

73. Barr RD. The role of the lymphocyte in haemopoiesis. Scott Med J 1979; 24: 267–72

74. Barr RD, Stevens CA. The role of autologous helper and suppressor T cells in the regulation of human granulopoiesis. Am J Hematol 1982; 12: 323–6

75. Gelfand EW, Dosch HM, Hastings B, Shore A. Lithium: a modulator of cyclic AMP-dependent events in lymphocytes? Science 1979; 203: 365–7

76. Stobo JD, Kennedy MS, Goldyne ME. Prostaglandin E modulation of the mitogenic response of human T cells. Differential response of T-cell subpopulations. J Clin Invest 1979; 64: 1188–203

77. Goodwin JS, Kaszubowski PA, Williams RC Jr. Cyclic adenosine monophosphate response to prostaglandin E2 on subpopulations of human lymphocytes. J Exp Med 1979; 150: 1260–4

78. Rossi GB, Migliaccio AR, Migliaccio G, et al. In vitro interactions of PGE and cAMP with murine and human erythroid precursors. Blood 1980; 56: 74–9

79. Gualtieri RJ, Berne RM, McGrath HE, et al. Effect of adenine nucleotides on granulopoiesis and lithium-induced granulocytosis in long-term bone marrow cultures. Exp Hematol 1986; 14: 689–95

80. Cohen MS, Zahkireh B, Metcalf JA, Root RK. Granulocyte function in patients receiving lithium carbonate. Adv Exp Med Biol 1980; 127: 335–46

81. Stein RS, Hanson G, Koethe S, Hansen R. Lithium-induced granulocytosis. Ann Intern Med 1978; 88: 809–10

82. MacGregor RR, Dyson WL. Inhibition of granulocyte adherence by lithium: possible relationship to lithium-induced leukocytosis. Adv Exp Med Biol 1980; 127: 347–55

83. Rothstein G, Clarkson DR, Larsen W, et al. Effect of lithium on neutrophil mass and production. N Engl J Med 1978; 298: 178–80

84. Cohen MS, Zahkireh B, Metcalf JA, Root RK. Granulocyte function during lithium therapy. Blood 1979; 53: 913–5

85. Capodicasa E, Russano AM, Ciurnella E, et al. Neutrophil peripheral count and human leukocyte elastase during chronic lithium carbonate therapy. Immunopharmacol Immunotoxicol 2000; 22: 671–83

86. Perez HD, Kaplan HB, Goldstein IM, et al. Effects of lithium on polymorphonuclear leukocyte chemotaxis. Adv Exp Med Biol 1980; 127: 357–70

87. Simchowitz L. Lithium movements in resting and chemotactic factor-activated human neutrophils. Am J Physiol 1988; 254: C526–C534

88. Reiser G, Lautenschlager E, Hamprecht B. Effects of colcemid and lithium ions on processes of cultured cells derived from the nervous system. In Borgers M, de Brabander M, eds. Microtubules and Microtubule Inhibitors. Amsterdam: 1982

89. Imandt L, Genders T, Wessels H, Haanen C. The effect of lithium on platelet aggregation and platelet release reaction. Thromb Res 1977; 11: 297–308

90. Siegel JN, Johnson RB Jr, Lowe RS, et al. Effects of lithium on neutrophil metabolism in vitro and on neutrophil function during therapy. Adv Exp Med Biol 1980; 127: 371–88

91. Mpanju O, Winther M, Manning J, et al. Selective cytotoxicity of lithium gamma-linolenic acid in human T cells chronically and productively infected with HIV. Antivir Ther 1997; 2: 13–9

92. Weetman AP, McGregor AM, Lazarus JH, et al. The enhancement of immunoglobulin synthesis by human lymphocytes with lithium. Clin Immunol Immunopathol 1982; 22: 400–7

93. Hart DA. Differential potentiation of in vitro lipopolysaccharide stimulation of B-lymphoid cells by lithium and ammonium ions. Cell Immunol 1982; 71: 159–68

94. Ishizaka S, Moller G. Lithium chloride induces partial responsiveness to LPS in nonresponder B cells. Nature 1982; 299: 363–5

95. Wilson R, Fraser WD, McKillop JH, et al. The 'in vitro' effects of lithium on the immune system. Autoimmunity 1989; 4: 109–14

96. Wilson R, McKillop JH, Crocket GT, et al. The effect of lithium therapy on parameters thought to be involved in the development of auto-immune thyroid disease. Clin Endocrinol (Oxf) 1991; 34: 357–61

97. Bray J, Turner AR, Dusel F. Lithium and the mitogenic response of human lymphocytes. Clin Immunol Immunopathol 1981; 19: 284–8

98. Fernandez LA, Fox RA. Perturbation of the human immune system by lithium. Clin Exp Immunol 1980; 41: 527–32

99. Hart DA. Lithium potentiates antigen-dependent stimulation of lymphocytes only under suboptimal conditions. Int J Immunopharmacol 1988; 10: 153–60

100. Sengar DP, Waters BG, Dunne JV, Bouer IM. Lymphocyte subpopulations and mitogenic responses of lymphocytes in manic–depressive disorders. Biol Psychiatry 1982; 17: 1017–22

101. Wahlin A, von Knorring L, Roos G. Altered distribution of T lymphocyte subsets in lithium-treated patients. Neuropsychobiology 1984; 11: 243–6

102. Crockard AD, Desai ZR, Ennis KT. Circulating T-cell subpopulations in lithium-associated granulocytosis. J Immunopharmacol 1984; 6: 215–26

103. Dosch HM, Matheson D, Schuurman RK, Gelfand EW. Anti-suppressor cell effects of lithium in vitro and in vivo. Adv Exp Med Biol 1980; 127: 447–62

104. Shenkman L, Wadler S, Borkowsky W, Shopsin B. Adjuvant effects of lithium chloride on human mononuclear cells in suppressor-enriched and suppressor-depleted systems. Immunopharmacology 1981; 3: 1–8

105. Greco FA. Lithium and immune function in man. Adv Exp Med Biol 1980; 127: 463–9

106. Fernandez LA, MacSween JM. Lithium and T cell colonies. Scand J Haematol 1980; 25: 382–4

107. Hart DA. Lithium, lymphocyte stimulation and the neuroimmune interface. In Gallicchio VS, ed. Lithium and the Blood. Basel: Karger AG, 1991: 46–67

108. Ghanta VK, Hiramoto NS, Solvason HB, et al. Conditioned enhancement of natural killer cell activity, but not interferon, with camphor or saccharin-LiCl conditioned stimulus. J Neurosci Res 1987; 18: 10–15

109. Fuggetta MP, Alvino E, Romani L, et al. Increase of natural killer activity of mouse lymphocytes following in vitro and in vivo treatment with lithium. Immunopharmacol Immunotoxicol 1988; 10: 79–91

110. Wu Y, Cai D. Study of the effect of lithium on lymphokine-activated killer cell activity and its antitumor growth. Proc Soc Exp Biol Med, 1992; 201: 284–8

111. Oh VM, Taylor EA. Effects of serum, lithium, ethacrynic acid, and low external concentration of potassium on specific [3H]-ouabain binding to human lymphocytes. Br J Clin Pharmacol 1987; 24: 681–4

112. Rapeport WG, Aronson JK, Grahame-Smith, DG, Harper C. The effects of serum, lithium, ethacrynic acid, and a low external concentration of potassium on specific [3H]-ouabain binding to human lymphocytes after incubation for 3 days. Br J Clin Pharmacol 1986; 22: 275–9

113. Gelfand EW, Cheung R, Hastings D, Dosch HM. Characterization of lithium effects on two aspects of T-cell function. Adv Exp Med Biol 1980; 127: 429–46

114. Scott IG, Poso H, Akerman KE, Andersson LC. Rapid activation of ornithine decarboxylase by mitogenic (but not by nonmitogenic) ligands in human T lymphocytes. Eur J Immunol 1985; 15: 783–7

115. Mustelin T, Poso H, Iivanainen A, Andersson LC. Myo-inositol reverses Li+-induced inhibition of phosphoinositide turnover and ornithine decarboxylase induction during early lymphocyte activation. Eur J Immunol 1986; 16: 859–61

116. Humes JL. Regulation of leukotriene formation in inflammatory cells. Ann NY Acad Sci, 1988; 524: 252–9

117. Young LT, Wang JF, Woods CM, Robb JC. Platelet protein kinase C alpha levels in drug-free and lithium-treated subjects with bipolar disorder. Neuropsychobiology 1999; 40: 63–6

34 Lithium in neuropsychiatry: results from brain imaging studies

E Serap Monkul, Jair C Soares

Contents Introduction • Magnetic resonance imaging findings • Magnetic resonance spectroscopy findings • Functional magnetic resonance imaging findings • Positron emission tomography and single photon emission computed tomography findings • Conclusions

INTRODUCTION

In vivo brain imaging methods provide powerful tools to examine the mechanisms by which lithium exerts its therapeutic effects. In this chapter, we reviewed studies that utilized magnetic resonance imaging (MRI), magnetic resonance spectroscopy (MRS), functional MRI (fMRI), positron emission tomography (PET) and single photon emission tomography (SPECT) to assess changes related to lithium treatment.

MAGNETIC RESONANCE IMAGING FINDINGS

Breeze *et al.*[1] reviewed relevant literature to determine whether lithium treatment resulted in increased prevalence of white matter hyperintensities in young adults with axis I psychiatric disorders, and did not find any significant correlation between lithium treatment and white matter hyperintensities. One longitudinal[2] and one cross-sectional study[3] examined the effects of chronic lithium treatment and reported increased total gray matter volumes in lithium-treated bipolar patients (Figure 34.1). Also, the cingulate volumes in lithium-treated bipolar patients were not significantly different from those of healthy comparisons, whereas untreated bipolar patients had decreased left anterior cingulate volumes compared with healthy controls and lithium-treated patients[4] (Figure 34.2). Recently, chronic lithium treatment has also been shown to increase gray matter volume in cortical brain regions in healthy controls[5]. Another recent

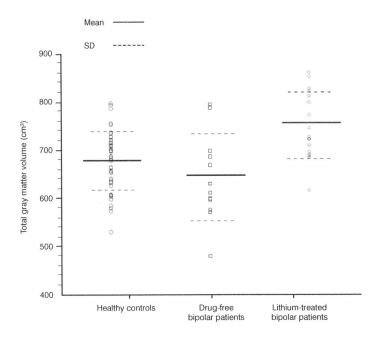

Figure 34.1 Lithium-treated bipolar patients had significantly larger gray matter volume compared with untreated bipolar patients and healthy controls (MANCOVA, age and gender as covariates, $p < 0.05$). From reference 3, with permission from Elsevier

anatomical MRI study[6] showed enlarged left hippocampus volumes in older (mean age 58 years) bipolar patients compared to healthy controls. The authors thought this increase in hippocampal volume might be associated with lithium use. These findings are thought to reflect neurotrophic effects of lithium with resulting neuropil increase.

MAGNETIC RESONANCE SPECTROSCOPY FINDINGS

Relatively few studies of treatment effects in bipolar disorder employed a longitudinal design using magnetic resonance spectroscopy (MRS) to evaluate lithium effects.

Lithium-induced changes in myoinositol

Moore et al.[7] examined the effects of lithium on the levels of myoinositol (12 depressed bipolar patients) and reported significant decreases in levels in the right frontal lobe after 5–7 days treatment with lithium, which persisted with chronic treatment (3–4 weeks). However, the decrease was observed prior to any change in patients' clinical state. The authors concluded that inositol depletion was not associated with the direct therapeutic effects of lithium, although lithium treatment may initiate a cascade of cellular events, first evidenced in changes in inositol, that lead to therapeutic benefit[7]. Davanzo et al.[8] reported a decrease in

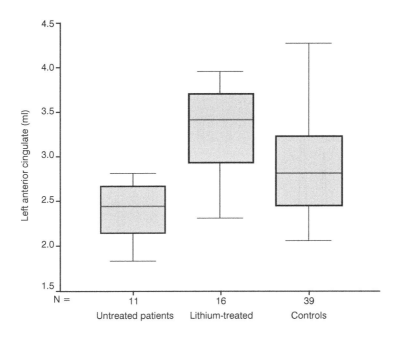

Figure 34.2 Left anterior cingulate volumes for untreated bipolar patients, lithium-treated bipolar patients, and healthy control subjects. Untreated patients presented significantly reduced volume when compared with lithium-treated patients and healthy control subjects. From reference 4, with permission from the Society of Biological Psychiatry

anterior cingulate myoinositol level following 1 week of lithium treatment in bipolar children, especially in lithium responders. However, in this study patients were receiving concomitant medications, which significantly confounded the interpretation of the findings. Silverstone *et al.*[9] used ^{1}H and ^{31}P MRS to examine the effects of lithium and valproate on metabolite concentrations of the frontal and temporal cortex in bipolar patients. They reported no difference in myoinositol level or phosphomonoesters (PME) concentrations between bipolar patients taking divalproex or lithium as compared to healthy controls, suggesting that administration of these

agents may normalize the phosphoinositol cycle in bipolar patients[9].

A recent longitudinal study by Friedman *et al.*[10] reported that lithium treatment of bipolar patients ($n = 12$, mean lithium treatment duration 3.6 ± 1.9 months) was associated with specific gray matter Glx (glutamate + glutamine + GABA) decreases and myoinositol increases, compared to valproate-treated bipolar patients and healthy controls. The authors concluded that this gray matter Glx decrease might be lithium's partial normalization effect of the previously hypothesized bioenergetic alterations of the redox state in unmedicated bipolar patients[11].

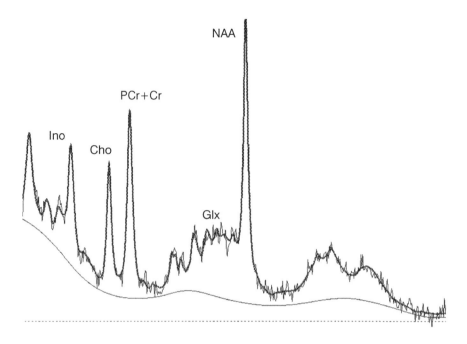

Figure 34.3 An *in vivo* ^{1}H MRS spectrum. Ino, myoinositol; PCr+Cr, phosphocreatine/creatine; Cho, choline; NAA, *N*-acetyl aspartate; Glx, glutamate + glutamine + GABA

N-acetyl aspartate and neurotrophic effects of lithium treatment

N-acetyl aspartate (NAA) is synthesized in mitochondria and reflects neuronal viability and function. It is one of the chemicals that can be measured with ^{1}H MRS (Figure 34.3). MRS findings of NAA response to lithium administration have been somewhat inconsistent. Lithium has been shown to increase NAA in frontal, occipital and temporal lobes of bipolar adults[12,13]. In a study involving healthy individuals, chronic (4 weeks) lithium treatment did not seem to change NAA concentration in the dorsolateral prefrontal cortex[14]. Davanzo *et al.*[8] reported no changes in NAA in bipolar children after 7 days of lithium treatment. A recent longitudinal study with bipolar patients on lithium or valproate treatment did not find any NAA changes[10]. Considering this discrepancy in findings, future studies will be needed to determine whether NAA is a robust marker for monitoring neurotrophic effects in the human brain *in vivo*.

Choline and phosphomonoesters related to membrane stabilization

One suggestion for lithium's mechanism of action is via its effects on choline metabolism, as it increases brain choline concentrations[15]. Lyoo *et al.*[16] administered choline as an adjunctive treatment for rapid-cycling bipolar disorder and assessed brain purine, choline and lithium levels using ^{1}H and ^{7}Li MRS in order to identify the role of oral choline supplementation in modifying energy metabolism in bipolar subjects. Although the group that was treated with choline showed a significant decrease in purine metabolite ratios from baseline compared to placebo, brain lithium level change was not a predictor of this change.

Brain and serum lithium levels

Studies have suggested that brain lithium levels may provide a better measure of predicting response and adverse effects than serum lithium levels. Brain lithium levels can be measured *in vivo* by ^{7}Li MRS. ^{7}Li MRS results have shown correlations (r^2) of 0.50–0.97 between brain and serum lithium levels[17–19]. Soares *et al.*[20] used ^{7}Li MRS to measure brain lithium concentration in bipolar patients and found no statistically significant correlation between serum and brain lithium levels, although patients on single daily dosing of ˉlithium had higher brain/serum lithium ratios than those on twice-a-day dosing. Moore *et al.*[21] compared brain/serum lithium ratios in children and adolescent bipolar patients with adult bipolar patients. They showed that the brain/serum lithium ratio increased with age. Younger patients had lower brain/serum lithium concentration ratios than adults, and the authors concluded that younger patients with bipolar disorder might need higher maintenance serum lithium levels than adults in order to achieve therapeutic brain lithium levels.

Effects of lithium on concentrations of amino acid neurotransmitters and brain high-energy phosphate metabolites

Both lithium and valproate decreased whole brain concentrations of aspartate, glutamate and taurine while brain concentrations of γ-aminobutyric acid (GABA) and alanine decreased following chronic sodium valproate administration but not following chronic lithium administration[22]. These findings indicate that lithium and sodium valproate share common effects on the concentrations of certain amino acid neurotransmitters in whole brain which may be related to their mechanisms of action in bipolar disorder. Yildiz *et al.*[23] observed a decrease in total nucleoside triphosphate levels in healthy controls with 7- and 14-day treatments, reflecting a lithium-induced alteration in brain high-energy phosphates.

Neuroimaging predictors of lithium response

Neuroimaging techniques may also help predict the response to lithium treatment. Although a recent review[1] did not find any significant correlation between lithium treatment and white matter hyperintensities, Kato and colleagues reported that white matter hyperintensities might be a positive predictor of lithium response[24]. The same group of investigators also reported that decreased intracellular pH was significantly associated with a positive lithium response, while increased phosphodiester and decreased phosphocreatine were associated with a poor lithium response[25]. The authors suggested that decreased intracellular pH and elevated phosphodiester levels might be related to white matter hyperintensities in bipolar disorder[26]. Another study[27] examined brain energy metabolism in lithium-resistant bipolar patients using the photic-stimulation paradigm in ^{31}P MRS. The phosphocreatine peak area ratio was significantly decreased after photic stimulation in lithium-resistant bipolar patients. The authors concluded that decreased phosphocreatine might be worthwhile as a negative predictor of lithium response. Ikeda and Kato[28] suggested that these findings might be compatible with mitochondrial dysfunction in lithium-resistant bipolar disorder, yet the above-mentioned findings need to be replicated in order to clarify the neurochemical correlates of lithium response in bipolar patients.

FUNCTIONAL MAGNETIC RESONANCE IMAGING FINDINGS

Bell *et al.*[29] assessed the effect of 14 days' pre-treatment with lithium and valproate on dextroamphetamine-induced changes in regional brain activity in healthy volunteers. This was a double-blind study in which volunteers received either 1000 mg sodium valproate ($n = 12$), 900 mg lithium ($n = 9$) or placebo ($n = 12$). Functional images were acquired using fMRI while subjects performed three cognitive tasks, a word generation paradigm, a spatial attention task and a working memory task. Pre-treatment with lithium attenuated dextroamphetamine-induced changes in the word generation paradigm and the spatial attention task, while pre-treatment with valproate attenuated the changes in the working memory task. The authors suggested that both lithium and valproate might have a similar effect on regional brain activation, through similar effects on phosphoinositol cycle activity.

POSITRON EMISSION TOMOGRAPHY AND SINGLE PHOTON EMISSION COMPUTED TOMOGRAPHY FINDINGS

Metabolic brain activity can be examined indirectly via PET and SPECT. A SPECT study of lithium in euthymic bipolar patients ($n = 14$) showed that its withdrawal was associated with a redistribution of brain circulation, with an increase in posterior perfusion and decrease in limbic areas, particularly the anterior cingulate cortex[30]. There was a correlation between the development of mania after

lithium withdrawal in some subjects and increased perfusion in the superior anterior cingulate[30].

CONCLUSIONS

New techniques from neuroimaging now allow *in vivo* examination of specific mechanisms involved in lithium's actions in the brain, as well as its pharmacokinetic effects. Lithium treatment may increase total gray matter volumes and NAA levels, possibly reflecting its neurotrophic effects. White matter hyperintensities may be a positive, and decreased phosphocreatine a potential negative, predictor of lithium response. Nonetheless, none of these available findings are currently at a point where they can be used to predict treatment response or help monitor treatment. There is great hope that as these studies advance further they will become tools to aid in the treatment of our patients.

REFERENCES

1. Breeze JL, Hesdorffer DC, Hong X, et al. Clinical significance of brain white matter hyperintensities in young adults with psychiatric illness. Harvard Rev Psychiatry 2003; 11: 269–83

2. Moore GJ, Bebchuk JM, Wilds IB, et al. Lithium-induced increase in human brain grey matter. Lancet 2000; 356: 1241–2

3. Sassi RB, Nicoletti M, Brambilla P, et al. Increased gray matter volume in lithium-treated bipolar disorder patients. Neurosci Lett 2002; 329: 243–5

4. Sassi RB, Brambilla P, Hatch JP, et al. Reduced left anterior cingulate volumes in untreated bipolar patients. Biol Psychiatry 2004; 56: 467–75

5. Monkul ES, Dalwani M, Nicoletti MA, et al. Brain gray matter changes after lithium

treatment: a voxel-based morphometry study in healthy individuals. Biol Psychiatry 2004; 55: 202S

6. Beyer JL, Kuchibhatla M, Payne ME, et al. Hippocampal volume measurement in older adults with bipolar disorder. Am J Geriatr Psychiatry 2004; 12: 613–20

7. Moore GJ, Bebchuk JM, Parrish JK, et al. Temporal dissociation between lithium-induced changes in frontal lobe myo-inositol and clinical response in manic–depressive illness. Am J Psychiatry 1999; 156: 1902–8

8. Davanzo P, Thomas MA, Yue K, et al. Decreased anterior cingulate myo-inositol/ creatine spectroscopy resonance with lithium treatment in children with bipolar disorder. Neuropsychopharmacology 2001; 24: 359–69

9. Silverstone PH, Wu RH, O'Donnell T, et al. Chronic treatment with both lithium and sodium valproate may normalize phosphoinositol cycle activity in bipolar patients. Hum Psychopharmacol 2002; 17: 321–7

10. Friedman SD, Dager SR, Parow A, et al. Lithium and valproic acid treatment effects on brain chemistry in bipolar disorder. Biol Psychiatry 2004; 56: 340–8

11. Dager SR, Friedman SD, Parow A, et al. Brain metabolic alterations in medication-free patients with bipolar disorder. Arch Gen Psychiatry 2004; 61: 450–8

12. Moore GJ, Bebchuk JM, Hasanat K, et al. Lithium increases N-acetyl-aspartate in the human brain: in vivo evidence in support of bcl-2's neurotrophic effects? Biol Psychiatry 2000; 48: 1–8

13. Silverstone PH, Wu RH, O'Donnell T, et al. Chronic treatment with lithium, but not sodium valproate, increases cortical N-acetyl-aspartate concentrations in euthymic bipolar patients. Int Clin Psychopharmacol 2003; 18: 73–9

14. Brambilla P, Stanley JA, Sassi RB, et al. 1H MRS study of dorsolateral prefrontal cortex in healthy individuals before and after lithium administration. Neuropsychopharmacology 2004; 29: 1918–24

15. Strakowski SM, DelBello MP, Adler C, et al. Neuroimaging in bipolar disorder. Bipolar Disord 2000; 2: 148–64

16. Lyoo IK, Demopulos CM, Hirashima F, et al. Oral choline decreases brain purine levels in lithium-treated subjects with rapid-cycling bipolar disorder: a double-blind trial using proton and lithium magnetic resonance spectroscopy. Bipolar Disord 2003; 5: 300–6

17. Komoroski RA. Applications of (7)Li NMR in biomedicine. Magn Reson Imaging 2000; 18: 103–16

18. González RG, Guimaraes AR, Sachs GS, et al. Measurement of human brain lithium in vivo by MR spectroscopy. Am J Neuroradiol 1993; 14: 1027–37

19. Plenge P, Stensgaard A, Jensen HV, et al. 24-Hour lithium concentration in human brain studied by Li-7 magnetic resonance spectroscopy. Biol Psychiatry 1994; 36: 511–16

20. Soares JC, Boada F, Spencer S, et al. Brain lithium concentrations in bipolar disorder patients: preliminary (7) Li magnetic resonance studies at 3 T. Biol Psychiatry 2001; 49: 437–43

21. Moore CM, Demopulos CM, Henry ME, et al. Brain-to-serum lithium ratio and age: an in vivo magnetic resonance spectroscopy study. Am J Psychiatry 2002; 159: 1240–2

22. O'Donnell T, Rotzinger S, Ulrich M, et al. Effects of chronic lithium and sodium valproate on concentrations of brain amino acids. Eur Neuropsychopharmacol 2003; 13: 220–7

23. Yildiz A, Moore CM, Sachs GS, et al. Lithium-induced alterations in nucleoside triphosphate levels in human brain: a proton-decoupled 31P magnetic resonance spectroscopy study. Psychiatry Res 2005; 138: 51–9

24. Kato T, Fujii K, Kamiya A, Kato N. White matter hyperintensity detected by magnetic resonance imaging and lithium response in bipolar disorder, a preliminary observation. Psychiatry Clin Neurosci 2000; 54: 11720

25. Kato T, Inubushi T, Kato N. Prediction of lithium response by 31P-MRS in bipolar disorder. Int J Neuropsychopharmacol 2000; 3: 835

26. Kato T, Murashita J, Kamiya A, et al. Decreased brain in tracellular pH measured by

31P-MRS in bipolar disorder: A confirmation in drug-free patients and correlation with white matter hyperintensity. Eur Arch Psychiatry Clin Neurosci 1998; 248: 3016

27. Murashita J, Kato T, Shioiri T, et al. Altered brain energy metabolism in lithium-resistant bipolar disorder detected by photic stimulated 31P-MR spectroscopy. Psychol Med 2000; 30: 10715

28. Ikeda A, Kato T. Biological predictors of lithium response in bipolar disorder. Psychiatry Clin Neurosci 2003; 57: 243–50

29. Bell EC, Willson MC, Wilman AH, et al. Lithium and valproate attenuate dextro-amphetamine-induced changes in brain activation. Hum Psychopharmacol 2005; 20: 87–96

30. Goodwin GM, Cavanagh JT, Glabus MF, et al. Uptake of 99mTc-exametazime shown by single photon emission computed tomography before and after lithium withdrawal in bipolar patients: association with mania. Br J Psychiatry 1997; 170: 426–30

35 Genetic factors and response to lithium treatment

Martin Alda, Paul Grof, Petr Zvolsky

Contents   Family and family-history studies of responders to lithium prophylaxis • Molecular genetic studies – are there 'genes for lithium response'? • Can investigations of lithium responders help identify genes for bipolar disorder? • Conclusions

FAMILY AND FAMILY-HISTORY STUDIES OF RESPONDERS TO LITHIUM PROPHYLAXIS

As lithium prophylaxis entered the mainstream of psychiatric treatment, the question of who responds and who does not became more and more important. This was especially so as the goal of prophylaxis is to prevent recurrences that are often difficult to anticipate because they can be separated by months or even years of spontaneous remissions. Yet, for clinical practice, it is relevant to identify as early as possible those who can benefit from the treatment and those who cannot. Among the clinical variables examined in this context was family history. Work of several research groups in the early 1970s suggested that patients with a family history of manic-depressive illness had significantly greater benefit from lithium than those with negative family histories[1,2]. Several subsequent studies agreed with these first observations[3–6]. The consensus was not unanimous, however, and several papers either could not find any difference between responders and non-responders[7,8], or found the opposite, that is subjects with a positive family history not responding as well[9,10].

The available published studies are summarized in Table 35.1. They can be divided into family studies in which a substantial majority or all of living relatives were examined in person, and family-history studies in which details of psychiatric morbidity in families were obtained by interviewing one or more selected family members.

It is apparent from the table that most reports found the above-mentioned association. How then do we reconcile these findings with the smaller number of disagreeing papers?

The discrepant findings have probably reflected differing methodologies, in particular in defining lithium responders and non-responders, and in diagnosing mood disorders.

Table 35.1 Family/family-history studies and response to lithium (Li)

Study	Type	Dependent variable	Probands	Treatment duration	Association of FH and Li response	Notes
Aronoff and Epstein, 1970[43]	FH	Family history of major psychiatric disorders (mood disorders, suicide or hospitalization)	7 R 5 NR	2 years on average	+	Positive FH more frequent in responders (5 out of 7) than in non-responders (1 out of 5)
Mendlewicz et al., 1973[1]	F	Family history of BD and UD	24 R 12 NR	6–37 months	+	More frequent history of BD in families of R
Zvolsky et al., 1974[2]	F	Rates of major psychiatric disorders in first-degree relatives	58 BD	>2 years	+	Higher rates in relatives of complete and partial responders
Prien et al., 1974[44]	FH	Response to lithium prophylaxis	48 R 43 NR	2 years	0	Better response in subjects with FH of BD (88% compared to 49% in FH group), but the results were not statistically significant
Svestka and Nahunek, 1975[45]	FH	Response to lithium prophylaxis	55 R 26 NR	1–7 years	+	FH of endogeneous psychoses and suicide more common in R
Dunner et al. 1976[7]	FH	Relapse rate on Li	52 R 44 NR	1–45 months	0	No effect of FH of BD or UD
Misra and Burns, 1977[9]	FH	Family history of affective disorders	9 NR	2–8 years	–	7 out of 9 NR had FH of AD; no R included in the sample
Zvolsky et al., 1979[46]	F	Rates of major psychiatric disorders in first-degree relatives	26 R 17 NR	> 7 years	+	Higher rates in relatives of R compared to NR
Mendlewicz, 1979[47]	F	Concordance rates in twins	24 R 18 NR	> 2 years	+	Higher concordance (both MZ and DZ) for R
Maj et al., 1984[3]	FH	Family history of BD, UD and other disorders	59 R 41 NR	2 years	+	More frequent FH of BD in relatives of R
Smeraldi et al., 1984[4]	F	Morbidity risks of AD in first-degree relatives	92 R 53 NR	> 3 years	+	Higher rates of AD in relatives of R

continued over

Table 35.1 *continued* Family/family-history studies and response to lithium (Li)

Study	Type	Dependent variable	Probands	Treatment duration	Association of FH and Li response	Notes
Mander, 1986[49]	FH	Likelihood of re-admission while on lithium	98 BD I, 48 treated with lithium	3.1 ± 2.4 years	0	FH+ in 30% (3/10) of relapsed subjects and in 32% (12/38) of the non-relapsed group
Abou-Saleh and Coppen, 1986[5]	FH	Affective Morbidity Index (AMI) during Li treatment	27 BD	2 years	+	Lower morbidity among patients with FH of BD or UD
Shapiro et al., 1989[48]	FH	Relapse rate on Li	117	2 years	0	Relapse rate on Li or imipramine unrelated to FH
Grof et al., 1994[6]	F	Morbidity risks of BD, UD and SZ in first-degree relatives	71 R 50 NR	3–20 years	+	Increased risk of BD in families of R; higher rates of SZ in families of NR
Engstrom et al., 1997[10]	F	Frequency of episodes on Li	51 familial (FH+) 47 non-familial (FH−)	13 ± 8 years in FH+; 11 ± 8 years in FH−	-	0.32 ± 0.44 in FH+ patients 0.58 ± 0.70 in FH− patients
Coryell et al., 2000[8]	F and FH	Morbidity risks of BD, UD, SZ and alcoholism in first-degree relatives	Grouped by morbidity on lithium (62 low, 55 medium, 69 high)	7.8 ± 5.8 years 5.7 ± 4.1 years 5.5 ± 4.5 years	0	No major differences between the groups

F, family study; FH, family-history study; R, responders; NR, non-responders; BD, bipolar disorder; UD, unipolar depression; AD, affective disorder; SZ, schizophrenia; FH+, family-history positive; FH−, family-history negative

For example, the earlier reports based their definition on a categorical approach (responder – non-responder) usually requiring long-term follow-up and evidence of high recurrence risk[6]. On the other hand, some of the more recent studies examined the rates of episodes before and during lithium treatment. In this case, especially in individuals observed for only a few years, variability of the natural clinical course could bias the results towards the null hypothesis. Furthermore, not all studies included subjects treated with lithium monotherapy (and according to a research protocol), introducing another source of 'noise' in the data.

In a way, this discussion parallels the discussion of the clinical heterogeneity of bipolar disorder, namely whether the response is distributed along a single continuum or whether it is possible to identify two separate groups: responders and non-responders. This point is discussed in detail in Chapter 14. Needless to say, no conclusive study has been done, although the comparisons of responders and non-responders as well as individual observations of an extremely favorable response in subjects with high morbidity recorded prior to lithium treatment appear to favor the two-group side.

Furthermore, the authors of this chapter pointed out elsewhere that at least some of the discrepancies not only in the family-history data, but also in the effectiveness of lithium in general could be explained by trends in diagnosis of mood disorders and diagnostic shifts among conditions considered in the differential diagnostic spectrum of mood disorders[11]. Specifically, the early success and resulting popularity of lithium may have led to overdiagnosis of mood disorders at the expense of psychotic disorder in the late 1970s[12]. This trend was subsequently reinforced by tightening of the diagnostic criteria for schizophrenia on one hand and loosening the criteria for mood disorders on the other in DSM-III and later

editions. Temporarily this was made even more complicated by the elimination of schizoaffective disorder in the DSM system. Since the 1990s we have witnessed a further expansion of the bipolar disorder spectrum, leading to an especially high reported prevalence of 'soft-spectrum' bipolar disorders and bipolar II disorder in particular[13]. Thus it appears that more subjects are now diagnosed with bipolar-spectrum disorders, who do not respond to lithium, but rather to anticonvulsants[14]. These same trends are likely to have an effect on the diagnoses in relatives, influencing the outcomes of family studies.

Another possibility to consider is that these are all chance results. That is, the null hypothesis of no association is true, but due to random fluctuations researchers obtain results pointing in different directions. Although this could be the case theoretically, the fact that the seemingly discrepant findings can be to a large extent explained by methodological differences, make this interpretation unlikely.

Finally, we cannot discount researcher bias. While the first studies would have been less likely to put weight on a conclusion in one direction rather than the other, the subsequent investigations may have been motivated by attempts to 'replicate' previous findings. However, it seems that the observed trend is the opposite – more recent studies reporting more contradictory findings than the earlier ones.

The debate about the relationship between psychiatric family history and the treatment response raises questions about the genetic (or rather familial) basis of the lithium response itself. Several small studies suggested that this could indeed be the case. For instance, Maj quotes his earlier observation of 11 pairs of relatives treated with lithium, of whom nine were concordant for the response[15]. A similar observation had been made earlier in a report on children of lithium responders[16]. Involving a moderately large sample, we investigated the response to lithium in relatives of responders and compared them with the response rates in unselected bipolar subjects[17]. The study supported the familial aggregation of a favorable response in families. Among the relatives, the rate of response was 67% in comparison with 35% responders in the comparison sample (odds ratio 3.71, 95% confidence interval 1.28–10.82).

MOLECULAR GENETIC STUDIES – ARE THERE 'GENES FOR LITHIUM RESPONSE'?

Since the late 1990s several studies investigated differences between responders and non-responders to lithium in a case–control manner. Ideally, such studies should also include a group of unaffected subjects. Possible differences could be related to the response itself or reflect differences with respect to specific subgroups of illness. Two genes attracted particular attention: the serotonin transporter gene and the inositol monophosphatase gene.

Serotonin transporter gene

The gene coding for the serotonin transporter is among the most commonly studied genes in psychiatry. It has been examined in connection with a number of clinical conditions as well as the response to antidepressants. With respect to bipolar disorder, earlier association studies could not find evidence of involvement of the gene in susceptibility to the illness itself. The most commonly investigated polymorphism of the gene is the insertion/deletion polymorphism in the promoter region. It has two variants, one commonly labeled as short (s) associated with lower transcriptional activity of the gene and the other one known as the long variant (l). Two studies suggested that the short allele may be associated with a poor response to lithium prophylaxis[18,19]. This is to some extent compatible with another study of antidepressant-induced mania[20]. However, there have been several other studies suggesting the contrary[21,22]. While the authors of the latter study considered their work to be a replication of their previous results[18], they could not find a poorer response in the ss individuals. These results can be interpreted in several ways – either as chance results or perhaps they could indicate a linkage disequilibrium of the studied marker with another functional polymorphism located nearby. Searches for such a polymorphism have not however, been successful.

Inositol monophosphatase gene

Another logical candidate gene for lithium responsiveness has been the gene for inositol monophosphatase (*IMPA*). The choice is obvious for two reasons. First, the enzyme is inhibited by lithium in therapeutic concentrations; it has been suggested that this blockade is the key to the mood-stabilizing properties of lithium[23]. Second, two genes, *IMPA1* and *IMPA2*, coding for inositol monophosphatases (IMPases) have been identified, with one of the genes, *IMPA2*, located in the chromosomal region 18p11.2. This region has been implicated by several linkage studies of bipolar samples, the first having been reported by Berrettini *et al.*[24]. However, none of the positive linkage reports has studied lithium responders. In fact, the only association and linkage studies of markers on chromosome 18 in lithium-responsive samples have been equivocal at best[25–27]. Furthermore, the two existing association studies of the *IMPA2* gene comparing responders and non-responders to lithium, one by Sjoholt *et al.*[28] and the other by Dimitrova *et al.*[29] have been negative.

Other candidate genes

A promising line of work links the response to the lithium to the mitochondrial gene *XBP1*. The gene is known to play a key role in the endoplasmic reticulum stress response. First, Kakiuchi *et al.* reported an association of the $-116C \rightarrow G$ polymorphism in the promoter region to bipolar disorder[30]. The polymorphism appears to be functional and those with the G allele show diminished expression of the gene. Interestingly, the impaired expression of the gene could be rescued by valproate but not by lithium *in vitro*. Subsequently, Masui *et al.* linked the same locus to response to lithium[31]. In their study patients who carried at least one C allele were more likely to respond to lithium. Taken together these two studies may be pointing to a subtype of illness associated with a lower expression of *XBP1* and *non-responsive to lithium*. It still remains to be shown whether these patients respond clinically to valproate.

Finally, there have been individual studies of numerous other candidate genes both positive and negative that remain non-replicated. The positive ones included genes for tryptophan hydroxylase[32], 10398 polymorphism in mitochondrial DNA[33], glycogen synthase kinase 3β[34], polymorphic inositol polyphosphate 1-phosphatase (INPP1)[35,36], phospholipase $C\gamma$ 1[37] and brain-derived neurotrophic factor[38]. The phospholipase $C\gamma$ gene has also been studied by Turecki *et al.* as a susceptibility gene for bipolar disorder responsive to lithium[39]. These investigators found similar allele frequencies in their cases, as did Lovlie *et al.* in the subgroup of responders[37], namely an increased frequency of the 'short' alleles of the same intronic dinucleotide-repeat marker.

Additionally, there have also been a number of negatives or inconclusive studies – these included dopamine receptor genes D2, D3, D4, as well as genes for the GABA receptor A1 subunit, serotonin receptors 5HT1A, 5HT2A, 5HT2C, COMT, MAO-A and G-β3 (for a more detailed review, see, for instance, reference 40).

The replicated findings are especially promising, but they also caution that the effects of any individual locus are relatively small and may not be practically applicable. The major promise of these findings is the possibility of better understanding the mechanisms involved in mood stabilization. Such an understanding could ultimately lead to a development of newer and specific treatments. On the other hand, the small effect size makes such findings less likely to be the sole or main factor in treatment decisions.

CAN INVESTIGATIONS OF LITHIUM RESPONDERS HELP IDENTIFY GENES FOR BIPOLAR DISORDER?

The clinical characteristics of patients who respond to lithium are very similar to what could be considered a typical or 'textbook' presentation of bipolar disorder. These are described in more detail elsewhere in this book (see Chapter 14). The specific clinical picture with a high degree of familiality, and low rates of co-morbid conditions led several research groups to suggest that such patients could represent a genetically more homogeneous form of bipolar disorder. This argument has been strengthened by several studies of the mode of inheritance as well. In 1984, Smeraldi *et al.*[4] tested several genetic models and found that the familial transmission of mood disorders in families of lithium responders was compatible with a major-gene effect. Similar conclusions were reached in two subsequent studies of two independent Canadian sets of families, in which both the best-fitting genetic model was autosomal recessive, with substantially weaker support for X-linked inheritance, and there was no evidence of a polygenic model with sex-specific thresholds[41,42]. It is important to point out that these studies do not constitute a proof of single-gene inheritance, but merely indicate that the observed familial transmission is compatible with such a model.

Since the mid-1990s several groups have started working more or less systematically with lithium-responsive probands in linkage and association studies. While results of these investigations are still preliminary, they support the view of lithium-responsive bipolar disorder as a distinct group. Specifically, in a series of linkage studies and two full genome scans, we have found no support for several of the previously reported linkage regions, namely 18p and 18q, 13q and 22q[26,27]. The negative findings fit the general picture of linkage findings in bipolar disorder with the chromosome 18 linkage, particularly convincing in families with co-morbid panic disorder, rapid cycling and high rates of bipolar II disorder, and evidence of linkage to chromosomes 13 and 22 being found in families with a high prevalence of psychotic symptoms. These differences suggest that there will probably be different genetic contributions to bipolar disorders of the classical, lithium-responsive type and to other subtypes in the bipolar spectrum that are more linked to co-morbidities and psychotic disturbances.

CONCLUSIONS

The promising initial findings of an association between a family history of bipolar disorder and a favorable long-term lithium response have become somewhat obscured by more recent family and family-history studies. However, these discrepancies could be explained by the phenotypic heterogeneity of mood disorders and may stimulate further molecular genetic research of more clinically homogeneous forms of the illness.

For future studies several useful lessons seem to have emerged from the largely discrepant findings. To proceed productively in genetic studies of lithium response, the designs will have to pay more attention to methodological challenges, in particular the variety of benefits lithium provides for psychiatric disorders, the phenotypic heterogeneity of bipolar disorders, the identification of true lithium responders, and the multivariate interaction of the involved clinical and biologic factors.

REFERENCES

1. Mendlewicz J, Fieve RR, Stallone F. Relationship between the effectiveness of lithium therapy and family history. Am J Psychiatry 1973; 130: 1011–13
2. Zvolsky P, Vinarova E, Dostal T, Soucek K. Family history of manic-depressive and endogenous depressive patients and clinical effect of treatment with lithium. Activ Nerv Suppl 1974; 16: 194–5
3. Maj M, Del Vecchio M, Starace F, et al. Prediction of affective psychoses response to lithium prophylaxis: the role of socio-demographic, clinical, psychological and biological variables. Acta Psychiatr Scand 1984; 69: 37–44
4. Smeraldi E, Petroccione A, Gasperini M, et al. The search for genetic homogeneity in affective disorders. J Affect Disord 1984; 7: 99–107
5. Abou-Saleh M, Coppen A. Who responds to prophylactic lithium? J Affect Disord 1986; 10: 115–25
6. Grof P, Alda M, Grof E, et al. Lithium response and genetics of affective disorders. J Affect Disord 1994; 32: 85–95
7. Dunner DL, Fleiss JL, Fieve RR. Lithium carbonate prophylaxis failure. Br J Psychiatry 1976; 129: 40–4
8. Coryell W, Akiskal H, Leon AC, et al. Family history and symptom levels during treatment for bipolar I affective disorder. Biol Psychiatry 2000; 47: 1034–42

9. Misra PC, Burns BH. 'Lithium non-responders' in a lithium clinic. Acta Psychiatr Scand 1976; 55: 32–8

10. Engstrom C, Astrom M, Nordqvist-Karlsson B, et al. Relationship between prophylactic effect of lithium therapy and family history of affective disorders. Biol Psychiatry 1997; 42: 425–33

11. Grof P, Alda M. Discrepancies in the efficacy of lithium. Arch Gen Psychiatry 2000; 57: 191

12. Stoll AL, Tohen M, Baldessarini RJ, et al. Shifts in diagnostic frequencies of schizophrenia and major affective disorders at six North American psychiatric hospitals, 1972–1988. Am J Psychiatry 1993; 150: 1668–73

13. MacQueen GM, Hajek T, Alda M. The phenotypes of bipolar disorder: relevance for genetic investigations. Mol Psychiatry 2005; 10: 811–26

14. Passmore M, Garnham J, Duffy A, et al. Phenotypic spectra of bipolar disorder in responders to lithium versus lamotrigine. Bipolar Disord 2003; 5: 110–14

15. Maj M. Clinical prediction of response to lithium prophylaxis in bipolar patients: a critical update. Lithium 1992; 3: 15–21

16. McKnew DH, Cytryn L, Buchsbaum MS, et al. Lithium in children of lithium-reponding parents. Psychiatr Res 1981; 4: 171–80

17. Grof P, Duffy A, Cavazzoni P, et al. Is response to prophylactic lithium a familial trait? J Clin Psychiatry 2002; 63: 942–7

18. Serretti A, Lilli R, Mandelli L, et al. Serotonin transporter gene associated with lithium prophylaxis in mood disorders. Pharmacogenomics J 2001; 1: 71–7

19. Rybakowski JK, Suwalska A, Czerski PM, et al. Prophylactic effect of lithium in bipolar affective illness may be related to serotonin transporter genotype. Pharmacol Rep 2005; 57: 124–7

20. Mundo E, Walker M, Cate T, et al. The role of serotonin transporter protein gene in antidepressant-induced mania in bipolar disorder. Arch Gen Psychiatry 2001; 58: 539–44

21. Del Zompo M, Ardau R, Palmas MA, et al. Lithium response: association study with two candidate gene [Abstract]. Mol Psychiatry 1999; 4: 66–7

22. Serretti A, Malitas PN, Mandelli L, et al. Further evidence for a possible association between serotonin transporter gene and lithium prophylaxis in mood disorders. Pharmacogenom J 2005; 4: 267–73

23. Berridge MJ. The biology and medicine of calcium signalling. Mol Cell Endocrinol 1994; 98: 119–24

24. Berrettini WH, Ferraro TN, Goldin LR, et al. Chromosome 18 DNA markers and manic-depressive illness: evidence for a susceptibility gene. Proc Natl Acad Sci USA 1994; 91: 5918–21

25. Turecki G, Alda M, Grof P, et al. No association between chromosome-18 markers and lithium responsive affective disorders. Psychiatr Res 1996; 63: 17–23

26. Turecki G, Grof P, Cavazzoni P, et al. Lithium responsive bipolar disorder, unilineality, and chromosome 18: a linkage study. Am J Med Genet 1999; 88: 411–15

27. Turecki G, Grof P, Grof E, et al. Mapping susceptibility genes for bipolar disorder: a pharmacogenetic approach based on excellent response to lithium. Mol Psychiatry 2001; 6: 570–8

28. Sjoholt G, Ebstein RP, Lie RT, et al. Examination of IMPA1 and IMPA2 genes in manic–depressive patients: association between IMPA2 promoter polymorphisms and bipolar disorder. Mol Psychiatry 2004; 9: 621–9

29. Dimitrova A, Milanova V, Krastev S, et al. Association study of myo-inositol monophosphatase 2 (IMPA2) polymorphisms with bipolar affective disorder and response to lithium treatment. Pharmacogenomics J 2005; 5: 35–41

30. Kakiuchi C, Iwamoto K, Ishiwata M, et al. Impaired feedback regulation of XBP1 as a genetic risk factor for bipolar disorder. Nat Genet 2003; 35: 171–5

31. Masui T, Hashimoto R, Kusumi I, et al. A possible association between the -116C/G single nucleotide polymorphism of the XBP1 gene and lithium prophylaxis in bipolar disorder. Int J Neuropsychopharmacol 2006; 9: 83–8

32. Serretti A, Lilli R, Lorenzi C, et al. Tryptophan hydroxylase gene and response to lithium

prophylaxis in mood disorders. J Psychiatr Res 1999; 33: 371–7

33. Washizuka S, Ikeda A, Kato N, Kato T. Possible relationship between mitochondrial DNA polymorphisms and lithium response in bipolar disorder. Int J Neuropsychopharmacol 2003; 6: 421–4

34. Benedetti F, Serretti A, Pontiggia A, et al. Long-term response to lithium salts in bipolar illness is influenced by the glycogen synthase kinase 3-beta -50 T/C SNP. Neurosci Lett 2005; 376: 51–5

35. Steen VM, Lovlie R, Osher Y, et al. The polymorphic inositol polyphosphate 1-phosphatase gene as a candidate for pharmacogenetic prediction of lithium-responsive manic-depressive illness. Pharmacogenetics 1998; 8: 259–68

36. Lovlie R, Berle JO, Steen VM. A role of the human inositol polyphosphate 1-phosphatase gene (INPP1) in lithium-treated bipolar disorder? Mol Psychiatry 1999; 4 (Suppl 1): S68

37. Lovlie R, Berle JO, Stordal E, Steen VM. The phospholipase C-γ1 gene (PLCG1) and lithium-responsive bipolar disorder: re-examination of an intronic dinucleotide repeat polymorphism. Psychiatr Genet 2001; 11: 41–4

38. Rybakowski JK, Suwalska A, Skibinska M, et al. Prophylactic lithium response and polymorphism of the brain-derived neurotrophic factor gene. Pharmacopsychiatry 2005; 38: 166–70

39. Turecki G, Grof P, Cavazzoni P, et al. Evidence for a role of phospholipase C-gamma1 in the pathogenesis of bipolar disorder. Mol Psychiatry 1998; 3: 534–8

40. Alda M. Pharmacogenetic aspects of bipolar disorder. Pharmacogenomics 2003; 4: 35–40

41. Alda M, Grof P, Grof E, et al. Mode of inheritance in families of patients with lithium

– responsive affective disorders. Acta Psychiatr Scand 1994; 90: 304–10

42. Alda M, Grof E, Cavazzoni P, et al. Autosomal recessive inheritance of affective disorders in families of responders to lithium prophylaxis? J Affect Disord 1997; 44: 153–7

43. Aronoff MS, Epstein RS. Factors associated with poor response to lithium carbonate: a clinical study. Am J Psychiatry 1970; 127: 472–80

44. Prien RF, Caffey EM, Klett CJ. Factors associated with treatment success in lithium carbonate prophylaxis: report of the Veterans Administration and National Institute of Mental Health Collaborative Study Group. Arch Gen Psychiatry 1974; 31: 189–92

45. Svestka J, Nahunek K. The result of lithium therapy in acute phases of affective psychoses and some other prognostical factors of lithium prophylaxis. Activ Nerv Sup 1975; 17: 270–1

46. Zvolsky P, Dvorakova M, Soucek K, et al. Clinical use of lithium salts from the genetic viewpoint. In Cooper TB, Gershon S, Kline NS, Schou M, eds. Lithium. Controversies and Unresolved Issues. Amsterdam: Excerpta Medica, 1979

47. Mendlewicz J. Prediction of treatment outcome: family and twin studies in lithium prophylaxis and the question of lithium red blood cell/plasma ratios. In Cooper TB, Gershon S, Kline NS, Schou M, eds. Lithium. Controversies and unresolved issues. Amsterdam: Excerpta Medica, 1979

48. Shapiro DR, Quitkin FM, Fleiss JL. Response to maintenance therapy in bipolar illness – effect of index episode. Arch Gen Psychiatry 1989; 46: 401–5

49. Mander AJ. Clinical prediction of outcome and lithium response in bipolar affective disorder. J Affect Disord 1986; 11: 35–41

36 Effects of lithium on behavior and cognition in animals and healthy humans

Robert H Belmaker, Alona Shaldubina, Yuly Bersudsky

Contents   Lithium effects on animal models of mania and depression • Lithium effects on cognition • Conclusions

LITHIUM EFFECTS ON ANIMAL MODELS OF MANIA AND DEPRESSION

Besides clinical or psychological studies, animal studies have been a mainstay of the study of lithium effects on behavior. These animal studies were reviewed in 1991[1] and again in 2003[2]. The overriding majority of studies in this field have used the concept of pharmacologically induced mania and depression and have attempted to show prevention by lithium. The usual agent for pharmacologic induction of mania has been amphetamine, although more specific and direct dopamine agonists such as quinpirole have also been used[3]. Reserpine or tetrabenazine to induce depression have also been studied[4]. A background concept has been the fact that low-dose amphetamine has effects primarily on open field activity, whereas higher-dose amphetamine causes stereotypy[5,6]. Dopamine blockers are well known to block both the low-dose hyperactivity and the high-dose stereotypy of amphetamine, and this fits their usefulness in both mania and schizophrenia[7]. Therefore, attempts have been made to look at the effect of lithium pre-treatment on low-dose amphetamine effects versus high-dose amphetamine effects, the hypothesis being that lithium as an antimanic agent will prevent the effects of low-dose amphetamine but, because it is devoid of true antipsychotic properties, it will not be able to affect amphetamine-induced stereotypy. Often an underlying biochemical hypothesis was that low-dose amphetamine released mostly serotonin and norepinephrine, whereas high-dose amphetamine released more dopamine. All of these assumptions, hypotheses and preconceptions are today viewed skeptically. They were heuristic as hypotheses that generated much good research; however, the yield of robust replicable data has been poor. Given the fact that modern studies of psychopharmacologic agents often require hundreds of patients to show statistically significant effects, it may not be surprising that animal studies with 10–15 rats in each group often come up with conflicting results. The heterogeneity of the amphetamine response is well known[8], and so the lithium response may also be heterogeneous in outbred rat strains[9,10].

Perhaps the most exciting advance in this field has occurred recently, in a paper by O'Brien et al.[11], who used a specific regimen of lithium administration to mice: mice received 0.2% lithium chloride in food for a period of 5 days, followed by 0.4% for an additional 10 days, and showed robust effects in the Porsolt forced swim test. Previous studies of lithium in the Porsolt forced swim test were equivocal, although Bourin's group[12,13] showed that lithium could reliably potentiate the effects of other antidepressants. The study of Bourin et al.[12,13] used an acute lithium dose, but it fit the preconceived notion that in the clinic lithium is an augmenter of the antidepressant response and not a powerful antidepressant itself. However, the paradigm of O'Brien et al.[11] suggests a powerful effect of lithium in the Porsolt forced swim test. This is unlikely to be an artifact, since activity in the Porsolt forced swim test requires an increase in struggling behavior. Previous concerns about lithium artifacts have usually pointed out that lithium patients experience some sense of malaise, muscle weakness and nausea. These would be unlikely to cause the reported effects in the Porsolt forced swim test.

We (Shaldubina et al., submitted) have been able to replicate the finding of O'Brien et al.[11] and have shown that it is dependent on blood levels of lithium. Blood levels greater than 1 mmol/l are necessary for the robust effect found by O'Brien et al.[11], whereas blood levels

of 0.7 mmol/l showed no effect in the Porsolt forced swim test. Many studies of chronic lithium in the past were satisfied with levels of 0.7 mmol/l on the average and even studies with higher blood levels had a significant proportion of the animals with blood levels below 0.7 mmol/l. This robust effect of lithium on the Porsolt forced swim test provides an opening for behavioral pharmacologic analysis in the future. For instance, questions can be asked such as whether pre-treatment with p-chlorophenylanine (PCPA), a serotonin synthesis inhibitor, will prevent the effect of lithium in the Porsolt forced swim test or whether presynaptic $5\text{-HT}_{1a/1b}$ or postsynaptic 5-HT_2 or β-adrenergic receptor agonists/antagonists will modulate this effect. A recent hypothesis of antidepressant action is induction of neurogenesis in the hippocampus. It could be an interesting question, whether TrkB (brain-derived neurotrophic factor (BDNF)) receptor agonists/antagonists will affect lithium's antidepressant effect in the Porsolt forced swim test. A key question would be whether other mood stabilizers such as valproate have a similar effect in this test. A remaining conundrum is whether the weight loss due to reduced appetite in chronically lithium-treated rats might cause increased activity in the Porsolt swim test. This needs to be performed by 'yoking' mice to others who are eating lithium and let them eat the same amount per day as do the lithium-treated animals. It is also possible to add a non-toxic bitter taste to the control food to reduce the food intake and to see whether this affects the Porsolt results. Our finding that the lithium effects in the Porsolt swim test require a blood level greater than 1 mmol/l is congruent with clinical reports that the antidepressant effects of lithium require higher blood levels than the prophylactic effect.

The effect of lithium to block hyperactivity in rats has also been given new impetus by a paper from Caron's group[14]. They injected dopamine transporter knock-out mice with lithium (50, 100 or 200 mg/kg) a half-hour after the mice were placed in an open field and found significant reduction in horizontal activity in mice injected with 100 and 200 mg lithium. This paradigm had previously been used by Nixon et al.[15] and positive results had also been found. However, in humans even very high doses of lithium do not have immediate effects in mania but clearly do have side-effects such as nausea and muscle weakness. Therefore, it is difficult to evaluate these acute effects reported by Caron's group[14], especially in light of the long history of contradictory results in this field. Several reports demonstrate inhibition of amphetamine-induced hyperactivity by acute and chronic lithium pre-treatment in rats and mice[6,10,16–21]. However, other publications show an absence of a lithium effect in this model[7,22–25].

It is possible to give amphetamine or methylphenidate to humans on chronic lithium, and many such studies have been carried out[9,26–29]. While some have claimed marked effects of lithium to attenuate the amphetamine-induced response, others have found no effect at all[28]. The numbers used in these studies were smaller than the large numbers of patients required to show a lithium effect in a clinical situation, and human heterogeneity may be the answer to these contradictory results. We await a clear paradigm that will give robust findings in the amphetamine hyperactivity model of mania in humans as in rodents. Perhaps the issue is the blood lithium levels, since these have varied greatly between studies; usually levels of 0.7 mmol/l have been considered sufficiently similar to human treatment to be an acceptable model. It is unclear why behavioral effects are so difficult to demonstrate, whereas biochemical effects of lithium to a challenge in normals controls are marked and highly replicable[30]. However, this may depend on how the fundamental actions of lithium are con-

ceptualized, e.g. within a strictly behavioral (psychological) context, or rather a neurochemical context. Thus, some authors suppose a general 'softening', 'deactualizing' effect of lithium in sensory processes[31–34]; and some, though not all, existing experimental findings point in such a direction[35,36]. In contrast, it has been shown unambiguously that lithium reduces exploratory and passive avoidance behavior in the rat[32,35,37], and there might be a link to such changes in sensory perception. It could also be speculated that the well-documented anti-aggressive effect of lithium in animals[38,39] might in some way be related to changes of sensory functions.

LITHIUM EFFECTS ON COGNITION

A completely different line of investigation has studied more subtle effects of lithium on the behavior and cognition of normal volunteers or patients. Judd et al.[40,41] studied normal volunteers for 2 weeks and found subtle decreases in energy levels and cognitive performance. Many clinicians assumed that these changes parallel early side-effects with lithium in patients, and that they may disappear after long-term treatment. Müller-Oerlinghausen et al., in a placebo-controlled double-blind trial of 24 normal healthy volunteers, gave lithium for 2 weeks[42]. The subjects were tested after 1 and 2 weeks using a quantitative electroencephalogram (EEG), psychological performance and mood scales. Lithium showed a decreased flicker fusion threshold and a slight change in mood toward depression. The resting EEG also showed changes[43]. These studies, while provocative, could be questioned as to whether they relate to the side-effects of lithium during the first weeks of treatment or the episode-preventive effect. The blood levels of the patients were about 0.5 mmol/l. It should be noted that EEG effects of lithium in both normal individuals and patients are marked compared to the behavioral effects of lithium, and it is difficult to understand this phenomenon within neurological terms of routine EEG diagnostics. These effects are also extraordinarily different and in many ways opposite to the effects of other mood stabilizers such as valproate and carbamazepine. The German research group[44,45] in its interpretation of the EEG findings refers to refined constructs of 'vigilance'. Within this concept the EEG changes may indicate a reduction of degrees of freedom as to the mental functions of lithium-treated patients.

In 1985/1986 Kropf and Müller-Oerlinghausen[46,47] published results using signal detection theory and assessed visual perception in 14 manic depression patients under their usual long-term lithium treatment and after a marked reduction in dosage. The findings indicated that lithium markedly antagonized the backward masking effect, so that it must be concluded that either visual persistence is shortened, or that visual perception starts earlier and is terminated earlier. Missing in these studies was an active comparator group with a small dose of diazepam or risperidone. This would have given some idea of the effect size and also its specificity. A further interesting control within the context of our present therapeutic armamentarium would be valproate, carbamazepine and lamotrigine effects. Although the interpretation of the authors appears at first glance to contradict data by Schou[48], who studied highly creative people and found that lithium did not seem to reduce creative productivity. Interviews with artists (writers, painters, musicians) revealed that, in contrast to popular beliefs, mania is not related to artistic productivity (Müller-Oerlinghausen, personal communication). Kropf and Mueller-Oerlinghausen suggested that, due to the restricted number of degrees of freedom (in

neurophysiological or neuropsychological terms), and to the improved capability to structure visual perception, a greater stability of experience and behavior would be achieved, which might be regarded as the onset of the prophylactic action in psychological terms.

Not so rarely, patients on lithium claim a deterioration of their memory functions. Various studies, therefore, have addressed this issue. Their outcome, depending on the methodology, is heterogeneous. Whereas Carlson et al.[49], Smigan and Perres[50], Pflug et al.[51] or Squire et al.[52] did not observe a change of memory functions, the findings by Jahuar et al.[53] point to a reduced speed of information processing. Rapp and Thomas[54] as well as Kropf and Müller-Oerlinghausen[55] demonstrated a reduction of short- and long-term memory. Kropf and Müller-Oerlinghausen interpret their findings, on a significant difference in free recall over 2 weeks in healthy volunteers given lithium for 2 weeks, as a change of spontaneous initial action and thereby the will to act.

CONCLUSIONS

There are several directions in which this field can go heuristically.

(1) Development of an entirely novel model. For instance, dogs are more difficult to study than rats and more expensive, and more ethical concerns are involved. However, male dogs exposed to the scent of vaginal secretions of a female dog in heat become hyperactive, aggressive and hypersexual and will not sleep or eat for days while under the influence of this scent. Since hypersexuality and hyperactivity are clearly parts of mania, and since a new love affair is a frequent stimulus for the onset of a manic episode, this model could have face

validity. The effects of lithium and other mood stabilizers on this model could indicate an important direction. The biochemical effects of the pheromones of female canines in heat on the brain of the male dog might also elicit important information.

(2) Recent papers[11,14] suggest that the classic field of study of lithium effects on amphetamine hyperactivity or on the Porsolt test might have been in the correct direction, and that the contradictory results might have been due to inadequate lithium dosing. A major effort is now underway to resolve whether this is the case. If so, studies of other mood stabilizers and the biochemical effects of higher-dose lithium in these models could rapidly lead to new information.

(3) An example of an incomplete model is the study of Bersudsky et al.[56] showing lithium inhibition of forskolin-induced hypoactivity. This study was based on the fact that lithium biochemically inhibits forskolin rises in cyclic AMP. The behavioral finding is therefore a bioassay of the chemical finding. However, to become a model it would need to be corroborated by a finding that forskolin induces hypoactivity or a depression-like syndrome in humans.

(4) Heuristic models of the action of lithium should not restrict themselves to purely neurochemical or neurophysiological concepts. A different and separate level of explanation not simply reducible to neurochemical constructs is psychology. Some interesting theoretical approaches in the past on how to explain in psychological terms the action of lithium on experience and behavior[32,45] should be re-evaluated and expanded with modern methodology.

REFERENCES

1. Kofman O, Belmaker RH. Animal models of mania and bipolar affective illness. In Soubrié P, ed. Anxiety, Depression and Mania. New York: Karger, 1991: 103–21

2. Einat H, Manji HK, Belmaker RH. New approaches to modeling bipolar disorder. Psychopharmacol Bull 2003; 37: 47–63

3. Shaldubina A, Einat H, Szechtman H, et al. Preliminary evaluation of oral anticonvulsant treatment in the quinpirole model of bipolar disorder. J Neural Transm 2002; 109: 433–40

4. Lerer B, Ebstein RP, Felix A, Belmaker RH. Lithium amelioration of reserpine-induced hypoactivity in rats. Int Pharmacopsychiatry 1980; 15: 338–43

5. Belmaker RH, Lerer B, Klein E, Hamburger R. The use of behavioral methods in the search for compounds with lithium-like activity. In: Levy A, Spiegelstein MY, eds. Behavioral Models and the Analysis of Drug Action. Amsterdam: Elsevier; 1982: 343–56

6. Borison RL, Sabelli HC, Maple PJ, et al. Lithium prevention of amphetamine-induced 'manic' excitement and of reserpine-induced 'depression' in mice: possible role of 2-phenylethylamine. Psychopharmacology (Berl) 1978; 59: 259–62

7. Ebstein RP, Eliashar S, Belmaker RH, et al. Chronic lithium treatment and dopamine-mediated behavior. Biol Psychiatry 1980; 15: 459–67

8. Tecce JJ, Cole JO. Amphetamine effects in man: paradoxical drowsiness and lowered electrical brain acitivity (CNV). Science 1974; 185: 451–3

9. Angrist B, Gershon S. Variable attenuation of amphetamine effects by lithium. Am J Psychiatry 1979; 136: 806–10

10. Gould TJ, Keith RA, Bhat RV. Differential sensitivity to lithium's reversal of amphetamine-induced open-field activity in two inbred strains of mice. Behav Brain Res 2001; 118: 95–105

11. O'Brien WT, Harper AD, Jove F, et al. Glycogen synthase kinase-3beta haplo-insufficiency mimics the behavioral and

molecular effects of lithium. J Neurosci 2004; 24: 6791–8

12. Bourin M, Hascoet M, Colombel MC, et al. Differential effects of clonidine, lithium and quinine in the forced swimming test in mice for antidepressants: possible roles of serotoninergic systems. Eur Neuropsychopharmacol 1996; 6: 231–6

13. Redrobe JP, Bourin M. Evidence of the activity of lithium on 5-HT1B receptors in the mouse forced swimming test: comparison with carbamazepine and sodium valproate. Psychopharmacology (Berl) 1999; 141: 370–7

14. Beaulieu JM, Sotnikova TD, Yao WD, et al. Lithium antagonizes dopamine-dependent behaviors mediated by an AKT/glycogen synthase kinase 3 signaling cascade. Proc Natl Acad Sci USA 2004; 101: 5099–104

15. Nixon MK, Hascoet M, Bourin M, Colombel MC. Additive effects of lithium and antidepressants in the forced swimming test: further evidence for involvement of the serotoninergic system. Psychopharmacology (Berl) 1994; 115: 59–64

16. Berggren U. Effects of chronic lithium treatment on brain monoamine metabolism and amphetamine-induced locomotor stimulation in rats. J Neural Transm 1985; 64: 239–50

17. Berggren U, Engel J, Liljequist S. The effect of lithium on the locomotor stimulation induced by dependence-producing drugs. J Neural Transm 1981; 50: 157–64

18. Berggren U, Tallstedt L, Ahlenius S, Engel J. The effect of lithium on amphetamine-induced locomotor stimulation. Psychopharmacology (Berl) 1978; 59: 41–5

19. Flemenbaum A. Lithium and amphetamine hyperactivity in rats. Differential effect on d and l isomers? Neuropsychobiology 1975; 1: 325–34

20. Hamburger R, Robert M, Newman M, Belmaker RH. Interstrain correlation between behavioral effects of lithium and effects on cortical cyclic AMP. Pharmacol Biochem Behav 1986; 24: 9–13

21. Lerer B, Globus M, Brik E, Hamburger R, Belmaker RH. Effect of treatment and withdrawal from chronic lithium in rats on stimulant-induced responses. Neuropsychobiology 1984; 11: 28–32

22. Arriaga F, Dugovic C, Wauquier A. Effects of lithium on dopamine behavioural supersensitivity induced by rapid eye movement sleep deprivation. Neuropsychobiology 1988; 20: 23–7

23. Cappeliez P, Moore E. Effects of lithium on an amphetamine animal model of bipolar disorder. Prog Neuropsychopharmacol Biol Psychiatry 1990; 14: 347–58

24. Fessler RG, Sturgeon RD, London SF, Meltzer HY. Effects of lithium on behaviour induced by phencyclidine and amphetamine in rats. Psychopharmacology (Berl) 1982; 78: 373–6

25. Pittman KJ, Jakubovic A, Fibiger HC. The effects of chronic lithium on behavioral and biochemical indices of dopamine receptor supersensitivity in the rat. Psychopharmacology (Berl) 1984; 82: 371–7

26. Flemenbaum A. Does lithium block the effects of amphetamine? A report of three cases. Am J Psychiatry 1974; 131: 820–1

27. Huey LY, Janowsky DS, Judd LL, et al. Effects of lithium carbonate on methylphenidate-induced mood, behavior, and cognitive processes. Psychopharmacology (Berl) 1981; 73: 161–4

28. Silverstone PH, Pukhovsky A, Rotzinger S. Lithium does not attenuate the effects of D-amphetamine in healthy volunteers. Psychiatry Res 1998; 79: 219–26

29. Wald D, Ebstein RP, Belmaker RH. Haloperidol and lithium blocking of the mood response to intravenous methylphenidate. Psychopharmacology (Berl) 1978; 57: 83–7

30. Ebstein R, Belmaker R, Grunhaus L, Rimon R. Lithium inhibition of adrenaline-stimulated adenylate cyclase in humans. Nature 1976; 259: 411–13

31. Johnson FN. Effects of lithium on information processing: evidence from memory and perceptual field changes in an incidental learning task. Lithium 1991; 2: 241–6

32. Johnson FN. Chlorpromazine and lithium: effects on stimulus significance. Dis Nerv Sys 1972; 33: 235–41

33. Hines G, Poling TH. Lithium effects on active and passive avoidance behaviour in the rat. Psychopharmacology 1984; 82: 78–82

34. Johnson FN. Dissociation of vertical and horizontal components of activity in rats treated with lithium chroride. Experientia 1979; 28: 533–5

35. Gray P, Solomon J, Dunphy M, et al. Effects of lithium on open field behaviour in 'stressed' and 'unstressed' rats. Psychopharmacology 1976; 42: 243–8

36. Smith DF. Effects of lithium on behaviour: critical analysis of a school of thought. Compr Psychiatry 1977; 18: 449–52

37. Wolthuis OL, de Vroome H, Vanwersch RAP. Automatically determined effects of lithium, scopolamine and methamphetamine on motor activity of rats. Pharmacol Biochem Behav 1975; 3: 515–18

38. Sheard MH. The effect of lithium and other ions on aggressive behaviour. Mod Probl Psychopharmacol 1978; 13: 53–68

39. Sheard MH. Clinical pharmacology of aggressive behavior. Clin Neuropharmacol 1984; 7: 173–83

40. Judd LL. Effect of lithium on mood, cognition, and personality function in normal subjects. Arch Gen Psychiatry 1979; 36: 860–6

41. Judd LL, Hubbard B, Janowsky DS, et al. The effect of lithium carbonate on affect, mood, and personality of normal subjects. Arch Gen Psychiatry 1977; 34: 346–51

42. Müller-Oerlinghausen B, Hamann S, Herrmann WM, Kropf D. Effects of lithium on vigilance, psychomotoric performance and mood. Pharmakopsychiatr Neuropsychopharmakol 1979; 12: 388–96

43. Ulrich G, Herrmann WM, Hegerl U, Müller-Oerlinghausen B. Effect of lithium on the dynamics of electroencephalographic vigilance in healthy subjects. J Affect Disord 1990; 20: 19–25

44. Müller-Oerlinghausen B. Psychological effects, compliance, and response to long-term lithium. Br J Psychiatry 1982; 141: 411–19

45. Müller-Oerlinghausen B. Towards a neuropsychological model of lithium action. Pharmacopsychiatry 1987; 20: 192–4

46. Kropf D, Müller-Oerlinghausen B. Assessment of visual perception by means of the signal detection theory in patients under lithium long-term treatment. Pharmacopsychiatry 1985: 102–3

47. Kropf D, Müller-Oerlinghausen B. Effects of lithium on visual perception in manic–depressive patients without acute symptomatology. Neuropsychobiology 1986; 15: 34–42

48. Schou M. Artistic productivity and lithium prophylaxis in manic–depressive illness. Br J Psychiatry 1979; 135: 97–103

49. Carlson GA, Rapport MD, Pataki CS, Kelly KL. Lithium in hospitalized children at 4 and 8 weeks: mood. J Child Psychol Psychiatry 1992; 33: 411–25

50. Smigan L, Perris C. Memory functions and prophylactic treatment with lithium. Psychol Med 1983; 13: 529–36

51. Pflug B, Hartung M, Klemke W. Die Beeinflussung von Befindlichkeit und Leistungsfähigkeit gesunder Versuchspersonen durch Lithiumcarbonat. Pharmacopsychiatry 1980; 13: 175–81

52. Squire LR, Judd LL, Janowsky DS, Huey LY. Effects of lithium carbonate on memory and other cognitive functions. Am J Psychiatry 1980; 137: 1042–6

53. Jahuar P, McClure I, Hillary C, Watson A. Psychomotor performance of patients on maintenance lithium therapy. Hum Psychopharmacol Clin Exp 1993; 8: 141–4

54. Rapp M, Thomas MR. Lithium and memory loss. Can J Psychiatry 1979; 24: 700–1

55. Kropf D, Müller-Oerlinghausen B. Changes in learning, memory, and mood during lithium treatment. Acta Psychiatr Scand 1979; 59: 97–124

56. Bersudsky Y, Patishi Y, Bitsch Jensen J, et al. The effect of acute and chronic lithium on forskolin-induced reduction of rat activity. J Neural Transm 1997; 104: 943–52

Part D

PRACTICAL ISSUES

37 Recommendations for the safe use of lithium

Anne Berghöfer, Paul Grof, Bruno Müller-Oerlinghausen

Contents Introductory remarks • Indications/patient selection • Contraindications • Necessary screening • Initiating lithium treatment • Clinical and laboratory monitoring • Adverse effects of lithium medication • Interactions: drugs and electroconvulsant therapy • High-risk patients • Duration of therapy: criteria for discontinuing therapy • Most common mistakes in lithium treatment

INTRODUCTORY REMARKS

The focus of this chapter is on long-term treatment because of its eminent importance. For the theoretical underpinnings of the recommendations summarized here, the reader is referred to the previous chapters of this book. For the most part, our recommendations are similar to those that have now become standard in Europe and North America[1–3]. Acute and prophylactic lithium therapy follow similar basic principles. The practical management of lithium treatment in manic patients differs in several respects, although only slightly, from the general prophylaxis guidelines.

INDICATIONS/PATIENT SELECTION

Prophylactic lithium treatment in affective disorders should be initiated only if (1) the probability that a patient will experience further episodes is very high; and (2) the social repercussions and severity of these episodes justify long-term pharmacological treatment. Early in the course of the illness, however, it is often difficult to estimate the probability of recurrence, and weigh the benefits and risks of lithium treatment in individual cases. Table 37.1 provides a summary of the most important indications for lithium treatment, and the issue is discussed in greater detail in Section B of this book (Clinical Applications).

Several sets of criteria have been developed to help physicians and patients decide when best to initiate lithium prophylaxis (see Chapters 8 and 10); the best known of these are based on a study conducted by Angst et al.[4,5].

They specify that long-term lithium treatment is indicated in patients who, following the index episode for which they received acute therapy, have experienced at least another recurrence:

Table 37.1 The most important psychiatric and medical indications for acute and long-term lithium treatment

Acute	Prophylactic
Bipolar depression and augmentation in unipolar depression	Recurrent depressive disorders
Manic episode	Bipolar affective disorder
	Schizoaffective psychosis
	Pathologic aggressive behavior
	Unipolar mania
Thyrotoxicosis	Cluster headache

(1) Within a 5-year period for unipolar depressive illnesses;

(2) Within a 4-year period for bipolar psychoses;

(3) Within a 3-year period for schizoaffective psychoses.

It should be noted here that these periods should include the year in which the index episode occurred.

Following these criteria, 70% of patients with unipolar and bipolar illnesses and 58% of those with schizoaffective psychoses experienced at least two further episodes over the following 5 years. Angst's selection criteria can help physicians estimate the probability of future episodes in individual patients. In order to weigh the benefits and risks of therapy, however, it is necessary to determine:

(1) The severity and impact of previous episodes;

(2) The specific risks and contraindications of lithium therapy (and of its alternatives);

(3) The patient's acceptance of long-term treatment.

Details on how to select patients for successful long-term lithium treatment can be found in Chapter 14.

Over the past 10 years, research has confirmed that lithium has anti-suicidal effects, over and above its mood-stabilizing properties. Clinicians should thus strongly consider initiating lithium treatment in patients with mood disorders accompanied by a high risk of suicide (see Chapter 15).

In order to integrate these findings on lithium's anti-suicidal effect in routine care, the algorithm in Figure 37.1 has been developed. This figure illustrates the use of the discriminating criterion 'suicidal behavior in the patient's history'. It implies that lithium should be preferred to any other treatment option in patients with a history of suicidal behavior even if lithium would not be the first choice in terms of episode prevention. The figure suggests an operationalized procedure if the primary lithium medication has not been found successful in terms of episode prevention[6].

In recent years the use of lithium as an adjunctive acute therapy in the management of treatment-resistant depression (i.e. lithium

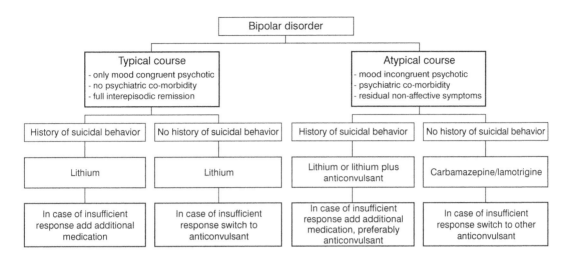

Figure 37.1 Algorithm for selecting the first-line prophylactic treatment in individual patients with bipolar disorder and for selecting a second-line drug in case the initial treatment fails

augmentation) has grown in importance (see Chapter 11).

CONTRAINDICATIONS

Contraindications to therapy with lithium are listed together with the drug's side-effects in Table 37.2 and are discussed in greater detail in the relevant chapters of this book. The only absolute contraindications to lithium are acute renal failure or acute myocardial infarction.

Relative contraindications include renal disorders accompanied by a reduced glomerular filtration rate (GFR), such as glomerular nephritis, which leads to a decrease in the renal clearance of the drug and thus a rise in serum lithium levels. Pre-existing renal tubular disorders can be aggravated by lithium treatment (Chapter 21).

Because lithium itself can lead to ataxia and muscle weakness (see Chapter 23), lithium therapy should be avoided in patients with cerebellar disorders or myasthenia gravis. Lithium is relatively contraindicated in patients with psoriasis, as the drug can lead in some patients to a worsening of symptoms (see Chapter 25).

Clinically manifest hypothyroidism can be aggravated by lithium therapy. Nevertheless, treatment with lithium is still possible as long as the condition has been stabilized through hormonal substitution treatment and the patient is monitored very closely. Lithium should not be used in patients with Addison's disease, as this illness leads to abnormally low blood sodium levels. When combined with a low-sodium diet or with diuretics (see Chapter 21), lithium can lead to toxic serum lithium concentrations due to increased reabsorption of lithium by the kidneys.

In the case of (major) surgery or anesthesia, lithium should be discontinued approximately 48 hours before the procedure in order to prevent complications resulting from drug interactions, e.g. between lithium and muscle relaxants, or electrolyte disturbances related to

Table 37.2 Absolute and relative contraindications to lithium

	Absolute	Relative	Additional conditions indicating special caution
Renal	Acute renal failure	Disorders with decreased glomerular filtration rate, tubular disorders	
Cardiovascular	Acute myocardial infarction	Cardiac rhythm disorders ('sick sinus' syndrome)	Arterial hypertension
Neurologic		Cerebellar disorders Myasthenia gravis	Cerebral sclerosis Dementia Epilepsy Parkinson's disease
Dermatologic		Psoriasis	
Endocrine		Hypothyroidism Addison's disease	
Gynecologic		Pregnancy, first trimester	Pregnancy, second and third trimesters Childbirth Breastfeeding
Hematologic		Myeloid leukemia	
General		Low-sodium diet Anesthesia/surgery	Diarrhea Vomiting Fever
Medication		Diuretics	Antiphlogistics Muscle relaxants Anesthesia Anticonvulsants Tetracyclines Spectinomycin ACE inhibitors Methyldopa Neuroleptics

ACE, angiotensin converting enzyme

the surgery itself. A substantial reduction in fluid intake prior to surgery can be especially dangerous. As soon as postoperative fluid and saline intake have returned to their normal levels, lithium therapy can usually be reinitiated at the same dosage.

Another relative contraindication to lithium therapy is myeloid leukemia, because lithium itself can lead to mild leukocytosis (see Chapter 33).

Pregnancy, childbirth, breastfeeding

Owing to a potentially elevated risk of teratogenic effects, lithium should be administered during the first trimester of pregnancy only if a patient's clinical history indicates that interrupting lithium therapy would lead to a severe relapse, endangering the patient's or the child's well-being, or if previous episodes were therapy-resistant. Because lithium is excreted in breast milk in variable concentrations, newborns should be breastfed only if lithium's concentration in milk does not exceed 10–15% of the lithium plasma level. Breastfeeding should be discontinued immediately if a baby fails to grow properly or exhibits unusual behavior or symptoms, such as diarrhea or abnormal drowsiness (see Chapter 18 for details).

NECESSARY SCREENING

As with most long-term treatments, before a patient starts lithium therapy it is important to obtain a full history and conduct a comprehensive psychiatric and medical evaluation. The examining clinician should also pay special attention to the patient's dermatologic status, body weight and neck size. It is also import to consider the patient's history of medication intake and his or her readiness to accept long-term pharmacologic treatment.

The most important laboratory tests before starting long-term lithium treatment are:

- Serum creatinine and creatinine clearance (see below);
- Dehydration test with DDAVP (vasopressin) to determine renal concentrating capacity;
- Triiodothyronine (T_3), thyroxine (T_4) and thyroid stimulating hormone (TSH) levels;
- Fasting glucose levels;
- Complete blood count;
- Electrocardiogram (ECG).

Either before or soon after lithium prophylaxis has been successfully initiated (i.e. in general within 3 months of starting long-term therapy), the patient's renal concentration capacity should be determined using the DDAVP test. This test is fast and easy to perform and will provide the physician with a reference value in the event that the patient experiences nephrologic problems at a later time. Undoubtedly, physicians will frequently encounter markedly reduced urinary osmolality in the process, which is due to the effect of lithium on water reabsorption (described in more detail in Chapter 21). Instead of determining creatinine clearance directly, it is more suitable and more precise in most cases to estimate creatinine clearance using the so-called Cockcroft equation[7]:

$$\text{Clearance of creatinine (Cl}_{Crea}) = \frac{(140 - \text{age}) \times \text{body weight [kg]}}{72 \times \text{serum creatinine [mg/dl]}}$$

(in women: $\text{Cl}_{Crea} \times 0.85$)

INITIATING LITHIUM TREATMENT

Lithium is a drug with a relatively small therapeutic index, like theophylline or cyclosporine. As a result, its dosage must be carefully tailored to the individual patient. Its dosage must be assessed and monitored, usually by performing serial serum lithium measurements. Pharmacokinetic tests to predict the dose of lithium needed for the intended serum lithium level are available. For long-term lithium treatment, these tests can be very valuable because the result is not dependent on patient compliance, unlike routine lithium level monitoring (Chapter 28).

It takes a variable length of time (from weeks to months) before lithium achieves a satisfactory stabilizing effect. After the patient has been thoroughly briefed on the use of the drug*, and after the necessary examinations have been performed (Table 37.3), treatment with one of the available lithium preparations can be initiated (listed in Table 37.4).

Currently there are a number of different lithium salts available worldwide, such as lithium carbonate, lithium sulfate, lithium citrate and lithium acetate. For efficacy, it does

---

* Schou's pocket treatment guide[8], developed especially for patients and their relatives, is well-suited for this purpose

Table 37.3 Examinations before and during lithium therapy

Before therapy	During therapy
History, psychiatric and medical assessment	Check on dosage, compliance and possible side-effects (e.g. thirst, nocturia, polyuria, tremor, weight gain)
Physical and neurologic examination	Check for goiter
Intake of other medication and chemicals	Intake of other medication and chemicals
Laboratory tests	*Laboratory tests*
Serum creatinine, estimate of creatinine clearance (Cockcroft equation)	Serum lithium level monitoring, first month weekly, first year monthly, later every 3 months
Dehydration test with DDAVP (vasopressin) to determine renal concentrating capacity	Every 6–12 months estimate of creatinine clearance (Cockcroft equation)
T_3, T_4, TSH in blood	T_3, T_4, TSH in blood
Fasting blood glucose levels	serum electrolytes including. calcium in blood
Complete blood count	complete blood count
Electrolytes including calcium in blood	ECG
ECG	
	Every 1–2 years renal concentrating capacity (DDAVP test)

T_3, triiodothyronine; T_4, thyroxine; TSH, thyroid stimulating hormone; ECG, electrocardiogram

not matter which type of lithium salt is used, as it is the lithium component of the salt – the lithium ion – that is effective. Indeed, the various lithium salts all have similar pharmacokinetics and exhibit only marginal differences from a practical point of view (see Chapter 28). In contrast, there are a number of important differences between the pharmacokinetics of conventional (i.e. rapidly absorbed) and slow-release preparations. Studies on the quality of the different preparations are available (see Chapter 28). It should be noted that some of the preparations marketed as sustained release formulations do not satisfy the pharmaceutical criteria for such compounds[9].

Lithium aspartate, which still holds a certain share of the market in Germany, has not been subjected to sufficient clinical research and thus cannot be recommended for lithium prophylaxis.

In the lithium preparations listed in Table 37.4, the amount of lithium ranges from 3.2 to 16.2 mmol/tablet. Overdosage or underdosage can result if these differences are not taken into account. Expressing the lithium content of a preparation as millimoles of lithium per tablet is more appropriate than indicating milligrams of lithium salt per tablet (still common in the USA). If lithium therapy is initiated during a symptom-free interval, the clinician can begin by administering 8–24 mmol/day, divided into two or three daily doses, depending on the age, creatinine clearance and body weight of the patient. In order to avoid initial side-effects that could negatively influence the patient's acceptance of lithium prophylaxis, treatment should begin with as low a daily dose as possible and then increased until an optimal dose is found.

As with many other drugs, lithium tablets are often prescribed to be taken 'three times a

Table 37.4 Currently marketed lithium preparations

Brand name	Country (ISO codes)	Producer	Salt	Amount of salt (mg/tablet)	Amount of lithium (mmol/tablet)	Release
Camcolit	BE, GB, NL, ZA	Norgine	Carbonate	400	10.8	TAB
Camcolit	GB, ZA	Norgine	Carbonate	250	6.8	TAB
Camcolit-400	GB	Norgine	Carbonate	400	10.8	Slow release
Carbolith	CA	ICN	Carbonate	300	8.1	Conventional
Carbolith	CA	ICN	Carbonate	600	16.2	Conventional
Carbolith	CA	ICN	Carbonate	150	4.1	Conventional
Carbolithium	IT	Elan	Carbonate	150	4.1	KAP
Carbolithium	IT	Elan	Carbonate	300	8.1	KAP
Carbolitium	BR	Eurofarma	Carbonate	300	8.1	TAB
Cibalith-S	USA	Ciba-Geigy	Citrate	752 in 5 ml	8.0 in 5 ml	Syrup
Contemnol	CZ	Slovakofarma	Carbonate	500	13.5	Slow release
Duralith	CA	Janssen	Carbonate	300	8.1	Slow release
Eskalith	USA	GlaxoSmithKline	Carbonate	300	8.1	Conventional
Eskalith	USA	GlaxoSmithKline	Carbonate	450	12.2	Slow release
Eskalith CR	USA	GlaxoSmithKline	Carbonate	300	8.1	Slow release
Lentolith	ZA	Mer-National	Carbonate	400	10.8	Slow release
Leukominerase	DE	Biosyn	Carbonate	150	4.0	Conventional
Li 450 'Ziethen'	DE	Ziethen	Carbonate	450	12.2	Slow release
Liskonum	GB	GlaxoSmithKline	Carbonate	450	12.2	Slow release
Litarex	CH	Dumex	Citrate	564	6.0	Slow release
Litarex	CH, DK, NL	Alpharma	Citrate	564	6.0	Slow release
Lithane	CA, USA	Pfizer	Carbonate	300	8.1	Conventional
Lithane	CA, USA	Pfizer	Carbonate	150	4.1	Conventional
Lithicarb	AU	Protea	Carbonate	250	6.8	Conventional
Lithiofor	CH	Lab. Vifor S.A.	Sulfate	660	12.0	Slow release
Lithiofor	GR	Nikolakopoulos	Sulfate	660	12.0	Slow release
Lithionit	SE, NO	Astra Zeneca	Sulfate	330	6.0	Slow release
Lithionit	SE, NO	Astra Zeneca	Sulfate	660	12.0	Slow release
Lithium Apogepha	DE	Apogepha	Carbonate	295	8.0	Conventional
Lithium Aspartat	DE	Köhler-Pharma	Aspartate	500	3.2	Conventional
Lithium carbonicum	CZ	Slovakofarma	Carbonate	300	8.1	Conventional

continued over

Table 37.4 *continued*   Currently marketed lithium preparations

Brand name	Country (ISO codes)	Producer	Salt	Amount of salt (mg/tablet)	Amount of lithium (mmol/tablet)	Release
Lithium carbonicum	PL	GlaxoSmithKline Pharmaceuticals S.A.	Carbonate	250	6.8	Conventional
Lithiumkarbonat	DK	OBA Pharma Aps	Carbonate	300	8.1	Conventional
Lithium Phasal	GB	Pharmax	Carbonate	300	8.1	Slow release
Lithobid	USA	Ciba-Geigy	Carbonate	300	8.1	Slow release
Lithonate	USA	Solvay	Carbonate	300	8.1	Conventional
Lithonate	GB	Approved Prescr	Carbonate	400	10.8	TAB
Lithotabs	USA	Solvay	Carbonate	300	8.1	Conventional
Lithuril	TR	Kocak	Unknown		8.1	KAP
Lito	FIN	Orion	Carbonate	300	8.1	TAB
Manialith	AU	Muir & Neil	Carbonate	250	6.8	Conventional
Maniprex	BE	Wolfs	Carbonate	500	13.5	TAB
Maniprex	BE	Wolfs	Carbonate	250	6.8	DRA
Milithin	GR	Minervapharm	Carbonate	300	8.1	KAP
Neurolepsin	AT	Kwizda F. Joh.	Carbonate	300	8.1	Conventional
Neurolithium	CH	Pharmafactory	Gluconate	1000	4.9	Phial
Neurolithium	FR	Labcatal	Gluconate	1000	4.9	Phial
Neurolithium	CH	Pharmafactory	Gluconate	2000	9.9	Phial
Neurolithium	FR	Labcatal	Gluconate	2000	9.9	Phial
Priadel	CH	Aventis	Carbonate	400	10.8	Slow release
Priadel	AU	Protea	Carbonate	400	10.8	Slow release
Priadel	BE, GB, NL, PT, NZ	Aventis	Carbonate	400	10.8	Slow release
Priadel	GB	Aventis	Carbonate	200	5.4	Slow release
Priadel Liquid	GB	Delandale	Citrate	520 in 5 ml	5.5 in 5 ml	Phial
Quilonorm	CH	Doetsch Grether	Azetate	536	8.1	Conventional
Quilonorm retard	AT	GlaxoSmithKline	Carbonate	450	12.2	Slow release
Quilonorm retard	CH	Doetsch Grether	Carbonate	450	12.2	Slow release
Quilonum	DE	GlaxoSmithKline	Azetate	536	8.1	Conventional
Quilonum retard	DE	GlaxoSmithKline	Carbonate	450	12.2	Slow release
Quilonum retard	ZA	Richelin	Carbonate	450	12.2	Slow release
Teralithe	FR	Aventis	Carbonate	250	6.8	TAB
Teralithe LP	FR	Aventis	Carbonate	400	10.8	Slow release

TAB, tablet; KAP, capsule ; DRA, sugar-coated tablet (dragée)

day', although this is due more to medical habit than any scientific considerations. With moderate daily doses, twice-daily regimens (morning and evening) are entirely feasible. This is important, as clinical experience has shown that patients often forget their lunchtime dose, or are reluctant to take their medication while at work. It does not appear to play an important role if the lithium pills are taken before, during, or after a meal. If a patient complains of gastrointestinal discomfort, it may be helpful to check whether taking the medication after a meal can reduce these side-effects. In any case, it is important that patients take the pills with a sufficient amount of water or other liquids. In fact, clinicians should ensure that patients have sufficient liquid intake even when they do not complain of increased thirst after taking their medication.

The decision about whether a patient would be better served by a conventional or a slow-release preparation can usually be made during the course of treatment after having assessed the side-effects. Several side-effects such as a tremor are less pronounced when slow-release preparations are used. It has not yet been proved whether one of the two types of preparation (conventional or slow-release) might lead more frequently to renal changes (see Chapter 21). On the other hand, preparations with very long release periods release lithium in the distal colon, leading to diarrhea in some patients. In such cases, switching to a conventional preparation can often bring immediate relief (see below).

There is a relatively simple way to adjust the dose of lithium to the patient's individual renal clearance. After 1 week of the patient's taking a particular dose with full compliance, the serum lithium level should be measured 12 ± 1 h after the last dose has been taken. The dose requirement can then be estimated proportionally. For example, if the measured serum lithium level is 0.4 mEq/l and the intended blood concentration is 0.8 mEq/l, then the daily dose has to be doubled. This will most often be between 20 and 30 mmol/day, but is subject to considerable interindividual variations. In older and smaller patients, particularly women, a dose of 8–12 mmol/day is often sufficient due to reduced GFR and lithium clearance. Following lithium intoxication, lithium clearance may be reduced for a period of weeks or even months, in which case a lower dose of lithium may be sufficient.

CLINICAL AND LABORATORY MONITORING

The need to assess serum lithium levels regularly

To ensure the safety of lithium prophylaxis, patients need to be carefully screened, well monitored (in particular by serum lithium levels, see Table 37.5) and educated about the principles of lithium treatment. Monitoring serum lithium levels is an important part of the process. Checking lithium levels regularly is necessary not only to determine adequate dosing and patient compliance, but also to recognize any reduction (deterioration) in kidney function, should this occur. If the dose has not been changed and patient compliance is high, but the serum lithium level nevertheless rises, there can mainly be two reasons: a change in sodium balance (i.e. a negative balance in comparison to earlier tests due to sweating, diarrhea, or diuretics, for example), or a reduced GFR. Whatever the case, the physician must not only readjust the dose of lithium, but also determine the root cause of the rise in lithium concentrations (e.g. laboratory error, pharmacy error, patient taking a wrong lithium preparation, increased compliance on the advice of relatives).

Table 37.5 Recommended standardized serum lithium levels and frequency of monitoring

---

Ranges of serum lithium levels

In general: 0.6–0.8 mEq/l
In cases of resistance to prophylaxis or impending recurrence, or acute mania: up to 1.2 mEq/l
Danger zone starts at: 1.5 mEq/l
The diagnosis of lithium toxicity is primarily clinical, supported by high serial lithium levels

Frequency of serum lithium monitoring

First month of treatment: weekly
Later: every 6–8 weeks
In patients who are physically healthy, responding well and educated about lithium: every 3–6 months
In special situations (e.g. in non-compliant patients, patients exhibiting sodium imbalance, postpartum): more frequent checks

---

Frequency of serum lithium level monitoring

Following the initiation of lithium prophylaxis, serum lithium levels must be checked on a weekly basis. Later, serum level monitoring should be performed approximately once per month during the first year of treatment and subsequently every 6–8 weeks, with the intervals between checks not exceeding 3 months. It should be noted that after every change in lithium dose, it takes approximately 1 week before a new equilibrium is established between body tissues and the intravascular compartment. The intervals within which serum levels should be checked will vary depending on the compliance of the patient, on any side-effects, and on a variety of attendant circumstances, such as individual sodium levels or the use of concomitant medications. If a pharmacokinetic lithium test has been performed prior to lithium treatment, serum lithium levels may be checked less frequently. Any depletion of sodium, whether it be due to reduced sodium intake or sodium loss, reduces the renal clearance of lithium and carries with it a greater risk of intoxication.

Recommended serum lithium concentrations

In general, for most patients a serum lithium level of 0.6–0.8 mmol/l is recommended for lithium prophylaxis. In older patients, in most women, and in patients who are particularly sensitive to side-effects, it may be advisable to reduce lithium levels to below 0.6 mmol/l. However, it appears that concentrations below 0.4 mmol/l are rarely effective. Nevertheless, not all elderly patients necessarily require lower serum levels. In the elderly, it is important to determine empirically which lithium level is most effective while still maintaining tolerability.

In younger patients, on the other hand – and in particular in young men – higher levels up to 1.1 mmol/l may be needed at times for a satisfactory outcome. Patients who take all their daily lithium in a single dose may also require relatively higher serum lithium levels. Frequently, an unsatisfactory response to prophylaxis is simply due to the fact that no attempt was made to stabilize the patient on a slightly higher than average dose (e.g. 0.9–1.1 mEq/l). Statistically, there is of course a greater risk of undesirable side-effects at these higher concentrations[10]. Higher serum concentrations (up to 1.2 mmol/l) are rarely necessary in the context of prophylactic treatment. Serum levels above 1.2 mmol/l lead only to an increase in undesirable side-effects, not in efficacy.

Optimum lithium dose

The optimum dose for lithium prophylaxis differs greatly from patient to patient, not only because of wide interindividual variations in the renal clearance of the drug, but also because of variance in patients' response to treatment. On the average, the optimum daily dose will lie somewhere between 20 and 30 mmol; however, there are extreme cases in which daily doses of 8 or 72 mmol have been prescribed! In order to determine the optimum dose, it is necessary to comply with the following three requirements:

(1) Keeping in mind that scientific studies have shown there to be an association between serum lithium levels and the frequency of desirable and undesirable effects;

(2) Ensuring that the number and severity of undesirable effects remain as low as possible;

(3) Achieving a clinical outcome that also motivates the patient to continue with prophylactic treatment.

The difficulty in doing so, however, is that the side-effects of the medication may appear rather quickly, whereas the benefits of prophylaxis often take a year or more to become apparent. Because of this, clinicians have little choice but to rely on the dose and serum level recommendations in the literature and to reduce serum lithium concentrations as soon as dose-related side-effects appear. If a relapse should subsequently occur, the physician should attempt to find an acceptable compromise in agreement with the patient while taking into account all attendant circumstances. It may be that the patient is willing to tolerate side-effects such as mild diarrhea, rather than experience another relapse. This will undoubtedly hold true in cases where the severity of such side-effects can be reduced (e.g. by administering beta receptor blockers to treat lithium-induced tremor). Additionally, it has often been observed that the adverse event that led to the original dose reduction will either not recur, or will be milder, when the previous serum concentration is reestablished. If, however, an acceptable benefit–risk relationship cannot be achieved from the point of view of the patient, the patient's relatives and the physician, it may be necessary to consider another pharmacologic option (see below). Combining an antidepressant with a sub-therapeutic dose of lithium should generally not be considered an acceptable alternative.

Even at the same dose, serum lithium levels vary intra- and interindividually. As can be seen in Table 37.6, this variability is not only due to differences in patient compliance. Owing to lithium's long elimination half-life, it is not necessary that the drug be taken at exactly the same time every day, although doing so is recommended as it may improve compliance. A few hours' difference does not present a problem. What is important, however, is that, prior to serum lithium assessment, patients take their last dose 12 ± 1 h before blood is drawn[8].

Missed doses

If a patient misses a dose, it is important that he or she does not double the dose of lithium, whether at the time the next dose is to be taken, or at all during the next day, as this may not be safe. Missed doses are compensated for over the course of several days by the pharmacokinetics of lithium salts. It is important that patients provide physicians with accurate information about their compliance with therapy, otherwise it is

Table 37.6 Causes of intraindividual fluctuations in lithium serum levels

---

Irregular drug intake (poor compliance)

Changes in the length of time between last drug intake and blood sampling (12-h interval)

Changes in lithium absorption due to:
    diarrhea (caused by gastrointestinal infections and/or lithium-induced intestinal disorder)
    vomiting
    co-medication

Changes in renal excretion due to:
    diuretic or antiphlogistic agents or other co-medication (often left unmentioned by patients when these are prescribed by other physicians)
    low-sodium diet, other unbalanced diets
    dehydration (hot weather, sports, sauna, fever, diarrhea)
    intercurrent renal disease

---

impossible to interpret the clinical relevance of the serum lithium level.

Monitoring for side-effects

During every visit, patients should be asked whether they have experienced any side-effects, especially thirst, polyuria, tremor, memory or cognitive difficulties, skin changes, or diarrhea. If side-effects are seen that may suggest lithium toxicity, such as coarse tremor, increased thirst, a sudden onset of diarrhea, or slurred speech, the physician must immediately check the serum lithium levels. The use of ion-sensitive electrodes can be convenient in such situations, as they allow serum lithium to be measured right away in the doctor's office (i.e. in the presence of the patient). If the concentrations are abnormally high, then the lithium dose must be reduced or stopped and the patient must be sent for another lithium serum level check soon.

Laboratory monitoring during lithium prophylaxis

Serum creatinine level should be monitored at least every 6–12 months. Serum calcium level should be monitored every 6–12 months due to the risk of hyperparathyroidism during lithium treatment (see Chapter 22). The patient's thyroid hormone status should be checked by measuring serum T_3, T_4 and basal TSH once a year.

A mild increase in TSH levels without any clinical signs of hypothyroidism does not necessarily need to be treated. However, distinctly elevated TSH levels should prompt physicians to check TSH more often. Patients with antibodies have an increased risk of developing acute hypothyroidism. Therefore, it is reasonable to assess MAK (thyroid microsome antibodies) and TAK (thyroid globulin antibodies) levels before initiating lithium therapy. The thyroid should be palpated and neck size measured on a regular basis, although according to a more recent publication these measures are of limited value and ultrasound screening of the thyroid is recommended (Bauer *et al.*, submitted for publication). Thyroid hormone levels should be monitored every 6 months during the first 3 years, and subsequently every 12 months (see Chapter 22).

A complete blood count (or at least a leukocyte count) should be performed every 6–12 months. In many patients, lithium therapy induces mild leukocytosis. It is important to be informed about spontaneous fluctuations in leukocyte counts during lithium therapy so as to recognize hematological changes in the blood picture that are not due to lithium, should they develop.

Occasional ECGs are recommended for documenting the status quo during lithium therapy in the event that other medical complaints make further ECGs necessary for diagnosis. Electroencephalograms (EEGs) also play an important role in monitoring for lithium intoxication. Medical comorbidity during lithium treatment should be carefully monitored. Cardiac rhythm disorders must be monitored by frequent ECGs. Bradycardia – especially sick sinus syndrome – represents a relative contraindication to lithium (see Chapter 25).

In patients with arterial hypertension, low-salt diets should not be used, and diuretics should be administered cautiously. Furthermore, in renal hypertension and diabetes mellitus, the late renal sequelae of each disease must be taken into account. In cases of cerebral sclerosis, dementia and other psycho-organic disorders, lithium – even at therapeutic levels – can induce disorientation and other neurotoxic symptoms (see Chapter 23). Because of this, serum lithium levels should be kept as low as possible, especially when neuroleptic drugs are administered at the same time.

In patients with epilepsy, frequent EEG monitoring is indicated during lithium therapy. The frequency of grand mal seizure can be either increased or decreased by lithium. Combined treatment with lithium and anticonvulsives is feasible. Lithium therapy may aggravate the symptoms of Parkinson's disease (Chapter 23).

ADVERSE EFFECTS OF LITHIUM MEDICATION

Given that the patients and the dosage are properly selected and monitored, serious long-term side-effects of lithium are infrequent. Because lithium ions influence a large number of important biochemical processes (see Section C, Pharmacology and mechanisms), lithium has a potential to induce a relatively wide spectrum of adverse reactions in a variety of organ systems. Tables 37.7 and 37.8 provide an overview of the most important psychiatric and somatic changes that may be observed during lithium therapy.

When considering side-effects, it is important to distinguish between: (1) acute and long-term changes; and (2) the relatively common symptoms that can appear during the normal course of lithium prophylaxis, and the rare, intense symptoms indicative of lithium intoxication.

Shortly after lithium therapy is initiated, a number of adverse effects can appear, although these frequently subside within 1–2 weeks. These include nausea, abdominal pain, more frequent stools, hand tremors, increased thirst and more frequent urination. These complaints may or may not persist during the course of long-term therapy. By the same token, other complaints, such as psoriasis, may not appear until after many years of treatment. It is surprising that – in contrast to other psychotropic drugs – the subjectively experienced effects of lithium are, on the average, so minimal that some patients even doubt that they are receiving an active form of treatment. Occasionally, patients complain of functional fatigue or weariness that is difficult to distinguish from residual depressive symptoms. The absence of mild manic fluctuations (which patients may have experienced as pleasant), or the attenuation of hypomanic states on lithium, may cause patients to regret having begun

Table 37.7 Adverse effects of lithium salts

Organ system	Symptoms	Remarks/therapy
Neurologic/ psychiatric	Fine tremor of the fingers	Frequent side-effect. Therapeutic options: dose reduction, change of dosing intervals, beta-receptor blockers
	Muscle weakness	More likely at start of therapy
	Memory impairment	
Gastrointestinal	Nausea	Often at start of therapy
	Vomiting	Diarrhea and vomiting can be signs of lithium intoxication
	Abdominal pain	
	Diarrhea	
Cardiovascular	Changes in ECG	Reversible. Non-specific changes are not dangerous
	Flattening of T wave	
	Inversion of T wave	
	Arrhythmias	Very rare. More frequent in patients with pre-existing heart disease
	First-degree atrioventricular (AV) block	Regular ECG monitoring
	Sick-sinus syndrome, ventricular extrasystoles	Discontinuation of lithium. Remember: lithium is contraindicated in cases of sick sinus
	Second- and third-degree AV block, bundle-branch block	
Renal	Polyuria, polydipsia, reduced concentration capacity (e.g. by thirst test, DDAVP test)	Reversible on discontinuation. Management options: dose reduction, diuretics (with caution)
	Reduced glomerular filtration rate	Rare
Metabolism, electrolytes and water balance	Weight gain	Frequent. Consider low caloric diet with normal sodium intake
	Edema	Rare. Caution when administering diuretics
Endocrine	Euthyroid goiter	Common. Suppressive therapy with L-thyroxine
	Rise of TSH, hypothyroidism	More common in women
	Hyperparathyroidism with hypocalcemia	Infrequent. Check serum calcium
Hematologic	Moderate leukocytosis	Common. Reversible
Dermatologic	Acne	Treat as usual
	Hair loss	Rare (check for hypothyroidism)
	Psoriasis	Can be exacerbated; may be a relative contraindication

Table 37.8 The frequency of adverse effects of lithium therapy according to long-term studies

Symptom	Frequency (%)	
	Dresden cohort (Felber1993[14]) (n = 850)	Cohort study in Denmark[15–17] (n = 236)
No symptoms		40
Thirst	25	
Tremor	23	15
Goiter	22	
Nausea	14	
Weight gain	10	73
Diarrhea	8	6
Fatigue	3	
Edema	2	
Psychological disturbances*		9

* Includes memory defect, impaired concentration, fatigue, libido disorders, apathy

therapy, leading them to interrupt an otherwise successful prophylactic treatment. Some patients also complain, either of their own accord or when asked specifically by their physician, of memory difficulties (see Chapter 23). Because the adverse psychiatric effects of proper lithium treatment are generally quite mild, patients should be considered fit to drive and operate motor vehicles. The most important adverse somatic effects, which can appear very soon after initiating therapy, include:

(1) Excessive thirst, which for some patients can be very troublesome. It tends to occur immediately after medication intake and is often accompanied by polyuria, which can prevent patients from sleeping through the night without waking. Researchers assume that this excessive thirst is due to lithium's effect on the thirst center in the central nervous system.

(2) Often considerable weight gain (8–10 kg), the precise cause of which has yet to be

determined (see Chapter 24). In addition to a high-calorie diet, the consumption of too many high-calorie soft drinks (due to increased thirst) can contribute to weight gain in lithium patients. As a result, patients should receive good nutritional counseling (recommendations: diluted tea, mineral water, sugar-free chewing gum, jelly babies/gummy bears, or dried fruit, etc.) and check their weight regularly. However, patients should be strongly discouraged from embarking on self-designed or fad diets, as these can lead to reduced sodium intake and thus increased side-effects or even lithium intoxication.

(3) Fine tremor of the fingers, which can be aggravated by emotional stress, posing particularly troublesome social or work-related difficulties. In the latter case, beta-receptor blockers, such as propranolol or pindolol, can be used to attenuate the symptoms (see Chapter 23).

(4) Diarrhea or, more precisely, loose stools occur most frequently when slow-release

preparations are used. Abdominal pain and nausea have also been reported, especially at the beginning of lithium treatment. Increased gastrointestinal symptoms can be an indication of impending lithium intoxication. Patients with frequent stools who are unable to switch to a different lithium preparation, or whose symptoms do not respond to such a switch, may experience relief with the intermittent use of anti-diarrheal agents such as loperamide. (Charcoal tablets are ineffective.) It must be taken into account that the serum lithium levels may rise when the diarrhea has stopped, possibly necessitating a reduction in the dose of lithium.

Tremors, thirst and diarrhea – the relative frequencies of which can be seen in Table 37.8 – are dependent on the dose of the drug. In many patients, the intensity of these symptoms decreases in the course of treatment, whereas in others they never occur at all. On the other hand, an unexpected aggravation of these symptoms might indicate impending lithium intoxication. In such cases, the patient's serum lithium levels must be checked immediately. When doing so, it is important to keep in mind that the symptoms of lithium intoxication can continue even after lithium levels appear to have normalized.

The most important symptoms of lithium intoxication, which must be strictly avoided because of the risk of kidney and cerebellar damage, are listed in Table 37.9. If the intoxication was not preceded by a change in dose, it might be attributed to a decrease in the renal clearance of the drug or increased, but unreported compliance. Possible causes of such a decrease are summarized in Table 37.10. Long-term somatic changes during lithium therapy affect, above all, thyroid and kidney function.

Thyroid function

Because lithium is a thyreostatic compound, it leads to an increase in basal TSH levels and can cause thyroid enlargement. In the clinical setting, physicians need to differentiate between: diffuse euthyroid goiter; manifest hypothyroidism with or without goiter; and pathologic hormonal changes (i.e. above all, any increase in TSH levels and thyroid antibody titers without clinically manifest symptoms).

In the case of euthyroid goiter, suppressive therapy with 50–100 µg L-thyroxine per day is recommended. Lithium treatment can be continued during this time. True hypothyroidism or myxedema are rare. When they do occur, they appear most frequently in

Table 37.9 Symptoms of lithium intoxication

Excessive thirst

Coarse tremor

Diarrhea

Hyperreflexia, myoclonus

Sluggishness, somnolence, coma

Slurred speech, ataxia

EEG: general changes, lowered threshold of convulsion

Parkinson syndrome, dyskinesia

Table 37.10 Causes of lithium intoxication

Renal insufficiency
Dehydration and sodium deficiency resulting, for example, from:
    low-caloric diet
    profuse sweating, fever
    change of nutritional or liquid intake during manic or depressive phase
    gastrointestinal infections accompanied by diarrhea and/or vomiting
Reduced renal lithium clearance due to:
    antirheumatic drugs
    thiazide diuretics
Co-administration with neuroleptics (increased neurotoxicity?)

women with pre-existing thyroid disease. Clinical hypothyroidism must be examined and treated by skilled internists. In these cases, too, lithium therapy may be continued, or at least re-initiated following an interruption.

Kidney function

The effects of lithium on kidney function are described in detail in Chapter 21. It is a well-known fact that lithium salts can lead to a reduction in renal concentrating capacity and thus to a condition that resembles insipid diabetes. At the lithium levels recommended today (i.e. 0.6–0.8 mEq/l) this condition occurs less frequently than before, when higher levels were used; nevertheless, it can have practical consequences insofar as polyuric patients are at especially high risk of developing lithium intoxication if they do not compensate by increasing their liquid intake or if they are suffering from sodium depletion (Table 37.11). These high-risk patients must therefore be monitored carefully clinically and with frequent standardized serum lithium levels. (See also the remarks above concerning the importance of routine laboratory and other tests, as well as Table 37.11.)

The majority of studies indicate that the GFR is not altered considerably by lithium administration. The most important way to avoid renal damage is to ensure that even lithium sub-intoxication is not allowed to occur. It is essential to be alert to any signs of impending lithium intoxication and to act immediately should they appear. In order to achieve the necessary level of alertness, doctors should repeatedly provide patients and their relatives with clear and comprehensive information about lithium treatment.

In the above sections we have discussed only the most important adverse side-effects of lithium therapy. For more detailed information, refer to the relevant chapters of this book. For more specific questions, readers may contact the following institution, which has at its disposal an excellent and continually updated register of scientific literature on lithium and lithium therapy (see Chapter 41):

Lithium Information Center
Dean Foundation
2711 Allen Boulevard
Middleton, WI 53562
USA
Tel: +1 608 827-2390
Fax: +1 608 827-2399

Table 37.11 Tests needed to help reduce risk of kidney damage

Before starting therapy	Goal: recognizing risk patients To achieve this: renal history, renal function
At beginning of therapy	Goal: monitoring baseline renal concentration value To achieve this: concentration text with DDAVP
During therapy	Goal: avoiding even the slightest lithium intoxication Therefore: • Regular monitoring of lithium serum levels • Caution in patients with polyuria, because risk of intoxication is higher • In case of unexplained increase in lithium levels: perform nephrological diagnostics • If renal concentration capacity is markedly reduced and lithium levels increase: discontinue medication. In case there is no remission of symptoms, a kidney biopsy may be necessary

INTERACTIONS: DRUGS AND ELECTROCONVULSANT THERAPY

Lithium clearance can be negatively influenced not only by diuretics, but also by certain antirheumatic medications such as diclofenac or indometacin, or by angiotensin converting enzyme (ACE) inhibitors (see Chapter 21; also Table 37.12).

In manic patients with psychomotor agitation, it is often impossible to do without neuroleptic drugs, at least at the beginning of treatment. This is due to the fact that the therapeutic effect of lithium does not become evident until approximately 1 week after the initiation of therapy. Concurrent (or sequential) therapy with neuroleptics and lithium is possible and represents a common approach in clinical practice. Although the risk of neurotoxic symptoms with this combination of drugs is occasionally exaggerated in the literature, it is nevertheless recommended that patients be monitored closely and EEGs be performed when higher doses of neuroleptics are used in the context of increased serum lithium levels.

For this indication, serum lithium may be set at a level of up to 1.2 mEq/l for a short period of time. Higher serum lithium concentrations are not generally recommended. A more rapid increase in dose is possible as long as the serum level is monitored at close intervals (i.e. every 2–3 days).

The effects of concurrent use of electroconvulsant therapy (ECT) and lithium have not been studied sufficiently. Whereas Wheeler Vega et al.[11] do not recommend this combination, the APA Task Force Report on ECT, 2nd edition[12] emphasizes the risk of neurotoxic reactions and suggests reduction of ECT energy and lithium dosage. Case reports underline the need for special attention when ECT is used to treat a severe breakthrough episode in a patient with ongoing lithium long-term treatment[13].

HIGH-RISK PATIENTS

At this point it should be noted once again that elderly individuals are to be regarded as high-risk patients, despite the fact that lithium

Table 37.12 The most important interactions between lithium salts and non-psychotropic drugs

	Mechanism

Thiazide and possibly also loop diuretics
    Antirheumatics (e.g. diclofenac, indometacine; not aspirin)
    ACE inhibitors (e.g. captopril, enalapril)
	Reduce lithium clearance
	(→increased risk of lithium intoxication)

Iodine salts (highly dosed)	Increase goitrogenic effect of lithium
Narcotics, muscle relaxants	Their effect is increased by lithium

prophylaxis can be beneficial in this group. Undesirable side-effects are not unusual even at relatively low serum lithium concentrations in elderly patients.

Women who continue lithium therapy during pregnancy should be monitored very closely. It is absolutely essential to take frequent serum samples and adjust the lithium dose and/or dose schedule, especially in the period immediately prior to delivery. This is due to increased lithium clearance during pregnancy and a markedly decreased clearance during delivery (i.e. back to the patient's pre-pregnancy level). Starting in the 16th week of pregnancy, ultrasound examinations should be performed in specialized clinics.

DURATION OF THERAPY: CRITERIA FOR DISCONTINUING THERAPY

When weighing the benefits and risks of lithium therapy during the course of treatment, physicians and patients may consider discontinuing lithium prophylaxis if: the outcome of long-term treatment has been disappointing or negative; serious side-effects occur; or lithium therapy becomes no longer indicated (due to pregnancy or intermediate diseases). The long-term remission of symptoms during lithium

therapy is the most common reason behind patients' desire to discontinue treatment. After lithium treatment has been terminated, however, the absence of prophylactic protection allows the disease to resume its natural course.

Other reasons why patients may ask their psychiatrist to discontinue lithium therapy – even when the physician–patient relationship is excellent – are discussed in more detail in Chapter 38. Two factors appear to be important when the issue of therapy discontinuation becomes a subject of discussion between the patient and his/her psychiatrist:

(1) For both parties it is important that the reasons for terminating therapy be made as clear as possible. What are the patient's motives for stopping therapy, and what are the physician's motives for agreeing to this decision?

(2) The medical records documenting the course of therapy should allow both parties to judge whether prophylaxis was a complete or partial success, or even a clear failure.

Experience has shown that it may take years to determine the success of treatment, and it is important to inform patients about this beforehand. Doctors should avoid initiating lithium prophylaxis if the patient is not willing from the start to continue therapy for a sufficient period of time. It is, of course, an entirely different situation if undesirable side-effects occur and force the patient to terminate therapy. However, even in cases where, for example, 3 years of therapy have been well monitored, therapeutic success can be judged only if there is sufficient documentation of the course of illness prior to the initiation of prophylaxis. Understandably, this is often a problem for patients and physicians alike.

According to recent findings, discontinuing lithium therapy abruptly can trigger acute and severe relapses of manic, depressive and schizoaffective psychoses in some patients (see Chapter 38). This appears to apply in particular to patients who never achieved complete psychological stabilization while on lithium and whose residual symptoms require adjunctive treatment with antidepressants or neuroleptics (see Chapter 14). When attempting to discontinue lithium treatment that has lasted for a number of years, the dose should be reduced gradually over the course of several months, notwithstanding the differentiation discussed in Chapter 14. If the patient's psychiatric condition remains stable over the course of several months at the lower dose, then the attempt can be made to discontinue treatment altogether. If, however, there is an increase in psychopathologic symptoms, the dose must be increased to its original level. Naturally, serious side-effects, pregnancy, or severe intermediate diseases may require that a patient discontinue therapy abruptly. This, it should be noted, does not always lead to immediate relapse.

If the decision is eventually made to discontinue lithium treatment, patients should nevertheless be required to continue their regular, scheduled doctor's visits so that their progress can be monitored. This is the only way to determine if the decision was justified and if any changes in treatment strategy need to be made.

In patients with affective psychoses, or schizoaffective psychoses of the bipolar type, the high risk of serious recurrence implies that discontinuing therapy, even if it has been only partially successful in the individual patient, is usually contraindicated, and particularly so if the patient has an elevated suicide risk (see Chapter 15). Furthermore, if a patient is still experiencing an illness episode of mild intensity while on lithium treatment, attempting to discontinue the medication is generally not recommended.

MOST COMMON MISTAKES IN LITHIUM TREATMENT

The most common mistakes made by physicians in the management of lithium therapy, from the perspective of the authors' clinical experience, are listed in Table 37.13. Before discontinuing lithium therapy because of its alleged non-effectiveness, physicians should always determine whether lithium treatment has been sufficiently optimized. Suggestions for optimization are listed in Table 37.14.

Table 37.13 Most frequent and serious mistakes made by physicians in the treatment of lithium patients

Failure to make the correct diagnosis

Discontinuing prophylaxis too early, before stabilization may be achieved

Unintentionally fostering non-compliance

Exaggerated notions of lithium therapy as a particularly toxic compound

Overdosing

Failure to recognize signs of lithium toxicity

Failure to consider the anti-suicidal effects of lithium

Unnecessary addition of other psychopharmaca (danger of destabilization)

Carelessness with regard to the necessary clinical and laboratory tests

Failure to differentiate between antipsychotic and prophylactic effects

Table 37.14 Steps towards optimizing lithium therapy in cases of non-response

Providing patients and relatives with clear and helpful information on lithium treatment

Establishing a workable concept of illness

Encouraging patients to cooperate with their physician

Increasing serum lithium levels

Checking and improving patient compliance

Diagnosis and treatment of co-morbidities

Combination treatment with cognitive behavioral therapy or IP/SRT

Addition of other mood stabilizers

REFERENCES

1. American Psychiatric Association. Practice guideline for the treatment of patients with bipolar disorder (revision). Am J Psychiatry 2002; 159 (Suppl): 1–50

2. Grunze H, Kasper S, Goodwin G, et al; WFSBP Task Force on Treatment Guidelines for Bipolar Disorders. The World Federation of Societies of Biological Psychiatry (WFSBP) guidelines for the biological treatment of bipolar disorders, part III: maintenance treatment. World J Biol Psychiatry 2004: 5: 120–35

3. Yatham LN, Kennedy SH, O'Donovan C, et al; Canadian Network for Mood and Anxiety Treatments. Canadian Network for Mood and Anxiety Treatments (CANMAT) guidelines for the management of patients with bipolar disorder: consensus and controversies. Bipolar Disord 2005; 7 (Suppl 3): 5–69

4. Grof P, Angst J, Karasek M, Keitner G. Patient selection for long-term lithium treatment in clinical practice. Arch Gen Psychiatry 1979; 36: 894–7

5. Angst J. Ungelöste Probleme bei der Indikationsstellung zur Lithiumprophylaxe

affektiver und schizoaffektiver Erkrankungen. Biblthca Psychiatr 1981; 161: 32–44

6. Müller-Oerlinghausen B, Felber W, Berghöfer A, et al. The impact of lithium long-term medication on suicidal behavior and mortality of bipolar patients. Arch Suicide Res 2005; 9: 307–19

7. Cockcroft DW, Gault MH. Prediction of creatinine clearance from serum creatinine. Nephron 1976; 16: 31–41

8. Schou M. Lithium Treatment of Manic Depressive Illness: A Practical Guide. New York and Basel: Karger, 2004

9. Heim W, Oelschläger H, Kreuter J, Müller-Oerlinghausen B. Liberation of lithium from sustained release preparations. A comparison of seven registered brands. Pharmacopsychiat 1994; 27: 27–1

10. Gelenberg AJ, Kane JM, Keller MB, et al. Comparison of standard and low serum levels of lithium for maintenance treatment of bipolar disorder. N Engl J Med 1989; 321: 1489–93

11. Wheeler Vega JA, Mortimer AM, Tyson PJ. Somatic treatment of psychotic depression: review and recommendations for practice. J Clin Psychopharmacol 2000; 20: 504–19

12. American Psychiatric Association. The Practice of Electroconvulsive Therapy: Recommendations for Treatment, Training, and Privileging: A Task Force Report of the American Psychiatric Association, 2nd edn. Washington, DC: American Psychiatric Association, 2001

13. Sartorius A, Wolf J, Henn FA. Lithium and ECT – Concurrent use still demands attention: Three case reports. World J Biol Psychiatry 2005; 6: 121–4

14. Felber W. Rezidivprophylaxe affektiver Erkrankungen mit Lithium. Multicenter-Studie Lithiumtherapie bei 850 Patienten. Regensburg: S Roderer, 1993

15. Schou M, Vestergaard P. Prospective studies on a lithium cohort. 2. Renal function. Water and electrolyte metabolism. Acta Psychiatr Scand 1988; 78: 427–33

16. Vestergaard P, Schou M. Prospective studies on a lithium cohort. 1. General features. Acta Psychiatr Scand 1988; 78: 421–6

17. Vestergaard P, Poulstrup I, Schou M. Prospective studies on a lithium cohort. 3. Tremor, weight gain, diarrhea, psychological complaints. Acta Psychiatr Scand 1988; 78:

38 Latency, discontinuation and re-use of lithium treatment

Ross J Baldessarini, Leonardo Tondo, Gianni L Faedda, Adele C Viguera, Christopher Baethge, Paola Salvatore, Irene M Bratti, John Hennen

Contents Introduction • Latency to prophylactic treatment • Lithium discontinuation • Lithium re-treatment • Conclusions

INTRODUCTION

This chapter summarizes clinical and research findings and recommendations pertaining to prophylactic treatment with lithium in patients with manic–depressive disorders: (1) delay in starting treatment; (2) discontinuing ongoing maintenance treatment; and (3) re-treatment following discontinuation. There has been substantial progress in recent years in understanding these important components of long-term prophylactic treatment with lithium salts. Several basic ideas were included in the initial report on lithium to treat mania by John Cade in 1949, which opened the modern era of psychopharmacology[1]. In his report of ten cases, the duration of preceding recurrent or chronic manic or manic-depressive illness ranged from 2 to 30 years in eight patients. In four cases, lithium was discontinued for a variety of clinical reasons, usually abruptly, followed by relapse within an average of 4 weeks. In three cases, lithium treatment was re-started with evident clinical benefit. These few, very early and informal observations in possibly selected cases suggested (1) that lithium could be effective even in prolonged and severe manic-depressive illness; (2) that continued treatment might prevent recurrences, that stopping ongoing treatment, especially abruptly, was followed by early relapse; and (3) that re-starting treatment could again be clinically effective.

LATENCY TO PROPHYLACTIC TREATMENT

As reviewed in other chapters of this volume, maintenance treatment in bipolar disorders, alone or in combination with other modern antimanic or mood-stabilizing agents, usually is not successful in providing complete protection from future morbidity[2,3]. Such imperfect prophylaxis makes it worthwhile to identify factors that predict response to long-term prophylaxis with lithium or other treatments. A potentially important predictive factor is history, including either the number of prior manic-depressive episodes or the time from illness-onset to the start of sustained, long-term treatment. The research on this topic is not extensive for lithium, and is limited for alternative treatments. Nevertheless, the findings with lithium are instructive and generally hopeful.

Effect of pre-treatment episode count

In 2003, we carried out a systematic review of the research available on this topic[4]. By computer-assisted searching, we identified 28 reports (1967–2003) with data on prior illness episode counts versus response to lithium given over an average of 3.8 years in 3091 adult patients with various types of manic-depressive illness[5–32]. The studies identified varied greatly in methods, diagnostic criteria, and measures of clinical outcome. Nevertheless, in 19/28 studies (68%), we found no support for the hypothesis that a larger number of prior episodes would predict an inferior response to treatment with lithium, given essentially as a monotherapy in most studies.

Effect of treatment latency

In a second 2003 analysis[33], we identified 11 studies[5,16,24,26,28,32,33–37] of 1485 adult manic-depressive patients, with information on the time (mean ± SD, 9.6 ± 1.3 years) from illness-onset to the start of long-term prophylactic treatment based primarily on lithium, lasting an average of 5.4 ± 3.1 years. In testing for relations between treatment-latency and clinical responses, we found that earlier treatment was strongly associated with greater pre-treatment illness

intensity, scored as the proportion of weeks ill or annual episode-recurrence rate. This inverse relationship of shorter latency and greater pre-treatment morbidity gave the impression that earlier intervention led to greater relative reduction of morbidity (before- versus during-treatment contrast). Instead, the relationship indicated that greater morbidity drove earlier treatment, with the risk of a misleading impression that earlier treatment led to greater clinical improvement. In support of this interpretation, pre-treatment episode count was no longer significantly related to latency when corrected for pre-treatment morbidity using multivariate regression methods.

In addition, we considered a large sample of 750 patients with various types of manic-depressive illnesses (84% DSM-IV bipolar I or II), most of whom (87%) were maintained on prophylactic treatment with lithium for an average of 5.0 ± 5.3 years[33]. The data considered were pooled from our collaborative studies in European mood disorder centers in Germany and Sardinia[26,31,38]. Delay from illness-onset to the start of long-term treatment averaged 9.2 ± 9.0 years in women and 7.5 ± 8.5 years in men ($p = 0.01$). Treatment latency was shortest among men diagnosed with bipolar I disorder and longest in women with bipolar II conditions marked by depression with hypomania. This contrast indicates that clinical presentation, and well-known sex differences in help-acceptance, probably determine the timing of diagnosis and intervention to a great extent. As expected from our preceding analysis indicating that earlier treatment was strongly associated with greater pre-treatment illness intensity[33], we found strong relationships of greater pre-treatment morbidity (estimated as episodes/year, hospitalizations/year, hospitalized days/year, or approximate weeks ill/year) with shorter treatment-latency – again indicating earlier intervention with more severe illness. For example, treatment-latency was strongly, inversely correlated with pre-treatment morbidity as episodes/year (non-parametric correlation, $r_s = -0.66$), or proportion-of-time-ill ($r_s = -0.67$; both $p < 0.0001$). As noted, the strong relationship of greater pre-treatment morbidity to shorter treatment-latency precludes fair assessment of *changes* in morbidity before versus during treatment, which would lead to the almost certainly invalid impression that earlier intervention produced greater improvement.

Importantly, there was no relationship between treatment latency and various measures of morbidity *during* prophylactic treatment (e.g., per cent time ill vs. latency, $r_s = 0.03$, $p = 0.38$; Figure 38.1). Moreover, when 253 patients who experienced no major recurrences of mania or depression during maintenance treatment (only 34% of the sample) were

compared to 112 patients who were ill more than half of the time during treatment (15% of patients), there was no difference in latency to treatment (8.3 ± 9.0 vs. 8.6 ± 9.2 years; $p = 0.80$)[33]. This lack of difference further supports the finding that latency to treatment has little effect on response to lithium treatment.

Finally, in a recent analysis[39] from the same Berlin and Cagliari samples[26,31,38], we found that morbidity in the 2 years prior to starting long-term maintenance treatment was very similar among patients in the longest versus shortest quartiles of latency to the start of treatment. This finding further supports our proposal that illness characteristics proximate to interventions greatly determine the timing of treatment, whether a period of relatively severe

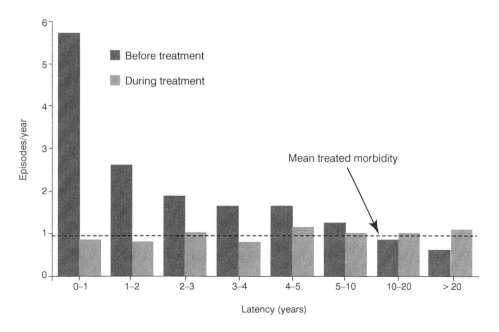

Figure 38.1 Morbidity (episodes/year) before starting and during long-term prophylactic treatment in 750 manic-depressive patients from Berlin or Cagliari versus years of latency from estimated illness-onset to start of maintenance treatment. Note that pre-treatment morbidity appears to decrease with longer latency ('dilution' effect), whereas morbidity during treatment (horizontal dashed line) is unrelated to latency. Adapted from data reported by Baethge *et al.* (2003)[33] as described in the text

morbidity occurs after a brief or prolonged course of lifetime illness.

The illness progression hypothesis

The concept that manic-depressive illness usually follows a progressive or accelerating course, in that episode frequency appears to increase over time, and wellness intervals to shorten, was first proposed by Emil Kraepelin in 1899[40]. However, Eliot Slater later pointed out in the 1930s that this impression rests heavily on a fundamental sampling artifact, such that persons who tend to cycle more rapidly appear more often so as to enrich sub-samples with higher episode counts[41,42]. This error can be corrected by comparing illness course (length of onset-to-onset cycles or of wellness intervals between acute episodes) in subjects matched for episode counts, by considering trends within individual subjects, or by use of multivariate analyses that control for episode count[42].

In a review of 38 studies reported over the past century, we were surprised to learn that conclusions pertaining to the cycle-acceleration hypothesis have varied markedly, even with consideration of the problem of selection bias (Salvatore and Baldessarini, manuscript in preparation, 2006). Approximately one-third of the studies found no evidence of cycle-acceleration, another third found acceleration, and the findings were inconclusive in a remaining third.

We also analyzed illness-course among nearly 200 American and European bipolar I disorder patients followed prospectively for several years from illness onset, and treated clinically[43]. In most cases, cycle length was highly variable over time and consistent trends were difficult to define. Nevertheless, we found that the relationship of cycle length versus cycle count analyzed as a rate (slope) function by within-subject regression methods was almost randomly distributed, with an excess of cases clustered around the null slope of zero, indicating neither acceleration nor slowing; 30–40% showed an accelerating course (negative slope, consistent with the concept of 'kindling' by analogy to progressive worsening in some forms of experimental epilepsy), and another quarter to one-third had lengthening cycles or wellness intervals (positive slope) as the cycle count increased. These findings are consistent with the view that cycle length may shorten in a substantial minority of manic-depressive patients but that highly variable and chaotic course patterns within and among individual patients appear to be the rule[33]. Indeed, the high variability of illness course may contribute to the lack of strong relationships between history and treatment response just summarized.

Rapid cycling

Another illness-course factor that we have considered as a predictor of treatment response is rapid cycling, defined as at least four discrete DSM-IV episodes of mania or depression within 12 months prior to starting long-term maintenance treatment with lithium. In an analysis involving 360 bipolar I ($n = 218$) and II disorder ($n = 142$) patients at Centro Bini, a collaborating Sardinian mood disorder center, we verified that rapid cycling was more prevalent among bipolar II than type I patients (31% vs. 6%) and among women versus men (18% vs. 12%)[44]. Rapid cycling did not appear to be a constant course feature in most cases. Somewhat surprisingly, rapid cycling had a limited impact on treatment response, as measured by latency of first recurrence, overall recurrence frequency, or proportion of time ill. This limited interaction with recent cycling rate and response to lithium may reflect conservative use of antidepressants in bipolar disorder patients at that center. Nevertheless, rapid-cycling was associated with nearly 3-fold excess of depressive recurrences and with somewhat less chance of full protection against illness during treatment[44].

The impression that rapid cycling is followed by less favorable responses to treatment with lithium was sustained in a more recent review of published reports that compared various measures of clinical outcome among rapid-cycling and non-rapid-cycling bipolar disorder patients[45]. However, contrary to widely accepted impressions, treatment response appeared to be even less favorable among rapid-cycling patients treated with various anticonvulsant drugs with antimanic or proposed mood-stabilizing effects than with lithium[45].

Conclusions about history and treatment response

The preceding reviews and analyses did not support the expectation that more prolonged manic-depressive illness, with more recurrences and longer delay of prophylactic treatment, particularly with lithium, might yield inferior responses to treatment. Indeed, a striking observation was that individual responses to long-term treatment with lithium showed marked variation, and virtual chaos, among individual patients – ranging from complete protection from major recurrences in a substantial minority to being virtually continuously unwell over several years in a smaller minority[33]. The lack of an orderly relationship of history (latency or episode count) to response to lithium prophylaxis may seem inconsistent with the view that bipolar and other forms of manic-depressive illness appear to be 'progressive' in many patients, leading to an expectation that more episodes of untreated illness, or delay of prophylaxis, would yield inferior outcomes. However, the prevalence of cycle acceleration appears to be limited to a minority of cases, and not a general characteristic of the natural history of bipolar

disorder. Finally, it is important to emphasize that the optimistic conclusion that response to lithium prophylaxis appears to be independent of history does not gainsay the clinical importance of early identification and intervention in the various forms of manic-depressive disorder.

LITHIUM DISCONTINUATION

Interruption of effective long-term treatment with lithium occurs very commonly. Discontinuation can be associated with: (1) adverse effects of treatment; (2) pregnancy; (3) patients' unwillingness to continue treatment following prolonged well-being or relatively minor side-effects; (4) patient non-adherence to recommended treatment; (5) clinician dissatisfaction with response and electing to try alternative treatments; and (6) experience during controlled therapeutic trials involving switching from lithium to placebo or alternative active treatments. Despite high prevalence of discontinuation of lithium prophylaxis[3], there is surprisingly little research-based information about the impact of such changes on clinical status or on the long-term course of bipolar disorders, although there is some information about short-term effects. A number of studies have provided evidence that stopping long-term treatment with lithium, especially abruptly or rapidly, leads to an unnaturally increased risk of early relapse[25,46–51] and a markedly increased risk of suicidal acts[52,53]. We have hypothesized that such effects may reflect the impact of treatment-discontinuation as a 'pharmacodynamic stressor'[3,54].

In a seminal review, Suppes et al.[46] concluded that lithium discontinuation was followed by a high rate of early recurrences in bipolar I disorder patients, that mania appeared earlier than depression, and that the risk was much higher than expected from cycling rates before starting lithium. Indeed, the median time to recurrence

(5 months) following lithium discontinuation was nearly seven-times shorter than spontaneous interepisode cycling intervals before maintenance treatment in some of the same patients. We have updated this overview in the next section.

Reports on the effects of discontinuing lithium

We reviewed the available literature for reports on outcomes following discontinuation of lithium, based on 25 reports (1949–2004) identified by computer-assisted literature searching[1,5,49,55–76] (Table 38.1). The studies are highly heterogeneous in patient sampling, design and conditions of discontinuation, but they yield several important overall observations. They involved 760 manic-depressive patients (50% bipolar) treated continuously with lithium at mean serum concentrations of 0.6–0.8 mEq/l over an average of 4 years, including randomized trials in 11 of the 25 studies. After stopping lithium either abruptly or in an unstated manner, 71% of subjects (428/605) became ill again within 4 months, at an overall estimated rate of 17%/month, with new manic (and rare mixed-state) episodes as the majority (71%) polarity.

Effects of discontinuation rate

We have proposed that evidence supporting the effect of an iatrogenically based pharmacodynamic stressor would include a higher relapse risk following abrupt or rapid (< 2 weeks) discontinuation of lithium, in contrast to gradual dose-reduction over at least several weeks[47,49]. Consistent with this criterion, we found several studies involving gradual discontinuation of lithium, typically over several weeks, in which the risk of early illness recurrence was much lower (63/155, 41%). The recurrence rate, at only 2.2%/month, was nearly

eight-times lower than was found in other studies summarized in Table 38.1.

The time-to-first-recurrences after discontinuing lithium treatment was considerably shorter than typical intervals of untreated bipolar illness, which averaged about one episode per year, and was lower during long-term maintenance treatment[77]. Consistent with this impression, in a large sample of bipolar disorder patients ($n = 230$) during at least 5 years of illness history without maintenance treatment[26], we found an average of 1.19 ± 1.56 episodes/year, suggesting a cycling interval of 10.1 ± 7.7 months, which is nearly three-times longer than the reported average of 3.9 months to a new episode of illness after stopping lithium rapidly or abruptly (Table 38.1). These crude comparisons suggest that stopping maintenance treatment with lithium may increase recurrence risk to levels much higher than are suggested by average cycling rates in untreated bipolar illness.

We have found such a contrast in several independent samples of bipolar disorder patients who discontinued lithium[47,78,79]. An example of the difference in impact of rapid versus gradual discontinuation of lithium prophylaxis is shown as a survival analysis (Figure 38.2). This analysis, involving 227 Sardinian patients with either type I or type II bipolar disorder indicates a 4-fold earlier median time to initial recurrence of mania or depression (6.0 vs. 24 months) after abrupt or rapid versus gradual discontinuation, with an intermediate latency (18 months), as expected, among another 31 patients in whom the rate of discontinuing lithium was not known precisely (Table 38.2, see legend). It is also noteworthy that most of the difference in recurrence risk was found within several months after discontinuation lithium, whereas the survival functions from 1 to 5 years were parallel, with virtually identical rates that probably reflect the natural history of untreated bipolar disorder.

Table 38.1 Studies of lithium discontinuation

Study	Design	Dx	Mean age	Cases (n)	Treated (mos)	[Li+] (mEq/l)	Relapsed (n)	Manic (%)	Relapse risk (%)	Follow-up (mos)	Relapse rate (%/mo)
Rapid or unspecified discontinuation											
Cade, 1949[1]	Open	BPD	50.2	4	3.8	—	4	100.0	100.0	1.00	100.0
Baastrup et al., 1967[5]	Open	MAD	45.5	25	3.2	0.95	22	77.8	88.0	3.20	27.5
Baastrup et al., 1970[55]	RCT	MAD	50.0	39	48.0	1.05	21	33.3	53.8	5.00[a]	10.8
Melia, 1970[56]	RCT	BPD	49.6	9	9.0	—	7	—	77.8	2.67	29.1
Small et al., 1971[57]	RCT	MAD	42.4	5	22.4	—	4	75.0	80.0	0.89	89.9
Cundall et al., 1972[58]	RCT	BPD	53.7	9	29.0	—	7	71.4	77.8	6.00[a]	13.0
Hullin et al., 1972[59]	RCT	MAD	46.0	18	40.0	1.00	6	—	33.3	6.00[a]	5.6
Fyrö and Petterson, 1977[60]	RCT	MAD	50.0	9	52.8	0.60	9	66.7	100.0	2.67	37.5
Lapierre et al., 1980[61]	Open	BPD	37.5	20	33.7	—	4	100.0	20.0	0.31	64.5
Klein et al., 1981[62]	RCT	MAD	43.0	21	46.8	0.68	11	—	52.4	0.47[a]	>100
Christodoulou & Lykouras, 1982[63]	RCT	MAD	47.3	18	27.8	0.93	3	33.3	16.7	0.50[a]	33.3
Margo and McMahon, 1982[64]	RCT	MAD	49.2	4	19.0	0.63	4	100.0	100.0	0.25	>100
Sashidaran and McGuire, 1983[65]	Open	MAD	46.3	22	90.3	—	16	56.3	72.7	13.3	5.5
Mendlewicz et al., 1984[66]	RCT	MAD	—	14	60.0	—	12	—	85.7	12.0[a]	7.1
Goodnick, 1985[67]	Open	BPD	33.2	12	49.2	0.95	0	—	0.0	0.75[a]	0.0
Mander, 1986[68]	Open	BPD	34.0	29	29.0	—	15	—	51.7	6.53	7.1
Mander and Loudon, 1988[69]	RCT	BPD	52.7	7	117.6	0.80	7	100.0	100.0	0.50	>100
Koukopoulos et al., 1995[70]	Open	MAD	45.0	110	146.4	0.59	89	72.0	80.9	4.86	16.6
Baldessarini et al., 1999[49]	Open	BPD	40.0	112	50.0	0.62	108	53.7	96.4	6.00	15.3
Viguera et al., 2000[71]	Open	BPD	32.6	60	47.3	0.75	38	—	54.3	8.00	6.8
Cavanagh et al., 2004[72]	Open	BPD	55.6	14	13.0	0.70	12	50.0	85.7	7.42	1.3
Yazici et al., 2004[73]	Open	BPD	41.0	23	72.0	—	19	—	82.6	7.00	11.8
Katantaris et al., 2004[74]	Open	BPD	15.0	21	2.0	0.90	10	—	47.6	0.50[a]	95.2
Total/average ± SEM (n = 23 studies)	52.2% Open	52.2% BPD	43.6 ±1.9[b]	605	44.0 ±7.5[b]	0.80 ±0.04[b]	428	70.7	70.7	4.26	16.6[c]
Gradual discontinuation											
Molnar et al., 1988[75]	Open	BPD	37.0	6	69.6	—	2	—	33.3	8.00	4.2
Baldessarini et al., 1999[49]	Open	BPD	40.0	84	50.0	0.60	34	45.5	40.5	24.0	3.6
Viguera et al., 2000[71]	Open	BPD	32.6	35	47.3	0.75	13	—	37.1	20.0	1.9
Fahy and Lawlor, 2001[76]	Open	MAD	77.6	21	23.1	0.37	11	—	52.4	7.80	6.7
Yazici et al., 2004[73]	Open	BPD	41.0	9	72.0	—	3	—	77.8	1.00	33.3
Total/average ± SEM (n = 5 studies)	100% Open	80.0% BPD	45.6 ±8.1[b]	155	52.4 ±8.9[b]	0.57 ±0.11[b]	63	45.5	40.6	18.9	2.15[c]

a, Months (mos) of study; b, weighted average; c, note: the pooled relapse rate is 7.7-times higher after rapid/unspecified vs. gradual discontinuation

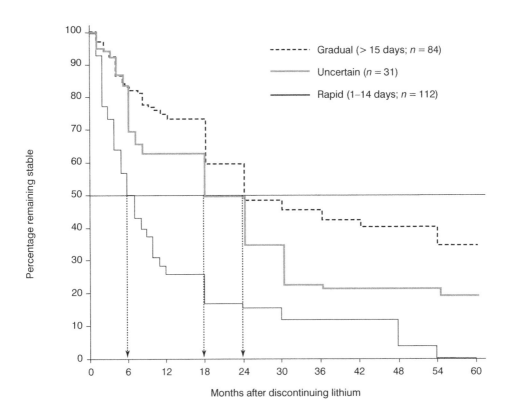

Figure 38.2 Survival analysis of 227 Sardinian bipolar disorder patients discontinued from 4 years of maintenance treatment with lithium as a virtual monotherapy, rapidly (1 day to 2 weeks; $n = 112$), gradually (>2 weeks; $n = 84$), or at uncertain rates ($n = 31$). Data are percentage of patients remaining well versus months after discontinuing lithium for clinical indications and excluding cases involving emerging hypomania or depression at the time of discontinuation. Note that the median (light horizontal line) times to illness recurrence (vertical light dotted arrows) were about 6 months after rapid discontinuation versus 24 months after gradual discontinuation (a 4-fold difference), and an intermediate 18 months after uncertain rates of discontinuation. Adapted from data summarized previously by Baldessarini et al. (1999)[49]

Moreover, this separation of risk functions between years 1 and 5 supports the interpretation that slow discontinuation of lithium not only delayed recurrence, but *reduced* risk related to early effects of what we hypothesize to represent as iatrogenic, pharmacodynamically based risk[47,49,79].

We also considered findings from the same studies to clarify how specific types of bipolar disorder or other factors influence the effects of the rate of discontinuing lithium treatment[47,49,79]. Bipolar I patients, discontinued rapidly, became ill again nearly 2 months earlier than type II patients. In addition, the difference in time to

Table 38.2 Computed weeks to 50% recurrence risk after discounting lithium abruptly or rapidly versus gradually

Measure	Rapid	Gradual	Risk ratio
Diagnostic type			
Any bipolar disorder	24.0 ± 4.8	96.0 ± 27.3	4.00
Bipolar I patients	20.0 ± 3.7	72.0 ± 21.9	3.60
Bipolar II patients	28.0 ± 4.6	156 ± 89.6	5.57
Illness type			
First mania	8.0 ± 1.9	40.0 ± 9.1	5.00
First depression	24.0 ± 3.7	68.0 ± 13.8	2.83

Data are computed weeks to 50% risk ± SE, among 117 bipolar I and 79 bipolar II patients, discontinued abruptly or rapidly (n = 112) versus gradually (n = 84), based on Kaplan–Meier survival analysis

An additional 31 cases involving uncertain discontinuation rates had an intermediate latency to any first recurrence, at 72.0 ± 9.6 weeks

Adapted from previously summarized data[49]

recurrence among bipolar II patients after gradual versus rapid discontinuation was greater than among bipolar I patients (5.6 vs. 3.6-fold), based largely on a prolonged latency to recurrence among bipolar II patients who discontinued lithium gradually (Table 38.2). In addition, we found little association between risk of recurrence after stopping lithium and sex, current age or age at onset of illness, duration of illness, morbidity during treatment, or duration of treatment[49].

Regarding types of morbidity found after stopping lithium treatment, we found a 4-fold greater overall risk of first illness recurrences within 12 months of stopping treatment abruptly or rapidly versus gradually, with similarly large differences in risk for DSM-IV mania, bipolar major depression, and rates of hospitalization (Figure 38.3). Following rapid discontinuation of lithium, the latency to recurrence of mania (8 weeks) was three times shorter than to depression (24 weeks; Table 38.2). An important observation was that rates of life-threatening suicidal acts and completed suicides were more than twice as great soon after rapid discontinuation (Figure 38.3)[53]. These findings support the conclusion that the impact of abrupt or rapid discontinuation of

ongoing lithium prophylaxis presents broad risks for all types of morbidity and an increased potential for suicidal mortality as well, and in both type I and II bipolar disorder patients.

It is important to emphasize that our studies of the rate of discontinuing lithium were clinical, naturalistic and retrospective in nature. Now that the impact of rapid treatment discontinuation is better known, conducting similar studies prospectively and under randomized conditions might be desirable scientifically, but would present major ethical challenges. It is also important to emphasize that, in the reported analyses of effects of the rate of discontinuing lithium, subjects were similar in sex distribution, age and psychiatric histories[47,78,79]. Moreover, we attempted to exclude subjects who were hypomanic, depressed, or dysthymic at the time of discontinuing treatment, since impending illness can lead to impaired judgment and increase the risk of non-adherence to recommended treatment just when it is most needed[47,78,79]. The most often encountered reason for stopping treatment was the patient's refusal to continue, typically following several years of affective stability (55% of cases), often with a wish to try alternative treatments later if

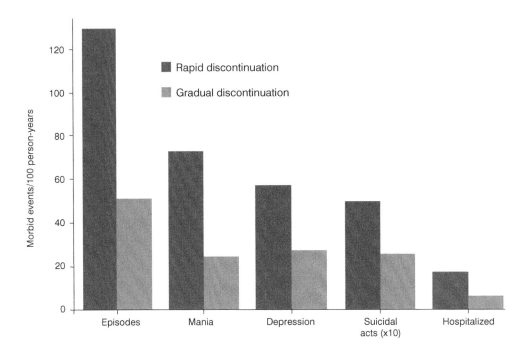

Figure 38.3 Impact of discontinuing lithium prophylaxis rapidly versus gradually, as shown in Figure 38.2, as illness events per 100 patients in 1 year after discontinuation of treatment (morbidity as per cent/year), for all recurrences (differing 2.7-fold), mania (2.8-fold), major depression (2.6-fold), suicidal acts (multiplied by 10 to facilitate representation; 2.1-fold) and hospitalization (2.6-fold). Adapted from data summarized previously by Baldessarini *et al.* (1999)[49]

needed (another 24%); other reasons included pregnancy or clinically significant adverse effects ascribed to treatment (21%)[47,78,79].

There is also suggestive evidence that even sharp reductions of lithium dose and serum concentrations[80,81] or use of every-other-day treatment regimens[82] may be sufficient to induce increased risk of illness recurrences in some bipolar disorder patients. We suggest, therefore, that any elective changes in treatment, including dose reductions as well as complete discontinuations, be done as gradually as seems feasible, and with close clinical monitoring for early indications of impending illness.

Discontinuing treatment during pregnancy and postpartum

A particularly complex circumstance in which discontinuation of lithium or other psychotropic medicines is common, and typically abrupt or rapid, is in anticipation of, or early in, pregnancy. We found that 42 pregnant and 59 age-matched non-pregnant women diagnosed with DSM-IV bipolar disorders followed similar patterns of recurrence during pregnancy or an equivalent follow-up time[71]. Recurrence rates during 10 lunar months were, respectively, 56% and 58% in pregnant vs. non-pregnant women, with latencies to 50% risk of first recurrence of major episodes of mania or depression of 30 versus 24 weeks. These similarities of risk-by-time suggest either that pregnancy has a limited effect on recurrence risk among women of childbearing age with bipolar disorder, or that the impact of treatment discontinuation is a much greater risk factor.

That pregnant women do differ in recurrence risk, at least in the early postpartum period, was supported by an additional observation that, among women who remained stable during pregnancy, 76% became ill within 6 months of delivery, at a high rate of about 14%/month, whereas age-matched non-pregnant women continued to experience risk similar to themselves earlier, or to pregnant women, at about 5–6% per month.

Such findings, and other studies of treatment and treatment-discontinuation in the perinatal period[83] are encouraging major reassessments of comprehensive risk–benefit considerations pertaining to the clinical care of women and their offspring during pregnancy and the neonatal period. There is an emerging, much greater appreciation of the high maternal morbid risks of interrupting ongoing maintenance treatment with lithium or other psychotropic agents, with unknown, but potentially deleterious additional effects on fetal and neonatal development[83]. This altered view encourages greater willingness to treat women during and following pregnancy, with due consideration of the potential impact on fetal and neonatal development, of both maternal illness and its treatment. Such treatment can include use of lithium following establishment of fetal cardiac and major blood vessel morphology in the first trimester of pregnancy, when exposure to lithium *in utero* has a 10–15-fold increased risk of inducing malformation of the tricuspid valve with variable cardiac septal defects (Ebstein's anomaly; at c. 1/1500 live births) that can often be diagnosed during pregnancy and corrected surgically in infancy[84].

Indeed, lithium appears to be much safer even from the start of pregnancy than certain anticonvulsants, including divalproex and carbamazepine, which have been associated with high rates of fetal spina bifida and increased risk of craniofacial anomalies[85].

Effects of discontinuing other psychotropic agents

We have also developed evidence that rapid discontinuation of ongoing maintenance treatment with antipsychotic drugs may also lead to an excess early risk of relapse or recurrences in chronic psychotic disorders[86]. This impression is supported by differences between abrupt or rapid versus gradual discontinuation or stopping long-acting agents including depot prodrug esters[86]. We have also found major increases in early risk of relapse or excerbation in unipolar major depressive patients maintained on antidepressant treatment[87]. Surprisingly, the risk involved tended to *increase* with longer antidepressant treatment, suggesting a possible pharmacodynamic dependency effect rather than an expected improvement in clinical stability with longer treatment[87]. However, antidepressant trials involving comparisons of rapid vs. gradual discontinuation of antidepressants are not available[87]. Moreover, effects of discontinuing mood-stabilizing agents other than lithium, including anticonvulsants and modern antipsychotic drugs, particularly as a function of the rate of discontinuing, have not yet been studied in bipolar disorder patients[3].

LITHIUM RE-TREATMENT

The first account on the outcome of re-treatment with lithium following its discontinuation was in Cade's original report on lithium in mania[1]. In his series of manic patients treated with lithium, three patients (cases 1, 6 and 10) who relapsed within 7 weeks after stopping treatment all responded again within 2 weeks after lithium was re-started. Several later reports commenting incidentally on clinical response after re-starting lithium all found that clinical benefits returned with re-treatment[57,61,76]. Small et al.[57] reported that all of five patients responded again within 6 weeks of re-starting lithium treatment at an unstated time after having stopped treatment. Lapierre and collaborators[61] also noted that all of four patients who discontinued lithium and relapsed within several weeks again improved after re-starting treatment. Fahy and Lawlor[76] encountered relapses among 11 patients following gradual discontinuation of lithium given as an adjunctive treatment, and nine of these showed clinically beneficial effects soon after re-starting treatment.

Very few reports have focused on clinical response to lithium, re-started after its discontinuation, as a primary outcome measure. These include reports of five cases evidently selected for refractoriness to lithium re-treatment among an unstated number of bipolar disorder patients who had previously responded well to lithium[88,89]. Maj et al. found that, among 54 bipolar disorder patients, 18.5% who had previously been maintained episode-free on lithium therapy for prolonged periods experienced some morbidity during a year of re-treatment after discontinuing, suggesting possible loss of benefit[90]. In a study of long-term prophylaxis with lithium in manic-depressive patients, Berghöfer and Müller-Oerlinghausen found no loss of benefit during re-treatment following discontinuation among 23/24 manic-depressive patients who had responded favorably to previous trials of lithium[91]. Also, in a cohort of 86 bipolar disorder patients who had tolerated and shown benefit to lithium treatment averaging 4.6 years, we found only minor losses of benefit during second, or even later re-trials of lithium averaging 4.1 years; however,

during re-treatment, 13% more patients required adjunctive medications, and 5% fewer were maintained without any recurrences[92,93]. Finally, Coryell et al.[94] also found no appreciable difference in the effectiveness of lithium during secondary long-term treatment trials in 28 patients.

It should be emphasized that, despite their suggestions that losses of long-term benefits of lithium prophylaxis are neither large nor universal, the kinds of study just summarized are subject to a notable selection bias. That is, patients included for analysis may be over-represented by those who tolerated and showed sufficient benefit of both initial and repeated trials of lithium as to remain in treatment for prolonged periods.

The possibility of some loss of benefit of lithium treatment after one or more interruptions or discontinuations, and the more general question of whether repeated interruptions or changes in long-term maintenance treatment with lithium or other alternative treatments may have an adverse impact on the course of bipolar disorder, both require further study[50,95,96]. These are particularly pressing questions since many, if not most, patients with bipolar disorder undergo multiple changes in treatment and many are variably adherent to recommended treatment, over years of follow-up.

CONCLUSIONS

The findings summarized in this chapter support several conclusions that have important clinical implications. First, benefit from prophylactic treatment with lithium does not appear to be precluded by even prolonged delay from illness onset, or by a rising number of illness recurrences. We recommend that, in evaluating such relationships, care should be taken to avoid the potential confound of earlier intervention following more severe illness. This association can result in a misleading impression that earlier intervention produces greater relative gains. Instead, assessment of morbidity or wellness during treatment can avoid such artifacts.

Even though these conclusions are optimistic about the potential benefit of even long-delayed treatment with lithium, it remains clinically essential to identify cases of bipolar disorder as early as possible and to attempt to minimize the secondary clinical, co-morbid, social and economic consequences of prolonged, untreated manic-depressive illness, and particularly in efforts to prevent the extraordinarily high risks of suicide that often appear early in the course of manic-depressive illness[52,53,97].

We also reviewed extensive evidence that interruptions of long-term maintenance treatment with lithium can provoke major increases in early risk of recurrences of all phases of manic-depressive illness, as well as major increases in rehospitalization rates and costs, and in risk of suicides and attempts, particularly within the initial 3–6 months after discontinuing treatment. This reaction to lithium discontinuation does not appear to be dependent on the duration of treatment prior to discontinuation. It seems clear that slowing the rate of discontinuation, when clinically feasible, can markedly limit the risks involved. We have proposed that this phenomenon – not unique to lithium, but to be expected with virtually any long-sustained psychotropic treatment – can be understood as a response to an iatrogenically based pharmacodynamic stressor based on removal of a neuropharmacologically active agent from a central nervous system in a drug-adapted state.

It is also important to emphasize that almost all experimental therapeutic studies involving long-term maintenance treatment involve discontinuing a treatment found to be effective initially, to an alternative treatment or to a placebo. Such changes, involving discontinuation of treatment, can produce marked differences in clinical outcomes. Yet, these may not fairly represent comparative effectiveness of treatments, owing to the impact of increased relapse risk associated with the stressor of treatment discontinuation. The concept is that stopping treatment is not the same as not treating.

In addition, the available evidence suggests that response to lithium does not undergo major losses on secondary re-trials following one or more interruptions of long-term treatment is limited. Finally, the potential impact of repeated changes or interruptions of long-term treatment in manic-depressive disorders requires study.

ACKNOWLEDGMENT

Preparation of this chapter was supported, in part, by a grant from the Bruce J. Anderson Foundation and the McLean Hospital Private Donors Research Fund for Psychopharmacology (RJB), as well as by research grants from NARSAD (LT and PS). The chapter is dedicated to the memory of our late collaborator and colleague, Dr. John Hennen.

REFERENCES

1. Cade JFJ. Lithium salts in the treatment of psychotic excitement. Med J Aust 1949; 2: 349–52

2. Baldessarini RJ, Tondo L, Hennen J, Viguera AC. Is lithium still worth using? An update of selected recent research. Harvard Rev Psychiatry 2002; 10: 59–75

3. Baldessarini RJ, Tarzi FI. Pharmacology of psychosis and mania. In Brunton LL, Lazo JS, Parker KL et al., eds. Goodman and Gilman's The Pharmacological Basis of Therapeutcs, 11th edn, Ch 18. New York: McGraw-Hill, 2005

4. Bratti IM, Baldessarini RJ, Baethge C, Tondo L. Preteatment episode count and response to lithium treatment in manic-depressive illness. Harvard Rev Psychiatry 2003; 11: 245–56

5. Baastrup PC, Schou M. Lithium as a prophylactic agent: its effect against recurrent depressions and manic-depressive psychosis. Arch Gen Psychiatry 1967; 16: 162–72

6. Angst J, Weis P, Grof P, et al. Lithium prophylaxis in recurrent affective disorders. Br J Psychiatry 1970; 116: 604–13

7. Coppen A, Noguera R, Bailey J, et al. Prophylactic lithium in affective disorders. Lancet 1971; 2: 275–9

8. Dunner DL, Fieve RR. Clinical factors in lithium carbonate prophylaxis failure. Arch Gen Psychiatry 1974; 30: 229–33

9. Prien RF, Caffey EM, Klett CJ. Factors associated with treatment success in lithium carbonate prophylaxis: report of the Veterans Administration and National Institute of Mental Health collaborative study group. Arch Gen Psychiatry 1974; 31: 189–92

10. Dunner DL, Fleiss JL, Fieve RR. Lithium carbonate prophylaxis failure. Br J Psychiatry 1976; 129: 40–4

11. Kocsis JH, Stokes PE. Lithium maintenance: factors affecting outcome. Am J Psychiatry 1979; 136: 563–6

12. Sarantidis D, Waters B. Predictors of lithium prophylaxis effectiveness. Progr Neuropsychopharmacol 1981; 5: 507–10

13. Abou-Saleh MT. Platelet MAO, personality and response to lithium prophylaxis. J Affect Disord 1983; 5: 55–65

14. Maj M, Del Vecchio M, Starace F, et al. Prediction of affective psychoses response to lithium prophylaxis. Acta Psychiatr Scand 1984; 69: 37–44

15. Abou-Saleh MT, Coppen A. Who responds to prophylactic lithium? J Affect Disord 1986; 10: 115–25

16. Bouman TK, Niemantsverdriet-van Kampen JG, Ormel J, Slooff CJ. The effectiveness of lithium prophylaxis in bipolar and unipolar depressions and schizoaffective disorders. J Affect Disord 1986; 11: 275–80

17. Mander AJ. Clinical prediction of outcome and lithium response in bipolar affective disorder. J Affect Disord 1986; 11: 35–41

18. Page C, Benaim S, Lappin F. A long-term retrospective follow-up study of patients treated with prophylactic lithium carbonate. Br J Psychiatry 1987; 150: 175–9

19. Gelenberg AJ, Kane JM, Keller MB, et al. Comparison of standard and low serum levels of lithium for maintenance treatment of bipolar disorder. N Engl J Med 1989; 321: 1489–93

20. Maj M, Pirozzi R, Kemali D. Long-term outcome of lithium prophylaxis in patients initially classified as complete responders. Psychopharmacology 1989; 98: 535–8

21. Aagaard J, Vestergaard P. Predictors of outcome in prophylactic lithium treatment: a 2-year prospective study. J Affect Disord 1990; 18: 259–66

22. O'Connell RA, Mayo JA, Flatow L, et al. Outcome of bipolar disorder on long-term treatment with lithium. Br J Psychiatry 1991; 159: 123–32

23. Stefos G, Bauwens F, Staner L, et al. Psychosocial predictors of major affective recurrences in bipolar disorder: a 4-year longitudinal study of patients on prophylactic treatment. Acta Psychiatr Scand 1996; 93: 420–6

24. Kusalic M, Engelsmann F. Predictors of lithium treatment responsiveness in bipolar patients: a two-year prospective study. Neuropsychobiology 1998; 37: 146–9

25. Maj M, Pirozzi R, Magliano L, Bartoli L. Long-term outcome of lithium prophylaxis in bipolar disorder: a 5-year prospective study of 402 patients at a lithium clinic. Am J Psychiatry 1998; 155: 30–5

26. Baldessarini RJ, Tondo L, Hennen J, Floris G. Latency and episodes before treatment: response to lithium maintenance in bipolar I and II disorders. Bipolar Disord 1999; 2: 91–7

27. Franchini L, Zanardi R, Smeraldi E, Gasperini M. Early onset of lithium prophylaxis as a predictor of good long-term outcome. Eur Arch Psychiatry Clin Neurosci 1999; 249: 227–30

28. Kulhara P, Basu D, Mattoo SK, et al. Lithium prophylaxis of recurrent bipolar affective

disorder: long-term outcome and its psycho-social correlates. J Affect Disord 1999; 54: 87–96

29. Yazici O, Kara K, Ucok A, et al. Predictors of lithium prophylaxis in bipolar patients. J Affect Disord 1999; 55: 133–42

30. Swann AC, Bowden CL, Calabrese JR, et al. Mania: differential effects of previous depressive and manic episodes on response to treatment. Acta Psychiatr Scand 2000; 101: 444–51

31. Baethge C, Smolka MN, Gruschka P, et al. Does prophylaxis-delay in bipolar disorder influence outcome? Results from a long-term study of 147 patients. Acta Psychiatr Scand 2003; 107: 260–7

32. Baldessarini RJ, Tondo L, Hennen J. Latency and episodes before treatment: effects on pretreatment morbidity but not response to lithium maintenance in bipolar I and II disorders. Bipolar Disord 2003; 5: 169–79

33. Baethge C, Baldessarini RJ, Bratti IM, Tondo L. Prophylaxis-latency and outcome in bipolar disorders. Can J Psychiatry 2003; 48: 449–57

34. Seretti A, Lattuada E, Franchini L, Smeraldi E. Melancholic features and response to lithium prophylaxis in mood disorders. Depress Anxiety 2000; 11: 73–9

35. Maj M, Pirozzi R, Magliano L. Late non-response to lithium prophylaxis in bipolar patients: prevalence and predictors. J Affect Disord 1996; 39: 39–42

36. Garcia-López A, Ezquiaga E, Nieves P, Rodriguez-Salvanés E. Factores predicters de requesta al litio en pacientes bipolares en seguimiento a largo plazo. Actas Esp Psiquiatr 2001; 29: 327–32

37. Goldberg JF, Ernst CL. Features associated with the delayed initiation of mood stabilizers at illness onset in bipolar disorder. J Clin Psychiatry 2002; 63: 985–91

38. Baethge C, Gruschka P, Berghofer A, et al. Prophylaxis of schizoaffective disorder with lithium or carbamazepine: outcome after long-term follow-up. J Affect Disord 2004; 79: 43–50

39. Baldessarini RJ, Tondo L, Baethge CJ, et al. Effects of treatment latency on response to maintenance treatment in manic–depressive disorders. Bipolar Disord 2005; in press

40. Trede K, Salvatore P, Baethge C, et al. Manic-depressive Illness: evolution in Kraepelin's Textbook, 1983–1926. Harvard Rev Psychiatry 2005; 13: 155–78

41. Slater E. Zur Periodik des manisch-depressiven Irreseins. Z Gesamte Neurol Psychiatrie 1938; 162: 794–801

42. Oepen G, Salvatore P, Baldessarini RJ. On the periodicity of manic–depressive insanity by Eliot Slater (1938): translation and commentary. J Affect Disord 2004; 78: 1–9

43. Baldessarini RJ, Salvatore P, Oepen G, et al. Course of manic-depressive illness: is there progressive cycle-shortening? (Poster/Abstract). Proceedings of the Annual Meeting of the ACNP, San Juan, PR, December, 2002

44. Baldessarini RJ, Tondo L, Hennen J. Effects of rapid cycling on response to lithium maintenance treatment in 360 bipolar I and II disorder patients. J Affect Disord 2000; 61: 13–22

45. Tondo L, Hennen J, Baldessarini RJ. Meta-analysis of treatment responses of rapid-cycling and non-rapid-cycling bipolar disorder patients. Acta Psychiatr Scand 2003; 104: 4–14

46. Suppes T, Baldessarini RJ, Faedda GL, Tohen M. Risk of recurrence following discontinuation of lithium treatment in bipolar disorder. Arch Gen Psychiatry 1991; 48: 1082–8

47. Faedda GL, Tondo L, Baldessarini RJ, et al. Outcome after rapid vs. gradual discontinuation of lithium treatment in bipolar mood disorders. Arch Gen Psychiatry 1993; 50: 448–55

48. Johnson RE, McFarland BH. Lithium use and discontinuation in a health maintenance organization. Am J Psychiatry 1996; 153: 993–1000

49. Baldessarini RJ, Tondo L, Viguera AC. Discontinuing lithium maintenance treatment in bipolar disorders: risks and implications. Bipolar Disord 1999; 1: 17–24

50. Davis JM, Janicak PG, Hogan DM. Mood stabilizers in the prevention of recurrent affective disorders: a meta-analysis. Acta Psychiatr Scand 1999; 100: 406–17

51. Franks MA, Macritchie KN, Young AH. The consequences of suddenly stopping

psychotropic medication in bipolar disorder. Clin Approaches Bipolar Disord 2005; 6: 11–17

52. Müller-Oerlinghausen B, Muser-Causemann B, Volk J. Suicides and parasuicides in a high-risk patient group on and off lithium long-term medication. J Affect Disord 1992; 25: 261–9

53. Tondo L, Baldessarini RJ, Hennen J, et al. Lithium treatment and risk of suicidal behavior in bipolar disorder patients. J Clin Psychiatry 1998; 59: 405–14

54. Goodwin GM, Cavanagh JTO, Glabus MF, et al. Uptake of [^{99}Tc]-exametazime shown by SPECT before and after lithium withdrawal in bipolar patients: associations with mania. Br J Psychiatry 1997; 170: 426–30

55. Baastrup PC, Poulsen JC, Schou M, et al. Prophylactic lithium: double blind discontinuation in manic–depressive and recurrent-depressive disorders. Lancet 1970; 2: 326–30

56. Melia PI. Prophylactic lithium: a double-blind trial in recurrent affective disorders. Br J Psychiatry 1970; 116: 621–4

57. Small JG, Small IF, Moore DF. Experimental withdrawal of lithium in recovered manic–depressive patients: a report of five cases. Am J Psychiatry 1971; 127: 1555–8

58. Cundall RL, Brooks PW, Murray LG. A controlled evaluation of lithium prophylaxis in affective disorders. Psychol Med 1972; 2: 308–11

59. Hullin RP, McDonald R, Allsopp MN. Prophylactic lithium in recurrent affective disorders. Lancet 1972; 1: 1044–6

60. Fyrö B, Petterson U. A double blind study of the prophylactic effect of lithium in manic–depressive disease. Acta Psychiatr Scand 1977; 53 (Suppl): 17–22

61. Lapierre YD, Gagnon A, Kokkinidis L. Rapid recurrence of mania following lithium withdrawal. Biol Psychiatry 1980; 15: 859–64

62. Klein HE, Broucek B, Greil W. Lithium withdrawal triggers psychotic states. Br J Psychiatry 1981; 139: 255–6

63. Christodoulou GN, Lykouras EP. Abrupt lithium discontinuation in manic–depressive patients. Acta Psychiatr Scand 1982; 65: 310–14

64. Margo A, McMahon P. Lithium withdrawal triggers psychosis. Br J Psychiatry 1982; 141: 407–10

65. Sashidharan SP, McGuire RJ. Recurrence of affective illness after withdrawal of long-term lithium treatment. Acta Psychiatr Scand 1983; 68: 126–33

66. Mendlewicz J. Lithium discontinuation in bipolar illness: double-blind, prospective, controlled study. In Corsini GU, ed. Current Trends in Lithium and Rubidium Therapy. Lancaster, UK: MTP Press, 1984: 135–41

67. Goodnick PJ. Clinical and laboratory effects of discontinuation of lithium prophylaxis. Acta Psychiatr Scand 1985; 71: 608–14

68. Mander AJ. Is there a lithium withdrawal syndrome? Br J Psychiatry 1986; 149: 498–501

69. Mander AJ, Loudon JB. Rapid recurrence of mania following abrupt discontinuation of lithium. Lancet 1988; 2: 15–17

70. Koukopoulos A, Reginaldi D, Minnai G, Serra G, Pani L, Johnson FN. The long-term prophylaxis of affective disorders. In Gessa G, Fratta W, Pani L, Serra G, eds. Depression and Mania: From Neurobiology to Treatment. New York: Raven Press, 1995: 127–47

71. Viguera AC, Nonacs R, Cohen LS, et al. Risk of discontinuing lithium maintenance in pregnant vs. nonpregnant women with bipolar disorders. Am J Psychiatry 2000; 157: 179–84

72. Cavanagh J, Smyth R, Goodwin GM. Relapse into mania or depression following lithium discontinuation: a 7-year follow-up. Acta Psychiatr Scand 2004; 109: 91–5

73. Yazici O, Kora K, Polat A, Saylan M. Controlled lithium discontinuation in bipolar patients with good response to long-term lithium prophylaxis. J Affect Disord 2004; 80: 269–71

74. Kafantaris V, Coletti DJ, Dicker R, et al. Lithium treatment of acute mania in adolescents: a placebo-controlled discontinuation study. J Am Acad Child Adolesc Psychiatry 2004; 43: 984–93

75. Molnar G, Pristach C, Feeney MG, Fava GA. A pilot study of managed lithium discontinuation. Psychopharmacol Bull 1988; 24: 217–19

76. Fahy S, Lawlor BA. Discontinuation of lithium augmentation in an elderly cohort. Int J Geriatr Psychiatry 2001; 16: 1004–9

77. Tondo L, Baldessarini RH, Floris G. Long-term effectiveness of lithium maintenance treatment in types I and II bipolar disorders. Br J Psychiatry 2001; 178 (Suppl): 184–90

78. Baldessarini RJ, Tondo L, Faedda G, et al. Effects of the rate of discontinuing lithium maintenance treatment in bipolar disorders. J Clin Psychiatry 1996; 57: 441–8

79. Baldessarini RJ, Tondo L, Floris G, Rudas N. Reduced morbidity after gradually discontinuing lithium in bipolar I and II disorders: a replication study. Am J Psychiatry 1997; 154: 551–3

80. Waters B, Lapierre YD, Gagnon A, et al. Determination of the optimum concentration of lithium for the prophylaxis of manic–depressive disorder. Biol Psychiatry 1982; 17: 1323–9

81. Perlis RH, Sachs GS, Lafer B, et al. Effect of abrupt change from standard to low serum levels of lithium: a reanalysis of double-blind lithium maintenance data. Am J Psychiatry 2002; 159: 1155–59

82. Jensen HV, Plenge P, Mellerup ET, et al. Lithium prophylaxis of manic–depressive disorder: daily lithium dosing schedule vs. every second day. Acta Psychiatr Scand 1995; 92: 69–74

83. Viguera AC, Cohen LS, Baldessarini RJ, Nonacs R. Managing bipolar disorder in pregnancy: weighing the risks and benefits. Can J Psychiatry 2002; 47: 426–36

84. Cohen LS, Friedman JM, Jefferson JW, et al. A reevaluation of risk of in utero exposure to lithium. JAMA 1994; 271: 146–50

85. Dodd S, Berk M. The pharmacology of bipolar disorder during pregnancy and breastfeeding Expert Opin Drug Safety 2004; 3: 221–9

86. Viguera AC, Baldessarini RJ, Hegarty JM, et al. Clinical risk following abrupt and gradual withdrawal of maintnenace neuroleptic treatment. Arch Gen Psychiatry 1997; 54: 49–55

87. Viguera AC, Baldessarini RJ, Friedberg J. Risks of interrupting continuation or maintenance treatment with antidepressants in major depressive disorders. Harvard Rev Psychiatry 1998; 5: 293–306

88. Post RM, Leverich GS, Altshuler L, Mikalauskas K. Lithium-discontinuation-induced refractoriness: preliminary observations. Am J Psychiatry 1992; 149: 1727–9

89. Bauer M. Refractoriness induced by lithium discontinuation despite adequate serum lithium levels (Letter). Am J Psychiatry 1994; 151: 1522

90. Maj M, Pirozzi R, Magliano L. Nonresponse to reinstituted lithium prophylaxis in previously responsive bipolar patients: prevalence and predictors. Am J Psychiatry 1995; 152: 1810–11

91. Berghöfer A, Müller-Oerlinghausen B. No loss of efficacy after discontinuation and reinstitution of long-term lithium treatment? In Gallicchio VS, Birch NJ, eds. Lithium: Biochemical and Clinical Advances. Cheshire, CT: Weidner Publishing, 1996: 39–46

92. Tondo L, Baldessarini RJ, Floris G, Rudas N. Effectiveness of restarting lithium treatment after its discontinuation in bipolar I and bipolar II disorders. Am J Psychiatry 1997; 154: 548–50

93. Baldessarini RJ, Tondo L. Recurrence risk in bipolar manic-depressive disorders after discontinuing lithium maintenance treatment: an overview. Clin Drug Invest 1998; 15: 337–51

94. Coryell W, Solomon D, Leon AC, Akiskal HS, Keller MB, Scheftner WA, Mueller T. Lithium discontinuation and subsequent effectiveness. Am J Psychiatry 1998; 155: 895–8

95. Maj M. The effect of lithium in bipolar disorder: a review of recent research evidence. Bipolar Disord 2003; 5: 180–8

96. MacQueen G, Joffe RT. The clinical effects of lithium discontinuation: the debate continues. Acta Psychiatr Scand 2004; 109: 81–2

97. Tondo L, Isacsson G, Baldessarini RJ. Suicide in bipolar disorder: risk and prevention. CNS Drugs 2003; 17: 491–511

39 Compliance with long-term lithium treatment

Per Vestergaard, Krista Nielsen Straarup, Kenneth Thau

Contents   Introduction • Concepts and definitions • The importance of patients' compliance • Non-compliance: the size of the problem • Factors associated with lithium non-compliance • Prevention of non-compliance with lithium • Compliance with lithium treatment among health-care providers • Conclusion

INTRODUCTION

Patients' compliance with medical treatment regimens is far from complete. This is true for medicine in general[1], for treatment of most psychiatric disorders[2] and for lithium treatment of bipolar disorder patients in particular[3]. Jamison, in her pioneering research into the subject of compliance with long-term lithium treatment, reviewed comprehensively the state of the art in 1990 in her textbook on manic-depressive illness[3]. This chapter offers brief summaries of the position in 1990 and reviews significant contributions to the knowledge of compliance with lithium acquired during the following 15 years.

CONCEPTS AND DEFINITIONS

Until 1990 the concept of 'compliance' prevailed over 'adherence'. The situation has changed during the past 15 years and now the two concepts are used interchangeably, apparently with an increasing preference for 'adherence'[4]. Both concepts, however, connote the patients' acceptance of recommended health behaviors[5]: taking the pills as prescribed, keeping appointments as agreed and staying in treatment as expected. In this text the authors have decided to apply 'compliance' as the concept that describes the health behaviors under study. Other concepts offered are concordance (between patient and doctor) 'suggesting a more egalitarian view of relationship between prescribing and medicine-taking, between patient and prescriber'[6] and drop-out, which describes the extreme opposite of good compliance: the patient leaving treatment prematurely without his doctor's consent. It should be kept in mind that, when patients comply, as opposed to dropping out, they rarely do so completely but often only partially or intermittently[3]. Even drop-out from treatment may retrospectively prove to be an intermittent non-compliance when the patient later resumes treatment.

THE IMPORTANCE OF PATIENTS' COMPLIANCE

Non-compliance with lithium is considered one of the main reasons for the unsatisfactory gap between lithium efficacy and effectiveness[7]. Efficacy of lithium in randomized, placebo-controlled studies is approximately 60%[8] as opposed to effectiveness, which in daily clinical use is often reported at levels between 20 and 40%[9]. Although lack of patient compliance may explain the majority of the efficacy–effectiveness gap, compliance among health-care professionals plays an important role, ranging from lack of dedication to treatment policies to clear-cut sabotage. The importance of care-givers' attitudes will be dealt with in a later section.

The consequences of patients' non-compliance are, besides a reduced quality of life for both patients and relatives, a significant increase in re-admittance to hospital[4] and a significant risk of premature death due to suicide[10].

NON-COMPLIANCE: THE SIZE OF THE PROBLEM

Rates of lithium non-compliance vary in 12 studies reported by Jamison[3] from 18 to 53% and, in a recent review of compliance with medication for affective disorders, a median prevalence of 41% was given[4]. In lithium-treated cohorts at the Aarhus University Psychiatric Clinic non-compliance rates between 20 and 40% have been reported during the past 15 years[11–13]. The estimates of non-

compliance from the Aarhus clinic are rather conservative, since essentially total non-compliance in the form of drop-out from treatment in consecutively admitted patients (intention to treat) was reported. Dropping out of treatment is a reliable and easy-to-obtain measure of non-compliance which, however, does not record more subtle aspects of compliance behavior. Other ways of estimating compliance behavior include objective measures such as pill count and determination of serum and urine drug concentrations[14] and subjective measures such as patient inquiries with formal questionnaires or less formal interviews[4,13].

FACTORS ASSOCIATED WITH LITHIUM NON-COMPLIANCE

Table 39.1[3,4,11,15–19] shows a list of illness, patient- and treatment-related factors that are associated with lithium non-compliance. These factors emerge from a rather large body of research conducted over the past 30 years, research which is partly epidemiologic, identifying predictor variables in cohorts of non-compliant patients and partly qualitative, identifying factors associated with patients' attitudes[3,4,11,16–20].

Illness-related factors that predict lithium non-compliance involve the severity (a high number of previous admissions to hospital) and complexity of illness with the appearance of psychotic symptoms, cognitive dysfunctions and co-morbidity with personality disorders and substance abuse[3,4,11,19].

Patient-related factors associated with lithium non-compliance include the patient's irrational concept of his illness: it does not exist, it is of minor importance, it will disappear without treatment, it represents an asset, providing him with both creativity and productivity. Some non-compliant patients also report missing the well-being of manic highs;

Table 39.1 Illness, patient and treatment factors associated with lithium non-compliance (from references 3, 4, 11, 15–19)

Illness
High number of previous admissions to hospital
Co-morbidity with personality disorders and
    substance abuse
Psychotic symptoms and cognitive dysfunctions

Patient
Denial of illness
Missing manic highs and creativity
Resisting mood control from medication
Feeling stigmatized because of medication
Fear of lithium-induced side-effects
Lack of social support
Feeling well – no need for continuous treatment

Treatment
Side-effects of lithium
Complexity of treatment regimen
Availability and affordability of health care
Continuity of care

they resist the notion of their mood being controlled with medication – irrational views often supported by their peers[3]. Some patients may fear lithium-induced side-effects which they have heard of but not (yet) experienced. This fear may in some patients exceed the trouble with existing side-effects[4]. Finally, some patients want to discontinue their treatment because they feel well and see no need for further treatment[3].

Aspects of lithium treatment itself may be associated with non-compliance. Most often mentioned by both clinicians and patients are lithium-induced side-effects, which appear in 50–75% of all patients and some of which are extremely troublesome[3]. In a rank order of side-effects associated with lithium non-compliance, Jamison mentioned memory problems as number one, weight gain as number two, and tremor and lack of coordination as number three. It has, however, been difficult to substantiate memory impairment in experimental studies of lithium (see Chapter 36). Polyuria, tiredness, blurring of senses, blurred vision and nausea followed as the next five side-effects[3]. Also, more general treatment factors known from somatic medicine operate in lithium treatment, such as the complexity of the treatment regimen (for lithium the regular control of serum lithium levels with blood sampling), the availability and affordability of the health-care system and the continuity of care offered to the patient[1,5].

A fourth factor that not infrequently contributes to patients' non-compliance is lack of knowledge, lack of enthusiasm or the clear-cut sabotage of treatment which the patient may encounter with various health workers who are unaware of the seriousness of bipolar illness, the treatment methods and options, but still feel compelled to voice an attitude towards the treatment in disrespect of both the patient and his treating physician[7]. An obvious occasion for treatment sabotage occurs when a woman with bipolar illness decides to become pregnant and hears advice from doctors, nurses or midwives such as: 'Stop lithium, you don't want to hurt your child, do you?' This spontaneous 'advice' substitutes for a serious and well-informed discussion of the pros and cons of continued lithium treatment during pregnancy[21] see also Chapter 18.

A recent study on medication-prescribing pattern for patients with bipolar I disorder in hospital settings showed that doctors' adherence to published practice guidelines was poor. The results of the study suggested that between one-third and two-thirds of patients with bipolar I disorder were discharged from hospitals on medications not generally recommended by current practice guidelines[22].

PREVENTION OF NON-COMPLIANCE WITH LITHIUM

Prevention of non-compliance is an extremely important issue for health-care providers who wish to secure their bipolar patients a maximum of treatment efficacy with lithium. The above-mentioned factors associated with lithium non-compliance offer a guide to efforts that will provide enhanced compliance.

It is important to identify and treat effectively the present illness episode and any interfering co-morbidity such as personality disturbances and substance abuse. Both pharmacologic means and various psycho-therapeutic programs, some of which will be detailed below, are relevant[20]. If treatment efforts are reduced before the patient is completely well, that is if the patient is not yet in a neutral mood, if psychotic symptoms, cognitive defects and other residual sympto-matology still prevail, the danger of non-compliance and the ensuing recurrence of a full-blown episode is imminent.

A change of negative, irrational and fearful attitudes in both the patient and his family is an important step towards better compliance. Information and knowledge about the illness and the treatment and comfort when fear and anxiety prevail is provided through different psychotherapeutic interventions. Knowledge and information is addressed by psycho-educational programs and – together with emotional issues – by different kinds of psychotherapy, cognitive, behavioral or inter-personal or psychodynamic[23–26]. In everyday practice the distinction between the various programs is often blurred, and different pro-grams are deliberately mixed in order to secure patients a maximum benefit. Psychosocial interventions are often initiated with a psycho-educational program which later will be followed by a psychotherapeutic program with focus on either cognitive or more psycho-dynamic methods.

Psychoeducational and psychotherapeutic approaches against non-compliance are often embedded in programs that address the psychological treatment of bipolar illness comprehensively[24,26]. The program may be part of the patient's individual treatment and less formal, or it may be part of well-organized, well-structured group psychotherapy which follows a schedule with specific sessions dealing with specific issues, one of them being the identification and prevention of non-compliance. Psychotherapeutic interventions for bipolar illness will, whether or not they are specifically aimed towards compliance, tend to enhance compliance, because any effort that serves the attachment of the patient to the health provider will enhance compliance.

A list of compliance-enhancing issues often dealt with in formal group psychoeducational programs is presented in Table 39.2[23–26].

Non-compliance is also related to treatment factors such as physical and cognitive side-effects. Side-effects may well subside with even a subtle lowering of the serum lithium level; with serum levels below $0.7–0.8$ mmol/l, side-effects usually are few and not very bothersome[12]. If side-effects do occur in spite of low serum lithium levels, hand tremor may be prevented with the prescription of beta-blocking agents, hypothyroidism with the prescription of levo-thyroxine, and weight gain with careful instructions about diet and exercise (Chapter 24). Some side-effects (e.g. gastro-intestinal) may dominate during the first month of treatment, and it is important that both doctors and patients know that they will be most likely to be experienced as less trouble-some after a short period of time. The blurring of senses and moderate cognitive side-effects (Chapter 37), which some patients do experience for months or years, may be a subject

Table 39.2 Psychological interventions for lithium non-compliance: important treatment issues (from references 23–26)

Facts about bipolar illness and lithium treatment: identification and modification of patients' (and relatives') concepts and misconcepts about the illness and the pharmacotherapy

Risk associated with treatment withdrawal

The influence of alcohol and street drugs on symptoms and treatment outcome

Early recognition of symptoms and warning signals

Establishment and maintenance of supporting social relations

Assessment of the pros and cons of taking medication

for the psychoeducational or psychotherapeutic efforts mentioned above. Furthermore, once-a-day dosing with slow-release lithium tablets may for many patients be more convenient than frequent dosing with conventional tablets, thus enhancing compliance. Blood sampling for the determination of serum lithium levels may scare some patients away from lithium treatment, but for most patients (and their doctors) the monitoring of serum lithium levels may serve as a convenient framework for their regular encounters and serve as an opportunity for discussions of other relevant clinical issues.

Not only may specific aspects of treatment, such as the lithium-induced side-effects, compromise compliance with treatment. More general factors, such as the geographical distance between patient and health-care provider, the continuity of staff and the physical environment in the offices, may prove important for establishing a stable and enduring relationship between the patient and the doctor and his staff. The general need for good health care is best met through well-educated general practitioners who have easy access to secondary-care specialized facilities such as lithium clinics or affective disorder hospital units[7].

COMPLIANCE WITH LITHIUM TREATMENT AMONG HEALTH-CARE PROVIDERS

Compliance among health-care providers has become an important issue, since new research reveals that patients are not always offered the treatment they need, that the necessary treatment is not given according to the generally accepted treatment guideline or policies and, finally, that health-care providers at times interfere negatively with treatments their patients are receiving in other settings[7,22]. In order to combat professional non-compliance, continuous medical education for both general practitioners and specialists is mandatory and ethical codes for doctors', nurses' and clinical psychologists' behaviors should be vigorously enforced. Through advocacy groups and the increasing acceptance of patients' rights to complain, patients today are hopefully better armed against such behavior of health-care providers.

CONCLUSION

Good compliance with lithium treatment is a precondition for a successful outcome of long-term prophylactic treatment of bipolar disorder patients.

In a narrow sense 'compliance' refers to the patient's ability and willingness to take his medicine (lithium) as prescribed by the doctor. In a broader sense the promotion of compliance with drug treatments has come to mean any measure that enhances the effectiveness of the drug in question, and prevention of non-compliance to mean combating against any obstacle to a successful treatment, be it co-morbidity, misconceptions, side-effects, an insufficient health service or incompetent health-care providers. In this way the compliance issue has brought into focus not only possible shortcomings of the drug and the health system which delivers the drug but also the many subtle issues relating to patient's health beliefs and attitudes towards his illness and the treatment, issues which clearly influences treatment outcome.

Psychological interventions, be they psycho-education, cognitive, interpersonal or psychodynamic therapy, have proven helpful in the effort to change health beliefs and attitudes and enhance compliance. Thus, psychotherapy has entered the stage of bipolar illness through the back door. Psychotherapy and education have served the enhancement of compliance, but today psychotherapy of bipolar patients also includes issues such as the patients' recognition of stressful triggers of illness, their ability to accept and cope with chronic illness and their maintenance of helpful relationships with peers and relatives.

Prevention of patients' non-compliance has been integrated into psychotherapy of bipolar illness, prevention of doctors' non-compliance has led to the development of treatment policies and guidelines and hopefully insufficient health systems will be replaced by systems with good general care and access to specialized facilities for the difficult-to-treat bipolar patients.

REFERENCES

1. Haynes RB, Taylor DW, Sackett DL. Compliance in Health Care. Baltimore: University Press, 1979
2. Verdoux H, Lengronne J, Liraud F. Medication adherence in psychosis: predictors and impact on outcome. A 2-year follow-up of first-admitted subjects. Acta Psychiatr Scand 2000; 102: 203–10
3. Jamison KR. Medication compliance. In Goodwin FK, Jamison KR, eds. Manic-depressive Illness. Oxford: Oxford University Press, 1990; 746–62
4. Lingam R, Scott J. Treatment non-adherence in affective disorders. Acta Psychiatr Scand 2002; 105: 164–72
5. Wright EC. Non-compliance – or how many aunts has Matilda? Lancet 1993; 342: 909–13
6. Mullen PD. Compliance becomes concordance. Br Med J 1997; 314: 691
7. Guscott R, Taylor L. Lithium prophylaxis in recurrent affective illness. Efficacy, Effectiveness and Efficiency. Br J Psychiatry 1994; 164: 741–66
8. Burgess S, Geddes J, Hawton K, et al. Lithium for maintenance treatment of mood disorders Cochrane Database Syst Rev 2001; (3): CD003013
9. Vestergaard P. Treatment and prevention of mania: a Scandinavian perspective. Neuropsychopharmacology 1992; 7: 249–59
10. Brodersen A, Licht RW, Vestergaard P, et al. Sixteen-year mortality in patients with affective disorder commenced on lithium. Br J Psychiatry 2000; 176: 429–33
11. Aagaard J, Vestergaard P. Predictors of outcome in prophylactic lithium treatment: a 2-year prospective study. J Affect Disord 1990; 18: 259–66
12. Vestergaard P, Licht RW, Brodersen A, et al. Outcome of lithium prophylaxis: a prospective follow-up of affective disorder patients assigned to high and low serum lithium levels. Acta Psychiatr Scand 1998; 98: 310–15
13. Licht RW, Vestergaard P, Rasmussen N-A, et al. A lithium clinic for bipolar patients: 2-year outcome of the first 148 patients. Acta Psychiatr Scand 2001; 104: 1–4
14. Linden M, Schussler G, Müller-Oerlinghausen B. Clinical trial of a test stick to control patient compliance under nomifensine treatment. Br J Psychiatry 1982; 140: 50–4
15. Harvey NS. The development and descriptive use of the lithium attitudes questionnaire. J Affect Disord 1991; 22: 211–19
16. Colom FC, Vieta E, Martínez-Arán A, et al. Clinical factors associated with treatment non-compliance in euthymic bipolar patients. J Clin Psychiatry 2000; 61: 549–55

17. Fleck DE, Keck PE, Corey KB, et al. Factors associated with medication adherence in African American and white patients with bipolar disorder. J Clin Psychiatry 2005; 66: 646–52

18. Greenhouse WJ, Meyer B, Johnson SL. Coping and medication adherence in bipolar disorder. J Affect Disord 2000; 59: 237–41

19. Schumann C, Lenz G, Berghöfer A, et al. Non-adherence with long-term prophylaxis: a 6-year naturalistic follow-up study of affectively ill patients. Psychiatry Res 1999; 89: 247–57

20. Vieta E. Improving treatment adherence in bipolar disorder through psychoeducation. J Clin Psychiatry 2005; 66 (Suppl l): 24–9

21. Yonkers KA, Wisner KL, Stowe A, et al. Management of bipolar disorder during pregnancy and the postpartum period. Am J Psychiatry 2004; 161: 608–20

22. Lim Z, Tunis L, Edel WS, et al. Medication prescribing patterns for patients with bipolar I disorder in hospital settings: adherence to published practice guidelines. Bipolar Disord 2001; 3: 165–73

23. Cochran SD. Preventing medical non-compliance in the outpatient treatment of bipolar affective disorders. J Consult Clin Psychol 1984; 52: 873–8

24. Colom F, Vieta E, Sánchez-Moreno J, et al. Psychoeducation in bipolar patients with comorbid personality disorders. Bipolar Disord 2004; 6: 294–8

25. Scott J, Tacchi MJ. A pilot study of concordance therapy for individuals with bipolar disorders who are non-adherent with lithium prophylaxis. Bipolar Disord 2002; 4: 386–2

26. Basco MR, Rush AJ. Cognitive–behavioral Therapy for Bipolar Disorder. New York: Guilford Press, 2005

40 Lithium intoxication: signs and treatment

Frank Martens

Contents Factors leading to intoxication • Epidemiology of poisoning • Diagnostic routines • Laboratory and technical diagnostic • Differential diagnosis • Treatment • Monitoring • Case vignettes

FACTORS LEADING TO INTOXICATION

Lithium toxicity typically occurs in one of three scenarios: acute overdose in a patient who does not normally take the drug; acute overdose in a patient chronically taking lithium; or chronic toxicity resulting from accumulation of the drug during therapeutic use. Lithium load and the duration of exposure to this load determine the extent of the intoxication[1,2].

Acute overdose

Acute poisoning typically occurs in a household member of a patient treated with lithium. Symptoms and clinical course of the intoxication under these circumstances differ from an acute overdose in patients who are treated with lithium chronically. This acute intoxication usually carries less risk and patients have milder symptoms than are observed in other forms of lithium poisoning, since the elimination half-life is shorter in lithium-naive individuals and distribution into the central nervous system (CNS) needs some time[3]. The main symptoms in this situation are nausea, emesis and diarrhea and may be confused with a gastrointestinal (GI) disorder. Patients do not usually have significant neurologic manifestations, despite high serum lithium levels during the first 12 hours or more after ingestion. Serum lithium concentrations as high as 9.8 mEq/l without significant toxicity have been reported after acute overdose[1]. However, neurotoxicity may develop over the subsequent 24–48 hours, even as serum levels fall[1]. An acute overdose of at least 1.08 mEq lithium/kg body weight is required to produce potentially toxic lithium levels.

Acute overdose in chronic therapy

Acute on chronic poisoning occurs in patients treated with lithium chronically who take an overdose. This ingestion may be intentional in a suicide attempt or accidental, especially in patients with bipolar disorders who are in a depressive phase, although the frequency of suicide attempts by ingestion of lithium is very low. Their clinical course is usually similar to that of individuals with acute ingestions, but a smaller dose may be required to produce severe intoxication depending on the preingestion lithium level. Often, patients present with symptoms of CNS and cardiac toxicity.

Chronic toxicity

Toxicity occurs in patients receiving lithium chronically whose dosage has been increased or whose excretion is decreased. A family member or therapist, because of neurologic symptoms, typically brings patients with chronic intoxication to medical attention. There is usually a recent history of excessive fluid loss caused by diuretics, gastroenteritis, fever, fasting before surgery or renal insufficiency unknown until now, due to interstitial nephritis, glomerulonephritis, tubular necrosis or other diseases of the kidneys, which in rare cases might also be related to long-term lithium therapy[4,5] (see also Chapter 21). Other diseases such as anorexia, cystic fibrosis, liver cirrhosis, congestive heart failure, diabetes insipidus or diabetes mellitus may also be responsible for a lithium overload. Drug interactions with, for example, angiotensin converting enzyme (ACE) inhibitors, cyclosporine, loop diuretics and thiazides, non-steroidal anti-inflammatory drugs, carbamazepine or a decreased dietary sodium intake also precipitate conditions of poisoning[1,2]. Toxic symptoms may be present even when concentrations appear to be within the recommended therapeutic range[6]. Understanding of the mechanism of lithium intoxication requires knowledge of the basic pharmacology of lithium, which is covered in Chapter 27.

EPIDEMIOLOGY OF POISONING

As most countries have no obligations to register intoxications due to pharmaceuticals, information about the epidemiology of such poisonings are published by poison information centers and in case series of various hospitals. Lithium intoxication is a rare event, compared with other causes of intoxication. The Ontario regional poison information center found 205 cases of lithium poisoning, compared to approximately 91 250 cases of intoxication due to other poisons, in one year. Acute overdose was found in 6% and acute on chronic in 85%; chronic poisoning was diagnosed in 9% of the cases[7]. Over a 10-year period, 304 cases were detected from the poison information center in Marseille[3]. Meltzer and Steinlauf in Tel Aviv, Israel found nine cases during a 10-year period in their hospital[8]. Chen *et al*. identified 78 patients with intoxication over a period of 3.5 years in the Taipei City Psychiatric Center[9]. The 2003 annual report of the American Association of Poison Control Centers recorded 5296 exposures to lithium as a pharmaceutical (0.4% of all exposures to pharmaceuticals): 76% occurred in persons over 19 years; 78% had to be treated in a health-care facility; no toxicity occurred in 23.8%; and minor, moderate or major toxicity occurred in 31.8, 36.5 and 7.7%, respectively[10]. Tuohy and Shemin described a case series of 56 patients over a 12-year period. Intentional overdose was found in 75% of the patients with a mean ingestion dose of 11.3 g (probably corresponding to 305 mEq Li$^+$) and inadvertent toxicity in 25% with an ingestion dose of 1.4 g (probably corresponding to 305 mEq Li$^+$), respectively[11]. In a case series of 81 patients who were admitted to a toxicological intensive care unit in Paris, France over a period of 9.5 years, 77.8% were classified as deliberate acute on chronic and 22.2% as chronic intoxication, respectively[12]. In our own experience, approximately ten cases in 30 years were observed in the intensive care unit (ICU).

DIAGNOSTIC ROUTINES

History and physical examination

The diagnosis of lithium poisoning can be difficult, because symptoms are often non-specific, and as many as one-third of patients are victims of chronic lithium intoxication and are usually unaware that their symptoms are related to lithium. Lithium intoxication should be primarily suspected in any lithium-treated patient but also in other psychiatric patients who are confused, ataxic or tremulous. The history should include the type of lithium preparation ingested, the drug amount and time since ingestion as well as the use of other medications (e.g. over-the-counter), recent illnesses and baseline level of functioning. It is important to distinguish between acute toxicity, chronic toxicity and acute toxicity in a patient on chronic lithium therapy. During physical examination, particular attention should be focused on vital signs, cardiovascular status and neurologic involvement.

Signs and symptoms

Clinical findings in cases of intoxication are symptoms of the CNS (tremor, ataxia, nystagmus, choreoathetosis, photophobia, lethargy, agitation, fascicular twitching, confusion, signs of cerebellar dysfunction, and in severe cases seizures and coma), symptoms of the cardiovascular system (sinus bradycardia, hypotension), symptoms of the GI tract (nausea, vomiting, diarrhea) and changes in metabolism (hypernatremia, azotemia, leukocytosis).

Neurologic symptoms are commonly used to grade the degree of severity of lithium intoxi-cation. Mild symptoms include nausea, vomiting, lethargy, tremor and fatigue. Symptoms of moderate intoxication are confusion, agitation, delirium, tachycardia, occasional heart blocks and hypertonia. Coma, seizures, hyperthermia and hypotension characterize severe intoxication. People chronically on lithium who took an overdose or have increases of their lithium levels for other reasons cannot tolerate much of an increase in serum lithium as they already have a significant amount of drug in their body. In these cases, levels that are even slightly above normal can coincide with developing symptoms. CNS symptoms occur only if significant amounts of lithium have entered the CNS. It usually takes a week of regular dosing to achieve significant CNS levels. Therefore, CNS symptoms are most likely to occur in patients chronically on lithium who overdose or show increased lithium blood levels for other reasons. The most severe cases from a study in Marseille had suicide attempts with acute-on-chronic intoxication, where 56% of these patients had to be managed in an ICU, 5% needed hemodialysis, 10% had cardiac (repolarization disturbances) or neurologic (seizures) complications, and 2% died[3]. Table 40.1 summarizes symptoms and blood concentrations in (chronic) lithium poisoning.

Signs after acute ingestion in persons naive to lithium

Following acute ingestion individuals not currently on lithium present with symptoms of the GI tract or of the cardiovascular system. GI symptoms such as nausea, vomiting and diarrhea are common. Cardiovascular side-effects are usually mild, and manifest as non-specific electrocardiogram (ECG) changes, such as ST-T flattening and T-wave inversion. These persons rarely develop serious symptoms in overdose, even though their levels are quite high. Accidental ingestions, even with children,

Table 40.1 Symptoms and blood levels in chronic lithium intoxication (from references 8, 13, 14, 16, 27, 36)

System	Mild (according to reference 27) (1.5–2.5 mEq/l)	Serious (2.5–3.5 mEq/l)	Life-threatening (>3.5 mEq/l)
Neurologic	Fine tremor Apathy Fatigue Muscle weakness Hyperreflexia Incontinence Gait abnormality	Coarse tremor Dysarthria, slurred speech Tinnitus Ataxia Hypertonia Myoclonus	Stupor Seizures Coma Fasciculations Spasticity Rigidity Choreoathetosis Paresis Paralysis
Gastrointestinal	Nausea Vomiting Diarrhea	Nausea Vomiting Diarrhea	Nausea Vomiting Diarrhea
Cardiovascular	T-wave changes, bradycardia Sinoatrial block, atrioventricular block I°	T-wave changes, bradycardia Sinoatrial block, atrioventricular block I° QRS prolongation	T-wave changes, bradycardia Sinoatrial block, atrioventricular block I° Hypotension, collapse Ventricular dysrhythmias
Renal			Renal failure
Thyroid (hypofunction)	Usually not in acute poisoning		

could be considered as less severe situations[3]. Serum levels following acute lithium ingestion correlate poorly with intracellular lithium levels and clinical symptoms. The mean amount ingested in the Ontario series was found in the range of 8–364 mEq with a mean of 97 mEq of non-extended-release formulations[7].

Signs in chronic or acute on chronic intoxication

Relatively mild intoxications cause anxiety, tremor, ataxia, nystagmus, choreoathetosis, photophobia and lethargy. At higher levels of intoxication agitation, fascicular twitching, confusion, nausea, vomiting, diarrhea and signs of cerebellar dysfunction may predominate. Severe toxicity is characterized by worsening neurologic dysfunction (seizures, coma) and cardiovascular instability (sinus bradycardia, hypotension, QT prolongation and tachyarrhythmias such as torsade de pointes). In the Ontario series, patients with acute on chronic overdose took 16–1216 mEq with a mean of 211 mEq of lithium; in seven patients sustained-release preparations were used. Patients with chronic intoxication took a mean daily dose of 35 mEq of lithium. These patients presented with an initial blood level of 2.4 mEq/l, which fell to 2.3 mEq/l after 6 hours. All were symptomatic and their creatinine level was elevated in 13 out of 19 patients[7].

LABORATORY AND TECHNICAL DIAGNOSTIC

In all patients an ECG should be recorded and the lithium blood level should be checked. Also, blood urea nitrogen (BUN), serum chloride, carbon dioxide, creatinine, blood glucose, serum potassium and serum sodium should be assessed from blood drawn early to check the level of intoxication and renal function. Most laboratories report therapeutic serum lithium levels to be between 0.6–0.8 and 1.2–1.5 mEq/l measured 12 hours after the last lithium dose[8,9,13,14]. It is important to use specimen tubes without lithium heparin, because this can falsely elevate the levels.

Serum lithium levels during chronic treatment should ideally be assessed in blood drawn about 12 hours after the last therapeutic dose to avoid falsely elevated results. Owing to its distributional phase, serum lithium levels assessed too soon after an acute ingestion can be misleading. Reported cases of minimally symptomatic patients with serum levels of 9.3 mEq/l exist, reflecting high serum but low tissue levels[15]. After acute ingestions there is a relatively poor correlation between initial serum levels and systemic toxicity. Serum lithium levels can rise for up to 3–4 days after admission following acute ingestions in patients naive to lithium. Generally, clinical symptoms are more reliable than serum lithium levels, but there is no clinical variable that accurately predicts which patients will deteriorate[13].

Lithium level assessment should be repeated at frequent (i.e. 2–4-hour) intervals after acute overdose until peak levels are observed or elevated levels are falling below the toxic range and the patient becomes asymptomatic. In chronic intoxications concentrations of 1.5–3.0 mEq/l are associated with mild or moderate toxicity. Severe poisoning and death may occur with serum concentrations greater than 3–4 mEq/l[1,16,17], but a Canadian study questioned the value of the Hansen and Amisen classification to predict either morbidity or mortality in lithium poisoning[7].

Elevated BUN and creatinine reflect renal insufficiency and suggest that intoxication results from gradual accumulation of lithium rather than acute ingestion. Patients who have a history or present with coma or seizures should be tested for elevated serum creatine phosphokinase and myoglobinuria. In lithium-induced nephrogenic diabetes insipidus usually urine is diluted with a low measured osmolality relative to serum. The diagnosis is confirmed by lack of adequate response to a test dose of vasopressin. Leukocytosis sometimes seen in patients taking lithium is a non-specific finding and does not reflect severity of intoxication. A reduced or absent anion gap* may be indicative of lithium intoxication.

Plain radiographs of the abdomen may reveal radiopaque lithium tablets after acute ingestion but a negative radiograph does not rule out an acute ingestion.

DIFFERENTIAL DIAGNOSIS

Altered mental status is detected in many diseases and should be considered in discussing differential diagnosis as well as conditions such as hypoxia, hypoglycemia, hypothermia or hyperthermia, electrolyte disorders, CNS

---

*Anion gap is defined as the interval between the sum of routinely measured cations (Na$^+$, sodium; K$^+$, potassium) minus the sum of the routinely measured anions (Cl$^-$, chloride; HCO$_3^-$, bicarbonate) in the blood: (Na$^+$ + K$^+$) − (Cl$^-$ + HCO$_3^-$). A normal anion gap is 12 ± 2 mEq/l. A high anion gap indicates metabolic acidosis. A low anion gap is relatively rare, but may occur from the presence of unmeasured cations (e.g. in hypercalcemia, hypermagnesemia, multiple myeloma, lithium poisoning[18])

infection, head trauma and intracranial bleeding. Hyperthermia and muscle rigidity occurring in a patient who is also taking antipsychotic medication may suggest a neuroleptic malignant syndrome. Other drug intoxications should be considered, especially if CNS symptoms appear shortly after an acute overdose.

TREATMENT

Lithium poisoning may present in several different ways. However, the initial management is similar.

Supportive care

Diuretics, neuroleptics as well as lithium preparations must be discontinued. In hypoglycemic states, glucose should be given, orally or intravenously, depending on the level of consciousness. If the patient shows an altered mental status with decreased consciousness, the oral airway must be protected. Supplemental oxygen should be administered. Seizures should be treated with benzodiazepines.

If hypotension does not reverse despite initial volume repletion with normal saline (usually 1–2 l, children 10–20 ml/kg), the use of vasopressors (norepinephrine) is recommended. After correction of a volume depletion and re-establishing a normal blood pressure, patients should receive normal saline (0.9% NaCl) or half-normal saline (0.45% NaCl) intravenously to maintain a diuresis of approximately 100–150 ml/h. Under these conditions patients must be monitored to prevent hypernatremia, especially in those with underlying diabetes insipidus[15,19]. Lithium blood levels should be measured every 2–4 hours. If there is no constant decline in the concentration, the course is to decide whether further elimination enhancement (e.g. hemodialysis) is necessary[13].

Antidotes

There are no specific antidotes available[15].

Gastrointestinal decontamination

Gastrointestinal decontamination is indicated in individuals after ingestions exceeding 1.08 mEq/kg of lithium if this procedure can be maintained in the first hour after ingestion[20]. Emesis induced by ipecac syrup may be useful for immediate treatment on scene (e.g. children at home) if it can be given within a few minutes after exposure. Gastric lavage is the preferred method of gastric decontamination after an overdose within 1 hour after oral ingestion of lithium. Activated charcoal is indicated only if co-ingestion with organic drugs is suspected, because it does not bind the lithium ion[19,21]. Sodium polystyrene sulfonate does bind to lithium and may decrease its absorption, but may also cause hypokalemia[22,23]. Multiple doses of sodium polystyrene sulfonate may result in GI dialysis and further lower serum lithium levels, but this therapy is unproven in human subjects[22]. Whole-bowel irrigation with polyethylene glycol may be indicated after ingestion of large doses of sustained-release preparations of lithium[24].

Enhancement of elimination

In normal renal function, the kidneys clear lithium at a rate of 10–25 ml/min[25,26]. However, forced diuresis using normal saline failed to increase lithium excretion except in patients who presented with true volume depletion. Therefore, this therapy is not recommended, and can be dangerous[26–28].

Hemodialysis is the method of choice to enhance the elimination of lithium. Because of its low molecular weight, lack of protein binding, good water solubility, low volume of distribution and prolonged half-life, clearance rates of up to 150 ml/min are achievable[26]. Continuous venovenous hemofiltration or continuous venovenous hemodialysis with clearance rates of approximately 40–60 ml/min may be a substitute if hemodialysis is not available, but does not reduce lithium levels as quickly as hemodialysis, and the need for anticoagulation often limits its usefulness[26,29,30].

Dialysis

Compared with the human kidney, peritoneal dialysis has a smaller clearance rate of 9–15 ml/min of lithium and is not recommended for treating lithium poisoning[2]. Conventional hemodialysis can reduce plasma lithium concentration by 1 mEq/l per 4 hours of treatment[14,31]. High flux dialyzers should be capable of removing more lithium per hour, but there are few data to support this[32]. Hemodialysis should be performed using a bicarbonate and not an acetate bath, as lithium clearance from intracellular stores is reduced when an acetate bath is used[32]. The hemodialysis catheter should be left in place, because treatment must often be repeated, owing to a rebound after hemodialysis as the intracellular lithium exits cells and re-enters the bloodstream[33,34]. Lithium levels may also rise in patients who ingested a sustained-release lithium preparation due to continued lithium absorption from the GI tract. Thus, lithium levels must be checked frequently after hemodialysis has been completed.

Indications for hemodialysis

The decision to initiate hemodialysis in lithium intoxication should be guided by clinical signs and serum levels. It should be started immediately in any patient who presents with coma, convulsions, respiratory failure, deteriorating mental status, or renal failure, irrespective of serum lithium levels measured. In all other cases the decision should be made after 8–12 h following admission, based on serial lithium levels, renal function and the patient's overall clinical condition. Serum levels of >3.5–4 mEq/l in an acute ingestion; serum levels of >2.5 mEq/l in chronic ingestion and symptomatic patients or renal insufficiency; and serum levels of <2.5 mEq/l after ingestion of a large lithium dose, where rising blood levels are anticipated, may be helpful for decision-making[3,31,35]. Because hemodialysis is very effective at removing lithium from the blood and has minimal side-effects, priority should be given to it whenever any doubt exists about the effectiveness of alternative methods.

Patients on chronic lithium therapy are at higher risk for permanent harm from lithium poisoning than patients with acute poisoning, since intracellular lithium levels are thought to be responsible for irreversible toxicity. Thus, acutely poisoned individuals may not need hemodialysis until lithium levels reach 6–8 mEq/l. Typically, at least two hemodialysis treatments are necessary in patients requiring hemodialysis[14].

MONITORING

Frequent evaluation of vital signs and signs of neurologic toxicity, ECG monitoring and laboratory investigations (sodium, potassium, BUN, creatinine) are advised. Lithium levels should be measured every 2–4 h until therapeutic values are achieved or patients become asymptomatic.

CASE VIGNETTES

Two case vignettes will make clear what has been outlined above:

(1) History suggests an acute ingestion of a significant amount of lithium in an asymp-

tomatic patient, who is not on chronic lithium therapy. Initial lithium level confirms lithemia. How to proceed? Give supportive care as described and obtain serial levels every 2–4 h. If levels exceed 3.5–4 mEq/l, admit the patient to a monitor bed and institute extracorporeal detoxification. Otherwise proceed with saline to maintain a good diuresis and proceed with monitoring until lithium levels are in the therapeutic range and the patient is asymptomatic.

(2) The patient presents with a history of a trivial ingestion of a regular release product and does not show any signs of intoxication. Obtain an initial lithium level and a second level after 6 h. If the second level does not indicate the ingestion of a toxic amount (level <1.5 mEq/l) the patient may be evaluated by a psychiatrist. If, however, a patient presents after ingestion of a sustained-release preparation, admit the patient to a monitor bed and obtain serial lithium levels every 2–4 h for at least 48 h until the lithium concentration remains below 1.5 mEq/l[13].

REFERENCES

1. Amdisen A. Clinical features and management of lithium poisoning. Med Toxicol Adverse Drug Exp 1988; 3: 18–32
2. Okusa MD, Crystal LJT. Clinical manifestations and management of acute lithium intoxication. Am J Med 1994; 97: 383–9
3. Haro L, Roelandt J, Pommier P, et al. Circonstances d'intoxication par sels de lithium: expérience du centre antipoison de Marseille sur 10 ans. Ann Fr Anesth Réanim 2003; 22: 514–19
4. Lepkifker E, Sverdlik A, Iancu J, et al. Renal insufficiency in long-term lithium treatment. J Clin Psychiatry 2004; 65: 850–6
5. Markowitz GS, Radhakrishnan J, Kambham N, et al. Lithium nephrotoxicity: a progressive combined glomerular and tubulointerstitial nephropathy. J Am Soc Nephrol 2000; 11: 1439–48
6. Miao YK. Lithium neurotoxicity within the therapeutic serum range. Hong Kong J Psychiatry 2002; 12: 19–22
7. Bailey B, McGuigan M. Lithium poisoning from a poison control center perspective. Ther Drug Monitoring 2000; 22: 650–5
8. Meltzer E, Steinlauf S. The clinical manifestations of lithium intoxication. Isr Med Assoc J 2002; 4: 265–7
9. Chen KP, Shen WW, Lu ML. Implication of serum concentration monitoring in patients with lithium intoxication. Psych Clin Neurosci 2004; 58: 25–9
10. Watson WA, Litovitz TL, Klein-Schwartz W, et al. 2003 Annual Report of the American Association of Poison Control Centers Toxic Exposure Surveillance System. Am J Emerg Med 2004; 22: 335–404
11. Tuohy K, Shemin D. Acute lithium intoxication. Dialysis Transplant 2003; 32: 478–81
12. Montagnon F, Said S, Lepine JP. Lithium: poisonings and suicide prevention, Eur Psychiatry 2002; 17: 92–5
13. Sadosty AT, Groleau GA, Atcherson MM. The use of lithium levels in the emergency department. J Emerg Med 1999; 17: 887–91
14. Timmer RT, Sands JM. Lithium intoxication. J Am Soc Nephrol 1999; 10: 666–74
15. Benowitz NL. Lithium. In Olson KR, ed. Poisoning and Drug Overdose, 2nd edn. East Norwalk: Prentice-Hall International, 1994
16. Dyson EH, Simpson D, Prescot LF, et al. Self-poisoning and therapeutic intoxication with lithium. Hum Toxicol 1987; 6: 325–9
17. Simard M, Gumbiner B, Lee A, et al. Lithium carbonate intoxication: a case report and review of the literature. Arch Intern Med 1989; 149: 36–46
18. Jurado RL, Rio C, Nassar G, et al. Low anion gap. South Med J 1998; 91: 624–9
19. Mokhlesi B, Leikin JB, Murray P, Corbridge TC. Adult toxicology in critical care: Part II Specific poisonings. Chest 2003; 123: 897–922

20. Ellenhorn MJ, Barceloux DG. Lithium. In Medical Toxicology – Diagnosis and Treatment of Human Poisoning. New York: Elsevier Science, 1988

21. Favin FD, Klein-Schwartz W, Oderda GM, Rose SR. In vitro study of lithium carbonate adsorption by activated charcoal. J Toxicol Clin Toxicol 1988; 26: 443–50

22. Linakis JG, Savitt DL, Wu TY, et al. Use of sodium polystyrene sulfonate for reduction of plasma lithium concentrations after chronic lithium dosing in mice. J Toxicol Clin Toxicol 1998; 36: 309–13

23. Tomaszewski C, Musso C, Pearson RJ, et al. Lithium absorption prevented by sodium polystyrene sulfonate in volunteers. Ann Emerg Med 1992; 21: 1308–11

24. Smith SW, Ling LJ, Halstenson CE. Whole-bowel irrigation as a treatment for acute lithium overdose. Ann Emerg Med 1991; 20: 536–9

25. Drukker W, Parsons FM, Maher JF. Lithium. In Replacement of Renal Function by Dialysis, 2nd edn. Dordrecht: Martinus Nijhoff Publishers, 1986

26. Leblanc M, Raymond M, Bonnardeaux A, et al. Lithium poisoning treated by high-performance continuous arteriovenous and venovenous hemodiafiltration. Am J Kidney Dis 1996; 27: 365–72

27. Hansen HE, Amdisen A. Lithium intoxication: report of 23 cases and review of 100 cases from the literature. Q J Med 1978; 186: 123–44

28. Scharman EJ. Methods used to decrease lithium absorption or enhance elimination. J Toxicol Clin Toxicol 1997; 35: 601–8

29. Hazouard E, Ferrandiere M, Rateau H, et al. Continuous veno-venous hemofiltration versus continuous veno-venous hemodialysis in severe lithium self-poisoning: a toxicokinetics study in an intensive care unit. Nephrol Dialysis Transplant 1999; 14: 1605–6

30. Beckmann U, Oakley PW, Dawson AH, et al. Efficacy of continuous venovenous hemodialysis in the treatment of severe lithium toxicity. J Toxicol Clin Toxicol 2001; 39: 393–7

31. Jaeger A, Sauder P, Kupferschmitt T, et al. When should dialysis be performed in lithium poisoning? Clin Toxicol 1993; 31: 429–47

32. Peces R, Pobes A. Effectiveness of hemodialysis with high-flux membranes in the extra-corporeal therapy of life-threatening acute lithium intoxication. Nephrol Dialysis Transplant 2001; 16: 1301–3

33. Kerbusch T, Mathot A, Otten HMMB, et al. Bayesian pharmacokinetics of lithium after an acute self-intoxication and subsequent hemo-dialysis: a case report. Pharmacol Toxicol 2002; 90: 243–5

34. Clendeninn NJ, Pond SM, Kaysen G, et al. Potential pitfalls in the evaluation of the usefulness of hemodialysis for the removal of lithium. J Toxicol Clin Toxicol 1982; 19: 341–52

35. Zimmerman JL. Poisonings and overdoses in the intensive care unit: General and specific management issues. Crit Care Med 2003; 31: 2794–801

36. Dunner DL. Optimizing lithium treatment. J Clin Psychiatry 2000; 61 (Suppl 9): 76–81

41 The Lithium Information Center

James W Jefferson, John H Greist, Margaret G Baudhuin, Bette L Hartley, David J Katzelnick

Contents   Information • Staffing and funding • Additional activities of the Center • Conclusions

'Index learning turns no student pale,
yet holds the eel of science by the tail.'

Alexander Pope (1688–1744)
The Dunciad, Bk. I

The Lithium Information Center was established formally in 1975 at the University of Wisconsin Medical School in Madison, Wisconsin. It had its informal beginning somewhat earlier as one of us (JWJ) struggled to make organizational sense out of a rapidly expanding collection of abstracts, articles, chapters and books on the subject of lithium in medicine. The organizational powers of the computer were called into use (under the guidance of JHG) to bring order out of chaos. From this collaboration arose the Information Center, the goals of which were to acquire, organize, archive and disseminate as much as possible of the world's literature on lithium in medicine[1–5].

The Center and its staff moved from the University of Medicine Medical School to the Dean Foundation for Health, Research and Education in 1992, and to the current location at the Madison Institute of Medicine in 1998. Creation of the Bipolar Disorders Treatment Information Center in 1999 has allowed the scope of the Institute to expand to include information about alternatives to lithium.

At present, the Information Center has a library of over 40 400 references that can be computer-searched by title, word, author, subject heading, journal and year of publication. Each article is read by one of the medical librarians (MGB and BLH) and indexed according to over 9800 distinct subject/keyword headings. In recent years, most abstracts have been included with the bibliographic record. More importantly, the tedious process of optically scanning all the articles into the database is underway currently, which will allow for more secure archiving and also for electronic delivery through email.

INFORMATION

Information sources

Lithium-related materials are obtained from a vast array of sources including MEDLINE (National Library of Medicine), Current Contents and Personal Alert Service (ISI Thompson Scientific) and PsycINFO (American Psychological Association). Additional resources include journals and newsletters by subscription, meeting abstracts, posters, books and other publications.

Organization of information

The computerized program used to enter, store and search the database is a modification of PaperChase which was developed at the Beth Israel Hospital in Boston, Massachusetts[6]. The system, in use since 1975, is currently being updated to make it compatible with more modern computer programs and to provide enhancements, such as electronic updating for faster processing of new literature.

Dissemination of information

The Information Specialists have responded to over 45 000 requests from a wide range of individuals and organizations, including clinicians, pharmacists, basic scientists, patients, families, support groups, attorneys, pharmaceutical companies and the press.

While most information requests come from the USA and Canada, the Center's services have been utilized throughout the world with the growth of the Internet doing much to facilitate worldwide communications. Over the years, requests have come from all 50 states, Washington, DC, Puerto Rico, most Canadian provinces and at least 35 other countries.

A Literature Update Service is also available to clinicians, researchers and others interested in keeping up with the latest publications on lithium. For an annual subscription fee, an individual will receive a monthly listing of all new references added to the database.

In addition to responding to information requests, educational efforts also include exhibits for consumers and professionals at national and local meetings, and presentations to clinicians and patient advocacy groups.

Managing information requests

Because the database is both broad and deep, literature searches can be tailored to meet both general and highly specific information requests. While the National Library of Medicine Medical Subject Headings (MESH) are used for indexing articles, numerous additional subject headings were created by the Information Specialists to allow for greater search specificity than otherwise would be available (Table 41.1). Indeed, comparative searches of the Center's database versus MEDLINE consistently show a greater yield of useful information and exclusion of extraneous citations (false hits).

Here is how an Information Specialist might tailor a request from a clinician for information on lithium and the kidney (3873 citations), subheading *diabetes insipidus/polyuria* (1025 citations), subheading *treatment* (361 citations), final subheading *potassium-sparing diuretics* (61 citations).

Perhaps a researcher is updating a manuscript and wants information on lithium and the hippocampus (453 citations), by H Manji (25 citations), published only in 2004 (3 citations).

To address frequent requests in particular areas, the Information Specialists have prepared information packets that contain a compilation of pertinent literature. Examples include Lithium and Pregnancy, Lithium and Kidney Function, Lithium and Thyroid Function,

Table 41.1 Examples of specific lithium subject headings

Lithium Preparations – Comparison of

Lithium Preparations – Tablets vs. Capsules

Monitoring Procedures – Recommended Frequency

Dose: Single vs. Divided

Dose: Single – Largest Dose That Can Be Given

Serum Lithium Levels – Peak

Serum Lithium Levels – Postmortem

Blood Lithium Levels – Fetal

Red Blood Cell/Plasma Lithium Ratio

Red Blood Cell/Urine Lithium Ratio

Urine Volume/Lithium Clearance Ratio

Brain/Serum Lithium Ratio

Lithium Excretion – Influence of Affective State

Teratogenesis – Dose Relationship

Teratogenesis – Father Taking Lithium

Withdrawal of Lithium – Recommended Procedures

Withdrawal of Lithium – Abrupt vs. Gradual

Adverse Effects, Persisting After Lithium Withdrawal

Adverse Effects, Progression of After Lithium Withdrawal

Adverse Effects, Time to Onset

Poisoning, Persisting Adverse Effects

Poisoning, Risk Factors for Permanent Sequelae

Lithium and Weight Gain, and Lithium Poisoning. These packets are updated frequently as new information accrues, and new packets are created when required by demand.

The Center is able to provide requesters with copies of pertinent articles subject to constraints of copyright laws. A nominal fee is charged for the services.

STAFFING AND FUNDING

The current Medical Directors of the Center are JWJ and JHG (founders) and DJK. Two Medical Librarians (MGB and BLH) serve as Information Specialists with support from their staff.

The Madison Institute of Medicine is a not-for-profit organization supported by user fees, sales of patient information booklets, and donations and grants from a variety of sources.

ADDITIONAL ACTIVITIES OF THE CENTER

Aided to a large extent by the readily available comprehensive database, publications by the staff have included patient education booklets on bipolar disorder and lithium, divalproex, carbamazepine and oxcarbazepine[7–10] (in total, over 1.3 million copies of the booklets have been distributed), books[11,12], book chapters (for example, in references 13–16) and numerous journal articles.

The Center also keeps an extensive list of clinicians with expertise in bipolar disorder, and of support groups, and serves as a referral resource for patients seeking evaluation and treatment throughout the USA, Canada and several other countries.

CONCLUSIONS

While the Lithium Information Center is the most comprehensive database on the subject, there is a continuing need for ever-greater accessibility to published materials. This is especially true with regard to literature from other countries and in languages other than English. Also, there is a continuing need to increase worldwide awareness of the Center and its resources. The Internet is a major vehicle in this regard, but also of great value has been the ability to exhibit at the Annual Meeting of the American Psychiatric Association and other scientific conferences. The opportunity to contribute to this book provides yet another opportunity to increase awareness.

Contacting the Lithium Information Center

Information requests reach the Center by mail, telephone, facsimile (fax) and email. Turn-around time is usually less than 24 hours, with more urgent requests received during working hours addressed immediately.

The Center can be reached by telephone at 608-827-2470 (answering machine after hours), by fax at 608-827-2479, and by email at mim@miminc.org. The Internet website is www.miminc.org. The mailing address is Lithium Information Center, Madison Institute of Medicine, 7617 Mineral Point Road, Suite 300, Madison, WI 53717, USA.

REFERENCES

1. Jefferson JW, Greist JH, Marcetich JR. Searching the lithium literature. In Johnson FN, ed. Handbook of Lithium Therapy. Lancaster UK: MTP Press, 1980: 433–7
2. Baudhuin MG, Jefferson JW, Greist JH. The Lithium Information Center: an efficient information service. Pharmacol Biochem Behav 1984; 21 (Suppl 1): 109–11
3. Carroll JA, Greist JH, Jefferson JW, et al. Lithium Information Center: one model of a computer-based psychiatric information service. Arch Gen Psychiatry 1986; 43: 483–5
4. Jefferson JW, Greist JH, Baudhuin MG, et al. The lithium literature, an evolutionary tree reflecting scientific advances and pseudo-scientific retreats. In Birch NJ, Gallicchio VS, Becker RW, eds. Lithium: 50 Years of Psychopharmacology – New Perspectives in Biomedical and Clinical Research. Cheshire, CT: Weidner Publishing Group, 1999: 22–7
5. Jefferson JW, Greist JH, Baudhuin MG, et al. Lithium Information Center [in Japanese]. In Global Views on Psychiatry. Japan: Churchill Communications, 1998: 1–7
6. Horowitz GL, Bleich HL. PaperChase: a computer program to search the medical literature. N Engl J Med 1981; 305: 924–30
7. Jefferson JW, Greist JH. Lithium and Bipolar Disorder: A Guide, revised edn. Madison, WI: Lithium Information Center, Madison Institute of Medicine, 2004
8. Jefferson JW, Greist JH. Carbamazepine and Bipolar Disorder: A Guide, revised edn. Madison, WI: Lithium Information Center, Madison Institute of Medicine, 2005
9. Jefferson JW, Greist JH. Divalproex and Bipolar Disorder: A Guide, revised edn. Madison, WI: Lithium Information Center, Madison Institute of Medicine, 2005
10. Jefferson JW, Greist JH, Katzelnick DJ. Oxcarbazepine and Bipolar Disorder: A Guide. Madison, WI: Lithium Information Center, Madison Institute of Medicine, 2002
11. Jefferson JW, Greist JH. Primer of Lithium Therapy. Baltimore: Williams & Wilkins, 1977
12. Jefferson JW, Greist JH, Ackerman DL, et al. Lithium Encyclopedia for Clinical Practice, 2nd edn. Washington, DC: American Psychiatric Press, 1987
13. Jefferson JW, Greist JH. Lithium. In Sadock BJ, Sadock VA, eds. Kaplan & Sadock's Comprehensive Textbook of Psychiatry, 8th edn. Philadelphia: Lippincott Williams & Wilkins, 2005; 2: 2839–51
14. Jefferson JW. Lithium. In: Aronson JK, ed. Side Effects of Drugs Annual 27. Boston: Elsevier, 2004: 19–28
15. Jefferson JW. Lithium. In Dukes MNG, Aronson JK, eds. Meyler's Side Effects of Drugs, 14th edn. Amsterdam: Elsevier Science BV, 2000: 86–94
16. Jefferson JW, Greist JH. Lithium in psychiatric therapy. In Adelman G, Smith BH, eds. Encyclopedia of Neuroscience, 2nd edn.revised. New York: Elsevier, 1999: 1057–9

42 Economics of lithium prophylaxis in bipolar disorders

Anne Berghöfer

Contents   Cost of illness of bipolar disorder • Economic evaluations • Conclusion

COST OF ILLNESS OF BIPOLAR DISORDER

Bipolar disorders are among the mental health conditions with the highest health-care and social costs. In the USA, the total annual costs of these disorders have been estimated at US $45 billion[1], of which only 15% are due to direct medical expenses. These data are based on an assumed prevalence of bipolar illness of 1.3%, or 2 million patients.

From a health economics perspective, the burden of bipolar disorder can be attributed to eight primary factors: the early onset of illness, the high risk of recurrences, the large proportion of patients in inpatient treatment, the absence from work, the early retirement, the high risk of suicide, the high prevalence of somatic co-morbidity and the high rates of psychiatric co-morbidity[2,3].

The first category of costs includes the so-called direct costs of illness. These are typically defined as expenditures on medical and non-medical services. Direct medical costs are directly associated with health-care interventions such as hospitalizations, emergency room visits, outpatient psychiatric or other visits, medications and patient or family payments. Direct non-medical costs, on the other hand, are associated with the expense of social welfare services, as well as with legal fees and transportation expenses. The second category of costs includes indirect costs, which are defined as a loss of resources resulting from reduced productivity due to illness, disability, or death. Typical manifestations include unemployment, early retirement, absence from work, lost family productivity and premature mortality due to suicide. Today most analyses describe the different types of costs in a standardized manner according to the recommendations of the Panel on Cost-effectiveness in Health and Medicine[4]. The third category is that of intangible costs, which include the costs of pain and suffering resulting from illness or treatment. Put another way, intangible costs are reductions in quality of life.

Another approach to calculating the costs of bipolar disorders involves a lifetime cost simulation model. In the one study to use this approach to date, costs were estimated for a cohort of patients with onset of bipolar disorder in 1 year assuming an incidence of approximately 100 000 new cases per year. Total costs were estimated to be US $24 billion throughout the lifetime of this cohort. The range in costs was enormous, starting at US $11 000 for a case with a single manic episode and peaking at a staggering US $600 000 for a case with a chronic course[5].

From the perspective of American businesses, bipolar illness with a chronic course is the most expensive mental disorder, costing US $64 per employee per year[6]. These data stem from a multiemployer database that links data on medical care, prescriptions, absence from work and short-term disability. Simon and Unützer analyzed data on health-care utilization from a large health plan, comparing the direct costs incurred by bipolar patients versus individuals with other medical conditions[7]. The direct costs incurred by bipolar patients averaged US $3416 per year versus US $1462 for the typical medical outpatient or US $2570 for patients with major depression. Indeed, the direct costs incurred by patients with bipolar disorder were even higher than those with diabetes (US $3083), which is widely accepted as a chronic condition with an enormous economic impact.

These data from the USA are, for the most part, corroborated by cost of illness studies from several other countries. Although different health systems are notoriously difficult to compare, the economic burden appears to be of the same magnitude in most Western nations[8]. A recent study from the UK assumed a prevalence of bipolar illness in the UK of 0.8%

due to a lack of robust prevalence data; the total costs were estimated to be US $4 billion, 86% of which was attributable to indirect costs[9]. A large percentage of the total costs in the UK study also resulted from hospital admissions and day hospital visits, which accounted for more than 50% of the total direct costs. Prescription drugs, however, had only a relatively small impact (approximately 4%). Another study estimated that, in France, the hospitalization costs for manic episodes alone amounted to 3 billion euros[10].

In a study based on health-care services data in Germany, the annual costs of bipolar disorders in this country were found to be approximately 5.8 billion euros[11]. These costs comprised indirect costs caused by morbidity-related unemployment, suicide-related losses in productivity, work absenteeism and early retirement. The same study also showed that hospital stays for bipolar patients in Germany were twice as long as for other psychiatric patients. Indeed, the costs of inpatient care accounted for two-thirds of direct costs.

It should be noted, however, that the subject of indirect costs and how best to calculate them is controversial. The human capital approach to this issue involves measuring an individual's productivity in terms of market wages and therefore varies considerably between countries. However, this method tends to result in high estimations of indirect costs and distorts the contribution of household work or non-employed persons. Another approach is the friction cost method, which assumes that the loss of productivity due to illness is rapidly mitigated by replacement. This is relevant in countries with high unemployment rates, for example, and leads to substantially lower estimates of indirect costs. Taken together, however, the vast majority of health economic data indicate that diagnosing bipolar illness early and providing suitable long-term treatment may have an enormous impact on the direct and indirect costs of this particular illness.

ECONOMIC EVALUATIONS

Although some cost-of-illness analyses for various health-care systems have been published in recent years, there are still few comparative studies on the economic effects of current intervention strategies and in particular of true long-term prophylactic treatments in bipolar illness. The studies that are available tend to be health economic evaluations – mainly cost–benefit analyses that compare new drugs in acute and maintenance treatment up to 12 months. Most of these analyses were conducted in the context of efficacy studies on new drugs, such as atypical antipsychotics or mood stabilizers with lithium as the gold standard comparator, i.e. they are sponsored by individual manufacturers and cannot be considered as independent of potential commercial interests.

In acute antimanic treatment there is a great deal of data that can be used for economic evaluations[12,13]. Valproate use in acute mania may be associated with greater cost savings due to its more rapid onset of action, especially in patients with mixed mania or rapid cycling, but lithium may have greater cost savings in patients with classical mania.

Maintenance treatment

Several studies on the potential economic impact of optimal maintenance treatment have been conducted since the 1980s. Although they do not all meet today's methodological standards, each of these studies points to a potential for substantial savings in direct and indirect costs. Table 42.1[14–17] shows cost–benefit analyses from claims data on maintenance treatment of any kind (maximum 12 months)

Table 42.1 Analyses of maintenance therapy (up to 12 months) of bipolar disorder based on claims data comparing treatment with no treatment, or comparing different treatment strategies

Author	Comparison	Method	n	Results
Svarstad et al., 2001[14]	Adherent vs. non-adherent patients	cost-ben	67	Adherence to any therapy led to hospital cost savings of US $8044 per patient per year
Li et al., 2002[15]	Consistent long-term treatment vs. no long-term treatment	cost-ben	3349	Cost savings of US $5044 per patient per year primarily by reducing inpatient costs
Birnbaum et al., 2003[16]	Recognized vs. unrecognized	cost-ben	626	Accurate and timely diagnosis led to medical cost savings of US $4536 and indirect cost savings of US $672 per patient per year
Simons and Krishnan, 2004[17]	Lamotrigine maintenance vs. any treatment in comparable period before study setting	cost-ben	406	Lamotrigine initiation (switch or add-on) leads to medical cost savings of US $424 per patient per year

cost-ben, cost–benefit analysis

compared to no treatment. All of the studies listed in the table show a net saving in direct costs, which is primarily due to lower rates of inpatient treatment and a reduction in the number of relapses. These evaluations are not limited specifically to lithium treatment, but show rather that in the case of maintenance treatment basic components such as correct diagnosis and adherence to therapy play a greater cost-saving role than the specific effects of any drug.

Data from clinical trials in particular can be considered to be representative of a controlled treatment setting in which correct diagnosis and the monitoring of patients' adherence to therapy is paramount. As a result, analyses of these data are fundamentally different from analyses of claims data, the latter of which are representative of everyday clinical routine. Table 42.2[18–25] summarizes economic evaluations from clinical trials comparing a number of different treatments with each other, often with lithium as the gold standard comparator. The results suggest that, in most cases, there are only marginal differences in cost savings between lithium and the more recent treatment options when only monetary outcomes are taken into account (i.e. cost–benefit analyses). Until now, only one study has provided preliminary findings on cost–utility analyses that take into account the costs of a treatment in relation to the outcome in quality of life units in bipolar patients[18]. Utility values for health states of euthymia, depression and mania were derived from quality of life scores collected from clinical trials and published data. Lithium was the least costly option in terms of direct costs but lamotrigine provided the most quality adjusted life years. The incremental cost for lamotrigine compared to lithium was US $25 900. However, results from model simulations are prone to overrating or underrating assumptions which cannot completely be prevented by sensitivity analyses. Therefore, data which are collected pros-

pectively, and independently from manufacturers' interests, are urgently needed for further cost–utility analyses.

Long-term lithium treatment

Data on the economic impact of long-term treatment with lithium are sparse and heterogeneous. Nevertheless, they point to substantial savings that could be achieved by recognizing the illness more accurately and using lithium on a more widespread basis (Table 42.3)[26–29]. The calculations by Felber are based on a large cohort of patients on long-term lithium treatment in the former German Democratic Republic[27]. Among a set of various outcome parameters, inpatient and outpatient treatment, the use of medication, absence from work and early retirement were prospectively documented over an average observation period of 5 years. However, the studies by Wyatt and co-workers from the USA[26,29] and Lehmann et al. from Germany[28] are model calculations based on assumptions that were drawn from various sources. Lehmann et al. entered the following cost assumptions into the model: prevalence of patients in need of treatment based on the prescription frequency of lithium within the statutory health insurance; costs of lithium treatment based on the physician fee scale; reduction of absence from work based on the data by Felber and calculated according to the human capital approach[27]. Although the model is rough, it points at substantial savings to the society.

However, there are no long-term data on cost-effectiveness using outcomes such as saved life years, or cost–utility analyses based on quality of life adjusted life years. Analyses of this kind are expected from the large Systematic Treatment Enhancement Program for Bipolar Disorder (STEP-BD)[30] and from the Texas Medication Algorithm Project (TMAP)[31].

Table 42.2 Analyses of maintenance therapy (up to 12 months) in bipolar disorder based on data from clinical trial settings comparing different treatment strategies

Author	Comparison	Method	n	Results
Keck et al., 1996[19]	Lithium vs. valproate acute and maintenance. Decision analytic model based on assumptions from the literature	cost-ben	—	VAL medical costs 9% lower than lithium in overall patient sample. Cost savings greater for lithium in subgroup of classical mania
Dardennes et al., 1999[20]	Lithium vs. carbamazepine	cost-ben	37	Lithium direct cost savings of $790 per patient per year compared to CBZ
Namjoshi et al., 2002[21]	Olanzapine maintenance vs. any treatment in comparable period outside study setting	cost-ben	76	Medical cost savings of US $10 608 primarily by reducing inpatient costs
Revicki et al., 2005[22]	Lithium vs. valproate 12 months	cost-ben	?	VAL medical cost savings of US $1755 per patient per year vs. lithium (US $28 911 vs. US $30 666)
Simon et al., 2002[23]	Usual care vs. multifaceted intervention program	cost-eff	441	Ongoing
Zhu et al., 2005[24]	Olanzapine vs. valproate	cost-ben	147	OLA and VAL equal costs. Higher drug costs of OLA were offset by lower costs for other services
Calvert et al., 2005[25]	Lamotrigine vs. lithium/ olanzapine/no medication Markov model over 18 months	cost-eff	assumed 1000	LAMO US $2400 more expensive per episode avoided compared to lithium (ICER)
Calvert et al., 2005[18]	Lamotrigine vs. lithium Markov model over 18 months	cost-util	assumed 1000	LAMO incremental cost per QALY US $25 900 vs. lithium

OLA, olanzapine; VAL, valproate; LAMO, lamotrigine; CBZ, carbamazepine; cost-ben, cost–benefit analysis; cost-eff, cost-effectiveness analysis; cost-util, cost–utility analysis; ICER, incremental cost-effectiveness ratio; QALY, quality adjusted life year

Table 42.3 Economic evaluations on the impact of lithium long-term treatment versus no lithium treatment

Author	Method	Result
Reifman and Wyatt, 1980[26]	Cost–benefit projection model, prevalence based	Lithium saved US $4 billion in 10 years
Felber, 1981[27]	Cost–benefit analysis on 623 clinical trial patients	Lithium reduced direct and indirect costs by 60% each
Lehmann et al., 1997[28]	Cost–benefit projection model	Cost savings of US $3213 per year per patient
Wyatt et al., 2001[29]	Cost–benefit projection model, prevalence based	Lithium saved US $170 billion in 20 years (direct and indirect costs)

CONCLUSION

The current state of research on the economic burden of bipolar disorder consists of several cost-of-illness studies from various countries. Although comparisons are hampered by issues of disparate methodology, the available data are consistent insofar as they show the important role played by indirect costs. There are only a few comprehensive economic evaluations on the impact of long-term interventions in bipolar illness, and research on outcomes in terms of quality of life is sparse. Future studies should therefore assess the effect of long-term treatment on the development, in particular, of indirect costs and address the issue of quality of life.

The long-term treatment of bipolar disorder could result in substantial savings in economic and societal terms, assuming that state-of-the-art treatment is used on a widespread basis. However, this illness is still widely under-recognized, and the majority of patients do not receive long-term treatment in accordance with current guidelines. As a result, cost-effectiveness and cost–utility analyses are urgently needed to demonstrate to key decision-makers on both sides of the Atlantic the potential economic and social benefits of optimized intervention strategies in the treatment of bipolar disorder.

REFERENCES

1. Wyatt RJ, Henter I. An economic evaluation of manic–depressive illness – 1991. Soc Psychiatry Psychiatr Epidemiol 1995; 30: 213–19
2. Kleinman L, Lowin A, Flood E, et al. Costs of bipolar disorder. Pharmacoeconomics 2003; 21: 601–22
3. Simon GE. Social and economic burden of mood disorders. Biol Psychiatry 2003; 54: 208–15
4. Weinstein MC, Siegel JE, Gold MR, et al. Recommendations of the panel on cost-effectiveness in health and medicine. JAMA 1996; 276: 1253–8
5. Begley CE, Annegers JF, Swann AC, et al. The lifetime cost of bipolar disorder in the US: an estimate for new cases in 1998. Pharmacoeconomics 2001; 19: 483–95
6. Goetzel RZ, Hawkins K, Ozminkowski RJ, Wang S. The health and productivity cost burden of the 'top 10' physical and mental health conditions affecting six large US employers in 1999. J Occup Environ Med 2003; 45: 5–14
7. Simon GE, Unützer J. Health care utilization and costs among patients treated for bipolar disorder in an insured population. Psychiatr Serv 1999; 50: 1303–8
8. Hakkaart-van Roijen L, Hoeijenbos MB, Regeer EJ, et al. The societal costs and quality of life of patients suffering from bipolar disorder in the Netherlands. Acta Psychiatr Scand 2004; 110: 383–92
9. Das Gupta R, Guest JF. Annual cost of bipolar disorder to UK society. Br J Psychiatry 2002; 180: 227–33
10. de Zelicourt M, Dardennes R, Verdoux H, et al. Frequency of hospitalisations and inpatient care costs of manic episodes: in patients with bipolar I disorder in France. Pharmacoeconomics 2003; 21: 1081–90
11. Runge C, Grunze H. Jährliche Krankheits-kosten bipolarer Störungen in Deutschland, Annual costs of bipolar disorders in Germany. Nervenarzt 2004; 75: 896–903
12. Keck PE Jr, McElroy SL, Bennett JA. Health-economic implications of the onset of action of antimanic agents. J Clin Psychiatry 1996; 57 (Suppl): 13–18
13. Bridle C, Palmer S, Bagnall AM, et al. A rapid and systematic review and economic evaluation of the clinical and cost-effectiveness of newer drugs for treatment of mania associated with bipolar affective disorder. Health Technol Assess 2004; 8: 1–187
14. Svarstad BL, Shireman TI, Sweeney JK. Using drug claims data to assess the relationship of

medication adherence with hospitalization and costs. Psychiatr Serv 2001; 52: 805–11

15. Li J, McCombs JS, Stimmel GL. Cost of treating bipolar disorder in the California Medicaid (Medi-Cal) program. J Affect Disord 2002; 71: 131–9

16. Birnbaum HG, Shi L, Dial E, et al. Economic consequences of not recognizing bipolar disorder patients: a cross-sectional descriptive analysis. J Clin Psychiatry 2003; 64: 1201–9

17. Simons WR, Krishnan AA. The economic value of lamotrigine as a mood stabilizer: a US managed care perspective. Manag Care Interface 2004; 17: 44–9

18. Calvert N, Burch SP, Fu AZ, et al. The economic outcomes of treatments for bipolar I disorder. Bipolar Disord 2005; 7 (Suppl 2): 40

19. Keck PE Jr, Nabulsi AA, Taylor JL, et al. A pharmacoeconomic model of divalproex vs. lithium in the acute and prophylactic treatment of bipolar I disorder. J Clin Psychiatry 1996; 57: 213–22

20. Dardennes R, Lafuma A, Watkins S. [Prophylactic treatment of mood disorders: cost effectiveness analysis comparing lithium and carbamazepine] Encephale 1999; 25: 391–400 [French]

21. Namjoshi MA, Rajamannar G, Jacobs T, et al. Economic, clinical, and quality-of-life outcomes associated with olanzapine treatment in mania. Results from a randomized controlled trial. J Affect Disord 2002; 69: 109–18

22. Revicki DA, Hirschfeld RM, Ahearn EP, et al. Effectiveness and medical costs of divalproex versus lithium in the treatment of bipolar disorder: results of a naturalistic clinical trial. J Affect Disord 2005; 86: 183–93

23. Simon GE, Ludman E, Unutzer J, Bauer MS. Design and implementation of a randomized trial evaluating systematic care for bipolar disorder. Bipolar Disord 2002; 4: 226–36

24. Zhu B, Tunis SL, Zhao Z, et al. Service utilization and costs of olanzapine versus divalproex treatment for acute mania: results from a randomized, 47-week clinical trial. Curr Med Res Opin 2005; 21: 555–64

25. Calvert N, Burch SP, Fu AZ, et al. The cost-effectiveness of lamotrigine in the maintenance treatment of bipolar I disorder. Poster presented at the 6th Conference on Bipolar Disorder, Pittsburgh, 2005

26. Reifman A, Wyatt RJ. Lithium: a brake in the rising cost of mental illness. Arch Gen Psychiatry 1980; 37: 385–8

27. Felber W. Rezidivprophylaxe affektiver Erkrankungen mit Lithium und ihre Auswirkungen. Psychiatria Clin 1981; 14: 161–6

28. Lehmann K, Ahrens B, Müller-Oerlinghausen B. Pharmacoökonomie der Lithiumprophylaxe. [Pharmacoeconomics of lithium long-term treatment] In Müller-Oerlinghausen B, Greil W, Berghöfer A, eds. Die Lithiumtherapie, 2nd edn. Berlin: Springer Verlag, 1997: 457–65

29. Wyatt JR, Henter ID, Jamison JC. Lithium revisited: savings brought about by the use of lithium 1970–1991. Psychiatr Q 2001; 72: 149–66

30. Sachs GS, Thase ME, Otto MW, et al. Rationale, design, and methods of the systematic treatment enhancement program for bipolar disorder (STEP-BD). Biol Psychiatr 2003; 53: 1028–42

31. Kashner MT, Rush JA, Altshuler KZ. Measuring costs of guideline-driven mental health care: the Texas Medication Algorithm Project. J Ment Health Policy Econ 1999; 2: 111–21

Index

Printed and bound by CPI Group (UK) Ltd, Croydon, CR0 4YY

21/10/2024

01777095-0012